10 0229802 X

£80

97

D1346446

DATE DUE FOR RETURN

UNIVERSITY LIBRARY

2 9 APR 2014

GML 02

Principles and Practice of Immunoassay

SECOND EDITION

EDITED BY

Christopher P Price
David J Newman

© Macmillan Reference Ltd, 1991, 1997.

All rights reserved. No reproduction, copy or transmission of this publication may be made without written permission.

No paragraph of this publication may be reproduced, copied or transmitted save with written permission or in accordance with the provisions of the Copyright, Designs and Patents Act 1988, or under the terms of any licence permitting limited copying issued by the Copyright Licensing Agency, 90 Tottenham Court Road, London W1P 9HE.

Any person who does any unauthorised act in relation to this publication may be liable to criminal prosecution and civil claims for damages.

First edition published in the United States and Canada by Stockton Press, 1991.
Second edition first published in the United States and Canada by
STOCKTON PRESS, 1997
345 Park Avenue South, 10 Floor, New York,
NY 10010-1707.

ISBN 1-56159-145-0

A catalogue record for this book is available from the Library of Congress.

UNIVERSITY
LIBRARY
NOTTINGHAM

First edition published in the United Kingdom by Macmillan Publishers Ltd, 1991.
Second edition first published in the United Kingdom by
MACMILLAN REFERENCE LTD, 1997
25 Eccleston Place, London SW1W 9NF
and Basingstoke

Companies and representatives throughout the world.

ISBN 0-333-625048

Distributed by Macmillan Direct Ltd
Brunel Road, Houndmills, Basingstoke,
Hampshire RG21 6XS, UK

A catalogue record for this book is available from the British Library.

Typeset by Morton Word Processing Ltd, Scarborough
Printed in Great Britain by The Bath Press, Bath

CONTENTS

iii

FOREWORD

It is a pleasure to contribute a Foreword to the 2nd Edition of this book. The editors are to be congratulated on being able to produce an almost entirely new volume so soon after the publication of the first edition. The outstanding success of the first edition is witnessed by the sales achieved and the need for the publishers to carry out several reprints. I think it is also fair to say that the 'Principles and Practice of Immunoassay' has established itself as the major book of reference on this subject.

As the Editors state the general area of immunoassay technology has become one of the foremost approaches to clinical diagnosis (although it is by no means limited to this application). It continues to astonish me how basic and applied scientists have pushed the methodologies forward at such a pace that without reviews such as this volume those of us who wish to apply the techniques would not be abreast of the best techniques. I am also most impressed by the 'hard-headed' critiques supplied for some of the more fancy molecular biological approaches to the production of antibodies (or should we now call them 'binding reagents'?) The bench workers who mainly wish to measure something rather than to spend years on assay methodology may be influenced by the novelty of a new approach without appreciating its current limitations. By turning these pages he or she is soon brought down to earth with a review of what has actually been achieved.

The editors have been very brave in providing a look into the future of immunoassay. This is undoubtedly as realistic as any of us could be at the moment. Mischievously I look forward to the 3rd Edition in five years' time and the final chapter which analyses where they went wrong and why !

C N Hales
Professor of Clinical Biochemistry
University of Cambridge

LIST OF CONTRIBUTORS

Dr Lars I. Andersson
Research Scientist
Department of Bioanalytical Chemistry
Pharmaceutical and Analytical R & D
Astra Pain Control AB
S-151 85 Södertälje
Sweden

Dr Rene Arentzen
Dade International Inc.
Glasgow Research Laboratory, Site 707
Newark
DE 18714-6101
USA

Dr Geoff Barnard
Regional Endocrine Unit
Duthie Building, 1st Floor
Southampton University
Tremona Road
Southampton
SO16 6YD
UK

Dr William Bedzyk
Dade International Inc.
Glasgow Research Laboratory, Site 707
Newark
DE 18714-6101
USA

Dr Roger A. Bunce
Wolfson Applied Technology Laboratory
Wolfson Research Laboratories,
Queen Elizabeth Medical Centre
Edgebaston
Birmingham
B15 2TH
UK

Dr Lee Anne Cassidy
Dade International Inc.
Glasgow Research Laboratory, Site 707
Newark
DE 18714-6101
USA

Dr Frederick Chu
Division of Molecular Endocrinology
University College London Medical School
Mortimer Street
London W1N 8AA
UK

Dr Sue J. Danielson
Principal Scientist
Johnson & Johnson Clinical Diagnostics
Rochester
NY 14650-2101
USA

Dr Ray Edwards
Director, NETRIA
The Royal Hospitals NHS Trust
St Bartholomew's Hospital
51-53 Bartholomew Close
London EC1A 7BE
UK

Professor Roger P. Ekins
Division of Molecular Endocrinology
University College London Medical School
Mortimer Street
London W1N 8AA
UK

Dr Andrew J. T. George
Department of Immunology
Royal Postgraduate Medical School
Hammersmith Hospital
Du Cane Road
London W12 0NN
UK

Dr Eileen G. Gorman
700 Cheltenham Road
Wilmington
DE 19808-1507
USA

Dr James P. Gosling
Department of Biochemistry
National Diagnostic Centre
University College Galway
Galway
Ireland

Dr Jan Hall
Wolfson Applied Technology Laboratory
Wolfson Research Laboratories,
Queen Elizabeth Medical Centre
Edgebaston
Birmingham
B15 2TH
UK

Dr David A. Hilborn
Johnson & Johnson Clinical Diagnostics
Rochester
NY 14650-2101
USA

Dr John Kane
Department of Medicine (Clinical Biochemistry)
Clinical Sciences Building
Hope Hospital
Salford M6 8HD

Dr Robert Karlsson
Biacore AB (publ)
Rapsgatan 7
S754 50 Uppsala
Sweden

Dr Christine L. Knott
Hybritech Inc.
11095 Torryana Road
PO Box 269006
San Diego
CA 92196-9006
USA

Dr Larry J. Kricka
Director, General Chemistry Laboratory
Professor of Pathology & Laboratory Medicine
University of Pennsylvania Medical Center
7103 Founders Pavilion
3400 Spruce Street
PA 19104-4283
USA

Dr Kristine Kuus-Reichel
Hybritech Inc.
11095 Torryana Road
PO Box 269006
San Diego
CA 92196-9006
USA

Dr Ru-Shya Liu
Hybritech Inc.
11095 Torryana Road
PO Box 269006
San Diego
CA 92196-9006
USA

Dr Christopher R. Lowe
Director, Institute of Biotechnology
University of Cambridge
Tennis Court Road
Cambridge
CB2 1QT
UK

Professor Klaus Mosbach
Department of Pure and Applied Biochemistry
Chemical Center
University of Lund
PO Box 124
S-221 00 Lund
Sweden

Dr Denise Pollard-Knight
Divisional Director of Life Sciences
Scientific Generics
Harston Mill
Harston
Cambridge
CB2 5NH
UK

Dr Duncan R. Purvis
Technology Consultant
Scientific Generics
Harston Mill
Harston
Cambridge CB2 5NH
UK

Dr Peter R. Raggatt
Department of Clinical Biochemistry
Addenbrooke's Hospital
Hills Road
Cambridge
CB2 2QR
UK

Dr Haken Roos
Biacore AB
Rapsgaten 7
S 754 50 Uppsala
Sweden

Dr John Seth
Endocrine and Tumour Marker Section
Department of Clinical Biochemistry
The Royal Infirmary of Edinburgh
Lauriston Place
Edinburgh
EH3 9YW
UK

Dr Ulf-Haken Stenman
Head, Hormone & Tumour Marker Laboratory
Department of Clinical Chemistry
Helsinki University Central Hospital
Haartmaninkatu 2
SF-00290 Helsinki
Finland

Dr Garry H. Thorpe
Wolfson Applied Technology Laboratory
Wolfson Research Laboratories
Queen Elizabeth Medical Centre
Edgbaston
Birmingham
B15 2TH
UK

Dr Paul Treloar
Department of Medicine (Clinical Biochemistry)
Clinical Sciences Building
Hope Hospital
Salford
M6 8HD
UK

Dr Marc H. V. Van Regenmortel
Head, Immunochemistry Department
Institute of Molecular and Cellular Biology
CNRS
15 rue René Descartes
67084 Strasbourg Cedex
France

Dr Ian Weeks
Molecular Light Technology Research Ltd
Cardiff Business Technology Centre
Senyhenydd Road
Cardiff
CF2 4AY
UK

Dr Peter Wilding
University of Pennsylvania Medical Center
7103 Founders Pavilion
3400 Spruce Street
Philadelphia
PA 19104-4283
USA

Dr Robert L. Wolfert
Hybritech Inc.
11095 Torreyana Road
PO Box 269006
San Diego
CA 92196-9006
USA

Dr Peter J. Wood
Regional Endocrine Unit
Duthie Building, 1st Floor
Southampton University
Tremona Road
Southampton
SO16 6YD
UK

Professor Pankaj Vadgama
Department of Medicine (Clinical Biochemistry)
Clinical Sciences Building
Hope Hospital
Salford
M6 8HD
UK

LIST OF ABBREVIATIONS

AACC	American Association for Clinical Chemistry		CLIA-88	(US) Clinical Laboratory Improvement Amendments 1988
AAI	ambient analyte immunoassay		CMD	carboxymethyldextran
ABTS	2,2′-azino-di-[3-ethylbenzthiazoline-6-sulphonate]		CPG	controlled pore glass
AC	alternating current		CR_{50}	coefficient of crossreactivity
ACDU	automatic cell deposition unit		CRAb	chelating recombinant antibody
ACMIA	affinity column-mediated immunoassay		CRM	certified reference materials
ACT	α1-antichymotrypsin		CRP	C-reactive protein
ACTH	adrenocorticotrophic hormone		CSF	cerebrospinal fluid
AFP	alphafetoprotein		CT	computerised (axial) tomography
ALP, AP	alkaline phosphatase		CV	coefficient of variation
ALTM	all-laboratory trimmed mean		dAbs	antigen-binding variable-region domains
AMG	α2-macroglobulin		DCIP	2,6-dichloroindophenol
AMPPD	3,4-methoxyspiro(1,2-dioxetane-3,2′-tricyclo[3.3.1.1.3,7]decan)-4-yl phenyl phosphate		DELFIA	dissociation-enhanced lanthanide fluorescence immunoassay
ANS	8-anilino-1-naphthalene sulphonic acid		DMAB	3-(dimethylamino) benzoic acid
AP, ALP	alkaline phosphatase		DMSO	dimethylsulphoxide
APC	allophycocyanin		DNP	dinitrophenylaminocaproyldipalmitoylphosphatidylethanolamine
APRT	adenine phosphoribosyltransferase			
ARIS	apoenzyme reactivation immunoassay systems		DPASV	differential pulse anode-stripping voltammetry
ATCC	American Type Culture Collection		DPP	differential pulse polarography
ATP	adenosine triphosphate		dsFv	disulphide-stabilized variable fragment
ATR	attenuated total reflection		DTPA	diethylenetriamine pentaacetic acid
B	total binding		EA	enzyme acceptors
B_0	binding at zero concentration		EBV	Epstein–Barr virus
BAW	bulk acoustic wave		EC	electrochemical (detection)
BCIP	bromochloroindolyl phosphate		EC	European Community
BCR	Community Reference Bureau		ECBS	Expert Committee on Biological Standardisation
BFA	bifunctional antibodies		ED	enzyme donors
BIPM	International Bureau of Weights and Measures		ED_{50}	estimated dose for 50% maximum binding
BSA	bovine serum albumin		EG	oestrone-3-glucuronide
CA	cancer antigen		EIA	enzymeimmunoassay
CAP	College of American Pathologists (National Committee of)		ELISA	enzyme-linked immunosorbent assay
			EMIT	enzyme-multiplied immunoassay technique
CBG	cortisol-binding globulin		EMU	early morning urine
CCD	charge-coupled device		EQA	external quality assessment
CD	collisional deactivation		EQAS	external quality assessment schemes
CDC	Centers for Disease Control		FACS	fluorescence-activated cell sorting
CDI	carbodiimide		FAD	flavine adenine dinucleotide
CDR	complementarity determining region		FADP	flavin adenine dinucleotide phosphate
CEA	carcinoembryonic antigen		FCFD	fluorescence capillary fill device
CEDIA	cloned enzyme donor immunoassay		FDA	Food and Drug Administration
CELIA	competitive enzyme-linked immunoassay		FET	field-effect transistor
CFA	complete Freund's adjuvant		FETI	fluorescence excitation transfer immunoassay
CFCC	Canadian Federation for Clinical Chemistry		FIA	flow-injection analysis

FIA	fluoroimmunoassay
FITC	fluorescein isothiocyanate
FMIA	fluorescence modulation immunoassay
FPIA	fluorescence polarisation immunoassay
FSH	follicle-stimulating hormone
G6PDH	glucose-6-phosphate dehydrogenase
HAMA	human anti-mouse antibody
HAT	hypoxanthine, aminopterin and thymidine (growth medium)
HbA1c	haemoglobin A1c
hCG	human chorionic gonadotrophin
HGPRT	hypoxanthine : guanine phosphoribosyltransferase
HIV	human immunodeficiency virus
hK2	human kallikrein-2
HLA	human leukocyte antigen
HMFG	human milk fat globule
HPA	hydrophobic surface (sensor chip)
HPL	human placental lactogen
HPLC	high-performance liquid chromatography
HRP	horseradish peroxidase
HSA	human serum albumin
i.p.	intraperitoneal
i.v.	intravenous
IAEA	International Atomic Energy Agency (Vienna)
IC	internal conversion
ID-MS	isotope dilution–mass spectrometry
IEC	International Electrotechnical Commission
IEMA	immunoenzymometric assay
IFCC	International Federation of Clinical Chemistry
IFMA	immunofluorometric assay
Ig	immunoglobulin
IL-4	interleukin-4
IL-6	interleukin-6
INSTAND	Institute for Standardisation and Documentation in Medical Laboratories (Germany)
IOMI	International Organisation of Legal Metrology
IQC	internal quality control
IQ-FIA	substrate-labelled fluoroimmunoassay
IRMA	immunoradiometric assay
IRP	International Reference Preparation
IS	International Standards
ISC	intersystem crossing
ISFET	ion-selective field-effect transistor
ISO	International Organisation for Standardisation
N^1-ITC-benzyl DTTA Eu^{3+}	N^1-(p-isothiocyanato-benzyl)-diethylene triamine tetra-acetic acid-Eu^{3+}
IU	International Unit
IUPAC	International Union of Pure and Applied Chemistry
IUPAP	International Union of Pure and Applied Physics
IUPAZ	International Union of Pure and Applied Chemistry
IVD	*in vitro* diagnostic (products)
K_a, K_a	affinity constant (association)
K_d, K_d	affinity constant (dissociation)
k_a, k_a	association rate constant
k_d, k_d	dissociation rate constant
KLH	keyhole limpet haemocyanin
LAPS	light-addressable potentiometric sensor
LC	liquid chromatography
LCR	ligase chain reaction
LED	light-emitting diode
LH	luteinising hormone
LIS	laboratory information systems
LOCI	luminescent oxygen channelling assay
Lp(a)	lipoprotein a
LPS	lipopolysaccharide
MAb	monoclonal antibody
MBS	*m*-maleimidobenzoyl-*N*-hydroxysuccinimide ester
MBTH	3-methyl-2-benzothiazolinone hydrazone
MCIA	microcapsule immunoassay
MDD	minimum detectable difference
MDP	muramyldipeptide
MEM	minimal essential medium
MHC	major histocompatibility complex
MIA	molecularly imprinted sorbent assay
MIP	molecularly imprinted polymer
MoM	multiples of the median
MPL	monophosphoryl lipid A
M_r	relative molecular mass
MRI	magnetic resonance imaging
MT&S	Measurement, Testing and Standards
4-MUP	4-methylumbelliferyl phosphate
MUG	4-methylumbelliferyl-β-d-galactoside
NAD$^+$	nicotinamide adenine dinucleotide (oxidised)
NADH	nicotinamide adenine dinucleotide (reduced)
NCA	normal crossreacting antigen
NCCLS	National Committee of Clinical Laboratory Standardisation
NHS	*N*-hydroxysuccinimide
NIBSC	National Institute for Biological Standards and Control

NIH	National Institutes of Health		RZ	Reinzeitszahl number
NRL	Naval Research Laboratory		SA	streptavidin-coated (sensor chip)
OPD	o-phenylenediamine		SAF-1	Syntex adjuvant formulation
OTC	'over the counter'		SAM	self-assembled monolayer
PAP	prostatic acid phosphatase		SAW	surface acoustic wave
PBD	photothermal beam deflection (spectroscopy)		SCID	severe combined immunodeficient (mice)
PBL	peripheral blood lymphocyte		SD	standard deviation
PBS	phosphate-buffered saline		SDS	sodium dodecyl sulphate
PC	personal computer		sFv	single-chain variable fragment
PC	phosphorylcholine		SH	shear-horizontally (polarised)
PCP	phencyclidine		SHBG	sex hormone-binding globulin
PCR	polymerase chain reaction		SLFIA	substrate-labelled fluorescent immunoassay
PCS	photon correlation spectroscopy		SMCC	N-succinimidyl-4-(N-maleimidomethyl)cyclohexane-1-carboxylate
PDEA	2-(2-pyridinyldithio)ethaneamine hydrochloride			
PEG	polyethylene glycol		SPA	scintillation proximity assay
PG	pregnanediol-3-glucuronide		SpA	staphylococcal Protein A
PGLIA	prosthetic group labelled immunoassay		SPR	surface plasmon resonance
PIOP	paramagnetic iron oxide particles		SSBW	surface-skimming bulk wave
PMMA	polymethyl methacrylate		T_3	triiodothyronine
PMT	photomultiplier tube		T_4	thyroxine
PS	photothermal spectroscopy		TAS	total analytical system
PSA	prostate-specific antigen		µTAS	micro-total analytical system
$PS\beta_1G$	pregnancy-specific β_1-glycoprotein		TBG	thyroxine-binding globulin
PTFE	polytetrafluoroethylene		T-BSA	BSA derivatized with aryldiazirines
PTH	parathyroid hormone (parathormone)		^{99m}Tc	technetium-99m
PVDF	polyvinylidine difluoride		TDM	therapeutic drug monitoring
QA	quality assurance		TDM	trehalose dimycolate
QCM	quartz crystal microbalance		TE	transverse electric
RAC	repeat analytical controls		T_g	glass transition temperature
RBE	radiobiological effectiveness		THC	tetrahydrocannabinoid
RCB	recombinant-cell bioassay		TIRF	total internal reflection fluorescence (technique)
RER	response error relationship		TK	thymidine kinase
RES	reticuloendothelial system		TLC	thin-layer chromatography
RF	rheumatoid factor		TM	transverse magnetic (component of light)
RFIA	release fluoroimmunoassay		TMB	3,3′,5,5′-tetramethylbenzidine
RIA	radioimmunoassay		TSH	thyroid-stimulating hormone (thyrotrophin)
RM	resonant mirror		UK NEQAS	United Kingdom National External Quality Assessment Scheme
RMV	reference method value			
RP	relative potency		VDU	visual display unit
RPPHS	reference preparation for proteins in human serum = CRM470		WHO	World Health Organisation

Chapter 1

Introduction

Christopher P. Price and David J. Newman

Immunoassay is now the fastest-growing analytical technology in use for the detection and quantification of biomolecules in the diagnosis and management of disease. Along with the various chromatographic techniques, immunoassay is probably the most commonly used technology for the analysis of biomolecules; each technique, of course, has its individual merits. Thus, although chromatographic techniques can detect and quantify a family of compounds, the immunoassay is generally intended for the specific quantification of a single molecular species. It may also be argued that chromatographic techniques are capable of greater discrimination between chemical structures, and they are often used as the analytical tool that precedes the development of an immunoassay for a new diagnostic marker. A review of the technology available shows that immunoassays can be developed that use less complex equipment, allowing them to be used in a wider range of testing environments. Thus, immunolog- ical- and chromatographic assays should be considered as complementary techniques.

The immunoassay takes advantage of a natural phenomenon in order to generate a biological functional molecule: an antibody. However, the antibody is not the only biological molecule that can be used for the quantification of antigens; bioassays using whole cells, receptors, binding proteins and enzymes can all be used for the quantification of antigens, particularly small molecules. However, the latter 'complementary molecules' can only provide reagents for a limited range of molecules; furthermore, in many instances they do not offer the unique specificity that can be attained with an antibody while also having relatively low affinity constants.

THE ANTIGEN-ANTIBODY REACTION

An immunoassay is a quantitative technique that depends on the reaction between the molecule of interest, 'the antigen', and a complementary molecule, 'the antibody'. The antigen is so called because it is a molecule capable of eliciting an immune response when injected into an animal (in which it is treated as a foreign species). The nature of the immune response and the production of antibodies is discussed in Chapter 3.

The antigen can be a small molecule (a hapten), such as the steroid hormone cortisol (relative molecular mass, M_r, 362) or the drug theophylline (M_r 180), or it can be a large protein such as albumin (M_r 66,000) or ferritin (M_r 580,000). However, there is only one portion of the antigen that binds to the antibody; the **epitope** of the antigen binds with the **paratope** of the antibody. An antigen may contain several epitopes, but only be capable of binding one antibody molecule, the remaining surface of the molecule being unavailable for binding because of steric hindrance of the first antibody molecule; thus a small molecule may consist of a series of overlapping epitopes, although only one can function at any time. On the other hand, a large biomolecule will contain many epitopes and indeed copies of the same epitope; furthermore a large biomolecule will have many independent epitopes, i.e. it is capable of binding several antibody molecules at the same time (Van Regenmortel, 1992). The nature of the epitope and complementary paratope and the nature of the antigen-antibody reaction are discussed in Chapter 2.

MOLECULAR BIOCHEMISTRY OF ANTIGEN AND ANTIBODY

As the nature of the molecular chemistry of the antigen-antibody reaction becomes clear, the prospect of being able to engineer more unique molecules is evident. The first example of this was the organic chemistry applied to the production of an immunogen to enable production of antibodies against small molecules (haptens). A particular example was the production of steroid molecule immunogens that exposed or presented the unique element of the steroid molecule (Corrie, 1983).

The next innovation was the production of monoclonal antibodies, a development that has revolutionised the whole field of immunoassay (Köhler & Milstein, 1975). The two key benefits were: (1) the ability to isolate a cell producing a single antibody species and (2) immortalising of this cell by fusion with a tumour cell line to produce a hybridoma. The ability to isolate a single antibody has improved the specificity of assays and the consistency of reagent supply (*see* Chapter 3).

As our knowledge of the antigen-antibody reaction increased (especially our knowledge of the molecular chemistry of the antibody paratope), it is not surprising that the next development was that of molecular biological techniques for modification of the paratope structure to improve the characteristics of the antibody. The first of these developments was the production of single-chain antibodies, of particular interest to immunotherapists looking to use antibodies as a means of targeting drug delivery in the body (Bird *et al.*, 1988). However, the expression of a single-chain antibody in a bacterial expression vector facilitated (1) modification of the amino acid sequence of the antibody as well as (2) large-scale production of an immortalised antibody. The subject of antibody engineering and its capabilities are discussed in Chapter 4.

The manipulation of the epitope region to enhance the specificity of antibodies has been extended in the case of complex molecules by the use of peptides as antigens (Bidart *et al.*, 1990). It is not surprising therefore that, having learnt how to construct the epitope to improve antibody specificity, then the next challenge would be to synthesise the paratope (Mosbach and Ramström, 1996), ie. an antibody mimic. The core of this development is the knowledge of the complementarity of primary, secondary and tertiary molecular structures associated with epitope and paratope. The development of this new contribution to immunoassay technology is described in Chapter 7.

The complete synthesis of a paratope mimic and its use in quantitative analysis must call into question the use of the term 'immunoassay'. This should serve to remind us that there are other means of recognising the unique features of molecules, some by virtue of other properties such as spectra and catalytic activity, as well as molecular constitution and conformation. The reader is left to judge the relative merits of these alternative approaches after a detailed discussion of the various approaches to immunoassay in the following chapters.

CLASSIFICATION OF IMMUNOASSAYS

Although the complementarity between antigen and antibody may enable the recognition of an antigen in a complex biological matrix such as whole blood, serum or urine, the antibody will not readily allow characterisation of a molecule. Thus an antibody species can be used for the purification of an antigen, recognition of its presence in a complex mixture, and its quantification. However, all of these functions are dependent on proof of specificity, and thus the availability of a pure antigen. In this case, the term 'pure antigen' must encompass conformational as well as constitutional identity; in other words, if you purify an antigen to homogeneity you must recognise that you may alter its tertiary structure (quite common in the case of proteins) such that it differs from the antigen as it appears in the biological sample of interest. This topic is very pertinent to calibration of immunoassays and is discussed in Chapter 11. However, although antibodies can be used for the recognition of antigens and to which all the above arguments apply, the term immunoassay is confined to the use of antibodies for the quantification of antigens (or indeed the use of antigens for the quantification of antibodies). In this respect quantification encompasses assays that may appear qualitative by reporting a positive or negative result, but in fact use a cut-off value that is clearly defined (e.g. in drugs of abuse testing), through to a fully quantitative result.

In this respect, it is interesting to reflect on the idea that quantitative methods can be considered as either 'comparative' or 'analytical' (Ekins, 1976). The 'comparative' or 'functionally directed (specific)' assay is exemplified in a bioassay and the 'analytical' or 'structurally directed (specific)' assay is a more physicochemical assay in which a gravimetric (i.e. defined) amount or concentration of a single species is measured. Miyai (1985) pointed out, in his classification of immunoassays, that the term 'comparative' assay is also used in a general sense implying that an assay involving the use of a standard or reference material is comparative. He argued that the immunoassay, as a quantitative method was an 'analytical assay' technique that also used a standard. It could also be argued that an immunocapture assay, such as that for an enzyme using one antibody with detection of capture using the enzymes' activity, might constitute a gravimetric assay; this assumes that the specific activity of the enzyme is known and is preserved (in the case of both: (1) the process by which it was derived, i.e. purification protocol, etc.; and (2) the sample preparation for the quantitative assay).

Immunoassays can be classified according to a range of criteria including sample type, nature of analyte, assay conditions, etc., (Miyai, 1985; Gosling, 1990). The majority of approaches have been described for the quantification of antigens, although most are equally applicable in the case of assays for large molecules, for antibodies.

The three major criteria for classification that have the greatest influence on the performance that can be expected of an assay with regard to precision and sensitivity are: (1) the use of a limited or excessive reagent format; (2) the use of a homogeneous or heterogeneous format and (3) the use of a label or unlabelled assay format and then choice of label. The accuracy (or bias) of an assay will primarily, but not solely, depend on the characteristics of the complementary molecule (i.e. antibody in the case of an assay for antigen). The influence of factors other than the antibody (listed in Table 1) are discussed throughout this book at the most appropriate points.

Limited Reagent

In this assay format for determining the amount of antigen present, a limited amount of antibody is used (the so called 'limited reagent') which is insufficient to bind all of the antigen. A fixed amount of labelled antigen competes with the unlabelled antigen (from the sample) for the limited number of antibody binding sites. The concentration of unlabelled antigen can be determined from the proportion of labelled antigen that is bound to the antibody (or remains free). It is clearly important that the amounts of labelled antigen and antibody are kept constant, so that the amount of bound (or free) labelled antigen can be compared with a series of calibrators to obtain a quantitative result.

Sample		
	Nature of antigen	Size
		pI
		Hydrophobicity
	Matrix	Viscosity
		Presence of binding proteins
		Presence of unusual antibodies
		Presence of crossreacting species, e.g. metabolites
		Interference with label
Reagent		Immunoassay buffer pH, ionic strength
		Polymer enhancers
		Detergents
		Preservatives
Reaction environment		Temperature
		Mixing
		Sequence and speed of addition of reagents

Table 1 Factors that influence the design and performance of an immunoassay.

Excess Reagent

In this assay format, antigen binds to an excess of antibody; a variety of approaches has been developed to detect the bound antigen. The most common is the two-site immunometric assay (the so called 'sandwich' assay); in this approach, the first antibody in excess is coupled to a solid phase. The bound antigen is then detected with a second antibody labelled in a way that aids detection (e.g. by use of an enzyme, fluorophore, etc.). In this instance, the amount of labelled antibody captured on the solid phase (i.e. forming the sandwich) is directly proportional to the amount of antigen in the sample.

The delineation into 'limited' or 'excess' reagent assay has important practical consequences. First, as indicated earlier, the response in a limited-reagent competitive assay is highly dependent on the amount of labelled antigen and antibody present, as well as sample antigen concentration; therefore sample and reagent metering have an important bearing on assay precision. Second, and of more positive benefit, is the fact that a situation of antigen excess never arises because, as the amount of sample antigen increases, the amount of bound labelled antigen diminishes toward zero. Third, in a limited-reagent competitive assay the equilibrium constant is of vital importance because the sensitivity of the assay is determined by its value (Ekins *et al.*, 1968).

Conversely, in a situation where there is an 'excess' of reagent antibody, metering of reagent is less critical; however, the situation of antigen excess has finite limits and, when it occurs, leads to a 'hook effect' when both antibody reagents are added simultaneously; above a certain sample concentration the response is no longer proportional to concentration and indeed falls, with the consequence that a particular response may be given for two different

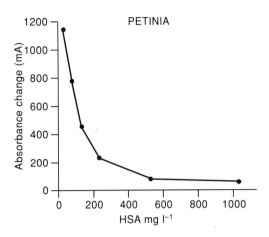
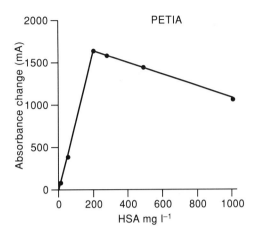

Figure 1 Examples of the calibration curves for the measurement of urine albumin using limited- and excess-reagent format. In this instance the examples are light-scattering immunoassays, the former, particle enhanced turbidimetric inhibition immunoassay (PETINIA) using human serum albumin coupled to a 70-nm latex particle together with a monoclonal antibody; the latter, particle enhanced turbidimetric immunoassay (PETIA) used a polyclonal antibody coupled to a 40-nm latex particle.

sample concentrations. This can produce aberrant low results for samples with a high antigen concentration, as for example in the case of a tumour marker assay when a very wide concentration range of analyte may be experienced. This problem can be overcome by the sequential addition of reagents. This situation necessitates careful design of the assay and recognition of the concentration at which a hook effect may occur. In practice the sensitivity of an excess reagent assay system is defined by the nonspecific binding and, to a lesser degree, by the 'activity' of the label. The calibration curves for limited- and excess-reagent assays are illustrated in Figure 1.

The benefits of the excess-reagent or immunometric assay were not available for the quantification of haptens until the development of anti-idiotypic antibodies (Barnard and Kohen, 1990; Altamirano-Bustamante *et al.*, 1991). Briefly, these assays involve the development of an antibody that recognises either hapten bound to antibody (but not free antibody, i.e. the occupied binding site itself) or free antibody (but not occupied antibody, i.e. the empty binding site itself).

Heterogeneous and Homogeneous

The use of either competitive or immunometric assays requires differentiation of bound from free label. This can be achieved either: (1) by separating bound from free label using a means of removing the antibody (heterogeneous assay) or (2) modulation of the signal of the label when antigen is bound to antibody compared to when it is free (homogeneous assay).

Heterogeneous There are many ways of separating bound from free label and these are discussed in Chapter 8. These can be briefly described in terms of: (1) precipitation of antibody; (2) coupling of antibody to a solid phase; and (3) chromatographic techniques.

In each case, the performance of the method is governed by: (1) the completeness of the separation, i.e. efficiency and lack of influence on the primary antigen-antibody equilibrium; (2) the efficiency of the washing to remove any unbound label; and (3) the level of nonspecific binding.

Homogeneous The need to separate free from bound label constitutes another analytical step (two steps if you include washing), which can influence method precision. Furthermore, it has proved a challenge to the automation of immunoassays and is probably one of the main stimuli for what has been a burgeoning development in homogeneous immunoassays over the past two decades. Indeed, Gorman *et al.* in Chapter 13 argue that researchers will continue to search for homogeneous assays with better sensitivity because of the greater simplicity of automation.

Miyai (1985) in his classification of immunoassays differentiates between direct modulation, indirect modulation and coupled modulation. In the case of direct modulation, binding of antibody to labelled antigen modulates a property of the label, e.g. enzyme activity, either decreasing or increasing the signal. Examples discussed elsewhere in this book include enzyme-multiplied immunoassay (EMIT, Chapter 15), fluorescence polarisation immunoassay (FPIA, Chapter 16) and luminescence enhancement or quenching (Chapter 17).

Indirect modulation is typified by the use of a cofactor or inhibitor as a label, the binding of antibody to labelled antigen influencing (generally inhibiting) the ability of the cofactor (etc.) to activate (etc.) an apoenzyme present in the reaction mixture. Coupled modulation describes an assay in which signal generation (e.g. fluorescence excitation) proceeds when the reactants are brought close together by the antigen-antibody binding.

There are many examples of homogeneous immunoassays and it is beyond the scope of this chapter to list them all, and they continue to be discovered. The reader is referred to previous reviews to get a flavour of the options, and this book to appreciate some of them in greater detail (Masseyeff *et al.*, 1993).

Immunoassays without Labels In which antigen molecules react with antibody molecules to form an immunoaggregate that can be detected by its turbidity. In its simplest form it is only applicable to large biomolecules and is discussed in Chapter 18. Effectively, the assay can be considered as a direct modulation homogeneous immunoassay, with the antibody acting as its own label. Greater sensitivity can be achieved by further labelling antibody with a particle, both types being reagent-excess assays (Price and Newman, 1993). The style of assay can be modified to a competitive format with its inherent benefits and pitfalls as mentioned earlier, by use of a labelled antigen. The role of antigen and antibody are reversed when designing an assay for the antibody.

Work Simplification The importance of sample and reagent metering in determining the accuracy and reproducibility of a method has led to many approaches to work simplification. This has encompassed the encapsulation of reagent components, the development of a complete unit-dose device requiring only the addition of diluent and sample, to the complete automation of all of the analytical steps. The emphasis of the work simplification, either in manufacture of a unit or in process automation, depends on the final use intended, the latter being favoured when a large throughput is called for. The topic of complete automation is discussed by Gorman *et al.* in Chapter 13. An alternative approach is to encapsulate the assay in a single-use device of which several examples are discussed in later chapters.

Immunosensors Although the term immunosensor can be used very broadly, even to include the use of an electrode to detect the product of an enzyme-label captured on a solid-phase sandwich assay (as discussed in part in Chapter 19, it should be reserved for a direct immunosensor device that detects the binding of antigen directly to the sensor surface (Morgan *et al.* 1996). As such, it is a true homogeneous immunoassay and, in Miyai's terms, reflects coupled modulation, i.e. the antigen is only sensed when close to the surface i.e. when bound to antibody (or vice versa when detecting antibody). The design of immunosensors is discussed in Chapter 19.

Immunochromatographic Systems In most instances this style of assay effectively embraces a heterogeneous immunoassay in a single operator step and, therefore, provides for the operator the simplicity of the homogeneous assay. However, in terms of design it is a true heterogeneous assay and must be optimised in those terms, e.g. the efficiency of removal of unbound label. The design of these apparently simple assays are described in chapters 21 and 22, illustrating the transition that has occurred with the effort made by the reagent manufacture to 'design out' the variability of the assay through encapsulation. This is further extended in Chapter 23 with the developments in microfabrication and the further benefits of miniaturisation.

The main market for these devices is for what is broadly called 'point-of-care' testing which might include 'over-the-counter' use. Clearly, the operators will in the main be less technically trained and therefore simplicity of operation is important. Early examples were developed with a urine sample in mind, the sample providing the diluent for the solubilisation and migration of the reagent. More recently there have been assays developed using a whole blood sample; clearly these are more demanding because of the more viscous nature of the matrix. Despite these apparent potential drawbacks, satisfactory performance has been demonstrated.

Methods of detection

Radioisotope, e.g. ^{125}I, ^{14}C

Enzyme, e.g. alkaline phosphatase

Enzyme cofactor, e.g. flavine adenine dinucleotide

Enzyme substrate, e.g. galactosyl umbelliferone

Fluorophore, e.g. fluorescein

Luminescent species, e.g. acridinium ester, luminol

Particle, e.g. latex, carbon sol

Metal ion, e.g. Au^{3+}

Ionophore, e.g. valinomycin

Table 2 Choice of labels in immunoassay (the examples are not exhaustive).

Colorimetry	Sensors:
Fluorometry	Potentiometric
Phosphorescence	Amperometric
Luminescence	Piezoelectric
Turbidimetry	Surface plasmon resonance
Nephelometry	Ellipsometry
Photon correlation	Total internal reflection
Photothermal	
Isotope counting	
Neutron activation	
Atomic absorption	

Table 3 Methods of detection used in immunoassay.

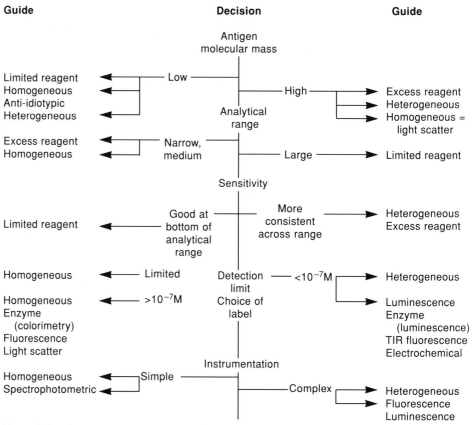

Figure 2 A typical practical decision tree for the design of an immunoassay format for an antigen. This is not exhaustive and variations may be introduced.

Quantification of the antigen-antibody reaction can be by visual assessment or using a variety of instrumentation. The choice of immunoassay format (limited or excess reagent), label and instrumentation can, all influence the characteristics of the assay with respect to detection limit, precision and analytical range (Kricka, 1994). The performance of the different types of immunoassay will be discussed in later chapters; however, a summary of the choice of labels and instrumentation used are given in Tables 2 and 3. This final variable is part of a practical design strategy which will be different for antigen and antibody quantification but can be illustrated briefly by the decision tree shown in Figure 2.

CONCLUSIONS

As our understanding of the antigen-antibody reaction has increased, so has our ability to use it for the quantitation of biomolecules. This has extended to the production of better antibodies (and antigens) as reagents, improved production methods and now synthesis of antibody-like molecules. In parallel, we have improved complementary components of the technology with a greater choice of labels and solid phases, yielding better sensitivity and reduced nonspecific binding.

What was originally a technique demanding expert skills and considerable dedication by the operator, has now been simplified by the manufacturer of diagnostics through automation and encapsulation in apparently simple devices. This apparent simplicity should not, however, mask the innovations that lie behind the technology and the need to understand its complexity to ensure that it is used in an appropriate fashion.

The chapters that follow describe the basic features of an immunoassay and the principles that underpin modern immunoassays to ensure that the user appreciates the strengths and limitations of the technology available.

REFERENCES

Altamirano-Bustamante, A., Barnard, G. & Kohen, F. (1991) Direct time-resolved fluorescence immunoassay for serum estradiol based on the idiotypic anti-idiotypic approach. *J. Immunol. Meth.* **138**, 95–101.

Barnard, G. & Kohen, F. (1990) Idiometric assay: A non-competitive immunoassay for small molecules typified by the measurement of serum estradiol. *Clin. Chem.* **36**, 1945–1950.

Bidart, J.-M., Troalen, F., Ghillani, P. *et al.* (1990) Peptide immunogen mimicry of a protein-specific structural epitope on human choriogonadotropin. *Science* **248**, 736–739.

Bird, R. E., Hardman, K. D. & Jacobson, J. W. *et al.* (1988) Single-chain antigen-binding proteins. *Science* **242**, 423–426.

Corrie, J. E. T. (1983) [125]Iodinated tracers for steroid radioimmunoassay: the problem of bridge recognition. In: *Immunoassay for Clinical Chemistry* (eds Hunter, W. M. & Corrie J. E. T.), pp. 353–357 (Churchill Livingstone, Edinburgh).

Ekins, R. P. (1976) General principles of hormone assay. In: *Hormone Assays and their*

Clinical Application 4th edn (eds Lorraine, J. A. & Bell, E. T.) pp. 1–72 (Churchill Livingstone, Edinburgh).

Ekins, R. P., Newman, B., O'Riordan, J. L. H. (1968) Theoretical aspects of 'saturation' and radioimmunoassay. In: *Radioisotopes in Medicine:* in vitro *Studies.* (eds Hayes, R. L., Goswitz, F. A. & Murphy, B. E. P.) pp. 59–100, (US Atomic Energy Commission, Oak Ridge, Tennessee).

Gosling, J. P. (1990) A decade of development in immunoassay methodology. *Clin. Chem.* **36**, 1408–1427.

Köhler, G. & Milstein, C. (1975) Continuous cultures of fused cells secreting antibody of predefined specificity. *Nature* **256**, 495–497.

Kricka, L. J. (1994) Selected strategies for improving sensitivity and reliability of immunoassays. *Clin. Chem.* **40**, 347–357.

Masseyeff, R. F., Albert, W. H. & Staines, N. A. (eds) (1993) Non separation methods (selected examples). In: *Methods of Immunological Analysis* Vol. 1: *Fundamentals,* pp. 389–475 (VCH, Weinheim).

Miyai, K. (1985) Advances in non-isotopic immunoassay. *Adv. Clin. Chem.* **24**, 61–110.

Morgan, C. L., Newman, D. J. & Price, C. P. (1996) Immunosensors: technology and opportunities in laboratory medicine. *Clin. Chem.* **42**, 193–209.

Mosbach, K. & Ramström, O. (1996) The emerging technique of molecular imprinting and its future impact on biotechnology. *Bio/Technology* **14**, 163–170.

Price, C. P., Newman, D. J. (1993) In: *Methods of Immunological Analysis* Vol.1: *Fundamentals* (eds Masseyeff, R. F., Albert, W. H. & Staines, N. A.) pp. 134–158, (VCH, Weinheim).

Van Regenmortel, M. H. V. (1992) *Structure of Antigens*, Vol. 1 (CRC Press, Boca Raton) p. 415.

Chapter 2

The Antigen–Antibody Reaction

Marc H. V. Van Regenmortel

INTRODUCTION

The term antigen refers to any entity, whether a cell, a macromolecular assembly or a single molecule, that can elicit an immune response in a competent host and be recognised by the products of that immune response. The ability to be recognised by antibodies is called antigenic reactivity, or antigenicity, and the ability to elicit a response, which depends on the potentialities of the host being immunised, is called immunogenicity. Note that immunogenicity is not an intrinsic property of a molecule but a relational property that has no meaning outside the context of the host. Mouse serum albumin is an antigenic protein that is immunogenic in the rabbit but not normally in the mouse because of the regulatory mechanism known as immunological tolerance to self.

The two properties of antigenicity and immunogenicity are clearly dissociated in the case of small antigens, i.e. so-called haptens that have a relative molecular mass (M_r) of about 2K or less. Molecules of this size are antigenic, i.e. they can bind specifically to antibodies, but they are not immunogenic unless conjugated to protein carriers (Frèche, 1993; Morel-Montero and Delaage, 1994).

Proteins and other chemical and biological entities owe their antigenic properties to the existence in higher vertebrates of an immune system endowed with the capacity to recognise and differentiate between a multitude of different structures. This recognition function is carried out by the specialised binding pockets of a family of proteins known as immunoglobulins. Over millions of years of vertebrate evolution, immunoglobulins have developed into exquisitely discriminating devices capable of recognising subtle differences between molecules. A single mouse is able to generate millions of different immunoglobulin specificities, each one arising from a unique combination of about 50 amino acid residues distributed on six loops complementary in shape and chemical composition to particular antigenic structures. These six hypervariable loops form the antibody combining site or paratope of the immunoglobulin molecule. The most common type of immunoglobulin (Ig) known as IgG contains two identical paratopes located at the surface of the molecule. Each paratope is able to bind specifically to an area of about 30 Å × 30 Å of its complementary antigen. This area of the antigen, which is specifically recognised by the paratope, is known as an antigenic determinant or epitope. The antibody nature of an immunoglobulin becomes established only after its complementary antigen has been identified. In the same way, the epitope nature of a small region of the antigen can be recognised only by means of an antibody molecule. Epitopes and paratopes are thus relational entities that can be defined only by their mutual complementarity and not by any intrinsic feature of each partner. The innumerable partnerships between individual epitope and paratope pairs form the basis of every immunoassay and it is the specificity of their interactions that gives immunological reactions their outstanding discriminating capacity.

The recognition function of antibody molecules is expressed by their capacity to bind in a reversible manner to antigen. Immunoglobulins also possess various other effector functions that are mediated by regions of the molecule that do not vary between individual antibodies (Nezlin, 1994). These other biological functions will not be discussed here because the only property of antibodies that is relevant in the context of immunoassays is their capacity to bind to antigens.

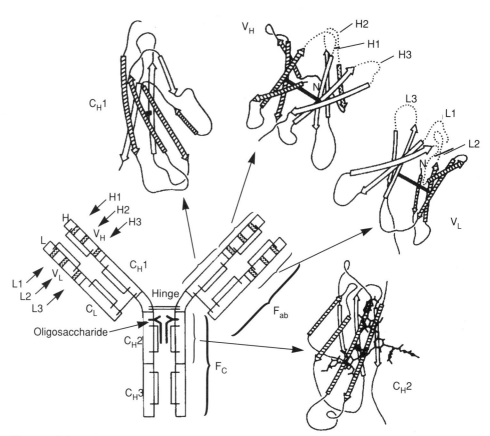

Figure 1 Schematic representation of an antibody molecule (human subclass IgG1). The homologous domains within the heavy (H) and light (L) chains are indicated, and the hypervariable segments within the variable (V) regions are shown. Inter- and intra-chain disulphide bridges are indicated by solid lines. The folding of the polypeptide chain within individual domains is also shown; the arrows represent strands of β-sheet, the solid bars are the intra-domain disulphide bridges, and the homologous four-stranded sheets of each domain are cross-hatched. The location of the hypervariable loop regions (H1–3, L1–3) may be seen within the V domains. An *N*-linked oligosaccharide chain covers part of the four-stranded face of each C_H2 domain. (From Sutton (1993) with permission.)

STRUCTURE OF IMMUNOGLOBULINS

Most immunoglobulins are found in the fraction of serum known as the gamma globulin fraction (on the basis of their electrophoretic mobility). All immunoglobulin molecules are hetero-dimers with a similar architecture consisting of four polypeptide chains linked by disulphide bridges: two identical large or heavy (H) chains of about 450–600 amino acid residues and two small or light (L) chains of about 220 residues. Sequence analysis of H and L chains and X-ray crystallography shows that each chain consists of homologous segments of about 110 amino acids that form independently folded domains (Figure 1) (Sutton, 1993). H and L chains all contain a variable region and a constant region, which are encoded by separate gene segments. The amino-terminal domain of both H and L chains differs in antibodies of different specificity and are called variable (V) regions. Within each V region, three segments exhibit hypervariability and constitute the complementarity-determining regions (CDR) of the immunoglobulin. The six CDRs form hypervariable loops at the ends of the two variable domains, which are labelled L1, L2 and L3 (L chain) and H1, H2 and H3 (H chain), respectively, in Figure 1.

The remaining domains in each chain are invariant and are called constant (C) regions. In the H chain of IgG, there are three constant domains called C_H1, C_H2 and C_H3. Between the C_H1 and C_H2 domains, there is an additional segment termed the hinge which contains the inter-heavy chain disulphide bridges and which confers a certain amount of flexibility on the molecule. The L chains contain a single constant domain called C_L.

Properties	IgG	IgM	IgA	IgD	IgE
H chain type	γ	μ	α	δ	ε
L chain type	κ or λ	κ or λ	κ or λ	κ or λ	κ or λ
Structure	H_2L_2	$(H_2L_2)_5$ + J chain	H_2L_2 and $(H_2L_2)_2$ + SC + J chain	H_2L_2	H_2L_2
Molecular mass	150×10^3	950×10^3	160×10^3	180×10^3	190×10^3
Sedimentation coefficient	7 S	19 S	7 and 11 S	7 S	8 S
Carbohydrate (%)	3	12	8	10	12
Approximate concentration in serum (mg ml^{-1})	10	1	2	0.04	0.0003
Ability to fix complement	+	+	–	–	–

Table 1 Properties of immunoglobulin classes.

In mammals there are five immunoglobulin classes or isotypes that differ in the sequence and carbohydrate content of their heavy chains. These five classes, known as IgG, IgM, IgA, IgD and IgE, contain heavy chains that are called γ, μ, α, δ and ε, respectively (Table 1). In contrast, the L chains are the same for all immunoglobulin classes, although there are two types of them, either lambda (λ) or kappa (κ). The λ and κ chains have different sequences and are usually free of carbohydrate (Nezlin, 1994). The ratio of κ/λ chains in human immunoglobulins and in mouse immunoglobulins is about 70:30 and 95:5, respectively. In mammals there are several IgG subclasses which differ in the structure of their H chains and in the length of the hinge and number of disulphide bridges linking the two H chains. In humans the subclasses are called IgG1, IgG2, IgG3 and IgG4, whereas in mice they are called IgG1, IgG2a, IgG2b and IgG3. In IgM and IgE, the hinge region of the H chain is replaced by an extra domain pair that holds the H chains together.

Immunoglobulins are glycoproteins that contain several carbohydrate chains, usually linked to H chains. Membrane forms of immunoglobulins have additional peptide segments at the carboxy-terminal ends of their H chains, which allow them to be embedded in cell membranes (Nezlin, 1994).

All immunoglobulins can be cleaved at the middle of their H chains by various proteases (Nezlin, 1994). Papain cleaves γ-chains at the N-terminal side of the disulphide bridges that keep the H chains together, thereby generating two Fab (fragment antigen binding) fragments and one Fc (fragment crystallisable) fragment (Figure 1). Each Fab fragment contains one of two identical combining sites of the immunoglobulin.

Pepsin cleaves γ-chains at the C-terminal side of the disulphide bridges and generates a single bivalent F(ab′)$_2$ fragment containing the two combining sites, as well as several smaller fragments of the C_H2 and C_H3 domains (pFc′). The pepsin-derived F(ab′)$_2$ can be dissociated into univalent Fab′ after reduction of the disulphide bridges. After removal of the reducing agent, spontaneous reoxidation of the bridges can occur which leads to the reappearance of bivalent F(ab′)$_2$. Hybrid F(ab′)$_2$ fragments can be obtained if Fab′ fragments from different antibodies are present in the mixture being reoxidised. The sensitivity of various IgG subclasses to proteolytic cleavage varies and depends on the length and sequence of their hinge regions (Nezlin, 1994). In exceptional cases pepsin digestion of immunoglobulins can yield a minimal antigen-binding fragment called Fv (Givol, 1991). The Fv fragment consists of only the variable regions of the H and L chains and retains the antigen-binding capacity of the parent immunoglobulin. Recombinant DNA technology now makes it possible to obtain Fv fragments in a routine manner (Plückthun, 1994).

IgG is the most abundant class of immunoglobulin in the serum of mammals and is synthesised predominantly by plasma cells after secondary exposure to antigen. IgM molecules are the predominant class of immunoglobulins during early phases of the immune response. IgM molecules consist of five subunits that resemble IgG molecules and are linked together by disulphide bridges (Table 1). Each pentameric IgM molecule is composed of 10 μ chains, 10 light chains and one joining (J) chain of M_r 15 × 10^3 which participates in the polymerisation process. Pentameric IgM molecules have 10 antigen-combining sites.

IgA molecules present in serum are usually in monomeric form. IgA is the dominant immunoglobulin found in secretions such as saliva, tears, breast milk and colostrum as well as in the mucus-containing fluids present in the respiratory passages and the gut. In secretions, IgA molecules are present as dimers and to a lesser extent as trimers and tetramers. Polymeric IgA contains a J chain and a secretory component of M_r 80 × 10^3.

STRUCTURE OF PARATOPES

Each immunoglobulin domain is folded such that it forms two β-pleated sheets of strands in antiparallel direction linked by a disulphide bridge. This characteristic folding pattern is known as the immunoglobulin fold. In the constant domains of H and L chains, one sheet is formed by three strands and the second by four strands. The V_L and V_H domains associate noncovalently to form a β-barrel structure which places the six CDR loops close to each other. The way in which the combining site of an antibody is built up from the juxtaposition of the six CDR loops is illustrated in Figure 2. The CDR loops vary not only in sequence but also in length from one antibody to the next (Lesk and Tramontano, 1993). For five of the hypervariable loops, there is only a limited number of main-chain conformations and these

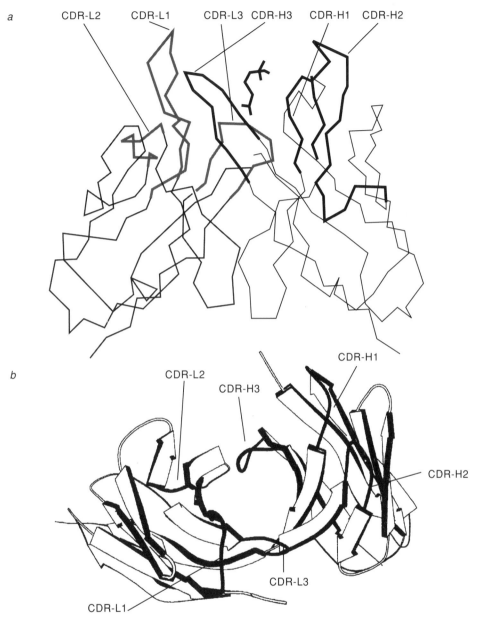

a

CDR-L2 CDR-L1 CDR-L3 CDR-H3 CDR-H1 CDR-H2

b

CDR-L2

CDR-H3

CDR-H1

CDR-H2

CDR-L3

CDR-L1

Figure 2 The hypervariable loops, as defined from sequence analysis shown for one antibody (the phosphorylcholine-binding McPC603 from mouse): *a*, from the side and *b*, from the top. (From Plückthun (1994) with permission.)

depend upon the nature of a few key residues. These commonly occurring main-chain conformations have been called canonical structures (Chothia *et al.*, 1989). The H3 loop is different from the other five loops in that it is sometimes quite long (up to 25 residues) and adopts a greater variety of structures. The range of length in residues of the other loops is: L1, 10–17; L2, 7; L3, 7–11; H1, 5–7 and H2, 9–12 (Rees *et al.*, 1994).

The existence of a limited number of canonical structures has made it possible to develop homology-based modelling methods for predicting the structure of antibody combining sites from primary structure data (Rees *et al.*, 1994). These methods allow the modelling of the main-chain conformations of the combining sites to about 1 Å resolution. Modelling the side chains, however, is a much more formidable problem for which no solution is yet in sight. Because molecular recognition of the epitope involves the side chains of the antibody combining site, this problem will need to be solved if the so-called rational design of antibodies with predetermined specificity is ever to become a reality.

Our knowledge of the structural basis of antigen-antibody interaction has been derived mainly from X-ray diffraction studies of complexes of monoclonal antibody fragments with their protein antigens (Padlan, 1994; Wilson and Stanfield, 1994; Braden and Poljak, 1995). The following features are characteristic of protein-antibody complexes:

1   An area of about 700–900 Å^2 of the antigen surface, made up of between 15 and 22 amino acid residues, is in contact with about the same number of residues of the antibody.

2   The paratopes consist of a limited number of residues originating from most or all of the CDRs of immunoglobulin molecules.

3   About half of the CDR residues implicated in the paratope are aromatic residues.

4   All protein epitopes identified so far are discontinuous and are made up of residues from between two and five separate regions of the antigen polypeptide chain.

Because of their small size, most haptens make fewer contacts with CDR residues, although this does not necessarily result in a smaller binding affinity provided the M_r of the hapten is above 400 (Chappey *et al.*, 1994). The types of interactions existing between epitopes and paratopes in complexes analysed by X-ray crystallography are listed in Table 2. Note that

Antibody (Fab)	Surface buried (Å)	Ligand	Relative molecular mass (M_r)	Surface buried (Å)	van der Waals contacts (side chains)	van der Waals contacts (main chains)	Hydrogen bonds; side chains	Hydrogen bonds; main chains	Ion pairs	K_a(l mol^{-1})
McPC603	151	Phosphocholine	169	138	54	4	3	–	2	1.7×10^5
4-4-20	338	Fluorescein	320	247	107	36	3	–	0	3.4×10^{10}
B1312	503	Myohaemerythrin peptide	818	439	113	27	13	2	2	–
17/9	488	Haemagglutinin peptide	1,055	418	143	36	14	1	1	5.0×10^7
D1.3	537	Lysozyme	14,000	541	110	18	14	2	0	2.0×10^8
HyHEL-5	744	Lysozyme	14,000	741	145	25	13	0	3	2.0×10^{10}
HyHEL-10	716	Lysozyme	14,000	759	180	21	19	1	0	5.0×10^9
NC41	822	Neuraminidase	50,000	838	154	20	13	1	0	–

Table 2 Examples of epitope-paratope interactions. For references, see Padlan (1994).

hydrophobic interactions are not considered to be direct epitope-paratope interactions because the hydrophobic effect actually drives the molecules towards each other by decreasing the unfavourable contacts existing between hydrophobic residues and water (van Oss, 1995) (see also below). The direct contacts comprise van der Waals interactions, hydrogen bonds and ion pairs. More than 90% of the hydrogen bonds involve side chains, whereas very few involve main-chain atoms. In the three anti-lysozyme antibodies of known structure, only about a quarter of the surface formed by the CDRs is in contact with the antigen. In these three antibodies, tyrosine and tryptophan residues contribute 155 of the 302 interatomic contacts between the antibodies and the antigen (Padlan, 1990). All paratopes contain a much greater frequency of aromatic residues than is usual at the surface of proteins. These aromatic side chains can make large rotations with little entropic cost and they contribute significantly to the binding energy (Mian *et al.*, 1991). In addition to CDR residues, a small number of framework residues are involved in the interaction with the epitope. The immense diversity of paratopes arises through the sequence and length variability of the CDRs, which leads to innumerable CDR conformations and side-chain dispositions.

Although the entire set of CDR residues of an immunoglobulin may be viewed as a potential binding pocket, each particular paratope is made up of only about one-third of these residues. The same immunoglobulin molecule may thus, for instance, harbour two totally independent subsites representing two paratopes for unrelated epitopes. Such a situation has been described in the case of an immunoglobulin that was able to bind phosphorylcholine and α-D-galactopyranoside concomitantly at two separate paratope subsites (Battacharjee and Glaudemans, 1978). A more frequent finding is that the different subsites present in the immunoglobulin binding pocket partly overlap, in which case binding to one epitope prevents a second epitope from being accommodated at a nearby location.

Because about two-thirds of the CDR residues of an antibody do not participate in the interaction with its complementary epitope, it is to be expected that immunoglobulins will be multispecific, i.e. that they will bind a disparate set of structurally related and unrelated ligands (Weininger and Richards, 1979). In view of this multispecificity, the relationship between an antibody and its antigen is never of an exclusive nature. This means that in addition to recognising the antigen against which it was elicited, an antibody will always bind to a variety of related antigens that share some structural features with the antigen used for immunisation (Roberts *et al.*, 1993). Usually the antibody will bind to its homologous antigen with higher affinity than to most heterologous antigens. However, it is not rare to find heterologous antigens to which the antibody binds more strongly than to the homologous immunogen. This phenomenon, known as heterospecific or heteroclitic binding, is observed whenever it is looked for in a systematic fashion, i.e. by testing the antibody against a series of closely related analogues of the immunogen (Al Moudallal *et al.*, 1982; Underwood, 1985; Harper *et al.*, 1987).

Heterospecificity can be of considerable practical use when attempts are made to obtain from a single hybridoma fusion experiment a set of monoclonal antibody reagents specific for the individual members of a family of related proteins (Frison and Stace-Smith, 1992). Heterospecificity results from the fact that the clonal selection of a B cell and its subsequent differentiation into an antibody-producing plasmocyte can be triggered by an immunogen endowed with only moderate affinity for the B cell receptor. The resulting antibodies will then react weakly with the homologous antigen but may show a higher affinity with structurally related epitopes that have greater complementarity with the antibody.

STRUCTURE OF EPITOPES

The antigenic reactivity of a protein is located in discrete regions of the molecule known as antigenic determinants or epitopes, which are recognised by the paratopes of certain antibodies. Initially, epitopes were classified as either sequential or conformational depending on whether or not they could be mimicked in active form by means of linear peptides (Sela, 1969). Antibodies to sequential epitopes were expected to bind to unfolded peptides that had not retained the original conformation present in the native protein, whereas antibodies to conformational epitopes were considered to be specific for this native conformation and to be unable to recognise the unfolded peptide.

At present, the most common way of classifying epitopes consists of distinguishing continuous and discontinuous epitopes. This distinction is based on whether the residues involved in the epitope are contiguous in the polypeptide chain or not. Continuous epitopes correspond to short peptide fragments of a few amino acid residues that can be shown to bind to antibodies raised against the intact protein. In contrast, discontinuous epitopes are made up of residues that are not contiguous in the sequence but are brought close together by the folding of the peptide chain. Although this classification is widely used, it should be stressed that the borderline between continuous and discontinuous epitopes is rather fuzzy. The region of a protein antigen recognised by the antibody is commonly described in terms of contiguous or noncontiguous amino acid residues, although it is in fact at the level of individual atoms that the binding process is taking place. Speaking of residues being in contact is actually misleading because it is unlikely that all or even most of the atoms of a given residue participate in the interaction. The distinction between the two types of epitopes is also made difficult because discontinuous epitopes very often contain several continuous stretches of a few contiguous residues. Conversely, so-called continuous epitopes tend to contain a number of indifferent residues that are not implicated in the binding interaction and that make the epitope, functionally speaking, discontinuous.

Whenever a short peptide of 3 or 6 residues is found to bind to an antibody, it will be called a continuous epitope even if it corresponds in reality only to a continuous stretch of residues within a more complex discontinuous epitope. Because the discontinuous nature of an epitope cannot be ascertained in the absence of tertiary structure information, it is common practice to call any antigenic peptide of less than 12 residues a continuous epitope.

It is usually considered that about 90% of all protein epitopes are discontinuous (Van Regenmortel, 1992; Jin and Wells, 1995). This is based on the observation that about 90% of antibodies raised against intact proteins do not react with any peptide fragment derived from the parent protein. When the protein is cleaved into fragments, the residues that constitute the discontinuous epitopes are mostly scattered on individual peptides. Only in a few cases will the linear peptide fragments harbour a sufficient number of residues from the original epitope to enable these peptides to bind to antibodies raised against the intact antigen. The percentage of anti-protein antibodies that truly recognise only a continuous stretch of a few residues in the protein is likely to be even less than 10%. The reason for this is that the criterion for considering epitopes as continuous is not genuine continuity in the interacting residues of the epitope but simply the presence of antigenic activity in peptides that may sometimes be as long as 12 residues.

Some authors have challenged the view that truly native proteins possess continuous epitopes recognised by antiprotein antibodies. It has been suggested (Laver *et al.*, 1990) that all so-called continuous epitopes correspond to 'unfoldons', i.e. unfolded regions of the protein antigen that crossreact only with antibodies specific for the denatured protein. Such antibodies may be present in antisera raised against the protein because it is likely that at least some of the molecules used for immunisation were denatured either before or after injection of the animal (Jemmerson, 1987). In reciprocal assays that use antibodies to peptides, the possibility cannot be excluded that the antibodies recognise some of the denatured molecules that are likely to be present in the antigen preparation. The interpretation that all crossreactions between peptides and proteins are due to antibodies to unfoldons arose because these crossreactions are usually detected in solid-phase immunoassays in which the immobilised protein antigen is known to be at least partly denatured (Darst, 1988; Spangler, 1991). However, there is no real justification for considering that all reported cases of crossreactivity between proteins and peptides are due to antibodies specific for the denatured form of the protein. There is good evidence, for instance, that antisera raised to peptides are able to neutralise the biological activity associated with the native form of proteins. In the case of viruses, it seems likely that anti-peptide antibodies are able to recognise the native state of the viral protein present in infectious virus particles although it is possible that some neutralising antibodies recognise unfolded regions of viral proteins (Van Regenmortel and Neurath, 1990). Although the proportion of elicited antibodies able to crossreact with short peptides and the parent protein is small, these antibodies are of considerable practical importance because of their use as immunological reagents for diagnosis and gene product detection (Van Regenmortel *et al.*, 1988; Leinikki *et al.*, 1993).

X-ray crystallographic studies of antigen-antibody complexes lead to the identification of so-called structural epitopes defined by the set of residues or atoms in the antigen considered to be in contact with atoms of the antibody. In general, contact is said to occur if the interatomic distance is less than 4 Å. This somewhat arbitrary cut-off point leads to an epitope size of 15–22 residues. Because the residues are allocated to the epitope on a purely structural basis, it is not clear how many of these residues contribute to the energy of interaction. Such information can be obtained only by activity measurements that analyse the change in binding affinity resulting from single residue substitutions (Kelley, 1994; Benjamin and Perdue, 1996). The recent introduction of biosensor instruments has greatly helped the quantitative measurement of binding interactions (Malmqvist, 1993; Kelley, 1994; Van Regenmortel, 1995b). Mutagenesis studies have shown that only 3–5 residues of the epitope defined in structural terms contribute significantly to the binding energy. Thus when the epitope is viewed as a functional entity, it appears to be much smaller than when it is defined on a structural basis. Substitutions in one of the few critical residues lead to a drop in affinity constant of 2–3 orders of magnitude whereas substitutions elsewhere in the contact region lead to smaller changes in affinity (Kelley, 1994; Benjamin and Perdue, 1996).

The contribution of individual amino acids to the antigenic activity of a peptide can also be established by replacement studies. A peptide replacement set is synthesised, for instance by the pepscan technique, in which each residue of the peptide is, in turn, replaced by the other 19 possible amino acids (Getzoff *et al.*, 1988; Geysen *et al.*, 1988; Rodda and Tribbick, 1996). When all the analogues are tested for antigenicity, it is found that some residues are critical for binding and cannot be replaced by any residue without impairing binding. Other residues can be replaced by any of the amino acids without affecting antigenic reactivity. It is usually assumed that indifferent, replaceable residues are not contact residues interacting with the antibody, although it is possible that their main-chain atoms interact with the paratope. On the other hand, replaceable residues may be important as scaffolding to position the essential contact residues at the correct location for binding.

In order to reach the level of binding affinity commonly observed in antigen-antibody

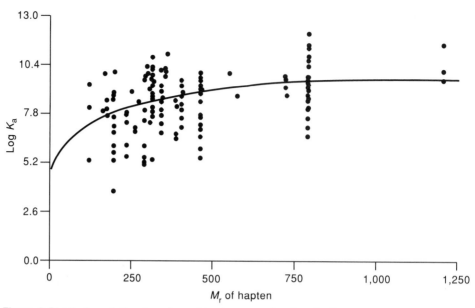

Figure 3 Distribution of K_a values for anti-hapten monoclonal antibodies versus the M_r of the native hapten compound. (From Chappey *et al.* (1994) with permission.)

interactions (affinity constant (K_a) values of 10^7–10^9 l mol^{-1}), it is necessary to have an intimate contact between only a few residues of the antigen and antibody. This conclusion agrees with the finding that increasing the size of haptens above a M_r of 400–500 (equivalent to four amino acid residues) does not lead to affinities higher than about 10^{10} l mol^{-1} (Chappey *et al.*, 1994; Morel-Montero and Delaage, 1994) (Figure 3). In the case of protein antigens, antibody affinity constants rarely exceed 10^{11} l mol^{-1}. This limit is probably due to the difficulty of achieving a very high degree of steric and chemical fit over epitope and paratope surfaces as large as 700–900 Å^2 (Van Regenmortel, 1995a). The relatively imperfect complementarity between the two surfaces is illustrated by the fact that many water molecules are retained at the interface where they fill the numerous cavities that are present (Bhat *et al.*, 1994).

The various approaches that have been used to localise epitopes in proteins have been discussed elsewhere (Van Regenmortel, 1992, 1994, 1996; Zegers *et al.*, 1995). As discussed above, it should be noted that different methods of analysis lead to different perceptions of the nature of epitopes. Depending on whether the probe used in the analysis is a free peptide, a conjugated peptide or a peptide immobilised on a solid phase, the same residues will not necessarily be found to be important for activity in different assays (Muller *et al.*, 1986).

PREDICTION OF EPITOPES

There is considerable controversy regarding the value of different algorithms for predicting the location of epitopes in proteins on the basis of one-dimensional sequence analysis. Antigenicity prediction attempts to identify in a protein sequence which linear peptide fragments are likely to crossreact antigenically with the intact protein. Antigenicity prediction is thus limited to the identification of continuous epitopes and cannot be applied to discontin-

nous epitopes, in spite of claims to the contrary (Hopp, 1993). In the absence of information on the tertiary structure of the protein, it is impossible to predict which noncontiguous residues along a sequence collectively make up a particular discontinuous epitope. If a prediction algorithm identifies a series of discontiguous residues along a sequence as being antigenic but fails to indicate which ones come together to form particular discontinuous epitopes, it does not amount to epitope prediction (Van Regenmortel and Pellequer, 1994).

Most antigenicity prediction methods analyse linear sequences in order to detect clusters of residues that are likely to be accessible at the surface of the protein. The prediction calculations are based on propensity scales for each of the 20 amino acids, which reflect properties such as hydrophilicity, accessibility and flexibility that have been associated with antigenicity. A window of seven residues along the sequence is commonly used in the analysis. The corresponding value of the scales is introduced at each of the seven residues and the arithmetical mean of the seven values is ascribed to the centre of the window. The window is moved along the entire sequence, leading to the construction of a prediction profile in the form of peaks and valleys (Pellequer *et al.*, 1994).

When the prediction efficacies of 25 different prediction scales were compared using 14 well studied proteins containing a total of 85 identified epitopes, it was found that various hydrophilicity and accessibility scales gave results that led to prediction that was 52–61% correct (Pellequer *et al.*, 1994). Two scales predicting turns were slightly more successful than the others and led to 70% correct antigenicity prediction (Pellequer *et al.*, 1993). Some authors have reported much higher scores of successful prediction (Hopp, 1993) but this is probably due to the use of unreliable criteria for assessing prediction efficacy (Hopp, 1994; Van Regenmortel and Pellequer, 1994). The low success rate of antigenicity prediction is due to the fact that predictions from sequence data reduce the complexity of epitopes, which always possess conformational features, to one-dimensional, peptide models. Another reason for the low success rate is that continuous epitopes nearly always contain indifferent replaceable residues whose side chains are not implicated in the binding interaction. When such residues are replaced by any of the other 19 amino acids, peptides are obtained that possess the same antigenic reactivity. Because the propensity scale value that is inserted at each indifferent residue corresponds to that of the residue that happens by chance to occupy that position in the sequence, it follows that considerable noise is introduced in the average value of the seven-residue window. The quality of the prediction is thereby considerably reduced.

One of the most common methods used for localising protein epitopes identifies which peptide fragments of the antigen are able to bind to antibodies raised against the intact protein. In view of the convenience and efficiency of solid-phase peptide synthesis (Atherton and Sheppard, 1989; Plaué *et al.*, 1990), synthetic peptides have mostly replaced natural peptide fragments as probes for epitope mapping. Various chemical strategies can be used to increase the level of conformational mimicry between peptide and intact protein (Vuilleumier and Mutter, 1992). Antibodies raised against peptide fragments of the protein can also be used to determine which linear regions of the polypeptide chain approximate to epitopes (Boersma and Van Regenmortel, 1994). The single most useful generalisation is that the N- and C-terminal regions of proteins tend to be located at the surface of proteins and that terminal peptides, therefore, are good candidates for raising anti-peptide antibodies that crossreact with the parent protein (Pellequer *et al.*, 1994).

THE PROCESS OF ANTIGEN-ANTIBODY INTERACTION

On a macroscopic level, protein molecules immersed in water tend to repel each other because of the hydrophilic nature of their surfaces. Because of the electron-donor character of the polar groups at the surface of the protein, the first layers of water molecules surrounding the protein tend to be oriented with the oxygen pointing outward. This orientation leads to hydrophilic repulsion when two protein molecules are brought close together, i.e. at a distance of 20–30 Å. This long-range force has to be overcome before specific binding can occur between complementary epitopes and paratopes (van Oss, 1995). In other words, the two reactants must attract each other at a distance of at least 30 Å with a specific energy of attraction large enough to overcome the repulsive hydrophilic force field. On a microscopic level, epitopes located on a protruding bend with a small radius of curvature are able to pierce this hydrophilic repulsion field.

The major forces in the primary attraction between epitopes and paratopes are hydrophobic and electrostatic interactions. Hydrophobic interaction is the propensity of nonpolar chains and groups to aggregate, when immersed in water. The driving force of the hydrophobic attraction lies in the free energy of cohesion of water caused by intermolecular hydrogen bonding among the water molecules. The term hydrophobic is somewhat misleading since it tends to give the impression that there is a repulsion between hydrophobic groups and water. In spite of their name, hydrophobic compounds actually do bind water molecules at an appreciable level, i.e. only 2 to 3 times less strongly than do hydrophilic compounds (van Oss, 1994). The nonpolar molecules tend to aggregate only because the interactions between water molecules and between various hydrophobic groups themselves are energetically more favourable than between hydrophobic groups and water molecules. The attraction between a hydrophilic and a hydrophobic entity can be considerable and is always stronger than between two repulsive hydrophilic groups. The strong hydrophobic nature of the CDRs in paratopes is thus well adapted to maximise binding with the predominantly hydrophilic groups found in epitopes.

Electrostatic interactions, also called salt bridges, between epitopes and paratopes are caused by one or more ionised sites on the epitope and ions of opposite charge on the paratope. The magnitude of the interaction is inversely proportional to the distance between the two charges and depends on the ionic strength of the liquid medium which controls the shielding effect of the diffuse ionic double layers surrounding the charged sites. In more dilute salt solutions, electrostatic interactions can exert their influence at a greater distance than they can in a solution of high ionic strength. As a first approximation, the free energy of attraction between a COO^- and a NH_2^+ group, at a distance of 3 Å in a medium with an ionic strength $\mu = 0.15$, is about -7 kcal mol^{-1} (van Oss, 1995).

Only after the primary binding has occurred through hydrophobic and electrostatic interactions will the epitope and paratope surfaces approach each other sufficiently to allow van der Waals interactions and hydrogen bonds to become operative. These van der Waals interactions occur between all atoms that are brought closely enough together. They are caused by a transient asymmetry of the electron distribution around one atom, i.e. a fluctuating dipole, which induces a complementary asymmetry in an adjacent atom. There is a marked increase in van der Waals attractions at short distances, although they usually represent less than 10% of the total interaction. As the atoms approach each other, the attractive forces are countered by repulsion between the electron clouds of the two atoms until the separation between the atoms has reached a minimum value defined as the sum of their van der Waals radii.

Hydrogen bonds result from the partial sharing of a hydrogen atom between two electro-negative atoms and exert their attraction at distances of 2–3 Å. The bond strength is maximal when the hydrogen atom is aligned in a straight line between the participating donor and acceptor atoms. Because of their short-range nature, hydrogen bonds cannot participate in the primary interaction between epitope and paratope and they become operative only in the secondary interaction when the partners have been brought close together. In the modelling of epitope-paratope interfaces based on crystallographic data, it is customary to fit optimally as many hydrogen bonds as possible, although it is a matter of debate how many of the possible hydrogen bonds are actually made (van Oss, 1994). The free energies associated with a single hydrogen bond range from –0.5 to –5.0 kcal mol⁻¹.

The interaction between antigen (Ag) and antibody (Ab) may be expressed as:

$$Ag + Ab \; \underset{k_d}{\overset{k_a}{\rightleftharpoons}} \; Ag - Ab \; complex$$

where k_a and k_d are the association and dissociation rate constants, respectively. At equilibrium, the affinity constant can be expressed as an association constant:

$$K_a = \frac{k_a}{k_d} = \frac{[Ag - Ab]}{[Ag]\,[Ab]} \quad (l \; mol^{-1})$$

or as a dissociation constant:

$$K_d = \frac{k_d}{k_a} = \frac{[Ab]\,[Ag]}{[Ag - Ab]} \quad (mol \; l^{-1})$$

It should be noted that the energy of antigen-antibody dissociation is usually higher than the energy of association because of the formation of additional secondary bonds. This phenomenon, known as hysteresis, implies that more energy is needed to dissociate most antigen-antibody bonds than is required to prevent their formation (van Oss, 1994).

It is important to realise that all antigen-antibody interactions are reversible and that the magnitude of the association and dissociation rate constants may directly influence the outcome of an immunoassay. The relationship between k_d values and the half-life of an interaction is presented in Table 3. From this table it is clear, for instance, that if a monoclonal antibody has a k_d value of 10^{-2} s^{-1}, it will be of little use in a solid-phase immunoassay because the antibody will become dissociated during the washing step of the assay. The advent of biosensor technology has made it possible to determine k_a and k_d values of antigen-antibody

Table 3 Relationship between dissociation rate constant (k_d) and half-life ($t_{1/2}$) of an interaction.

k_d (s^{-1})	$t_{1/2}$
10^{-1}	7 s
10^{-2}	70 s
5×10^{-3}	2.3 min
10^{-3}	11.5 min
5×10^{-4}	23 min
10^{-4}	1.9 hours
5×10^{-5}	3.8 hours
10^{-5}	19.2 hours
5×10^{-6}	1.6 days
10^{-6}	8 days

interactions with unprecedented ease and precision (Fägerstam and Karlsson, 1994; Granzow, 1994; Van Regenmortel, 1995b).

The free energy (ΔG) of antigen-antibody interactions can be derived from K_a by the equation:

$$\Delta G = -RT \ln K_a$$

where R is the molar gas constant (1.98 cal or 8.31 J K^{-1} mol^{-1}) and T is the absolute temperature in kelvin.

When the binding energy of single molecules is considered, the gas constant must be divided by Avogadro's number (6.02×10^{23}), to obtain the Boltzmann constant k.

$$\Delta G = -kT \ln K_a$$

In this case, ΔG is expressed as kT units per molecule pair (at 20°C or 293 K, 1 kT = 4 × 10^{-21} J).

From these equations, it follows that a 10-fold increase in binding affinity corresponds to a free energy change of 1.4 kcal mol^{-1} at 25°C. This means that K_a values of 10^5, 10^8 and 10^{11} l mol^{-1} correspond to a ΔG of −7, −11 and −15 kcal mol^{-1}, respectively. Note that the entire range of affinity constants normally encountered in antigen-antibody interactions does not differ by more than 8 kcal mol^{-1}.

The free energy change is composed of an enthalpic and an entropic term:

$$\Delta G = \Delta H - T\Delta S$$

where ΔH is the change in enthalpy (the heat of the reaction) and ΔS is the entropy (a term expressing the disorder produced by the reaction).

When K_a is measured at different temperatures, the enthalpy can be calculated from:

$$\frac{d \ln K_a}{dT} = \frac{\Delta H}{RT^2} \quad \text{or}$$

$$\ln \frac{K_1}{K_2} = \frac{\Delta H}{R}\left(\frac{1}{T_1} - \frac{1}{T_2}\right)$$

ΔH can then be obtained from the slope of $\ln K$ against $1/T$. It is also possible to obtain ΔH by calorimetric measurement of the heat of reaction (Kelley *et al.*, 1992; Jelesarov *et al.*, 1996). Recent calorimetric studies have shown that many antigen-antibody reactions are enthalpy driven and not driven by entropy as previously believed (Braden and Poljak, 1995; Schwartz *et al.*, 1995). This belief originated from the expectation that most hydrophobic interactions were likely to be entropic, as was observed in classical studies with alkanes (Tanford, 1973). However, studies with other hydrophobic compounds have shown that the hydrophobic interaction energy can often be enthalpic and that there is in fact no systematic pattern with respect to entropy or enthalpy (van Oss, 1995). In line with the earlier belief that antigen-antibody interactions were entropy driven, it was assumed that water molecules become extruded from the interface, thereby contributing to the rise in entropy. This seemed to agree with the initial crystallographic studies of antigen-antibody complexes done at medium resolution, which failed to reveal the presence of water molecules within the crystals (Davies *et al.*, 1990). However, when the complexes were studied at high resolution, it became obvious that a large number of water molecules could be present at the interface and that the interaction between epitope and paratope was not as tight as previously believed (Bhat *et al.*, 1994). The interstitial water molecules present at the interface represent residual water of hydration that is not expelled because of the imperfect steric complementarity between the two surfaces. In the absence of such interstitial water, the fit would be better and the bond between the two immunological partners would be much stronger.

For many years two competing explanatory models, the 'lock-and-key' and 'induced-fit' models, have been used to explain the mechanism of antigen-antibody recognition. According to the lock-and-key model, the two molecules interact as rigid bodies and the recognition is based on very precise steric and chemical complementarity without any deformation in either of the two partners. The induced-fit model assumes that conformational changes occur in one or both reactants which allow them to improve their complementarity and to form more stable complexes.

Most crystal structures of antibodies in their free and bound forms obtained in recent years have shown conformational rearrangements in the complexed antibody structure compared to the free form. These rearrangements include rotations of up to 16 degrees in the association of the variable antibody domains and displacements of up to 9 Å in CDR residues (Wilson and Stanfield, 1994). The structure of a bound peptide antigen can also vary considerably from that of the corresponding region in the cognate protein (Churchill *et al.*, 1994). It seems, therefore, that the induced-fit model is a better description of the recognition process that occurs between antigen and antibody molecules than the lock-and-key model.

EPITOPE-PARATOPE INTERACTIONS AND IMMUNOASSAY DESIGN

The specific interactions between epitopes and paratopes lie at the heart of every immunoassay. The law of mass action and the rate constants of the interaction (Table 3) determine the outcome of every assay. The reversible nature of antigen-antibody interactions can be visualised easily when two-site binding assays are carried out with biosensor technology (Saunal and Van Regenmortel, 1995). When the k_d of the immobilised first antibody is 10^{-2}–10^{-3} s^{-1}, approximately half of the trapped antigen will become dissociated during the 10 min of injection of the second antibody. This leads to a dynamic competition between the different antibodies that can be readily visualised with a biosensor instrument.

When mixtures of polyclonal antibodies are used, it is the antibodies with the highest affinity, i.e. those capable of interacting at the highest dilution, that will contribute most to the observed reaction. The equilibrium affinity constants of monoclonal antibodies lie in the range of 10^6–10^{10} l mol^{-1} (Van Regenmortel and Azimzadeh, 1994), which correspond to association and dissociation rate constants of $k_a = 10^4$–10^6 l mol^{-1} s^{-1} and $k_d = 10^{-2}$–10^{-4} s^{-1}, respectively (Foote and Eisen, 1995). When mixtures of monoclonal antibodies are used in an assay, circular complexes of two molecules of antibody and two of antigen tend to form, which leads to a considerable increase in the apparent affinity of the overall reaction (Moyle *et al.*, 1983).

As far as haptens are concerned, it should be remembered that they are not immunogenic by themselves and that anti-hapten antibodies are always obtained by immunising animals with hapten-carrier conjugates (Frèche, 1993). In addition to recognising the hapten, the antibodies obtained in this way will often also be directed to a few residues of the carrier protein or even to the coupling chemical moiety used for preparing the conjugate (Briand *et al.*, 1985). Adequate controls are therefore necessary to ensure that the assay is actually measuring the antibodies of interest.

The physicochemical principles underlying protein stability are clearly relevant when attempts are made to control the activity of antibodies in an immunoassay. Parameters such as pH, ionic strength, temperature and addition of dehydrating agents or organic solvents can be adjusted to favour either the association or dissociation of antigen-antibody complexes (van Oss, 1994). When protein antigens are adsorbed to plastic during a solid-phase assay, they tend to become at least partly denatured and they may then be recognised only weakly or not at all by antibodies specific for the native protein (Darst *et al.*, 1988; Spangler, 1991). One beneficial effect of this denaturation is that antibodies raised against peptide fragments of the protein will often react better with the protein immobilised on a solid phase than with the native protein in solution (Van Regenmortel, 1994). Hydrophobic antigens can be analysed and quantified by competitive inhibition immunoassay in the presence of various organic solvents. The binding ability of monoclonal antibodies tends to decrease as the concentration of organic solvent increases, although no loss in binding was observed when antibodies were suspended in mixtures of methanol with acetone, diethylether or benzene (Matsuura *et al.*,

1993). The antibody binding affinity usually decreases when the hydrophobicity of the organic solvent increases (Russell *et al.*, 1989) but this does not prevent useful assays from being carried out under these conditions.

Highly insoluble compounds, such as the immunosuppressive drug cyclosporin, can be readily assayed using specific antibodies. When this compound was dissolved from lyophilised powder in dimethyl sulphoxide or trifluoromethanol, and the solution was then diluted in an aqueous preparation of antibody, it was possible using biosensor technology to follow the conformational changes in cyclosporin (Zeder-Lutz *et al.*, 1995). These experiments suggested that the rate-limiting step of complex formation was determined by the interconversion between different cyclosporin conformers existing in solution. These results illustrate the influence of assay conditions on the binding properties of antigens.

REFERENCES

Al Moudallal, Z., Briand, J. P. & Van Regenmortel, M. H. V. (1982) Monoclonal antibodies as probes of the antigenic structure of tobacco mosaic virus. *EMBO J.* **1**, 1005–1010.

Atherton, E. & Sheppard, R. C. (eds) (1989) *Solid-phase Peptide Synthesis. A Practical Approach* (IRL Press, Oxford).

Benjamin, D. C. & Perdue, S. S. (1996) An analysis of site-directed mutagenesis in epitope mapping. *Methods: A Companion to Meth. Enzymol.* **9**, 508-515.

Bhat, T. N., Bentley, G. A., Boulot, G. *et al.* (1994) Bound water molecules and conformational stabilisation help mediate an antigen-antibody association. *Proc. Natl Acad. Sci. USA* **91**, 1089–1093.

Bhattacharjee, A. K. & Glaudemans, C. P. J. (1978) Dual binding specificities in MOPC 384 and 870 murine myeloma immunoglobulins. *J. Immunol.* **120**, 411–413.

Boersma, W. J. A., Haaijman, J. J. & Claassen, E. (1993) Use of synthetic peptide determinants for the production of antibodies. In: *Immunohistochemistry 2nd ed* (ed. Cuello, A. C.) pp. 1–77 (John Wiley & Sons, New York).

Braden, B. C. & Poljak, R. J. (1995) Structural features of the reactions between antibodies and protein antigens. *FASEB J.* **9**, 9–16.

Briand, J. P., Muller, S. & Van Regenmortel, M. H. V. (1985) Synthetic peptides as antigens: Pitfalls of conjugation methods. *J. Immunol. Meth.* **78**, 59–69.

Chappey, O., Debray, M., Niel *et al.* (1994) Association constants of monoclonal antibodies for hapten: Heterogeneity of frequency distribution and possible relationship with hapten molecular weight. *J. Immunol. Meth.* **172**, 219–225.

Chothia, C., Lesk, A. M., Tramontano, A. *et al.* (1989) Conformations of immunoglobulin hypervariable regions. *Nature* **342**, 877–883.

Churchill, M. E. A., Stura, E. A., Pinilla, C. *et al.* (1994) Crystal structure of a peptide complex of anti-influenza peptide antibody Fab 26/9: Comparison of two different antibodies bound to the same peptide antigen. *J. Molec. Biol.* **241**, 534–556.

Darst, S. A., Robertson, C. R. & Berzofsky, J. A. (1988) Adsorption of the protein antigen myoglobin affects the binding of conformation-specific monoclonal antibodies. *Biophys. J.* **53**, 533–539.

Davies, D. R., Padlan, E. A. & Sheriff, S. (1990) Antigen-antibody complexes. *Ann. Rev. Biochem.* **59**, 439–473.

Fägerstam, L. G. & Karlsson, R. (1994) Biosensor technology. In: *Immunochemistry* (eds van Oss, C. J. & Van Regenmortel, M. H. V.) pp. 949–970 (Marcel Dekker, New York).

Foote, J. & Eisen, H. N. (1995) Kinetic and affinity limits on antibodies produced during immune responses. *Proc. Natl Acad. Sci. USA* **92**, 1254–1256.

Frèche, J.-P. (1993) Strategy of immunogen production. In: *Methods of Immunological Analysis* (eds Masseyeff, R. F., Albert, W. H. & Stainess, N. A.) pp. 54–60 (VCH, Weinheim).

Frison, E. A. & Stace-Smith, R. (1992) Cross-reacting and heterospecific monoclonal antibodies produced against arabis mosaic nepovirus. *J. Gen. Virol.* **73**, 2525–2530.

Getzoff, E. D., Tainer, J. A., Lerner, R. A. *et al.* (1988) The chemistry and mechanism of antibody binding to protein antigens. *Adv. Immunol.* **43**, 1–98.

Geysen, H. M., Mason, T. J. & Rodda, S. J. (1988) Cognitive features of continuous antigenic determinants. *J. Molec. Recognition* **1**, 32–41.

Givol, D. (1991) The minimal antigen-binding fragment of antibodies. *Molec. Immunol..* **28**, 1379–1387.

Granzow, R. (ed.) (1994) Biomolecular interaction analysis. *Methods: A Companion to Meth. Enzymol.* **6**, 95–205.

Harper, M., Lema, F., Boulot, G. *et al.* (1987) Antigen specificity and cross-reactivity of monoclonal anti-lysozyme antibodies. *Molec. Immunol.* **24**, 97–108.

Hopp, T. P. (1993) Retrospective: 12 years of antigenic determinant predictions, and more. *Peptide Res.* **6**, 183–190.

Hopp, T. P. (1994) Different views of protein antigenicity. *Peptide Res.* **7**, 229–231.

Jelesarov, I., Leder, L. & Bosshard, H. R. (1996) Probing the energetics of antigen-antibody recognition by titration microcalimetry. *Methods: A Companion to Meth. Enzymol.* **9**, 533-541.

Jemmerson, R. (1987) Antigenicity and native structure of globular proteins: low frequency of peptide reactive antibodies. *Proc. Natl Acad. Sci. USA* **84**, 9180–9184.

Jin, L. & Wells, J. A. (1995) Mutational analysis of antibody binding sites. In: *Structure of Antigens* Vol. 3 (ed. Van Regenmortel, M. H. V.) pp. 21–36 (CRC Press, Boca Raton).

Kelley, R. F. (1994) Thermodynamics of protein-protein interaction studied by using BIAcore and single-site mutagenesis. *Methods: A Companion to Meth. Enzymol.* **6**, 111–120.

Kelley, R. F., O'Connell, M. P., Carter, P. *et al.* (1992) Antigen binding thermodynamics and antiproliferative effects of chimeric and humanised anti–p185[HER2] antibody Fab fragments. *Biochemistry* **31**, 5434–5441.

Laver, W. G., Air, G. M., Webster, R. G. *et al.* (1990) Epitopes on protein antigens: Misconceptions and realities. *Cell* **61**, 553–556.

Leinikki, P., Lehtinen, M., Hyöty, H. *et al.* (1993) Synthetic peptides as diagnostic tools in virology. *Adv. Vir. Res.* **42**, 149–186.

Lesk, A. M. & Tramontano, A. (1993) An atlas of antibody combining sites. In: *Structure of Antigens* Vol. 2 (ed. Van Regenmortel, M. H. V.) pp. 1–29 (CRC Press, Boca Raton).

Malmqvist, M. (1993) Surface plasmon resonance for detection and measurement of antigen-antibody affinity and kinetics. *Curr. Opin. Immunol.* **5**, 282–286.

Matsuura, S., Hamano, Y., Kita, H. *et al.* (1993) Preparation of mouse monoclonal antibodies to okadaic acid and their binding activity in organic solvents. *J. Biochem.* **114**, 273–278.

Mian, I. S., Bradwell, A. R. & Olson, A. J. (1991) Structure, function and properties of antibody binding sites. *J. Molec. Biol.* **217**, 133–151.

Morel-Montero, A. & Delaage, M. (1994) Immunochemistry of pharmacological substances. In: *Immunochemistry* (eds van Oss, C. J. & Van Regenmortel, M. H. V.) pp. 357–372 (Marcel Dekker, New York).

Moyle, W. R., Lin, C., Corson, R. L. *et al.* (1983) Quantitative explanation for increased affinity shown by mixtures of monoclonal antibodies: importance of a circular complex. *Molec. Immunol.* **20**, 439–452.

Muller, S., Plaué, S., Couppez, M. *et al.* (1986) Comparison of different methods for localising antigenic regions in histone H2A. *Molec. Immunol.* **23**, 593–601.

Nezlin, R. (1994) Immunoglobulin structure and function. In: *Immunochemistry* (eds van Oss, C. J. & Van Regenmortel, M. H. V.) pp. 3–45 (Marcel Dekker, New York).

Padlan, E. A. (1990) On the nature of antibody combining sites: Unusual structural features that may confer on these sites an enhanced capacity for binding ligands. *Proteins Struct. Funct. Genet.* **7**, 112–124.

Padlan, E. A. (1994) Anatomy of the antibody molecule. *Molec. Immunol.* **31**, 169–217.

Pellequer, J.-L., Westhof, E. & Van Regenmortel, M. H. V. (1993) Correlation between the location of antigenic sites and the prediction of turns in proteins. *Immunol. Lett.* **36**, 83–100.

Pellequer, J.-L., Westhof, E. & Van Regenmortel, M. H. V. (1994) Epitope prediction from primary structure of proteins. In: *Peptide Antigens: A Practical Approach* (ed. Wisdom, G. B.) pp. 7–25 (IRL Press, Oxford).

Plaué, S., Muller, S., Briand, J. P. *et al.* (1990) Recent advances in solid-phase peptide synthesis and preparation of antibodies to synthetic peptides. *Biologicals* **18**, 147–157.

Plückthun, A. (1994) Recombinant antibodies. In: *Immunochemistry* (eds van Oss, C. J. & Van Regenmortel, M. H. V.) pp. 201–236 (Marcel Dekker, New York).

Rees, A. R., Pedersen, J. T., Searle, S. M. J. *et al.* (1994). Antibody structure from X-ray crystallography and molecular modeling. In: *Immunochemistry* (eds van Oss, C. J. & Van Regenmortel, M. H. V.) pp. 615–650 (Marcel Dekker, New York).

Roberts, V. A., Getzoff, E. D. & Tainer, J. A. (1993) Structural basis of antigenic cross-reactivity. In: *Structure of Antigens* Vol. 2 (ed. Van Regenmortel, M. H. V.) pp. 31–53 (CRC Press, Boca Raton).

Rodda, S. J. & Tribbick, G. (1996) Antibody-defined epitope mapping using the mulitpin method of peptide synthesis. *Methods: A Companion to Meth. Enzymol.* **9**, 473-481.

Russell, A. J., Trudel, L. J., Skipper, P. L. *et al.* (1989) Antigen-antibody binding in organic solvents. *Biochem. Biophys. Res. Commun.* **158**, 80–85.

Saunal, H. & Van Regenmortel, M. H. V. (1995) Kinetic and functional mapping of viral epitopes using biosensor technology. *Virology* **213**, 462–471.

Schwartz, F. P., Tello, D., Goldbaum, F. A. *et al.* (1995) Thermodynamics of antigen-antibody binding using specific anti-lysozyme antibodies. *Eur. J. Biochem.* **228**, 388–394.

Sela, M. (1969) Antigenicity: Some molecular aspects. *Science* **166**, 1365–1374.

Spangler, B. D. (1991) Binding to native proteins by antipeptide monoclonal antibodies. *J. Immunol.* **146**, 1591–1595.

Sutton, B. J. (1993) Molecular basis of antibody-antigen reactions: Structural aspects. In:

Methods of Immunological Analysis (eds. Masseyeff, R. F., Albert, W. H. & Stainess, N. A.) pp. 66–79 (VCH, Weinheim).

Tanford, C. (1973) *The Hydrophobic Effect: Formation of Micelles and Biological Membranes* (John Wiley & Sons, New York).

Underwood, P. A. (1985) Theoretical considerations of the ability of monoclonal antibodies to detect antigenic differences between closely related variants, with particular reference to heterospecific reactions. *J. Immunol. Meth.* **85**, 295–307.

van Oss, C. J. (1994) Nature of specific ligand-receptor bonds, in particular the antibody-antigen bond. In: *Immunochemistry* (eds van Oss, C. J. & Van Regenmortel, M. H. V.) pp. 581–614 (Marcel Dekker, New York).

van Oss, C. J. (1995) Hydrophobic, hydrophilic and other interactions in epitope-paratope binding. *Molec. Immunol.* **32**, 199–211.

Van Regenmortel, M. H. V. (1992) Molecular dissection of protein antigens. In: *Structure of Antigens* Vol. 1 (ed. Van Regenmortel, M. H. V.) pp. 1–27 (CRC Press, Boca Raton).

Van Regenmortel, M. H. V. (1994) The recognition of proteins and peptides by antibodies. In: *Immunochemistry* (eds van Oss, C. J. & Van Regenmortel, M. H. V.) pp. 277–301 (Marcel Dekker, New York).

Van Regenmortel, M. H. V. (1995a) Transcending the structuralist paradigm in immunology. Affinity and biological activity rather than purely structural considerations should guide the design of synthetic peptide epitopes. *Biomed. Pept. Prot. Nucleic Acids* **1**, 109–116.

Van Regenmortel, M. H. V. (ed) (1995b) Uses of biosensors in immunology. *J. Immunol. Meth.* **183** (**special issue**), 3–182.

Van Regenmortel, M. H. V. (ed) (1996) Strategies for Mapping B-Cell Epitopes. *Methods: A Companion to Meth. Enzymol.* **9**, 465-558.

Van Regenmortel, M. H. V. & Azimzadeh, A. (1994) Determination of antibody affinity. In: *Immunochemistry*(eds van Oss, C. J. & Van Regenmortel, M. H. V.) pp. 805–828 (Marcel Dekker, New York).

Van Regenmortel, M. H. V., Briand, J. P., Muller, S. *et al.* (1988) *Synthetic Polypeptides as Antigens* (Elsevier, Amsterdam).

Van Regenmortel, M. H. V. & Neurath, A. R. (eds) (1990) *Immunochemistry of Viruses II. The Basis for Serodiagnosis and Vaccines* (Elsevier, Amsterdam).

Van Regenmortel, M. H. V. & Pellequer, J. L. (1994) Predicting antigenic determinants in proteins: Looking for unidimensional solutions to a three-dimensional problem? *Peptide Res.* **7**, 224–228.

Vuilleumier, S. & Mutter, M. (1992) Antigen mimicry with synthetic peptides. In: *Structure of Antigens* Vol. 1 (ed. Van Regenmortel, M. H. V.) pp. 43–54 (CRC Press, Boca Raton).

Weininger, R. B. & Richards, F. F. (1979) Combining regions of antibodies. In: *Immunochemistry of Proteins* (ed. Atassis, M. Z.) pp. 123–166 (Plenum, New York).

Wilson, I. A. & Stanfield, R. L. (1994) Antigen-antibody interactions: New structures and new conformational changes. *Curr. Opin. Struct. Biol.* **4**, 857–867.

Zeder-Lutz, G., Rauffer, N., Altschuh, D. *et al.* (1995) Analysis of cyclosporin interactions with antibodies and cyclophilin using the BIAcore. *J. Immunol. Meth.* **183**, 131–140.

Zegers, N. D., Boersma, W. J. A. & Claasen, E. (eds) (1995) *Immunological Recognition of Peptides in Medicine and Biology.* (CRC Press, Boca Raton).

Chapter 3

Development of Antibodies for Diagnostic Assays

Christine L. Knott, Kristine Kuus–Reichel, Ru–Shya Liu and Robert L. Wolfert

INTRODUCTION

Since the advent of hybridoma technology in 1975 there has been a slow but progressive change in the type of antibodies used in immunoassays (Köhler and Milstein, 1975, Gosling, 1990). Many early assays relied on the use of rabbit polyclonal antibodies, nearly 65% even in 1980 according to Gosling (1990), but since then monoclonal antibodies have become the predominant reagent, reaching the 50% mark by 1990. This pronounced change requires that the emphasis of this chapter is on the development of monoclonal antibodies, although polyclonal antibodies remain the immunoreagent of initial choice for early work on many new analytes and for particular assay technologies such as immunoaggregation.

Monoclonal antibody (mAb) technology has advanced considerably in the 20 years since the initial report by Köhler and Milstein (1975) of cell-cell fusion to immortalise B cells, producing antibodies of predefined specificities. In the past 10–15 years, mAbs have become an integral component in the arsenal of immunologists, chemists and clinicians. They have been used to dissect biological and chemical mechanisms and structures, and to characterise disease state processes. Monoclonal antibodies have had three major areas of application: research, diagnostics and therapeutics. Their use in manufacturing processes, including immunopurification, is also an area of great potential for the future. Although the development of a true therapeutic 'magic bullet' that could target and destroy a tumour has remained elusive, mAbs have been successfully used to 'image' tumours *in vivo* with radioisotopes. These approaches can detect tumours that are otherwise not detectable by other imaging methods such as computerised tomography, (CT) and magnetic resonance imaging (MRI). This use of mAbs will be extremely valuable to the surgeon to detect 'occult' lesions and metastatic sites distal to the primary tumour.

However, of all the applications for mAbs, the area in which they have made an indisputable impact on clinical medicine has been their use as 'analytical probes' for clinical diagnostics and research. In this chapter we will focus on the development of monoclonal antibodies for use in *in vitro* diagnostic testing and the measurement of analytes in cells, serum, urine, saliva and other biological specimens.

V_L coded by two DNA segments (multiple, different copies).

V_H coded by three DNA segments (multiple, different copies).

Combinatorial association of V_H and V_L.

Somatic mutation: driving force for affinity maturation in the immune system's response to antigenic challenge and stimulation (higher affinity results in greater protective immunity).

Table 1 Mechanisms of generating antibody diversity.

The capacity of the B cell repertoire to yield diverse antibodies with unique specificities is enormous (Table 1). This has enabled the development of immunoassays for hormones, peptides, steroids, drugs, lipoproteins, infectious organisms, autoantibodies and enzymes. Immunoassays for cancer antigens, with specificity for carbohydrate, lipid and protein structures (McCormack *et al.*, 1992b) have also been developed. The level of specificity, and thus selectivity, achievable by mAbs is truly remarkable. Monoclonal antibodies have been made that can differentiate between minute changes in molecular structure including single amino

Approaches	Examples/Comments
Immunogen manipulation	Conjugation to carrier protein
	Polylysine backbone
	Cationisation
Immunogen targeting	TcR, sIg, class I and II MHC
Immune system manipulation	Adjuvants
Enhancement	Immunopotentiators (MDP, liposomes, interleukins)
Suppression	Passive immunisation
	Neonatal tolerance
	Selective removal of clones
	Cyclophosphamide
Use of synthetic peptides	Detect single amino acid differences
	Must ensure antibody reactivity with native protein
Routes of immunisation	Intrasplenic
	Lymph node
	In vitro

Table 2 Strategies for production of monoclonal antibodies.

acid changes in proteins, oxidation states of lipids, stereoisomers and post-translational modification of identical gene products even down to a single glucose molecule. Several reports have shown the generation of mAbs to transition state compounds where the mAbs mimic the catalytic function of the associated enzyme (Lerner *et al.*, 1991; Posner *et al.*, 1994).

The goal of a mAb development programme, for the generation of reagents that will ultimately result in a diagnostic immunoassay, is to define the appropriate sensitivities, specificities, yields and chemistries required for the assay (Table 2). This can be accomplished by the selection of specific immunogens to generate the appropriate immune response in animals; through B cell immortalisation protocols that ensure stable production and a high yield of the mAb; by development of screening procedures that specifically select for the sensitivity and specificity required of the mAb for the application; and, finally, through the choice of a measurable target molecule. The selection of a mAb for a particular application is very important. We have observed that mAbs that were selected using techniques such as immunohistochemistry, immunoblotting, or fluorescence activated cell sorting (FACS) may not work in other applications such as serum-based diagnostic immunoassays. The reason for this may be attributed to the variability in concentration and form of the target molecule under different assay conditions. Depending on the assay and the source of the sample, the analyte may consist of native/conformational versus denatured/linear epitopes or may be 'free' versus complexed with another compound. For these reasons, the method for selection of the mAbs after fusion is very important. This aspect will be discussed here and in the chapter on Assessment of Antibodies (Chapter 6). Finally, practical questions must be addressed; these include the ability to create proteolytic fragments of the mAbs, to bind the mAbs to solid phases, or to label them with radioisotopic, fluorescent, chemiluminescent or enzyme reporter groups. This must be done while retaining the specificity and affinity of the mAb. Many of these issues, particularly those related to antibody purification, coupling chemistries and yield, are addressed in subsequent chapters.

In this chapter we review procedures for the production of polyclonal and monoclonal antibodies, the latter *in vivo* and *in vitro* with our primary focus on monoclonal antibody production in mice. Topics include immunisation parameters, cell selection, fusion techniques, mAb selection, cloning techniques and scale-up of antibody production. Besides proven techniques used to generate antigen-specific hybridomas, new and experimental procedures will be discussed.

THE IMMUNE RESPONSE

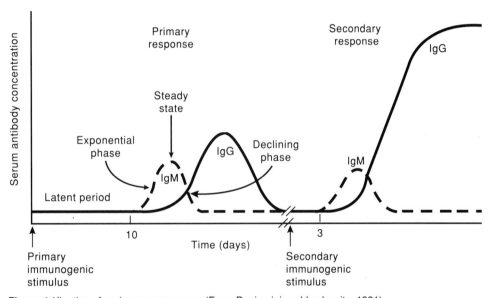

Figure 1 Kinetics of an immune response (From Benjamini and Leskowitz, 1991).

The immune response in mice (or any other mammal) leading to antigen-specific antibody production is a complex series of events that requires the interaction of T cells, B cells and antigen presenting cells. The kinetics of the immune response is outlined in Figure 1. The first encounter with antigen leads to the expansion of antigen-specific T and B lymphocytes and to the production of low levels of antibody. A second exposure to antigen produces a faster response and a higher level of production of antibody than the first exposure. These effects are the result of the expansion of the specific T and B cell clones that follow the first exposure to antigen. In T cell-dependent responses, antigen is processed by antigen presenting cells and is then presented to specific T cells. These T cells respond by proliferation and production of soluble lymphokines that stimulate antigen-specific B cells to proliferate and differentiate into plasma cells. The T and B cells respond to different epitopes on the antigen. For cell cooperation to occur, the two different epitopes must be present on the same molecule. T cell-independent antigens, such as polysaccharides, have many identical epitopes on each molecule and are capable of triggering B cells without significant help from T cells. IgM is the predominant antibody isotype produced in T cell-independent responses.

IMMUNISATION

There are many factors to consider in the immunisation of mice for the generation of antibody-producing spleen cells to be used for hybridoma production. These include selection of the strain of mice, adjuvant, form of immunogen, dosage of immunogen, immunisation schedule and route of immunisation.

A general protocol that has proved very successful in our hands is outlined below. It uses two strains of mice and two different adjuvants. In our experience, at least one of these four mouse-adjuvant combinations will result in the generation of a vigorous immune response to an antigen. The particular combination that produces the best immune response appears to be antigen-specific and is surprisingly variable from antigen to antigen, but highly reproducible. A discussion of the individual parameters follows.

Both BALB/c and A/J mice (3 per group) are immunised with the immunogen and either complete Freund's adjuvant (CFA) or alum adjuvants as follows:

Day 0 Inject 50 µg antigen containing 10% alum or emulsified with CFA, i.p. (intraperitoneally).

Day 14 Inject 25 µg antigen containing 10% alum or emulsified with incomplete Freund's adjuvant (IFA), i.p.

Day 28 Inject 25 µg antigen containing 10% alum or in PBS (for the CFA group), i.p.

Day 35 Bleed mice and titre sera for the presence of antigen-specific antibodies by enzyme-linked immunosorbent assay (ELISA).

Three days prior to fusion Inject 10 µg antigen in phosphate-buffered saline (PBS), i.v.

The mice may be bled on day 21, following the second injection of antigen, to determine the serum titre at that time. A third injection of antigen, prior to the final boost, may not be necessary. With certain antigens an i.v. (intravenous) final boost can be lethal, usually because the antigen is aggregated or is insoluble in a physiological solution. In this case, the final boost should be administered i.p.

Immunisation Parameters

Species and/or Strain of Animal

Most monoclonal antibodies produced for diagnostic or research applications are derived from the fusion of immune murine spleen cells with a murine myeloma cell line. The BALB/c mouse remains the most popular strain for this application. Other strains of mice, including A/J (Kuus-Reichel *et al.*, 1994), C57Bl/6 (Fernandez and Moller, 1991) and MLR (Shan *et al.*, 1994) have been successfully used for the production of antigen-specific hybridomas. Recently, Bcl–2 transgenic mice have been described as a source of immune murine spleen cells that resulted in increased antigen-specific hybridoma production (Knott *et al.*, 1996).

Other species of animals have been used for mAb production. These include rat (Hale *et al.*, 1987), hamster (Bright *et al.*, 1990), cow (Guidry *et al.*, 1986; Groves *et al.*, 1987; Tucker *et al.*, 1987; Kennedy *et al.*, 1988), rabbit (Yarmush *et al.*, 1980; Raybould and Takahashi,

1988; McCormack *et al.*, 1992a), sheep (Beh *et al.*, 1986; Flynn *et al.*, 1989), chimpanzee (Ehrlich *et al.*, 1988), swine (Raybould *et al.*, 1985; Lumanglas *et al.*, 1994), goat (Caparelli *et al.*, 1990), mink (Ufimtseva *et al.*, 1991) and human (Ehrlich *et al.*, 1988). A deterrent to the overall success of these non-murine sources is the lack of a species-specific fusion partner. Fusion between species, such as an immune rabbit spleen with a mouse myeloma, has met with limited success. The generation of heteromyeloma (mouse × rabbit, mouse × sheep) fusion partners may help to alleviate this problem.

Immunogen

The source and purity of the immunogen can greatly influence the outcome of immunisation protocols. Generally, the cleaner the antigen preparation, the greater the chance of recovering the antigen-specific hybridomas desired. However, it is not always possible to obtain milligram quantities of purified antigens. In these cases, alternative forms of immunogen may be successfully used.

In the case of antigens with low immunogenicity in mice, such as small peptides or highly phylogenetically conserved antigens, the use of carrier proteins can overcome the lack of immune response to the antigen alone. Some commonly used carriers include (KLH) keyhole limpet haemocyanin, (BSA) bovine serum albumin and thyroglobulin. Antigens are covalently coupled to the carrier through a variety of means (Burrin and Newman, 1991; Brinkley, 1992). The inclusion of the carrier as part of the immunogen provides an additional source for the induction of T cell help that is not present in the hapten alone. We routinely and successfully use KLH as a carrier for peptide antigens. Peptide:KLH ratios of 100:1 or greater will routinely generate vigorous immune responses in mice in the immunisation protocol outlined above. In addition to providing a source of T cell help, the inclusion of a carrier protein to an immunogen effectively increases the net mass of immunogen available. This property is very helpful when the antigen is scarce.

The elicitation of an immune response to antigens on cell surfaces has always been a challenge. Often, cell surface antigens are at a low density and cannot be readily purified in sufficient quantity for immunisation. Immunisation with whole cells for generation of an immune response to a cell surface antigen is complicated by the competition with other cell-associated antigens during the immunisation process, thus masking the desired antibody response. One approach to circumvent this problem is described by de Boer *et al.* (1992). Human CD40 antigen was expressed in baculovirus and used as the immunogen in mice. The mice responded to the human CD40 antigen. Because the antigen was produced in baculovirus and not associated with human proteins, human cells could be used for screening. Another approach was described by Tong *et al.* (1984) where immunisation with two different tumour cell lines on alternate weeks resulted in the production of more tumour-specific hybridomas than either line alone. This effect was attributed to the presence of crossreactive, tumour-specific determinants on the two cell lines.

A more conventional approach to the generation of antibodies to cell surface antigens is through the preparation of a crude membrane preparation that is subsequently used as the immunogen with CFA/IFA.

Route of Immunisation

Different routes of immunisation are more or less appropriate with different antigen preparations. Antigens administered with adjuvants, especially emulsions, are usually injected into mice intraperitoneally (i.p.). Multiple subcutaneous injections may also be used, particularly if you wish to develop an immune response in a lymph node near the site of injection. Foot-pad injections are helpful if the immune response is targeted to the popliteal lymph nodes. Intravenous (i.v.) injections are limited to aqueous antigens for understandable reasons. Intravenous injection of antigens that tend to aggregate or antigens dissolved in nonphysiological solutions, such as detergents, tend to result in the rapid decline of the mouse. Antigens administered i.v. are quickly cleared by the reticuloendothelial system (RES). The final boost before fusion of an immunised mouse is generally given i.v. three days prior to fusion to allow for rapid uptake of antigen into the spleen and rapid activation of antibody-forming cells in the spleen. Antigens prepared in liposomes are often administered i.v. to allow uptake of the antigen-containing liposomes by macrophages in the RES (Verma *et al.*, 1992). Antigen may also be administered orally. This route results in enhanced stimulation of the mucosal immune system and generation of IgA antibodies (Ruedl and Wolf, 1995; Vajdy and Lycke, 1995). Intrasplenic immunisation can be useful when only minute amounts of antigen are available for immunisation (Spitz, 1984; Nilsson and Larsson, 1992) and there is a need to deliver antigen directly to splenic B cells. Antigen may be delivered intrasplenically by injection (Spitz, 1984) or on an inert matrix such as nitrocellulose or a bead to provide an antigen depot (Nilsson and Larsson, 1992).

Adjuvants

Adjuvants are routinely used in immunisation protocols in mice for a variety of reasons. They can provide a depot for the immunogen at the site of injection allowing for slow and prolonged release of the immunogen in the animal. More importantly, they provide a means of enhancing the immune response to the antigen in question. The choice of adjuvants currently available to the researcher is somewhat overwhelming. A multitude of formulations providing different mechanisms of immune stimulation, as well as antigen delivery, are commercially available. A recent review by Vogel and Powell (1995) provides a concise and very informative overview of adjuvants and their actions. Because a complete overview of all the adjuvants available for the immunisation of mice is not practical here, we will confine ourselves to the more common adjuvant formulations used. It must be remembered that, in addition to the adjuvant composition, adjuvant activity is dependent on the properties of the immunising antigen (Claassen *et al.*, 1992; Nicklas, 1992; Verheul and Snippe, 1992).

Complete Freund's adjuvant (CFA) remains one of the most effective adjuvants for mouse immunisation, although its use in animals is currently in dispute because of its potentially serious side effects (see below). CFA is a mixture of 85% mineral oil and 15% emulsifier that contains 500 μg ml^{-1} of heat-killed and dried *Mycobacterium tuberculosis*. An antigen is prepared with CFA for injection by mixing an equal volume of aqueous antigen and CFA in two syringes coupled by a double luer-lock connector. The mixing creates a water-in-oil emulsion that is ready for injection. For a recent discussion on the preparation of water-in-oil antigen preparations see Moncada *et al.* (1993). The adjuvant properties of CFA result from the creation of an antigen depot with slow release of antigen at the site of injection and the immunostimulatory properties of *M. tuberculosis*. CFA generates an inflammatory response that invokes both antibody production and delayed-type hypersensitivity (Freund, 1956; Bomford, 1980). The active compound in *M. tuberculosis* is a peptidoglycolipid made of a polysaccharide esterified by mycolic acids and linked to a peptidoglycan fragment (Adam, 1985). The minimal adjuvant active compound is muramyldipeptide (MDP), first synthesised in 1975

(Adam, 1985). MDP is used as a component in many other adjuvant formulations (Allison and Byars, 1991).

Drawbacks to the use of CFA for mouse immunisation are the side-effects, which may include granulomas and abcesses at the site of injection, arthritis, amyloidosis, allergic reactions, splenomegaly and adhesions (Allison and Byars, 1991; Claassen *et al.*, 1992). In spite of these many side-effects, animals do not appear to be severely or chronically impaired, since food intake, bodyweight and locomotor activity are within normal limits for most of the post immunisation period (Claassen *et al.*, 1992).

Aluminium salts (aluminium hydroxide, aluminium phosphate, alum, alumina, Alhydrogel) are another class of adjuvants used for mouse immunisation. The use of aluminium salts as adjuvants is somewhat confusing because of the variety of preparations that have been described and the lack of standardisation and descriptive nomenclature. Different methods are used to prepare antigens with aluminium salts (Nicklas, 1992). In our laboratory we mix 100 µl aqueous antigen solution with 10 µl of Alumina C (Sigma 8628) suspension, vortex, rest for 5 minutes or more and inject. Alumina C contains $AlSO_4$ as the aluminium source. Aluminium salt preparations have high adsorptive capacity for antigens; 1 mg $Al(OH)_3$ will bind 50–200 µg protein (Nicklas, 1992). Thus, mixtures of antigens with aluminium salts provide a depot form of the antigen as well as immunomodulation by aluminium (Gupta, 1995). Unlike CFA, aluminium salts are not associated with serious side-effects and are the only approved adjuvants for use in humans (Nicklas, 1992; Vogel and Powell, 1995). Aluminium salts do not potentiate the cell-mediated immune responses that are observed with CFA (Ott *et al.*, 1992).

Development of adjuvants with the immunostimulatory capacity of CFA, without CFA's undesirable side effects, is an ongoing effort. The Ribi adjuvant system, composed of squalene, monophosphoryl lipid A (MPL) and trehalose dimycolate (TDM), has been shown to work as well as, if not better than CFA with some antigens (Lipman *et al.*, 1992). Syntex adjuvant formulation (SAF-1), composed of threonyl-MDP in an emulsion vehicle of squalene, Pluronic L121, polysorbate 80 and phosphate-buffered saline, is effective for the immunisation of mice to a variety of antigens (Allison and Byars, 1991, 1992; Kuus-Reichel *et al.*, 1994). These adjuvants take advantage of the immunostimulatory properties of bacterial byproducts (MPL, TDM, MDP) in oil preparations to create a potent adjuvant formulation without the serious side-effects of CFA. Synthetic lipopeptide–antigen conjugates have also been used to enhance immune responses to an antigen while avoiding the side-effects associated with CFA (Bessler and Jung, 1992). Lipopeptides are derived from the lipoprotein of Gram-negative bacteria and also provoke the immunostimulatory properties of bacterial byproducts with concomitant enhancement of the immune responsiveness to the conjugated antigen.

The isotype of antibody generated in mice to an antigen can be influenced by the choice of adjuvant. Immunisation with aluminium adjuvants is accompanied by stimulation of interleukin (IL-4) production and activation of Th2 subsets in mice resulting in enhanced IgG_1 and IgE responses (Kenney *et al.*, 1989; Vogel and Powell, 1995). Induction of IgG_{2a} antibodies, which are necessary for protection against plasmodium infection (Ten Hagen *et al.*, 1993), cell-mediated cytotoxicity (Allison and Byars, 1992) and tumour localisation *in vivo* (Buchegger *et al.*, 1992) is accomplished with SAF-1 (Allison and Byars, 1986; Kenney *et al.*, 1989), Ribi adjuvant (Gustafson and Rhodes, 1992) and CFA (Kenney *et al.*, 1989), and with a variety of oil-in-water or no-oil formulations, such as saponin, Pertussis and P1004 copolymer (Ten Hagen *et al.*, 1993). The preferential induction of IgG_{2a} antibodies with certain adjuvants suggests that the Th1 subsets in mice are stimulated, in contrast to the action of aluminium salts that preferentially induce IgG_1 production via activation of Th2 subsets (Mosmann and Coffman, 1989).

In general, the murine immune response to carbohydrate antigens results in the production of IgM or IgG_3 antibodies. Enhancement of serum antibody responses to polysaccharide–protein conjugates has been demonstrated by injecting the antigen with MPL (Schneerson *et al.*, 1991). Recovery of IgG-secreting hybridomas specific to a carbohydrate-rich tumour associated antigen was accomplished by careful screening of hybridomas for the desired isotype (Kuus-Reichel *et al.*, 1994).

The properties of antibodies produced under the influence of different adjuvants is also variable. CFA preferentially induces antibodies against denatured epitopes of proteins (Wolberg *et al.*, 1970) compared to Ribi or Quil-A (Kenney *et al.* 1989). Alum and Quil-A have been shown to induce antibodies with greater affinity for human serum albumin (HSA) than SAF-1, Ribi and CFA (Kenney *et al.* 1989).

There are many aspects to consider in the choice of adjuvant for use in the immunisation of mice for antibody production. It must be remembered that successful immunisation is not guaranteed by the selection of a single adjuvant, as the immune response is highly dependent on the antigen as well.

Polyclonal Antibodies

Polyclonal antibodies are useful reagents for a variety of immunochemical applications including immunohistochemistry, western blots and many immunoassays. Polyclonal antibodies offer the advantage of a simpler method of production with the disadvantage of the heterogeneous, and often crossreactive, binding properties of the antisera. As with all antibodies, polyclonal antisera need to be well characterised for the intended application.

Animal	Serum volume (ml)	Comments
Rabbits	500	Good choice for polyclonal antibody production even with limited antigen
Mice	2	Low serum volume. Many inbred strains available.
Rats	20	Some inbred strains available
Hamsters	20	Good choice for polyclonal antibody production when antigen is limited
Guinea Pigs	30	Hard to bleed
Chickens	50	Good for highly conserved mammalian antigens
Goats	litres	High serum volume. Multiple bleeds with additional antigen boosts

Table 3 Polyclonal antisera production.

Polyclonal antisera can be made in a variety of animals. Immunisation of different species of animals provides the possibility of generating antibodies with different reactivity profiles based on the differences in B cell repertoires in the different species. Genetically in-bred strains of animals are available for rodent and rabbit species that can provide a potentially more predictable immune response to a given antigen. In general, the same variables involved in the immunisation of mice for monoclonal antibodies also apply to other animal species. For example, the immunogenicity of the antigen, the choice of carrier protein, dose and route of immunisation and choice of adjuvant all need to be considered in polyclonal antibody production. The amount of antigen required for immunisation of larger animals is not directly proportional to the size of the animal. For example, similar total amounts of antigen can be used for immunisation of mice, rabbits and goats. Freund's adjuvants are probably the most commonly used adjuvants for polyclonal antibody production. Some characteristics of polyclonal antisera production in different animals are shown in Table 3.

Rabbits are a very popular choice for polyclonal antibody production because of their size (blood volume and ease of handling). A blood sample should be taken from the rabbit before immunisation and tested for reactivity to the immunising antigen to alleviate potential background reactivities that can interfere with applications using the antisera. A good description of rabbit polyclonal antisera production techniques is given by Harlow and Lane (1988).

Goats are used to make large quantities of polyclonal antisera. With appropriate antigen boosts, goats can produce high-titre polyclonal antisera for years. One procedure that has proved very successful requires injection by either intramuscular or subcutaneous routes of 25–200 μg of antigen emulsified in CFA on day 0 and day 30. This is followed by another injection of antigen with IFA on days 60 and 90. At 9 to 11 days after the last injection, the animal is bled and the serum titre determined for the antigen in question. Additional boosts can be made with IFA on a monthly basis. Antiserum is collected by plasmapheresis 9 to 11 days after the boost (R. Valenta, personal communication). Several goats are usually immunised to determine the animal that produces the highest-titre antibody.

Alternative Immunisation Protocols

Antigen Targeting

Antigens can be targeted to specific cells in the immune system. The combination of antigen with antibodies directed to T cell or B cell receptors (Hendrickson *et al.*, 1994) has been used to generate immune responses to specific antigens. Conjugation of an antigen to a cell receptor is thought to aid in the delivery of the antigen to the target cell. Whether the enhanced immune response is a result of specific targeting of antigen to a cell population or enhanced responsiveness as a result of the antigen being coupled to a carrier protein, is not entirely clear.

The incorporation of antigens into liposomes for immunisation has several potential advantages (Alving, 1991; Buiting *et al.*, 1992). Antigens can be attached to the outer surface, encapsulated within the internal aqueous spaces or reconstituted within the lipid bilayers of the liposomes. Liposomes are efficiently phagocytosed by macrophages, thus providing an effective means of antigen processing and presentation to the cells of the immune system. Antigens in liposomes can be combined with other adjuvants, growth factors and/or major histocompatibility complex (MHC) gene molecules to enhance the immune response to the antigen.

DNA Immunisation

Recently, immunisation of mice with plasmid DNA expression vectors that encode the protein of interest has been described. This approach is particularly suitable in situations where the protein is difficult to purify, or where the gene for the protein has been isolated but the protein has not yet been identified from a natural source (Barry *et al.*, 1994). Introduction of the plasmid DNA into the mouse has been accomplished via intramuscular injection using a pneumatic gun (Vahlsing *et al.*, 1994), intradermal injection (Raz *et al.*, 1994) and intramuscular injection (Manickan *et al.*, 1995; Michel *et al.*, 1995). Using this approach, mice have been immunised to hepatitis B surface antigens (Michel *et al.*, 1995), Herpes simplex virus (Manickan *et al.*, 1995) and influenza nucleoprotein (Raz *et al.*, 1994; Vahlsing *et al.*, 1994).

SCID–HU

Human antibodies can be produced by reconstitution of severe combined immunodeficient SCID mice with human peripheral blood lymphocytes (PBL's) (Mosier, 1990) or human fetal tissue (McCune *et al.*, 1988). The challenge in the production of human antibodies in this system is the production of human antibodies to unique antigens. Specifically, this refers to antigens to which the human donors have not been previously sensitised. Antigen-specific human antibodies can be raised to tetanus toxoid, hepatitis, human leukocyte antigens (HLA) and bacteriophage φX174 in systems where the donor lymphocytes were obtained from immunised or infected individuals (Mosier *et al.*, 1988; Niguma *et al.*, 1993; Nonoyama *et al.*, 1993). In contrast, reports of the generation of primary immune responses that result in naive B cell differentiation into antigen-specific IgG antibody-producing cells remain sparse (Walker and Gallagher, 1994; Mårtensson *et al.*, 1995). This system holds the promise of the generation of high-affinity human IgG antibodies for diagnostic and therapeutic applications. The procedures for consistent and reproducible production of these antibodies in SCID mice still required additional modification.

In Vitro Immunisation

In vivo immunisation techniques are routinely used to produce polyclonal sera and monoclonal antibodies. This method is not always successful, either because of insufficient quantity of antigen compared to that required for *in vivo* immunisation or lack of immunogenicity of the antigen. The use of *in vitro* immunisation techniques may overcome these problems (Koda and Glassy, 1990; Guzman *et al.*, 1993).

In vitro immunisation offers many potential advantages. *In vitro* immunisation procedures are performed outside the normal regulation of the immune system, so it may be possible to obtain an immune response to an antigen that is not normally immunogenic *in vivo* (Borrebaeck, 1989; Kolberg and Blanchard, 1991). Cell culture conditions and cell composition can be manipulated to obtain the antibody of desired specificity (Federspiel *et al.*, 1991; Uthoff and Boldicke, 1993). An *in vitro* immune response may also be elicited against weak or hazardous immunogens (Guzman *et al.*, 1993). The scale of the process is more focused, in that antigens are presented directly to the cells in the culture dish, thus requiring smaller amounts of antigen and fewer animals (Federspiel *et al.*, 1991). Finally, most *in vitro* immunisation procedures take less time, 5–10 days, compared to conventional *in vivo* immunisations that can take 21–28 days (Federspiel *et al.*, 1991).

There are also disadvantages to *in vitro* immunisation. The antibodies produced are generally of the IgM isotype (Guzman *et al.*, 1993; Uthoff and Boldicke, 1993). Because the procedure uses general tissue culture conditions, any additives, including the immunogen, must be sterile (Guzman *et al.*, 1993). Finally, *in vitro* immunisation conditions have not been adequately defined with regard to the timing, dosage and interaction of cytokines and other growth factor supplements (Koda and Glassy, 1990).

Protocols for *in vitro* immunisations are highly variable. Generally, naive BALB/c mice are used as a source of B cells. A single cell suspension is prepared from the whole spleen and antigen is added for varying amounts of time. Cells are collected and immortalised using a standard fusion technique or Epstein–Barr virus (EBV). The addition of T helper cell lines or media supplements, derived from mixed lymphocyte cultures, have driven B cells to produce antibodies of IgG isotypes (Federspiel *et al.*, 1991; Schilizzi *et al.*, 1992; Uthoff and Boldicke, 1993).

In vitro immunisation has been used to produce human antibodies where immunisation of humans is not practical for safety and ethical reasons. Sources of human B cells include spleen, peripheral blood and tonsils (Carroll *et al.*, 1990; Koda and Glassy, 1990). The problems encountered with *in vitro* immunisation using human cells are similar to those noted above. In addition, donor cell variation provides an added complication. The ability to produce high-affinity, antigen-specific human IgG antibodies routinely would provide a major advance in the potential use of human monoclonal antibodies, especially for therapeutic applications. Optimisation of *in vitro* immunisation systems, with regard to the addition of cytokines, growth stimulants, dosage and timing of antigen delivery, is under intense investigation.

Selection of Cells for the Production of Antigen-specific Hybridomas

Several methods have been used to enhance the selection of antigen-specific hybridomas. These methods have involved either the selection of antigen-specific B cells prior to fusion or selection of antigen-specific hybridomas after fusion.

Tomita and Tsong described a system where antigen-specific B cells were selected from immunised mouse spleens by binding B cells to biotinylated antigen followed by crosslinking of the B cell–antigen conjugate to avidin-coupled myeloma cells (Tomita and Tsong, 1990). Steenbakkers *et al.* (1993) describe a system to select antigen-specific B cells from the spleen cells of immunised mice by panning on antigen-coated dishes or rosetting specific B cells with antigen-coated magnetic beads. Kuus-Reichel *et al.* (1991) described a procedure to isolate hybridoma-forming cells from immune mouse spleens by fractionation of immune mouse B cells on a serum gradient where the fusible cells were recovered in the large cell population that comprised only 10% of the splenic B cell population. Post-fusion selection of antigen-specific hybridomas has been achieved using antigen-coated magnetic beads (Horton *et al.*, 1989; Ossendorp *et al.*, 1989). All of these procedures resulted in enrichment of the specific antibody-producing cells, resulting in more efficient hybridoma production and, in some cases, the generation of higher affinity antibodies (Ossendorp *et al.*, 1989).

FUSION TECHNIQUES

Fusion of Immune Spleen Cells with Myelomas

Immune spleen cells are obtained from mice that were immunised and given their final boost with an antigen 3 days prior to fusion. On the day of fusion, immune spleens are removed aseptically and teased into a single-cell suspension. The splenocytes or B cells are mixed with an appropriate fusion partner which is commonly a nonsecreting hybridoma or myeloma cell. The mixture of spleen cells and myelomas is mixed gradually with a polyethylene glycol solution (PEG 30–50%) to induce fusion. After $1\frac{1}{2}$ minutes, the cell suspension is slowly diluted in serum-free and then serum-containing media. The fused cells are cultured in growth medium containing hypoxanthine, aminopterin and thymidine (HAT), in which the hybridoma cells can survive whereas nonfused cells undergo apoptosis and die. After 5 days, hybridoma colonies are visible. The fusion plates are fed with fresh medium every 3–4 days, for 14–21 days, until the majority of wells show 80% confluent cell growth. The supernatants from wells with growing hybridomas are screened for specific antibody production by enzyme-linked immunoassay, radioimmunoassay, immunostaining or western blot. Once the desired antibody-secreting wells are identified, the corresponding hybridoma cells are expanded for cryopreservation and subcloned to ensure hybridoma stability and monoclonality.

Polyethylene glycol (PEG) is routinely used as the fusogen in hybridoma production. The mechanism of action of this agent is unknown but it is thought that PEG removes the hydration shell from cell surfaces, allowing a hydrophobic interaction between membrane lipids. Cell fusion occurs between adjacent cells. A 30–50% solution of 1,000–4,000 M_r PEG is commonly used. In our experience, a 35% solution of PEG 1,500 M_r gives reliable and consistent fusion efficiencies. Norwood *et al.* (1976) demonstrated that the addition of 10% dimethylsulphoxide (DMSO) to the fusion media can enhance the efficiency of PEG- mediated fusions.

Murine Fusion Partners

The selection of a suitable fusion partner for hybridoma production relies on two key factors. The myeloma cell line must not secrete any immunoglobulin and it must be deficient for enzymes, e.g. hypoxanthine: guanine phosphoribosyltransferase (HGPRT) or thymidine kinase (TK) that allow survival in HAT selection medium. There are many established murine myeloma cell lines available for fusing with splenocytes to form hybridomas. In our hands, the P3.653 myeloma cell line, available from the American Type Culture Collection (Bethesda, MD), has consistently yielded high-efficiency fusions. Additional fusion partners are listed below.

1   MOPC 21 (P3-X67Ag8): A spontaneous myeloma cell line from BALB/c mice, which was selected to be 8-azaguanine resistant (Köhler and Milstein, 1975). This cell line was used in the pioneering hybridoma development by Köhler and Milstein. It produces IgG₁ heavy and κ light chain antibodies. All other established myeloma cell lines were originated from this cell line.

2   SP2/0: Developed by fusing BALB/c B-lymphocytes with MOPC 21 myelomas. It does not secrete immunoglobulin and has been used very successfully in BALB/c spleen fusions (Shulman *et al.*, 1978).

3   NS-1: A subclone of MOPC 21. It synthesises κ light chain but does not secrete it. It has been successfully used in heterohybridoma systems (rat × mouse, human × mouse) (Köhler and Milstein, 1976).

4   P3.653: Isolated from MOPC by FACS. It does not express surface immunoglobulin (Kearney *et al.*, 1979).

5   FO: A subclone cell line of SP2/0 (Roth *et al.*, 1982).

6   S194: A cell line deficient in thymidine kinase myeloma that has been used in rat mono-clonal antibody development (Coffman and Weissman, 1981).

7   FOX-NY: A spontaneous mutant cell line derived from NS-1. It is deficient in both ade-nine phosphoribosyltransferase (APRT) and HGPRT enzymes (Taggart and Samloff, 1983). When FOX-NY cells are fused with immune splenocytes from an Rb (8.12) mouse, adenine, aminopterin, thymidine (AAT) and HAT selection can be used. It has been shown that there is an increase in hybrids developed using this system compared to the HAT system.

Cloning of Hybridomas

In order to stabilise cell growth and prevent overgrowth by nonsecreting cells in culture, it is crucial to subclone hybridomas as soon as possible after detection of specific antibody pro-duction. Three methods for subcloning are described.

Limiting Dilution

Limiting dilution is the most popular way of ensuring the monoclonality of selected hybrido-mas (Lefkovits, 1979). Hybridoma cells are serially diluted to a concentration of 5 cells per ml so that 200 μl will deliver 1 cell per well into a 96-well microtitre plate. In practice, we di-lute cells to deliver an average of 1/3 cell per well into wells containing 2×10^5 syngeneic spleen cells per well as a feeder layer. Spleen cell feeder layers provide growth factors and cell contact to support low-density hybridoma growth.

Soft Agar

Hybridoma cells can be subcloned using soft agar. In this technique, hybridoma cells are di-luted in nutrient medium containing 3% agarose and plated in Petri dishes. Colonies derived from single cells can be isolated and expanded. A disadvantage of this method is the technical skill required to pick individual colonies from the soft agar. In addition, some hybridomas may not grow as well in soft agar as in liquid culture.

FACS

Subcloning can be easily accomplished using a fluorescent-activated cell sorter (FACS) equipped with an automatic cell deposition unit (ACDU). The FACS can be set up to deliver one cell into each well of a 96-well plate. As with limiting dilution, we routinely use spleen cell feeder layers in the 96-well plates to support the growth of the single cells (Parks *et al.*, 1979).

Enhancement of Hybridoma Production

Many reports describe methods to enhance hybridoma growth and antigen-specific antibody production. As previously mentioned, the recovery of specific antibody producing cells can be increased by selection of cells on antigen-specific beads or through isolation of specific cell subpopulations. Simple depletion of T cells from murine spleens with anti-T cell antibody and complement or anti-T cell-coated magnetic beads markedly enhances the efficiency of hybri-doma production by eliminating most of the non-B cells from the fusion process.

The basal medium for hybridoma growth is minimal essential medium (MEM) supplemented with 10% foetal calf serum. Enrichment of hybridoma growth medium with a variety of compounds, including insulin (Bartal *et al.*, 1984), transferrin, additional glucose and glutamine, ethanolamine, linoleic acid, pyruvate, putrescine, selenite and 2-mercaptoethanol, have been reported to enhance hybridoma growth (Chang *et al.*, 1980; Murikami *et al.*, 1982).

Hybridoma growth factors are readily available from many commercial sources. These factors are usually conditioned medium obtained from cultures of primary or established murine or human cell lines, including macrophages, splenocytes, thymocytes, endothelial cells (Pintus *et al.*, 1983) and fibroblasts. These preparations probably contain a mixture of cytokines. Detailed analysis of the composition of the mixtures is not generally available from the manufacturers.

Feeder layers are very useful for supporting growth of hybridomas, especially at low cell densities. Feeder layers may be composed of splenocytes, macrophages, thymocytes, irradiated fibroblast cell lines (Long *et al.*, 1986) or cell lines treated with mitomycin-C (Butcher *et al.*, 1988). Feeder layers also provide a mixture of cytokines and cell contact to enhance hybridoma growth.

The frequency of antigen-specific antibody-producing cells can be expanded by *in vitro* treatment of B cells with mitogens such as lipopolysaccharide (LPS) + dextran sulphate (Woloschak and Senitzer, 1983; Horton *et al.*, 1989; Ossendorp *et al.*, 1989; Kuus–Reichel *et al.*, 1991), cell wall extracts from *Salmonella typhimurium* or different forms of lipid A, prior to fusion (Davis, 1988). Enhancement of hybridoma production by pretreating myeloma fusion partners with colcemid (Miyahara *et al.*, 1984), neuraminidase (Igarashi and Bando, 1990) and PEG (Orlik and Altaner, 1988) have also been described.

Another method useful for the expansion of antibody-producing cells involves adoptive transfer of spleen cells from an immunised mouse to several irradiated, syngeneic recipients (Kenny, 1981). The adoptively transferred mice are boosted with antigen and fused shortly after transfer of immune spleen cells. This procedure is extremely useful when limited amounts of antigen are available for primary immunisation or when only a limited number of mice are responsive to a particular antigen. It essentially increases the pool of immunised mice available for fusion.

Antibody Selection/Hybridoma Screening

Even using some of the selection and enrichment procedures outlined above to decrease the number of cells in a fusion, a typical fusion may contain a thousand or more wells to screen for antibody activity. For this reason, screening methods must lend themselves to rapid, automated approaches to ensure that the hybridoma wells can be screened before antibody-secreting clones are overgrown by nonproducing clones. We favour a microplate format to screen our hybridomas because it allows for direct transfer of the hybridoma supernatant from the fusion plates to the screening plates. Initial screens of the culture supernatants are often performed against the immunogen. Secondary testing will often determine antibody secretion levels by titration of the culture supernatants, and comparative affinity, by limiting target antigen concentration in the assay. Additional selection criteria may involve testing for cross reactivity of the antibody with homologous antigens, isotype analysis and epitope analysis, to determine compatibility with previously selected antibodies in sandwich assays. For a

Method	Characteristic	Points to Consider
RIA	(1) Typically antigen is labelled	Antigen may be damaged by labelling technique 'pure' form of antigen is required
	(2) Solution phase binding	Antigen presented in more 'native' conformation
	(3) Uses 'trace' amount of antigen in system	Limits amount of antigen required for assay
		Often can be designed for selection of highest-affinity mAbs
	5 - ^{125}I label used	May provide good sensitivity for selection of high-affinity mAb
		Poses biohazard, disposal issues
ELISA	Typically antigen is unlabelled; secondary Ab used to detect mAb	No labelling damage associated with antigen modification
		Pure antigen not required
	Solid-phase binding	Antigen may be denatured by adherence to hydrophobic plastic surface of microwell
	Uses excess antigen in system	Availability of sufficient quantity of antigen may be a problem
		May not select for highest-affinity mAbs

Table 4 Comparison of RIA vs. ELISA screening methods.

further description of affinity analysis and epitope binding, refer to the chapter on 'Assessment of Antibodies' (Chapter 6).

The choice of screening techniques is often driven by certain practical considerations, such as availability of proper detecting equipment and adequate supply of antigen. We have used RIAs and ELISAs to a significant extent for screening hybridomas. Table 4 summarises some of the variables that require consideration in selection of a screening assay. We have been able to address some of the issues presented in Table 4 by modifications of certain methods. For example, in place of a radioisotopic ^{125}I label, one may use fluorescent- or chemiluminescent-labelled antigens, to achieve many of the benefits of RIAs, without the problems associated with radioactive labels. Similarly, by use of biotin–avidin coupling of peptides or protein antigens to microwell surfaces, one can mitigate some of the denaturing effects of solid-phase binding ELISAs, while retaining many of its benefits.

Finally, in hybridoma screening protocols, selection of the appropriate screening antigen is of paramount importance. Screening on peptides offers the ease of defined chemistries and known linear epitope binding, but often does not select for mAbs that will bind conformational epitopes on the native molecule. Screening hybridoma supernatants on recombinant material is often preferred because of the availability of adequate quantities of purified material. When using recombinant material derived from *Escherichia coli*, yeast, or baculovirus, the appropriateness of post-translational modifications must be taken into consideration. Production of the antigen in suitable mammalian host cell systems is optimal, but is often encumbered with problems of low levels of expression. The most desirable antigen is the native protein derived from a natural biological source. This presumes the material can be purified in sufficient quantities for screening protocols, in the absence of other, potentially cross-reactive, antigens. In the final analysis, screening of the hybridoma supernatant and selection of the mAbs against the antigen target that most closely represents its presence in the clinical specimen, in a format that closely mimics the immunoassay design to be employed in the diagnostic application, will increase the likelihood of a successful mAb development effort.

ALTERNATIVE FUSION PROTOCOLS

Preparation of Bifunctional Antibodies

Bifunctional antibodies (BFA) offer the ability to target an effector molecule, such as a drug or radioisotope to specific target sites, by combining the specificity for both the effector molecule and the target antigen in one antibody molecule. This property has been used to target tumours with toxins (Honsa *et al.*, 1990), radioisotopes (Stickney *et al.*, 1991) or cytotoxic drugs (Corvalan *et al.*, 1988; Kuus-Reichel *et al.*, 1995) and to refocus effector T cells towards different cell targets (Xiang *et al.*, 1992). Bifunctional antibodies can be prepared by natural, chemical and recombinant techniques.

Natural Bifunctional Antibodies

Natural bifunctional antibodies refer to the fusion of an antigen-specific hybridoma with an immune spleen cell specific for a different antigen (trioma) or the fusion of two different antigen-specific hybridomas (quadroma). Both result in the generation of antibodies with dual specificity. The selection of triomas after fusion is essentially the same as a routine fusion using a HAT-sensitive cell line. The selection of quadromas after fusion is somewhat more complicated, as two different selection criteria are required to ensure the survival of only the fused cells. Each hybridoma used in the generation of a quadroma must be sensitive to a distinct site-specific, irreversible metabolic inhibitor, so that only fused cells comprising the two hybridomas will survive in culture. Metabolic inhibitors that have been used in quadroma production include ouabain, actinomycin D, cycloheximide and hydroxyurea andemetine (Colowick and Kaplan, 1979).

Chemical Bifunctional Antibodies

Bifunctional antibodies can be made by reducing two different intact antibodies into (Fab')$_2$ fragments and reassociating the two fragments using chemical coupling agents (Brennan *et al.*, 1985).

Recombinant Bifunctional Antibodies

Bifunctional antibodies may be produced by engineering two different antibody specificities into one molecule and modifying the constant heavy-chain regions so that, when expressed, the two half molecules with different specificities will recombine to form a whole molecule. Feasibility for this approach has recently been demonstrated by Carter (1995) and Yazaki *et al.* (1995).

Electrofusion

Electrofusion uses transient high-voltage electric fields instead of PEG to fuse cells together (Stenger *et al.*, 1988). Fusion is achieved by temporary disruption of cell membranes during exposure to critical electric field conditions. Zimmermann *et al.* (1980) called this phenomenon 'reversible electrical breakdown'. Electrofusion has been used in the generation of human monoclonal antibodies (Glassy, 1988) where the availability of primed B cells is low and insufficient for a PEG-mediated fusion. Advantages of this technique are the low cell numbers required for both the primed B cells and the fusion partners, and the high efficiency of hybrid generation. This technique requires special equipment and is not, in general, as popular as PEG fusions.

Epstein–Barr Virus – Mediated Fusion

Epstein–Barr virus (EBV) is a herpes virus that is the aetiological agent of infectious mononucleosis (Roder *et al.*, 1986). EBV infects only human and primate cell lines that bear EBV receptors. Its utility for monoclonal antibody production is, therefore, limited to production of human or primate antibodies.

EBV is a polyclonal B cell activator (Glasky and Reading, 1995). *In vitro*, infection of B lymphocytes leads to permanent stimulation of cell growth called transformation or immortalisation. Immortalisation preserves the characteristics of the original B cells, including EBV receptors, complement receptors, surface immunoglobulin and secretory immunoglobulin (Roder *et al.*, 1986).

A major disadvantage of EBV-transformed cells is the loss of antibody production in long-term cultures. Stable, antibody-producing cell lines are the exception rather than the rule. Another disadvantage is the low quantities of antibody produced, generally less than 1 μg ml^{-1} (Roder *et al.*, 1986).

Interspecies Fusions

Murine mAbs are frequently criticised for their lack of effector functions, such as the ability to fix complement, and for their low affinity compared to polyclonal antisera made in other species. Indeed, some substances that are poorly immunogenic in rodents produce significant responses in other animals. Interspecies fusions are needed to immortalise antibodies from species other than the mouse because myeloma cell lines are not routinely available from non-rodent species. Compared to mouse × mouse fusions, interspecies fusions have met with limited success because of the lack of suitable fusion partners to facilitate the formation of stable hybrids. The failure of such interspecies hybrids has been attributed to the instability of the heterohybrid and subsequent loss of relevant chromosomes required for immunoglobulin production. Several approaches have been used to address this problem. Heteromyelomas (mouse × other species) have been established for use as fusion partners in individual laboratories. Early and aggressive subcloning has been used to stabilise hybrids. Heterohybridomas have been produced from small laboratory animals (rabbit (Kuo *et al.*, 1984; Raybould and Takahashi, 1988; McCormack *et al.*, 1992), mink (Ufimtseva *et al.*, 1991)) and farm animals (cattle (Srikumaran *et al.*, 1983; Tucker *et al.*, 1987), goat (Capparelli *et al.*, 1990), sheep (Tucker *et al.*, 1981; Flynn *et al.*, 1989)) using these approaches.

Serum-free Fusion

Traditional fusion technology requires complete medium with serum supplements to support the growth of hybridoma cells. Serum is also required for subcloning of hybridoma cells to support low-density cell growth. We have found that interleukin-6 (IL-6) can be used as a serum replacement in fusion media. IL-6 has been shown to enhance the growth of hybridomas and stimulate antibody production by B cells (Hirano, 1991). Stable hybridoma cell lines were generated to peptide, protein and cell antigens using serum-free adapted P3.653 myelomas as the fusion partner and medium containing 300 U ml⁻¹ of IL-6. Our results indicate that, in general, the fusion efficiencies of serum-free IL-6-supplemented fusions are lower than the fusions using serum-containing media (40–60% versus 80–100%). However, in spite of the lower fusion efficiency, the number of antigen-specific clones generated using IL-6 is equal to or higher than fusions using serum supplements. The use of IL-6 instead of serum in the generation of monoclonal antibodies has several advantages. We are able to eliminate the costly need for serum in media by using IL-6 that is prepared in-house. In addition, we eliminate the need for time-consuming serum-free adaptation of hybridoma cell lines prior to transfer to hollow-fibre bioreactors, as well as the need for ascites production in mice.

SCALE-UP OF ANTIBODY PRODUCTION

In vivo Antibody Production

In vivo antibody production in the form of ascites is a common means to produce milligram-to-gram amounts of monoclonal antibodies. Although the amount of antibody produced in ascites can be variable and clone dependent, 2 to 20 mg ml⁻¹ of antibody can generally be recovered. Mice are the most commonly used animal for ascites production. The mouse strain used for ascites production must be compatible with the hybridoma cell line. BALB/c mice were originally, and still are, extensively used for ascites and monoclonal antibody production because of their propensity for spontaneous ascites production (Merwin and Algire, 1959). However, BALB/c mice do not always give the best immune response to a particular antigen and are therefore not always the best candidate for hybridoma production. BALB/c-derived hybridomas grow best in BALB/c mice. Hybridomas derived from other mouse strains, including A/J and C57Bl/6, or rat/mouse hybrids can be produced in nude or athymic mice. Nude mice lack functional T cells and are therefore unable to reject foreign cells because of H-2 incompatibility or xenogenicity.SCID mice have also been used for ascites production, but are generally too expensive for large-scale production runs (Pistillo *et al.*, 1992).

Priming mice prior to hybridoma cell injection can enhance ascites production. Commonly used primers are pristane or incomplete Freund's adjuvant (IFA) (Hoogenraad *et al.*, 1983; Brodeur *et al.*, 1984; Hoogenraad and Wraight, 1986; Gillette, 1987). Both primers, injected i.p., elicit a generalised inflammation of the cells in the peritoneum. With pristane, 0.5 ml is injected i.p. at least 2 weeks prior to injection of the hybridoma. We have found that any shorter priming period negates the benefits of the primer. IFA (0.3 ml) injected i.p. 3 days prior to the hybridoma is sufficient to prime the peritoneum for ascites production. In our experience, mice primed with IFA generally produce ascites faster than pristane-primed mice. However, this is clone dependent. Some clones produce less concentrated ascites with IFA than with pristane.

After priming, $1-2 \times 10^6$ viable hybridoma cells are injected i.p. Care should be taken that the hybridoma cells are healthy and in good condition at the time of injection. There are two major methods of collecting the ascites fluid from the mouse. A terminal collection is a one-time-only fluid accumulation; The mouse is killed and the ascites fluid is removed from the peritoneum. Tapping involves multiple collections of ascites fluid. A large-gauge sterile needle (18 gauge) is inserted into the peritoneum of the mouse, and the ascites fluid is drained out. This procedure can be repeated several times until the health of the mouse is compromised or the fluid volume diminishes. Then a terminal ascites accumulation ends the collection process. The success of each method is very clone dependent. Some clones produce very bloody ascites which has a severe impact on the health of the mouse. These clones rarely tap well and so a terminal collection is the method of choice. Other clones may tap 4–5 times and yield 3–4 ml per tap. Thus, each clone must be tested to determine which method will produce the greatest antibody yield (Keep *et al.*, 1984).

In vitro Antibody Production

The quantity of mAb produced in culture depends on the culture system used. The concentration of antibodies in static cell culture media ranges from 1 to 250 μg ml^{-1}. *In vitro* antibody production can be scaled up using fermentation techniques and bioreactors. These systems allow for production of gram-to-kilogram quantities of antibodies. In recent years, a wide range of cultivation systems for scale–up of antibody production from hybridomas have been developed. Fermenters range in size from 1 to 1,000 litres. Continuous culture or perfusion systems are smaller in size, but all systems have the similar optimisation requirements and

System	Name	Manufacturer	Cities, State	Yield
Hollow Fibre	Cell-Pharm Series	Unisyn	Hopkinton, MA	mg to grams
	Micro-mouse	Unisyn	Hopkinton, MA	mg
	Celex Maximizer	Celex	Minneapolis, MN	grams
	Technomouse	Integra Biosciences	Woburn, MA	mg
	CELLMAX	Cellco Inc.	Germantown, MD	mg
Fermenters	miniPERM (0.5–2 litres)	Heraeus Instruments	S. Plainfield, NJ	mg
	Omni-Culture (0.5–2 litres)	VirTis	Gardiner, NY	mg
	Virti-Culture (7.5–20 litres)	VirTis	Gardiner, NY	grams
	Celligen-Plus (2.5–7.5 litres)	New Brunswick Scientific	Fullerton, CA	grams
	Microlift (7.5–30 litres)	New Brunswick Scientific	Fullerton, CA	grams
	Cell Culture Fermenters (1–7 litres)	Applikon, Inc	Jamestown, RI	grams
	Biobench (7–20 litres)	Applikon, Inc	Jamestown, RI	grams
	Biopilot (20–200 litres)	Applikon, Inc	Jamestown, RI	grams

Table 5 *In vitro* antibody production systems.

are, to some degree, cell line dependent. Optimisation of growth conditions include: (1) defining optimal nutrient composition of growth media; (2) determining the cell tolerance for, or removal of, accumulated and possibly toxic metabolic by-products from the growth media; (3) optimising oxygen mass transfer in cultures; (4) determining cell sensitivity to shear, and physical and physiological constraints on cell growth; (5) process analysis and control; and (6) determination and maintenance of optimum cell density for antibody production. Examples of commercially available systems are shown in Table 5. A brief description of scaled–up *in vitro* production systems are as follows:

Batch and modified batch cultures (static cultures and fermentation)

In batch cultures, the temperature, pH and dissolved oxygen concentration are usually controlled, but no new media is added after culture initiation. Nutrients are depleted continuously, and inhibitory waste products accumulate. The batch culture yields the lowest cell densities in a given growth medium. Modified batch cultures are fed with new media continuously or intermittently. This improves cell concentration, cell viability and the overall length of time that the culture produces antibody (Lebherz, 1987).

Perfusion systems (hollow-fibre bioreactor and microencapsulation)

In these systems, the cells are physically retained in a container and continuous fresh medium is added while spent medium is removed without dilution of the media. The cell concentration in this system constantly increases until high density limits growth (VanBrunt, 1987).

Antibody Production in Transgenic Animals

The large-scale production of proteins in transgenic animals is under evaluation (Houdebine, 1994). In the future, this technique may be a valuable tool for the production of antibodies. Development of transgenic animals that produce recombinant proteins in the milk or blood still remains an arduous task, although steps are being taken to optimise the procedures. Transgenic animals that produce recombinant proteins in their milk produce µg to g per litre of the product from a predictable, high-yield source. Antibodies derived from the milk of transgenic animals should be relatively easy to purify and will have appropriate post-translational modifications compared to recombinant proteins produced by bacteria or other expression systems.

SUMMARY

In this chapter we have described some of the practical and theoretical considerations relevant to the generation and selection of monoclonal and polyclonal antibodies, with a particular emphasis on immunodiagnostic applications. Wherever possible, we have tried to relate this to experiences in our own antibody development centre. If one considers the number of variables associated with the proper selection of antigen preparations, immunisation schemes, fusion protocols and screening techniques, it is clear that embarking upon a full–scale monoclonal antibody development programme can be a costly and time-consuming endeavour. This is especially true for rare, poorly immunogenic or highly homologous antigenic substances.

However, the exquisite specificity and the high and uniform affinity provided by correctly selected mAbs, as well as the potential source of unlimited amounts of pure antibody reagents, has justified this investment in time and technology for many immunodiagnostic applications.

ACKNOWLEDGEMENTS

We would like to express our indebtedness to Ms Jean Shelton for her invaluable assistance in preparation of this chapter.

REFERENCES

Adam, A. (1985) *Synthetic Adjuvants*. (John Wiley & Sons, New York).

Allison, A. C. & Byars, N. E. (1986) An adjuvant formulation that selectively elicits the formation of antibodies of protective isotypes and of cell mediated immunity. *J. Immunol. Meth.* **95**, 157–169.

Allison, A. C. & Byars, N. E. (1991) Immunological adjuvants: Desirable properties and side-effects. *Mol. Immunol.* **28**, 279–284.

Allison, A. C. & Byars, N. E. (1992) Syntex adjuvant formulation. *Res. Immunol.* **143**, 519–525.

Alving, C. R. (1991) Liposomes as carriers of antigens and adjuvants. *J. Immunol. Meth.* **140**, 1–13.

Barry, M. A., Barry, M. E., & Johnston, S. A. (1994) Production of monoclonal antibodies by genetic immunisation. *Biotechniques* **16**, 616–619.

Bartal, A. H., Feit, C., & Hirshaut, Y. (1984). The addition of insulin to HAT medium (HIAT) enhances hybridoma formation *Int. Ass. of Biol. Standard.* **57**, 27–33 (Abstract).

Beh, K. J., Haynes, S. E. & Ward, K. A. (1986) Characterization of two mouse myeloma × sheep lymphocyte cell lines secreting sheep antibody. *Mol. Immunol.* **23**, 717–724.

Benjamini, E. & Leskowitz, S. (eds) (1991) *Immunology: A Short Course*. Chapter 10, p. 174 (Wiley–Lis, New York).

Bessler, W. G. & Jung, G. (1992) Synthetic lipopeptides as novel adjuvants. *Res. Immunol.* **143**, 548–553.

Bomford, R. (1980) The comparative selectivity of adjuvants for humoral and cell-mediated immunity. II. Effect on delayed-type hypersensitivity in the mouse and guinea pig, and cell-mediated immunity to tumor antigens in the mouse of Freund's incomplete and complete adjuvants, Alhydrogel, *Corynebacterium parvum*, *Bordetella pertussis*, muramyl dipeptide and saponin. *Clin. Exp. Immunol.* **39**, 435–441.

Borrebaeck, C. (1989) Strategy for the production of human monoclonal antibodies using *in vitro* activated B cells. *J. Immunol. Meth.* **123**, 157–165.

Brennan, M., Davison, P. F. & Paulus, H. (1985) Preparation of bispecific antibodies by chemical recombination of monoclonal immunoglobulin G1 fragments. *Science* **229**, 81–83.

Bright, S. W., Chen, T., Flebbe, L. M., *et al.* (1990) Generation and characterisation of hamster–mouse hybridomas secreting monoclonal antibodies with specificity for lipopolysaccahride receptor. *J. Immunol.* **145**, 1–7.

Brinkley, M. (1992) A brief survey of methods for preparing protein conjugates with dyes, haptens and cross–linking reagents. *Bioconj. Chem.* **3**, 2–13.

Brodeur, B. R., Tsang, P. & Larose, Y. (1984). Parameters affecting ascites tumour formation in mice and monoclonal antibody production. *J. Immunol. Meth.* **71**, 265–272.

Buchegger, F., Pälegrin, A., Hardman, N. *et al.* (1992) Different behaviour of mouse–human chimeric antibody F(ab′)₂ fragments of IgG1, IgG2 and IgG4 sub-class *in vivo. Int. J. Cancer* **50**, 416–422.

Buiting, A. M. J., van Rooijen, N. & Claassen, E. (1992) Liposomes as antigen carriers and adjuvants *in vivo. Res. Immunol.* **143**, 541–548.

Burrin, J. & Newman, D. (1991) Production and assessment of antibodies. In: *Principles and Practice of Immunoassay* (eds Price, C. P. & Newman, D. J.) (Stockton Press, New York).

Butcher, R. N., McCullough, K. C., Jarry, C. *et al.* (1988) Mitomycin C–treated 3T3/B (3T3/A31) cell feeder layers in hybridoma technology. *J. Immunol. Meth.* **107**, 245–251.

Capparelli, R., Del Sorbo, G. & Iannelli, D. (1990) Goat–mouse hybridomas secreting goat immunoglobulins. *Hybridoma* **9**, 149–155.

Carroll, K., Prosser, E. & O'Kennedy, R. (1990) Parameters involved in the *in vitro* immunization of tonsilar lymphocytes: Effects of rIL–2 and muramyl dipeptide. *Hybridoma* **9**, 81–89.

Carter, P. (1995) Knobs-into-holes engineering of antibody C$_H$3 domains for heavy chain heterodimerisation. *6th Annual International Conference on Antibody Engineering*, San Diego, (Abstract), San Diego, CA.

Chang, T. H., Steplewski, Z. & Koprowski, H. (1980) Production of monoclonal antibodies in serum free medium. *J. Immunol. Meth.* **39**, 369–375.

Claassen, E., de Leeuw, W., de Greeve, P. *et al.* (1992) Freund's complete adjuvant: An effective but disagreeable formula. *Res. in Immunol.* **143**, 478–483.

Coffman, R. L. & Weissman, I. L. (1981) A monoclonal antibody that recognises B cells and B-cell precursors in mice. *J. Exp. Med.* **153**, 269–279.

Colowick, S. P. & Kaplan, N. O. (1979) Cell Culture. *Meth. Enzymol.* **58**, 353–371.

Corvalan, J. R. F., Smith, W., & Gore, V. A. (1988). Tumour therapy with vinca alkaloids targeted by a hybrid–hybrid monoclonal antibody recognising both CEA and vinca alkaloids. *Int. J. Cancer.* **2**, 22–25.

Davis, W. C. (1988) Enhancement of myeloma B cell hybridoma outgrowth in primary cultures with B cell mitogens. *Periodicum Biologorum* **90**, 367–374.

de Boer, M., Conroy, L., Min, H. Y. *et al.* (1992) Generation of monoclonal antibodies to human lymphocyte cell surface antigens using insect cells expressing recombinant proteins. *J. Immunol. Meth.* **152**, 15–23.

Ghalich, P. H., Moustafa, Z. A., Juslice, J. C. *et al.* (1988) Human and primate monoclonal antibodies for *in vivo* therapy. *Clin. Chem.* **34**, 1681–1688.

Federspiel, G., McCullough, K. C., & Kihm, U. (1991) Production of monoclonal antibodies specific for African swine fever virus following *in vitro* primary immunisation of mouse splenocytes in the presence of stimulated T lymphocyte supernatants. *J. Immunol. Meth.* **145**, 71–81.

Fernandez, C. & Moller, G. (1991) The influence of T-cells on the immunoglobulin repertoire and the affinity maturation of the immune response against dextran B512 in C57BL/6 mice. *Scand. J. Immunol.* 33, 307–317.

Flynn, J. N., Harkiss, G. D. & Hopkins, J. (1989) Generation of a sheep × mouse heterohybridoma cell line (1C6.3a6T.1D7) and evaluation of its use in the production of ovine monoclonal antibodies. *J. Immunol. Meth.* 121, 237–246.

Freund, J. (1956) The mode of action of immunologic adjuvants. *Adv. Tuberc. Res.* 7, 130–148.

Gillette, R. W. (1987) Alternatives to pristane priming for ascitic fluid and monoclonal antibody production. *J. Immunol. Meth.* 99, 21–23.

Glasky, M. & Reading, C. (1995) Stability of specific immunoglobulin secretion by EBV-transformed lymphoblastoid cells and human–murine heterohybridomas. *Hybridoma* 8, 377–389.

Glassy, M. C. (1988) Creating hybridomas by electrofusion. *Nature* 333, 6173.

Gosling, J. P. (1990) A decade of development in immunoassay methodology. *Clin. Chem.* 36, 1408–1427.

Groves, D. J., Morris, B. A. & Clayton, J. (1987) Preparation of a bovine monoclonal antibody to testosterone by interspecies fusion. *Res. Vet. Sci.* 43, 253–256.

Guidry, A. J., Srikumaran, S. & Goldsby, R. A. (1986) Production and characterisation of bovine immunoglobulins from bovine × murine hybridomas. In: *Methods in Enzymology* (eds Colowick, S. P. & Kaplan, N. O.), pp. 244–265. (Academic Press, New York).

Gupta, R. (1995) Adjuvant properties of aluminium and calcium compounds. In: *Vaccine Design* (eds Powell, M. F. & Newman, M. J.), pp. 229–248 (Plenum Publishing, New York).

Gustafson, G. L. & Rhodes, M. J. (1992) Bacterial cell wall products as adjuvants: early interferon gamma as a marker for adjuvants that enhance protective immunity. *Res. Immunol.* 143, 483–488.

Guzman, J., Schoendon, G. & Blau, N. (1993) *In vitro* immunization with antigen directly blotted from SDS-polyaerylamide gels to polyvinylidine difluoride membranes. *J. Immunol. Meth.* 158, 37–47.

Hale, G., Cobbold, S. P., Waldmann, H. *et al.* (1987) Isolation of low-frequency class-switch variants from rat hybrid myelomas. *J. Immunol. Meth.* 103, 59–67.

Harlow, E. & Lane, D. (1988) Immunisations. In: *Antibodies: A Laboratory Manual* pp. 53–138. (Cold Spring Harbor Laboratory Press, New York).

Hendrickson, T. L., Wilson, G. S., Frazer, J. M. *et al.* (1994) Enhanced immunogenicity of leucine enkephalin following coupling to anti-immunoglobulin and anti-CD3 antibodies. *J. Immunol. Meth.* 172, 165–172.

Hirano, T. (1991) Interleukin-6. In: *The Cytokine Handbook* (ed. Thomson, A. M.) pp. 169–190 (Academic Press, New York).

Honsa, S., Ichimori, Y. & Iwasa, S. (1990) A human hybrid–hybridoma producing a bispecific monoclonal antibody that can target tumor cells for attack by *pseudomonas aeruginosa* exotoxin A. *Cytotechnology* 4, 59–62.

Hoogenraad, N., Helman, T. & Hoogenraad, J. (1983) The effect of pre-injection of mice with pristane on ascites tumour formation and monoclonal antibody production. *J. Immunol. Meth.* 61, 317–320.

Hoogenraad, N. J. & Wraight, C. J. (1986) The effect of pristane on ascites tumor formation and monoclonal antibody production. *Meth. Enzymol.* 121, 375–381.

Horton, J. K., Evans, O. M., Swann, K. *et al.* (1989) A new and rapid method for the selection and cloning of antigen-specific hybridomas with magnetic microspheres. *J. Immunol. Meth.* **124**, 225–230.

Houdebine, L (1994). Production of pharmaceutical proteins from transgenic animals. *J. Biotechnol.* **34**, 269–287.

Igarashi, M. & Bando, Y. (1990) Enhanced efficiency of cell hybridisation by neuraminidase treatment. *J. Immunol. Meth.* **135**, 91–93.

Kearney, J. F., Radbruch, A., Liesegang, B. *et al.* (1979). A new mouse myeloma cell line that has lost immunoglobulin expression but permits the construction of antibody-secreting hybrid cell lines. *J. Immunol.* **123**, 1548–1550.

Keep, P. A., Rawlins, G. A., Bagshawe, J. A. D. *et al.* (1984) Serial ascitic fluid tapping and monoclonal antibody yield in passaged mice. *Exp. Clin. Cancer Res.* **3**, 235–238.

Kennedy, H. E., Jones, B. V., Tucker, E. M., *et al.* (1988) Production and characterisation of bovine monoclonal antibodies to respiratory syncytial virus. *Virology* **69**, 3023–3032.

Kenney, J. S., Hughes, B. W. Masada, M. P. *et al.* (1989) Influence of adjuvants on the quantity, affinity, isotype and epitope specificity of murine antibodies. *J. Immunol. Meth.* **121**, 157–166.

Kenny, P. A. (1981) Enrichment and expansion of specific antibody-forming cells by adoptive transfer and clustering, and their use in hybridoma production. *Aust. J. Exp. Biol.* **59**, 427–437.

Knott, C., Reed, J. C., Bodrug. S. *et al.* (1996) Evaluation of Bc1.2/B cell transgenic mice (B6) for hybridoma production. *Hybridoma.* **15**, 365–371.

Koda, K. & Glassy, M. C. (1990) *In vitro* immunisation for the production of human monoclonal antibody. *Hum. Antibodies Hybridomas* **1**, 15–22.

Köhler, G. & Milstein, C. (1975) Continuous cultures of fused cells secreting antibody of predefined specificity. *Nature* **256**, 495–497.

Köhler, G. & Milstein, C. (1976) Derivation of specific antibody producing tissue culture and tumor lines by cell fusion. *J. Immunol.* **6**, 511–519.

Kolberg, J. & Blanchard, D. (1991) A mouse monoclonal antibody against glycophorin A produced by *in vitro* stimulation with human red cell membranes. *Immunol. Lett.* **30**, 87–92.

Kuo, M.-C., Sogn, J. A., Max, E. E. *et al.* (1984) Rabbit–mouse hybridomas secreting intact rabbit immunoglobulin. *Mol. Immunol.* **21**, 95–104.

Kuus-Reichel, K., Beebe, A. & Knott, C. (1991) Isolation of hybridoma forming cells from immune spleens by unit gravity sedimentation. *Hybridoma* **10**, 529–538.

Kuus-Reichel, K., Knott, C. L. McCormack, R. T. *et al.* (1994) Production of IgG monoclonal antibodies to the tumor-associated antigen CA-195. *Hybridoma* **13**, 31–36.

Kuus-Reichel, K., Knott, C., Sam-Fong, P. *et al.* (1995) Therapy of streptozotocin induced diabetes with a bifunctional antibody that delivers vinca alkaloids to IL–2 receptor positive cells. *Autoimmunity* **22**, 173–181.

Lebherz, W. B. (1987) Batch production of monoclonal antibody by large-scale suspension culture. In: *Commercial Production of Monoclonal Antibodies: A Guide for Scale–up* (ed Seaver, S. S.) pp. 93–102 (Marcel Dekker, New York).

Lefkovits, I. (1979) Limiting dilution analysis of cells in the immune system. In: *Immunological Methods* (eds Lefkovits, I. & Pernis, B.) pp. 355–370 (Academic Press, New York).

Lerner, R., Benkovic, S. & Schultz, P. (1991) At the crossroads of chemistry and immunology: Catalytic antibodies. *Science* **252**, 659–667.

Lipman, N. S., Trudel, L. J., Murphy, J. C. *et al.* (1992) Comparison in immune response potentiation and *in vivo* inflammatory effects of Freund's and Ribi adjuvants in mice. *Animal* **42**, 193–197.

Long, W. J. McGuire, W., Palombo, A. *et al.* (1986) Enhancing the establishment efficiency of hybridoma cells. Use of irradiated human diploid fibroblast feeder layers. *J. Immunol. Meth.* **86**, 89–93.

Lumanglas, A. L., Sadeghi, H., & Wang, B. S. (1994) Generation of heterohybridomas capable of releasing swine monoclonal antibody specific to porcine growth hormone. *Hybridoma* **13**, 237–240.

Manickan, E., Rouse, J. D., Yu, Z. *et al.* (1995) Genetic immunisation against herpes simplex virus. Protection is mediated by CD4+ lymphocytes. *J. Immunol.* **155**, 259–265.

Mårtensson, C., Ifversen, P., Borrebaeck, C. A. K. *et al.* (1995) Enhancement of specific immunoglobulin production in SCID–hu–PBL mice after *in vitro* priming of human B–cells with superantigen. *Immunology* **86**, 224–230.

McCormack, R., Liu, R., Darter, R., *et al.* (1992a) Generation and characterisation of stable rabbit monoclonal antibodies. *8th Int. Cong. of Immunol.* p. 442, workshop 70; poster 17. (Abstract) Budapest, Hungary.

McCormack, R. T., Ludwig, J. R., & Wolfert, R. L. (1992b) Advances in design, generation, and manipulation of monoclonal antibodies. In: *Immunochemical assays and biosensor technology for the 1990s* (eds Nakamura, R. M., Kasahara, Y. & Rechnitz, G. A. (pp. 57–82). American Society for Microbiology, (Washington DC).

McCune, J. M., Namikawa, R., Kaneshima, H. *et al..* (1988) The SCID–hu mouse: murine model for the analysis of human hematolymphoid differentiation and function. *Science* **241**, 1632–1639.

Merwin, R. M. & Algire, G. H. (1959) Induction of plasma cell neoplasms and fibrosarcomas in BALB/c mice carrying diffusion chambers. *Proc. Sci. Exp. Biol. Med.* **101**, 437–439.

Michel, M.-L., Davis, H. L., Schleef, M., *et al.* (1995) DNA–mediated immunisation to the hepatitis B surface antigen in mice: Aspects of the humoral response mimic hepatitis B viral infection in humans. *Proc. Natl Acad. Sci. USA* **92**, 5307–5311.

Miyahara, M., Nakamura, H. & Hamaguchi, Y. (1984) Colcemid treatment of myeloma prior to cell fusion increases the yield of hybridomas between myeloma and splenocyte. *Biochem. Biophys. Res. Commun.* **124**, 903–908.

Moncada, C., Torres, V. & Israel, Y. (1993) Simple method for the preparation of antigen emulsions for immunisation. *J. Immunol. Meth.* **162**, 133–140.

Mosier, D. E. (1990). Immunodeficient mice xenografted with human lymphoid cells: New models for *in vivo* studies of human immunobiology and infectious diseases. *J. Clin. Immunol.* **10**, 185–191.

Mosier, D. E., Gulizia, R. J., Baird, S. M. *et al.* (1988) Transfer of a functional human immune system to mice with severe combined immunodeficiency. *Nature* **355**, 256–259.

Mosmann, T. R. & Coffman, R. L. (1989) Heterogeneity of cytokine secretion patterns and functions of helper T-cells. *Adv. Immunol.* **46**, 111–147.

Murikami, H., Masui, H., Sato, G. H., *et al.* (1982) Growth of hybridoma cells in serum free medium: Ethanolamine is an essential component. *Proc. Natl Acad. Sci. USA* **79**, 1158–1162.

Nicklas, W. (1992) Aluminium salts. *Res. in Immunol.* 143, 489–494.

Niguma, T., DeVito, L. D., Grailer, A. P. *et al.* (1993) HLA–A2-specific antibody production in severe combined immunodeficient mice reconstituted with human peripheral blood leukocytes from HLA-presensitized donors. *Transplant. Proc.* 25, 239–240.

Nilsson, B. O. & Larsson, A. (1992) Inert carriers for immunisation. *Res. Immunol.* 143, 553–556.

Nonoyama, S., Smith, F. O., & Ochs, H. D. (1993) Specific antibody production to a recall or a neoantigen by SCID mice reconstituted with human peripheral blood lymphocytes. *J. Immunol.* 151, 3894–3901.

Norwood, T. H., Zeigler, C. J. & Martin, G. M. (1976). Dimethyl sulfoxide enhances polyethylene glycol–mediated somatic cell fusion. *Somatic Cell Genet.* 2, 263–270.

Orlik, O. & Altaner, C. (1988) Modifications of hybridoma technology which improve the yield of monoclonal antibody producing cells. *J. Immunol. Meth.* 115, 55–59.

Ossendorp, F. A., Bruning, P. F., Van den Brink, J. A. M. *et al.* (1989) Efficient selection of high-affinity B-cell hybridomas using antigen–coated magnetic beads. *J. Immunol. Meth.* 120, 191–200.

Ott, G. Van Nest, G. & Burke, R. L. (1992) The use of muramyl dipeptides as vaccine adjuvants. In: *Vaccine Research and Development* (eds Koff, W. C. & Six, H. R.) pp. 89–113 (Marcel Dekker Inc., New York).

Parks, D. R., Bryan, V. M., Oi, V. T. *et al.* (1979) Antigen-specific identification and cloning of hybridomas with a fluorescence-activated cell sorter. *Proc. Natl Acad. Sci. USA* 76, 1962–1966.

Pintus, C., Ransom, J. H. & Evans, C. H. (1983) Endothelial cell growth supplement: A cell cloning factor that promotes the growth of monclonal antibody producing hybridoma cells. *J. Immunol. Meth.* 61, 195–200.

Pistillo, M. P., Sguerso, V. & Ferrara, G. B. (1992) High yields of anti–HLA human monoclonal antibodies can be provided by SCID mice. *Hum. Immunol.* 35, 256–259.

Posner, B., Smiley, J., Lee, I. *et al.* (1994). Catalytic antibodies: Perusing combinatorial libraries. *Trends Biochem. Sci.* 19, 145–150.

Raybould, T. J. G., Wilson, P. J., McDougall, L. J. *et al.* (1985) A porcine–murine hybridoma that secretes porcine monoclonal antibody of defined specificity. *Am. Vet. Res.* 46, 1768–1769.

Raybould, T. J. G. & Takahashi, M. (1988) Production of stable rabbbit–mouse hybridomas that secrete rabbit mAb of defined specificity. *Science* 240, 1788–1790.

Raz, E., Carson, D. A., Parker, S. E. *et al.* (1994) Intradermal gene immunisation: the possible role of DNA uptake in the induction of cellular immunity to viruses. *Proc. Natl Acad. Sci. USA* 91, 9519–9523.

Roder, J. C., Cole, S. P. C. & Kozbor, D. (1986). The EBV-hybridoma technique. *Meth. Enzymol.* 121, 140–174.

Roth, R. A., Cassell, D. J., Wong, K. Y., *et al.* (1982) Monoclonal antibodies to the human insulin receptor block insulin binding and inhibit insulin action. *Proc. Natl Acad. Sci. USA* 79, 7312–7316.

Ruedl, C. & Wolf, H. (1995) Features of oral immunisation. *Int. Archs Allergy Immunol.* 108, 334–339.

Schilizzi, B. M., Kroesen, B.-J., The, T. H. *et al.* (1992) Increased production of antigen-specific B lymphocytes during *in vitro* immunisation using carrier-specific T helper hybridomas. *J. Immunol. Meth.* 153, 49–56.

Schneerson, R., Fattom, A., Szu, S. C., *et al.* (1991) Evaluation of monophosphoryl lipid A (MPL) as an adjuvant. Enhancement of the serum antibody response in mice to polysaccharide–protein conjugates by concurrent injection with MPL. *J. Immunol.* **147**, 2136–2140.

Shan, H., Shlomchik, M. J., Marshak-Rothstein, A. *et al.* (1994) The mechanism of autoantibody production in an autoimmune MRL/lpr mouse. *J. Immunol.* **153**, 5104–5119.

Shulman, M., Wilde, C. D., & Köhler, G. (1978) A better cell line for making hybridomas secreting specific antibodies. *Nature* **276**, 269–270.

Spitz, M. (1984) Intrasplenic primary immunisation for the production of monoclonal antibodies. *J. Immunol. Meth.* **70**, 39–43.

Srikumaran, S., Guidray, A. J., & Goldsby, R. A. (1983) Bovine × mouse hybridomas that secrete bovine immunoglobulin G1. *Science* **220**, 522–524.

Steenbakkers, P. G. A., van Wezenbeek, P. M. G. F., & Olijve, W. (1993) Immortalisation of antigen selected B cells. *J. Immunol. Meth.* **163**, 33–40.

Stenger, D. A., Kubiniec, R. T., Purucker, W. J. *et al.* (1988) Optimization of electrofusion parameters for efficient production of murine hybridomas. *Hybridoma* **7**, 505–518.

Stickney, D. R., Anderson, L. D., Slater, J. B. *et al.* (1991) Bifunctional antibody: a binary radiopharmaceutical delivery system for imaging colorectal carcinoma. *Cancer Res.* **51**, 6650–6655.

Taggart, R. T. & Samloff, I. M. (1983) Stable antibody-producing murine hybridomas. *Science* **219**, 1228–1230.

Ten Hagen, T. L. M., Sulzer, A. J., Kidd, M. R. *et al.* (1993) Role of adjuvants in the modulation of antibody isotype, specificity, and induction of protection by whole-blood stage plasmodium yoelii vaccines. *J. Immunol* **151**, 7077–7085.

Tomita, M. & Tsong, T. Y. (1990) Selective production of hybridoma cells: antigenic-based pre-selection of B lymphocytes for electrofusion with myeloma cells. *Biochim. Biophys. Acta* **1055**, 199–206.

Tong, A. W., Lee, J. & Stone, M. J. (1984) Characterization of two human small cell lung carcinoma-reactive monoclonal antibodies generated by a novel immunization approach. *Cancer Res.* **44**, 4987–4992.

Tucker, E. M., Clarke, S. W. & Metenier, L. (1987) Murine/bovine hybridomas producing monoclonal alloantibodies to bovine red cell antigens. *Anim. Genet.* **18**, 29–39.

Tucker, E. M., Dain, A. R., Wright, L. J. *et al.* (1981) Culture of sheep × mouse hybridoma cells *in vitro*. *Hybridoma* **1**, 77–86.

Ufimtseva, E. G., Galakhar, N. L., Matjakhina, L. D. *et al.* (1991) Mink–mouse interspecific hybridomas. *Hybridoma* **10**, 517–528.

Uthoff, S. & Boldicke, T. (1993) In vitro immunization of mouse spleen cells for the production of monoclonal IgG1 antibodies using an antigen-specific T helper cell clone (D.10.G4.1). *J. Immunol. Meth.* **166**, 165–175.

Vahlsing, H. L., Yankauckas, M. A., Sawdey, M. *et al.* (1994) Immunisation with plasmid DNA using a pneumatic gun. *J. Immunol. Meth.* **175**, 11–22.

Vajdy, M. & Lycke, N. (1995) Mucosal memory B-cells retain the ability to produce IgM antibodies 2 years after oral immunisation. *Immunology* **86**, 336–342.

VanBrunt, J. (1987) A closer look at fermentors and bioreactors. *Biotechnology* **5**, 10–15.

Verheul, A. F. M. & Snippe, H. (1992) Non-ionic block polymer surfactants as immunological adjuvants. *Res. Immunol.* **143**, 512–519.

Verma, J. N., Rao, M., Amselem, S., *et al.* (1992) Adjuvant effects of liposomes containing lipid A: Enhancement of liposomal antigen presentation and recruitment of macrophages. *Infect. Immun.* **60**, 2438–2444.

Vogel, F. R. & Powell, M. F. (1995) A compendium of vaccine adjuvants and excipients. In: *Vaccine Design: The Subunit and Adjuvant Approach* (eds Powell, M. F. & Newman, M.) pp. 141–228 (Plenum Publishing, New York).

Walker, W. & Gallagher, G. (1994) The *in vivo* production of specific human antibodies by vaccination of human–PBL–SCID mice. *Immunology* **83**, 163–170.

Wolberg, G., Liu, C. T., & Adler, F. L. (1970) Passive hemagglutination. II. Titration of antibody against determinants unique for aggregated denatured bovine serum albumin and further studies on gelatin. *J. Immunol.* **105**, 797–801.

Woloschak, G. & Senitzer, D. (1993) Effect of mitogenic stimulation of murine splenocytes on PEG-induced cell fusion. *Hybridoma*, **2**, 341–349.

Xiang, J., Pan, Z. Attah-Poku, S. *et al.* (1992) Production of hybrid bispecific antibody recognising human colorectal carcinoma and CD3 antigen. *Mol. Biother.* **4**, 15–23.

Yarmush, M. L., Gates F. T. III, Weisfogel, D. R. *et al.* (1980). Identification and characterisation of rabbit–mouse hybridomas secreting rabbit immunoglobulin chains. *Proc. Natl Acad. Sci. USA* **77**, 2899–2903.

Yazaki, P. J., Rathnachalam, R. & Moore, M. D. (1995) IgG heterodimer heavy chain assembly by charge interaction: insertion of a salt bridge in the C_H3 region. *6th Annual International Conference on Antibody Engineering* (Abstract), San Diego, CA.

Zimmermann, U., Vienken, J. & Pilwat, G. (1980). Development of a drug carrier system: electrical field-induced effects in cell membranes. *Bioelect. Bioeng.* **7**, 553–574.

Chapter 4

Antibody Engineering: Potential Applications for Immunoassays

Andrew J. T. George

INTRODUCTION

Over the past 20 years the increase in our knowledge of the structure and genetics of the immunoglobulin molecule, together with new recombinant DNA techniques, has allowed a massive expansion in genetic engineering of antibodies. This explosion has not yet had a major impact on the daily use of immunoassays, but it is likely over the next few years that more and more commercial and experimental immunoassays will use recombinant molecules. There are three main reasons why this might be the case.

1. DNA technology allows the properties of the antibody molecule to be altered, for example by fusion with enzymes, thus improving on the native molecules.

2. Recombinant antibodies can be produced in large amounts using a variety of expression systems, reducing their cost.

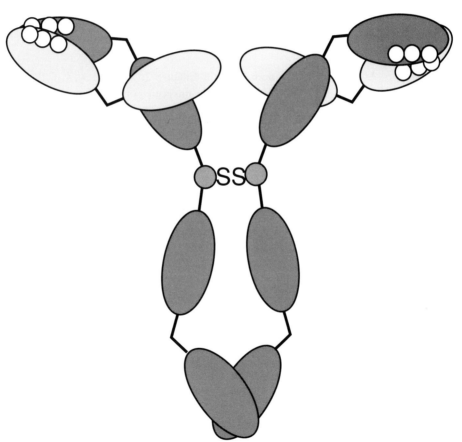

Figure 1 Structure of the IgG molecule. The structure of the IgG molecule is shown in terms of the domains that make up the heavy chain (dark shading) and light chain (light shading). The CDRs of the variable domains (V_H and V_L) are shown as white circles (note that their location is diagrammatic, rather than representing their structural location). A single disulphide bond linking the two heavy chains is indicated, although there are frequently multiple disulphide bonds in this region. For simplicity the disulphide bonds between the light and heavy chain, and the intra-domain bonds are not shown.

3. The development of phage technology allows the generation of antibodies with novel specificities that are unavailable using conventional polyclonal or hybridoma techniques.

It should be remembered, however, that much of the effort in antibody engineering has focused on improving the properties of the molecules for *in vivo* clinical use and thus is not of direct relevance to immunoassays (George *et al.*, 1994a; 1996; George and Epenetos, 1996). In this chapter I will briefly cover some of these developments, as they illustrate common themes in antibody engineering. It should also be noted that there are many cases where it is not appropriate to use genetic engineering to produce or modify antibody molecules; the more traditional techniques of immunisation and hybridoma technology, allied with chemical modification and conjugation, being more appropriate. There is a danger of being attracted to a technology not because of its utility, but because of its novelty. This temptation should be resisted. However there is little doubt that the genetic engineering of antibodies will become increasingly important, and so a basic understanding of its potential and the principles involved will be of use to any scientist or clinician involved in developing or using immunoassays.

ANTIBODY STRUCTURE

As is discussed in more detail in Chapter 2, and reviewed in (Padlan, 1994; Searle *et al.*, 1995) the structure of an antibody molecule consists of two different chains, the heavy and light chains (Figure 1). These chains are made up of domains, each of which contains approximately 110 amino acids in a characteristic structure consisting of antiparallel β-sheets that are held together by intra-chain disulphide bonds (Barclay *et al.*, 1993). One of the important features of these domains for engineering purposes is that they are essentially self contained units that fold independently. They can therefore be used as 'building blocks', which can be interchanged or added to at will. The chains of the immunoglobulin molecule are held together by inter-chain disulphide bonds. In addition they are held together by noncovalent interactions between the constant region domains.

The antigenic specificity of an antibody is conferred by the variable domains of the heavy (V_H) and light (V_L) chains. As in most systems (including immunoassays), the main property of interest of an antibody is its ability to bind antigen; most attention has thus been focused on this aspect of the molecule. Chemical cleavage of the molecule has led to the description of a number of antibody fragments that retain the ability to bind antigen, including the $(Fab')_2$, Fab', Fab and Fv fragments (Figure 2). Of these the Fv fragment, which consists of just the V_H and V_L domains, is the smallest. It has been produced by proteolytic cleavage of some immunoglobulin molecules (Inbar *et al.*, 1972). However, as discussed below, this is not a routine procedure and the resulting molecule is not stable.

Even though the Fv fragment is the smallest antigen-binding fragment, much of the sequence of the V_H and V_L domains is not involved in antigen binding, but rather it provides a structural scaffolding for the six complementarity determining regions (CDRs) which determine much of the specificity of the molecule. The CDRs (three for each V_H and V_L) form hypervariable loops that come together in three dimensions to form the antigen-binding site (Poljak *et al.*, 1973). The framework residues of the V_H and V_L domains in the region of the CDRs can influence antigen binding, either by direct interaction with antigen or by influencing the conformation of the hypervariable loops. Furthermore it has been shown that, at least in the human, the CDRs (with the exception of CDR3 of the heavy chain) exist in a lim-

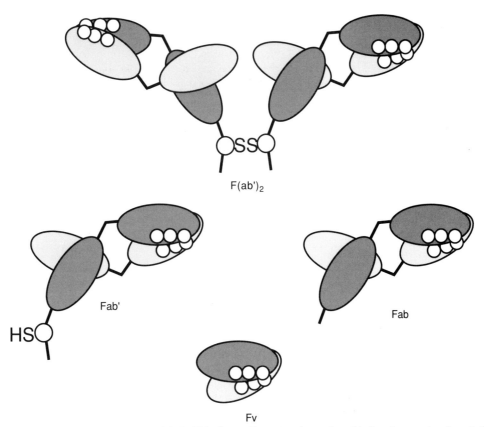

Figure 2 Enzymatic digestion of IgG. This figure illustrates the antigen-binding fragments of an IgG molecule that can be produced by enzymatic digestion. Thus the F(ab')$_2$ is made by pepsin digestion; this can then be reduced to yield the Fab' molecule. Fab fragments are made by papain digestion, which also produces the Fc fragment of the molecule (not shown). In some molecules it is also possible to generate Fv fragments, however these tend to be unstable

ited number of canonical structures, determined by conserved residues within the CDRs and framework regions (Chothia *et al.*, 1989; 1992; Tomlinson *et al.*, 1992; 1995). As a result the overall backbone structure of the antibody variable regions is restricted to a relatively small repertoire (seven in the case of the human V_H) (Chothia *et al.*, 1992; Tomlinson *et al.*, 1992) which carries the variable amino acids that provide antigen-binding diversity.

ANTIBODY GENETICS

One of the features of B cells is their ability to produce a vast repertoire of different antibody specificities. They do this by a combination of gene rearrangement, combinatorial diversity, imprecise joining and mutation. These processes are well reviewed elsewhere (Max, 1993), and so I will provide only a short summary in this section.

Immunoglobulin molecules are encoded by relatively complex gene loci. The locus for the human immunoglobulin κ light chain is shown in Figure 3. The locus consists of a large number of variable (V) and junctional (J) segments and one constant segment (C) (see Table

69

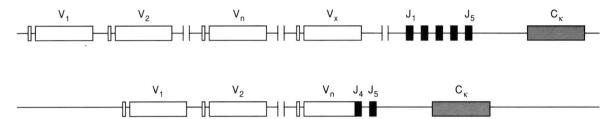

Figure 3 Organisation of the human κ chain locus. This figure schematically represents the κ chain locus, consisting of multiple V segments, 5 J segments and a single constant segment. The exons are indicated by rectangles, white for the V regions, black for the J and grey for the Cκ. During B cell maturation one of the V segments rearranges to splice with one of the J segments (in the case shown V_n rearranges to J_4). The figure is not to scale, and omits pseudo genes, promoters and enhancers that are found in this region. An accurate map of this region is available through the world wide web (Tomlinson *et al.*, 1996b) (http://www.mrc–cpe.cam.ac.uk/imt–doc/vbase–home–page.html).

	V_H	V_κ	V_λ
V segments	51	40	30
D segments	27	–	–
J segments	6	5	4
Location	14q32.3	2p11-12	22q11.2

Table 1 Human immunoglobulin gene loci. The number of functional V, D and J segments in the immunoglobulin loci of humans are shown. Nonexpressed genes or genes on the wrong chromosome are not counted. The numbers of V segments indicated show the maximum possible as, due to polymorphisms in the population, some individuals have fewer segments. Data for V_H and V_κ taken from Cook and Tomlinson, 1995; Tomlinson *et al.*, 1995. The number of V_λ segments is currently unpublished, and may be inaccurate by a couple of segments (I. Tomlinson, personal communication).

1). During maturation of a B cell the loci are rearranged, with one of the V segments combining with one J segment (Figure 3). When the novel, rearranged gene is transcribed into RNA, and the RNA is then processed to make messenger RNA, the intron sequences (including unused J exons) are spliced out, and the VJ gene segment is apposed to the C segment (Figure 4). Similar rearrangements are seen in the heavy chain locus, although the germline locus is more complex, consisting of D segments, as well as multiple constant regions, encoding the different immunoglobulin isotypes (Figure 5)(Cook and Tomlinson, 1995). The rearrangement of the V(D)J gene segments, together with the different combinations of heavy and light chains, contribute greatly to the diversity of antibody molecules. In addition, further sequence differences are generated by the junctional diversity caused by the imprecise nature of the recombination events.

It is of interest to note that much of the diversity is focused on the CDR3 region of the molecule. This is the region encoded by the V(D)J recombination events, and so has diversity as a result both of the different V(D)J segments used, and of the junctional diversity created between these segments. As a result the CDR3 (in particular of the heavy chain) shows the greatest heterogeneity in both sequence and length (Kabat *et al.*, 1991). For this reason some strategies to create artificial antibody repertoires have concentrated on the CDR3 region (in particular of the heavy chain), as will be discussed later in this chapter.

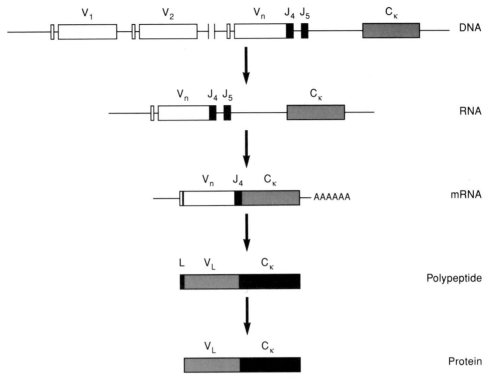

Figure 4 Transcription, translation and modification of the κ chain. In the B cell containing the rearranged κ chain locus the DNA is transcribed into RNA. This is processed to form mRNA by removal of the introns, and addition of the polyA⁺ tail to the molecule. This is then translated into the polypeptide chain at the ribosomes. The molecule is further modified by cleavage of the leader signal peptide (L) which directs synthesis to the endoplasmic reticulum. In addition the chain may be glycosylated (as is the heavy chain).

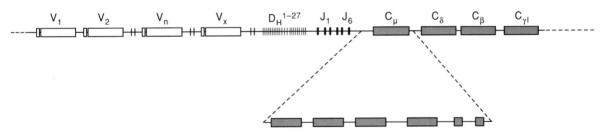

Figure 5 Organisation of the heavy chain locus. The heavy chain locus of immunoglobulin is more complex than the light chain locus because it contains multiple constant domains as well as an additional series of gene segments, the D regions. This diagram outlines the locus. For simplicity only four of the constant regions are shown (each indicated by a single rectangle); in reality (as indicated for C_μ) they consist of multiple exons. This diagram is not to scale. For a detailed map please refer to Cook and Tomlinson, 1995; Tomlinson *et al.*, 1996b.

Once the B cell has matured and encountered antigen, further diversity occurs by the process of somatic mutation. This essentially random process leads to the generation of novel variable region sequences, that can then be selected or rejected on the basis of their affinity to the antigen. Recently analysis of the sequence of germline and somatically mutated sequences in the human variable region genes has been performed, relating the sequence diversity with structural information on the antigen site (Tomlinson *et al.*, 1996a). Interestingly this has shown that, in the primary repertoire, diversity is focused at the centre of the antigen-binding site whereas, following somatic hypermutation, diversity spreads to regions at the periphery of the binding site that are largely conserved in the germline sequences. This suggests that germline diversity and somatic mutation are complementary processes that have been selected during evolutionary history to provide an efficient strategy for creating novel antigen-binding sites and exploiting the full potential diversity of variable region sequences (Tomlinson *et al.*, 1996a).

The outline given above of immunoglobulin genetics describes the situation seen in mouse and human. However, it should be noted that other species (e.g. chicken and rabbit) can use a process of gene conversion to generate diversity, in which insertion of nonfunctional V genes into a single functional V region generates novel sequences (Knight, 1992; Ratcliffe and Jacobsen, 1994).

Genetic Modification of Antibody Molecules

A large number of genetic modifications to antibody molecules has been made, and in this review I will concentrate on a few examples to illustrate what can be done. These modifications will be considered under three headings: modification of the immunoglobulin molecule, fusion of the molecule with other molecules or peptides, and the production of bivalent or bispecific molecules.

Modification of the Immunoglobulin Molecule

The domain structure of the antibody molecule has greatly facilitated its modification, as the ability of each domain to fold independently, forming a stable unit, allows the engineer to mix and match the domains with impunity, using them as individual building bricks (Plückthun, 1990; Winter and Milstein, 1991). Thus all the antibody fragments shown in Figure 2 can be made by genetic engineering, simply by deleting the unwanted domains from the gene construct. At the practical level this process is simplified by the gene structure of immunoglobulins, in which individual domains are encoded for by separate exons, allowing for simply 'cutting and pasting' of the exons.

Although IgG, F(ab′)$_2$, Fab′, Fab and Fv fragments can be produced in this manner, it is possibly more interesting to consider novel antibody molecules that are not available using conventional enzymatic manipulation of molecules (Winter and Milstein, 1991). Much of the impetus for this has been the attempt to produce less immunogenic antibodies for *in vivo* clinical use. The immunogenic nature of rodent monoclonal antibodies can lead to the production of a human anti-mouse antibody (HAMA) response in patients which not only limits the effectiveness of the therapy but also cause immune complex disease (Courtenay-Luck *et al.*, 1987, 1988). The first recombinant molecules to address this problem were chimeric antibodies, in which the variable domains of the murine antibodies are linked to human constant regions (Boulianne *et al.*, 1984; Morrison *et al.*, 1984; Neuberger *et al.*, 1985). The sequence of the resulting molecule is predominantly human and, as a result, the molecule is less immunogenic in patients (Khazaeli *et al.*, 1994). As an additional benefit the acquisition of a human Fc region improves the ability of the molecule to recruit human effector mechanisms. Clearly it is possible to choose any Fc region when designing such constructs, allowing one to modify the function of the resulting molecule.

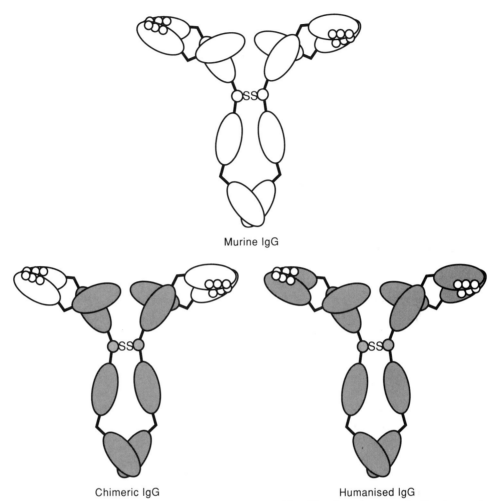

Figure 6 Modifications of IgG to reduce immunogenicity. The figure represents the two major approaches to reducing the immunogenicity of murine antibodies in humans. Murine-derived proteins are shown in white, human-derived proteins are shaded. In chimeric molecules the constant region domains of the murine antibody are replaced with human domains, whereas in humanised antibodies the entire molecule is human in origin, with the exception of the CDRs which retain their murine sequence.

In order to reduce the immunogenicity still further, Winter and colleagues developed the humanised antibody (Jones *et al.*, 1986; Reichmann *et al.*, 1988). In this construct the six CDRs of the murine antibody are attached to human variable regions, resulting in a molecule that is entirely human with the exception of the CDRs that confer antigenic specificity (Figure 6). The human variable regions are chosen on the grounds of sequence homology with the original murine antibody (Güssow and Seemann, 1991). In most cases the human framework hold the CDRs in the correct conformation, preserving the affinity of the antibody-Fv (sFv) for its antigen. In some cases it proves necessary to alter individual framework residues that interact with CDR residues and so contribute to the conformation of the antigen-binding site (Foote and Winter, 1992). A large number of humanised antibodies have been developed for clinical use, most notably CAMPATH 1H directed against CDw52 on lymphocytes (Hale *et al.*, 1988; Reichmann *et al.*, 1988; Isaacs *et al.*, 1992).

A final approach that has been used has been to 'veneer' or resurface the antibody. This elegant strategy involves identifying those variable region framework residues that lie on the surface of the molecule, and differ between mouse and human (Padlan, 1991). These residues can then be altered to change them into the human sequence. The result is variable domains that are human on the outside and rodent on the inside. Such molecules have now been produced and have been shown to retain the specificity of the parental cell (Pedersen *et al.*, 1994; Roguska *et al.*, 1994). These molecules should be similar to humanised antibodies in terms of their ability to be recognised by antibody during a human immune response against the antigen. However, it is possible that xenotypic 'internal' residues will act as T cell epitopes in the immune response, providing help for an anti-idiotypic humoral response. Further experimentation will be necessary to determine whether this theoretical problem is real, and whether this method has any advantages over humanisation in terms either of making the necessary constructs or the properties of the product.

At the other end of the scale (at least in terms of size) are constructs based on the Fv fragment of the antibody. These molecules exploit the small size of the Fv, which has a number of advantages for *in vivo* clinical use, including rapid clearance from the circulation and good penetration of solid tissue (reviewed in Huston *et al.*, 1993 and 1996). However, the Fv fragment has also become a convenient building block in making further recombinant molecules that have no need of the constant domains of immunoglobulin. In addition these molecules can frequently be produced in bacteria, potentially reducing their cost.

The Fv fragment can be readily produced using standard recombinant techniques by cloning and expressing the genes encoding the V_H and V_L domains (Skerra and Plückthun, 1988). However, the V_H and V_L domains are not covalently equilibrium attached and so, in solution, they tend to dissociate (the affinity (measured as the dissociation constant, K_D) of the two domains for each other is typically $\sim 10^{-10}$ mol l^{-1}, although this can vary depending on the se-

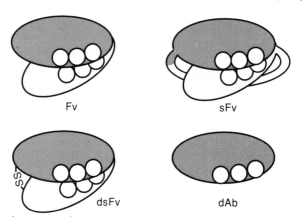

Figure 7 Engineered constructs based on the Fv fragment. The Fv fragment of an antibody is the smallest fragment that retains an intact antigen-binding site. However, it is unstable, because the V_H and V_L domains are free to dissociate in solution. Two strategies have been designed to overcome this. The first is to link the two domains with a peptide to generate a single-chain Fv (sFv). The second is to introduce cysteines at appropriate locations on the interface between the V_H and V_L domains, so that they form a disulphide bridge that holds the protein together (a disulphide-stabilised Fv (dsFv)). (The location of the bond shown in the figure is illustrative, and not meant to show the actual location). In addition it is possible to show antigen-binding properties with single domains derived from some Fv (dAb). Such molecules, however, tend to be sticky and aggregate, and so strategies are being developed in which residues that encourage aggregation are mutated.

quences of the CDR regions (Searle *et al.*, 1995)). There are two strategies to stabilise the molecule. The most common is to make single-chain Fv fragments (sFv, also frequently termed scFv), in which a peptide linker is used to bridge the amino terminus of one domain with the carboxy terminus of the second (Figure 7) (Bird *et al.*, 1988; Huston *et al.*, 1988). This linker prevents dissociation, and allows the construct to be encoded in a single gene, simplifying subsequent genetic modification. A large number of linkers have been produced, the most common of which is the 15 amino acid sequence ((Gly)4Ser)3, in which the glycines confer flexibility and the serines solubility (Huston *et al.*, 1988). However, although this peptide has a general use, the sequence of the linker can affect the properties of the molecule, including its expression, proteolytic stability and aggregation properties (Pantoliano *et al.*, 1991; Whitlow *et al.*, 1993; Desplancq *et al.*, 1994; Turner *et al.*, 1996).

The alternative approach to stabilising the interaction has been to introduce cysteine residues into the two variable domains, such that in the fully folded Fv molecule the two residues will be adjacent, and so able to form a disulphide bond (Glockshuber *et al.*, 1990; Brinkmann *et al.*, 1993). The presence of the disulphide bond prevents the dissociation of the domains, and the resulting disulphide-stabilised Fv (dsFv) may have advantages over some sFv in terms of aggregation, affinity and stability of the molecule (Glockshuber *et al.*, 1990; Reiter *et al.*, 1994a, b, c; Webber *et al.*, 1995). However, in some antibodies there is a need for the V_H and V_L domains to move relative to each other to accommodate the antigen (Stanfield *et al.*, 1993), and in such cases it is possible that dsFv will not have sufficient flexibility to allow such movement, thus reducing the affinity of the interaction.

Although Fv is the smallest antibody fragment that contains an intact antigen-binding site, there have been attempts to produce antigen-binding molecules that are smaller. Thus single variable region domains (particularly of the heavy chain) can show antigen-binding activity (termed dAbs) (Ward *et al.*, 1989) in a similar manner to antigen-binding activity that has long been recognised to occur with isolated heavy or light chains (Haber and Richards, 1966; Yoo *et al.*, 1967; Painter *et al.*, 1972). However, these molecules have a strong tendency either to dimerise or to aggregate. One intriguing possibility to overcome this tendency to associate noncovalently has been suggested by the finding that camel immunoglobulins do not contain a light chain, and so have just one variable region domain (Hamers-Casterman *et al.*, 1993). This opens the possibility of either using camel V_H domains on their own, or 'camelising' V_H domains of other species by altering the hydrophobic residues on the V_H–V_L interface into the residues seen in the camel molecule (Davies and Reichmann, 1994).

In addition, peptides derived fromu CDR regions of the molecule have shown antigen-binding properties (Williams *et al.*, 1989; Saragovi *et al.*, 1991). In most cases this binding has been of low affinity, and it is not clear how useful these will be for immunoassay reagents. However, covalent coupling of the peptides into multimeric structures can improve their affinity, and these molecules may have advantages over antibody-like molecules in terms of production costs and stability.

Techniques developed for antibody engineering have also been used with other members of the immunoglobulin gene superfamily. Thus, recombinant T cell receptors have been made, both as intact soluble molecules, fusion proteins and as single-chain and disulphide-stabilised Fv fragments (Gascoigne *et al.*, 1987; Lin *et al.*, 1990; Kurucz *et al.*, 1993; Corr *et al.*, 1994; Hilyard *et al.*, 1994; Reiter *et al.*, 1995).

Artificial antibody-like structures have also been developed, consisting of a 61- residue β-sheet structure (designed using V_H as a template). These molecules, termed minibodies, carry two CDRs which can bind antigen (Pessi *et al.*, 1993; Martin *et al.*, 1994). In addition, alternative, nonimmunglobulin-derived protein frameworks are being developed, for example the

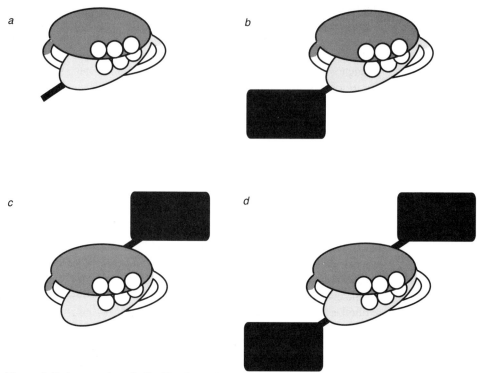

Figure 8 Fusion proteins of sFv. The figure illustrates several of the potential configurations between an sFv and a second effector molecule (shown in black). Thus fusions can be made with short peptides (*a*), or with molecules fused to the C terminus (*b*) or N terminus (*c*) of the molecule. In addition it is possible to fuse proteins to both termini of the sFv (*d*). In general the binding properties of the sFv are not affected by the fusion, although in individual molecules the effector domain may interfere with some of the CDRs. The properties of the effector molecule may be influenced by the configuration of the fusion. In some cases the introduction of a linker peptide between the two molecules, to space them, may improve their function.

four-helix bundle protein cytochrome B 562 has had two loops randomised to create CDRs, which have been selected for antigen-binding (Ku and Schultz, 1995). This opens up the possibility of generating totally artificial antigen binding molecules. It is not clear what role such molecules will have in immunoassays; however, it is possible that they will find specialised applications.

Modification of Immunoglobulin Function

The modification of the function of antibody-based molecules can be done in one of two ways. The first is to introduce into the antibody molecule small mutations. Thus, for example, mutations have been introduced that directly alter the ability of the Fc region of IgG to bind to C1q (Duncan and Winter, 1988) and Fc receptors (Duncan *et al.*, 1988). In most cases, however, this approach can only be used to modify a function of the molecule that is already existing. Perhaps the most exciting application of molecular biology is to endow the antibody molecule with totally novel functions. This can best be done by fusing the molecule with a peptide or protein that confers the desired function on the antibody (Figure 8). Such fusions are relatively trivial to create, and can be used to generate totally novel molecules. They can be carried out with any of the antibody species described above, although there is a certain elegance in using sFv-based molecules that contain the minimal antigen-binding site and are encoded for by a single gene, as fusions with these molecules will produce a single polypeptide chain that contains both antigen-binding and the function of the second molecule. In general such fusions can be N-terminal or C-terminal without affecting the binding of the sFv (though the function of the second molecule may require that the fusion be in a particular orientation) (Tai *et al.*, 1990; Batra *et al.*, 1991). Indeed fusions, have been made with molecules at both termini of the sFv (Figure 8) (Nicholls *et al.*, 1993a). In some cases the use of a peptide between the two proteins can help space them, preventing them from blocking each other's function.

Peptide Fusions

Fusions of antibody fragments with peptides have a number of uses. Thus they can be used as reagents in enzyme-linked immunosorbent assay (ELISA) or cell-staining methodologies, employing second stage anti-peptide reagents to detect the recombinant molecule (see for example Ward *et al.*, 1989; George *et al.*, 1994a, 1995b; Spooner *et al.*, 1994). This is of particular importance when using molecules such as sFv which lack the constant domains of the molecule recognised by most conventional anti-immunoglobulin reagents. The anti-peptide antibodies can also be used to capture the recombinant molecules, for example on the surface of a biosensor.

Similarly peptide fusions have been used to develop very convenient agglutination immunoassays for anti-viral antibodies, based on the use of an sFv-peptide fusion that has specificity for glycophorin A (expressed on human red blood cell membranes) and contains a 35 amino acid peptide derived from the gp41 surface glycoprotein of HIV (Lilley *et al.*, 1994). This fusion protein coats red blood cells and, in the presence of anti-HIV antibodies, causes their agglutination. This system could be readily adapted to detect antibodies directed against any peptide that can be fused to the sFv.

Fusion of peptides can also be used in the purification of recombinant molecules. Anti-peptide antibodies are being increasingly superseded for these purposes by the use of metal chelate affinity chromatography, in which a short sequence of histidine residues (frequently six) is incorporated into the molecule (Skerra *et al.*, 1991). These residues bind immobilised Cu^{2+}, Zn^{2+}, or Ni^{2+}, allowing the purification of the molecules either by reduction of the pH or by competition with imidazole. This approach has gathered considerable popularity owing to the high purity that can be achieved and the ease of the process (Casey *et al.*, 1995).

In addition peptides can be used that have a more direct function. Thus a short peptide sequence has been fused with sFv that has been designed to chelate technetium–99m (^{99m}Tc) within a N_3S coordination site (George *et al.*, 1995a). The resulting molecule can be readily labelled with the γ-emitting radiometal in a single-step reaction, yielding a highly stable product that retains the immunoreactivity of the original sFv. Although this approach was developed in order to generate an imaging agent, it could also be used in radioimmunoassays. The ability to label rapidly and easily a molecule to a high activity with a readily available isotope, in a site-specific manner, is attractive (George *et al.*, 1995a; Huston *et al.*, 1996). In addition the high activity of ^{99m}Tc should increase the sensitivity of such assays, while its short half-life will eliminate radioactive waste disposal costs.

Peptides can also be made that incorporate residues or sequences that allow conjugation or dimerisation with other molecules. Thus cysteinyl-containing peptides allow convenient, site-specific, conjugation with a range of molecules, such as biotin (Kipriyanov *et al.*, 1994).

77

Incorporation of appropriate peptide signal sequences can also allow the natural bio-synthetic machinery of the expression system to modify the molecule. Thus sequences that are naturally tagged with lipid can be used (Keinänen and Laukkanen, 1994; Laukkanen et al., 1995), for example, to incorporate the molecule into liposomes. Such liposomes are being developed for immunoassay purposes by labelling them with a variety of molecules, such as europium, that can be detected with high sensitivity (Laukkanen et al., 1995).

Fusions with Proteins

Fusion of antibody molecules with whole effector molecules was pioneered by Neuberger and colleagues who linked the V_H region of an antibody (and part of the constant region) with both staphylococcal nuclease and the C-terminal portion of the c–myc oncogene (Neuberger et al., 1984). Following coexpression with the appropriate light chain they were able to de-monstrate antigen-binding activity from the antibody component, together with the appropri-ate enzymatic or immunoreactive properties of the fusion partner. The generation of such fu-sion proteins has several advantages over the chemical conjugation of the two proteins; these include a homogeneous, molecularly defined product, the lack of a chemical linker that may affect function (or immunogenicity) of the molecules, and prevention of the loss of function frequently associated with chemical approaches. Furthermore the recombinant nature of the product allows access to the various expression systems, as described below, allowing produc-tion of large amounts of protein.

Since the production of the first antibody fusion proteins, a massive number of such mole-cules have been developed, including fusions with toxins (Chaudhary et al., 1989), protein A fragments (Tai et al., 1990; Gandecha et al., 1992), transmembrane regions (Eshhar et al., 1993), metal-binding proteins (Das et al., 1992; Sawyer et al., 1992), cytokines (Savage et al., 1993; Boleti et al., 1995), cell surface molecules such as CD4 (Traunecker et al., 1991), and enzymes. Enzyme fusions have included enzymes of potential therapeutic benefit (e.g. fibroly-tic agents (Holvoet et al., 1991; Yang et al., 1994) or prodrug activators (Bosslet et al., 1992; Goshorn et al., 1993; Rodrigues et al., 1995) and enzymes capable of driving colorimetric assays (Kohl et al., 1991; Wels et al., 1992; Ducancel et al., 1993; Gandecha et al., 1994; Weiss and Orfanoudakis, 1994; Burioni et al., 1995). Clearly the development of this latter type of antibody-enzyme fusion has potential for the use of immunoassays, for example in ELISA-type assays, but these molecules are not yet in widespread use. This is because, at pre-sent, the investment of time and effort in generating the fusion is not warranted by the advantages of the recombinant product. It is likely that, as antibody engineering techniques become simplified, this situation will change and that the cost-benefit analysis will favour the production of such molecules.

Enzyme-antibody fusions have the most direct application for immunoassays. However, in-direct interactions can also be used. Antibody fragments have been fused with molecules such as calmodulin (Neri et al., 1995a), streptavidin (Dübel et al., 1995) or protein A (Tai et al., 1990; Gandecha et al., 1992, 1994), which interact with other molecules (calmodulin-binding peptides, biotin or immunoglobulins) and so can be readily adapted for immunoassay purposes.

Bispecific or Bivalent Antibodies

Genetic engineering techniques can also be applied to generate bispecific antibodies, which have a dual specificity. These molecules have been predominantly developed for therapeutic

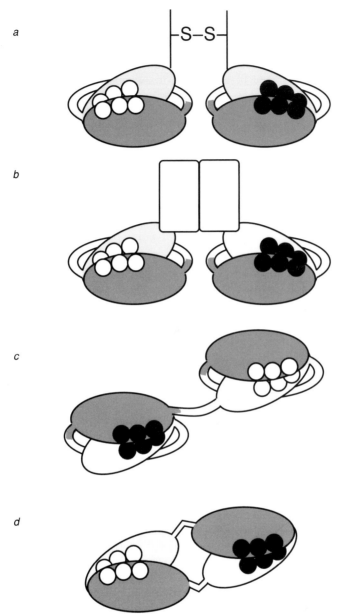

Figure 9 Bispecific sFv. There are a number of bispecific molecules that can be generated from sFv. The different specificities of the antigen-binding sites is indicated by different shadings of the CDRs. The molecules can be made by crosslinking of sFv fused to peptides that include cysteine residues (*a*). In this figure the crosslink has been shown as a disulphide bond, although it is possible to introduce other chemical conjugates between the molecules. The dimerisation of the sFv can be encouraged by use of dimerisation domains, such as leucine zippers (*b*) that encourage homo- or hetero-dimerisation. In addition the two sFvs can be made on a single polypeptide chain (*c*), making a single chain bispecific antibody. Finally diabodies (*d*) can be generated which use two peptide chains, each containing two variable regions. These domains can associate to form a molecule that contains two antigen-binding sites. This figure illustrates the production of bispecific antibodies. It is also possible to use similar approaches to generate monospecific, but bivalent, species. Many of these species could or have been made using other recombinant antibody fragments, such as dsFv and Fab molecules.

purposes, for example to target cytotoxic agents to tumour cells (George, 1995). However, they have also been used to capture enzymes and fluorochromes in immunocytochemistry and ELISAs (Milstein and Cuello, 1983; Karawajew *et al.*, 1988; Wognum *et al.*, 1989; Kontseko-va *et al.*, 1992). There are a number of methods for generating such molecules using recombi-nant techniques, as illustrated in Figure 9 for sFv (but also applicable to other immunoglobu-lin fragments). It should be noted that, in addition to generating bispecific antibodies, the same approaches can be used to generate bivalent antibodies from monovalent Fab or sFv molecules, with the consequent increase in functional affinity inherent in the avidity gain of binding. Perhaps the simplest is to use a cysteinyl-containing peptide to crosslink the two mo-lecules (Cumber *et al.*, 1992; Adams *et al.*, 1993). Dimerisation can be encouraged by fusion of the molecules to amphiphilic helices that naturally dimerise (Pack and Plückthun, 1992). Use of similar domains that preferentially heterodimerise (such as the leucine zippers encoded by *jun* and *fos*) will encourage the formation of bispecific heterodimers (Kostelny *et al.*, 1992). In addition the bispecific sFv can be encoded on a single polypeptide chain, with an additional linker between the two sFv components (Gruber *et al.*, 1994; Hayden *et al.*, 1994; Mallender and Voss, 1994; Kurucz *et al.*, 1995). A most interesting development of this has been the generation of CRAbs (Chelating Recombinant Antibodies), in which the two sFvs have specificity for different epitopes on the same molecule (Neri *et al.*, 1995b). These mole-cules show a very high affinity and, consequently, specificity for their antigen and may be of great use in the generation of novel agents for immunoassays. An alternative is to generate 'diabodies' which consist of two polypeptide chains, each with one V_H and one V_L region (Hollinger *et al.*, 1993; Whitlow *et al.*, 1994). The two chains dimerise such that the V_H of one chain associates with the V_L of the other, and *vice versa*. The formation of diabodies is dependent on the length of the linker; the use of short linkers encourages the formation of the diabody as it prevents the two domains on a single polypeptide chain from associating.

Other Constructs

All the constructs mentioned above have utilised the antigen-binding site of the antibody. However, there is one class of molecule being increasingly used that consists of a fusion between a protein and the Fc region of immunoglobulin (Capon *et al.*, 1989) (Figure 10). Such immunoglobulin fusion proteins are almost a routine research tool, taking advantage of the Fc region to aid purification and detection of the fusion protein. Among such molecules that have been made are cytokine receptors. The high affinity of the receptors for cytokines makes them natural reagents to quantify cytokine levels, and the Fc region can be used to de-tect the fusion protein using protein A or anti-immunoglobulin antibodies.

The discussion above may seem to present a bewildering set of constructs that can be or have been, generated. The essential point is that the use of antibody fragments (in particular the sFv) allows novel molecules to be built up in a modular way, using the antibody fragment as one of the building blocks. Thus, if one has the need to make a particular fusion for a particular assay system it should be possible to design and make it.

PRODUCTION OF RECOMBINANT ANTIBODIES

It is clearly necessary to consider how best to produce the recombinant antibody molecule, once the genetic engineering on the molecule has been performed. The choice of which

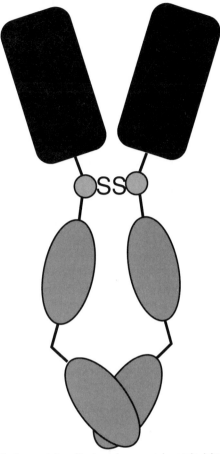

Figure 10 Immunoglobulin fusion proteins. Fusion of a second protein (shown in black) to the Fc region of immunoglobulin yields an immunoglobulin fusion protein. The Fc portion aids purification and detection of the molecule, and can also improve the pharmacokinetic properties of the molecule for *in vivo* use.

expression system will be dictated by such factors as the necessity for post-translational modification, the difficulty in folding the molecule, the yield and purity of the expression system and the costs involved. Other factors that may prove to be important are regulatory concerns and the availability of local expertise in appropriate expression systems. However, the ability to produce high yields at relatively low cost can be one of the advantages of recombinant antibody technology. In addition the use of defined expression systems, with cloned DNA constructs, should increase the confidence of regulatory agencies in the safety and precise nature of the product.

The major problem in expression is not to make large amounts of the protein, but to achieve correct folding of the molecule. This involves forming the proper disulphide bonds, and the correct secondary and tertiary structure of the molecule. In addition post-translational modification (for example glycosylation) may be necessary. There is an enormous number of different expression systems available, and this review is not the place to cover them in detail (see Ge *et al.*, 1995; Huston *et al.*, 1995; Morrison *et al.*, 1995). However, I will give an overview of the major systems, highlighting the advantages and disadvantages of each.

Prokaryotic expression (expression in bacteria, normally *E. coli*) is perhaps the most popular approach. The advantages are obvious: the bacteria grow very rapidly, the medium is very inexpensive, a large proportion of the total protein can be the recombinant product, the process is rapidly scaled up and, in laboratories that are used to DNA manipulation, all the necessary expertise and equipment for growing bacteria are readily available. However, there are disadvantages. Bacteria are unable to glycosylate proteins, so if carbohydrates are essential for function (e.g. IgG) then an alternative expression system is needed. In addition the recombinant proteins are normally made in the cytoplasm in inclusion bodies. The cytoplasm is a reducing environment, and so the resulting molecules are unfolded and need to be refolded before use. The ease of refolding recombinant proteins varies depending on the complexity of the molecule, and may need to be optimised for individual antibodies. For a review of the different refolding techniques available see Huston *et al.*, 1995.

An alternative is to use the secretory apparatus of the bacteria to encourage refolding. In Gram-negative bacteria (including *E. coli*) the periplasm is the space that lies between the inner and outer membrane of the cell. It is an oxidising environment, and also contains a number of chaperonin-type molecules that help in the refolding of proteins (Wülfing and Plückthun, 1994). Attachment of an appropriate leader sequence to the molecule directs the nascent polypeptide chain into the periplasm (Better *et al.*, 1988; Skerra and Plückthun, 1988). This has proved a highly successful method for producing recombinant antibodies, with the protein being collected either directly from the periplasm (Ge *et al.*, 1995) or, in cases where the outer membrane becomes leaky, from the culture supernatant (Ward *et al.*, 1989). However, the success of this approach is highly dependent on the antibody molecule, with some being obtained at high yield and others at vanishingly low yield. In many cases it is possible to increase the amount of antibody obtained by relatively simple refolding techniques which help solubilise material that has precipitated in the periplasm (George *et al.*, 1994b; Huston *et al.*, 1995). In addition relatively minor alterations in the sequence of the molecule can dramatically improve the yield (Deng *et al.*, 1994; Ayala *et al.*, 1995; Knappik and Plückthun, 1995).

Bacterial expression systems may appear to have drawbacks and require time and expertise to obtain the best results. However, if successful they are easy to use and also capable of producing very high yields of recombinant antibody. Thus, in one study (following optimisation of the culture and induction systems) several grams per litre of a F(ab')$_2$ molecule could be produced (Carter *et al.*, 1992).

If prokaryotic expression is not suitable or successful then the use of eukaryotic systems is called for. These can be divided into yeast, insect and mammalian expression systems. Yeast is a convenient 'half-way house', combining many of the advantages of bacteria (inexpensive and rapid to grow) with a protein secretory system that is capable of glycosylation and contains more chaperonin-type molecules. Several antibody fragments have been successfully produced in yeast (Horwitz *et al.*, 1988). However, the yeast cell is still very different from a mammalian cell, and the glycosylation patterns are different. Insect systems, especially baculovirus expression systems in which the gene is carried by the viral particle to infect the insect cell lines transiently, are very popular for producing large amounts of recombinant proteins. They have been used for antibody fragments (Hasesmann and Capra, 1990; Bei *et al.*, 1995), and may be useful in some circumstances, as they are capable of more sophisticated glycosylation of the protein, and have very efficient protein export pathways.

However, these eukaryotic cells lack the specialised protein-processing pathways available in mammalian cells (in particular B cells) for refolding antibodies. It is possible to use either transient transfection (for example into COS cells) to produce the antibody, or permanent transfection (for example in myeloma cells) (Dorai *et al.*, 1994; Jost *et al.*, 1994; Morrison *et al.*, 1995). The advantage of transient transfection is that it allows rapid evaluation of the activity of the molecule. However, yields are low. The generation of permanent cell lines is more labour-intensive, requiring selection systems. However, the yields can be very high, especially following amplification.

It should be noted that the use of mammalian cell expression systems does not guarantee success, especially with 'artificial' antibodies that have unnatural effector regions or fragments. In such cases modification of the antibody may increase the yield. Thus, in one example an sFv was not produced in an active form in a mammalian expression system until a glycosylation site was introduced into the protein (Jost *et al.*, 1994).

In addition to the expression systems described above, there are a number of specialised systems that may be useful in some circumstances. Thus, antibody fragments can be expressed in plants (Hiatt *et al.*, 1989; Whitelam *et al.*, 1994), a potentially useful commercial source, and also totally *in vitro*, using rabbit reticulocyte lysates (Nicholls *et al.*, 1993a).

In summary, the use of expression systems can produce high yields of active protein. However, the amount of work and effort involved in getting good yields should not be underestimated. Some antibodies will work very well, and will refold or be secreted with no problems, but many antibodies are difficult, and need a lot of attention.

Cloning and Isolation of Antibody Variable Region Genes

In order to engineer antibodies genetically it is necessary to isolate the genes encoding the variable regions of the molecule. This can be done either by isolating the genes from a pre-existing hybridoma, or by using phage display technology to obtain novel antibody specificities from a library. The cloning of V regions has been greatly simplified by the use of approaches based on the polymerase chain reaction (PCR) to amplify the variable region genes from complementary DNA of rodent, human and other species (Orlandi *et al.*, 1989). This uses oligonucleotide primers at the 5′ and 3′ end of the gene fragments to amplify the gene and, as a consequence, is extremely rapid and easy. There are a number of strategies that can be adopted in the design of primers. Thus, degenerate oligonucleotides have been designed that are complementary to conserved sequences at the 5′ and 3′ ends of the variable region genes, and panels of primers have been made that are specific for individual J segments and V region gene families. In addition it is possible to use primers specific for the constant regions and leader sequences of the genes (Orlandi *et al.*, 1989; Sastry *et al.*, 1989; Larrick and Fry, 1991; Marks *et al.*, 1991b; Dübel *et al.*, 1992; Nicholls *et al.*, 1993b; Ward *et al.*, 1993).

Phage Display Technology

Possibly the most exciting prospect for immunoassays in the field of antibody engineering is the production of novel antibody specificities using phage display technology (reviewed in Winter *et al.*, 1994). This allows not only an alternative to polyclonal and hybridoma technology, but also the ability to isolate novel specificities not available using these conventional approaches.

For a full understanding of phage display technology it is necessary to understand something about the structure and life cycle of the filamentous bacteriophages used in this work. This family of phage (which includes the well known M13 phage) have a single-stranded DNA genome enclosed by many copies (~2,700) of the major coat protein (pVIII), which forms a long tube approximately 1 μm in length and 6–7 nm in diameter. At either end of the molecule are the minor coat proteins pVII, pIX, pVI and pIII (approximately 5 copies each) (Model and Russel, 1988).

Filamentous phage infect male (F⁺) bacteria that are capable of erecting a sex pillus (normally used to pass genetic material between plasmids). The pIII protein binds to the tip of the pillus, which then collapses, during which the phage particle enters the cell (Model and Russel, 1988). Once infected by a phage, the bacteria are unable to produce sex pilli, preventing infection of bacteria by more than one phage (Model and Russel, 1988).

Inside the cell the single-stranded DNA is converted to double-stranded DNA, and the viral genes are then copied to make the coat proteins and other molecules needed for DNA replication. Single-stranded copies of the DNA are made, and extruded through the inner and outer membranes, picking up the coat proteins in the periplasm to make free phage particles. These are made on a continuous basis (several hundred phage particles per cell per generation) without lysing the cell, which can continue to divide, albeit at a reduced rate (Sambrook *et al.*, 1989).

Phage display was originally developed by George Smith (from the University of Missouri), who showed that it was possible to make fusions between a peptide and the pIII minor coat protein (Smith, 1985). The resulting phage display the peptide on their surface, and phage bearing the appropriate peptide can be isolated from a library of random sequences by panning with an antibody (Scott and Smith, 1990). This approach was extended by Winter's group, who showed that it was possible to fuse an antibody fragment (sFv) onto the pIII to generate phage displaying the antibody on their surface (McCafferty *et al.*, 1990) (Figure 11). The original experiments used an antibody directed against lysozyme, and showed that it was possible to purify the sFv-bearing phage from normal phage by affinity chromatography on a lysozyme column.

The next step was to make a library of antibody specificities, so that one could have many phage expressing a large range of antibodies. The original library was obtained by using PCR to amplify V_H and V_L encoding regions from the cDNA derived from spleens of mice immunised with phenyloxazolone. The phenyloxazolone antigen was then used to affinity-isolate phage-bearing antibodies of the appropriate specificity (Clackson *et al.*, 1991) (Figure 11).

These early experiments proved the principle that phage display could be used to isolate novel antibodies. Since then there have been considerable developments in the technology. These have included the source of the variable region genes used to make the library, different constructs that can be used in the library and strategies to increase the affinity of the resulting antibodies for the antigen. The selection of the antibodies can be done either on a column (McCafferty *et al.*, 1990), by panning to antigen immobilised onto plastic surfaces (Barbas *et al.*, 1991; Marks *et al.*, 1991a), antigen expressed on cell surfaces (Marks *et al.*, 1993; de-Kruif *et al.*, 1995) or in fluid phase, using biotinylated antigen (Hawkins *et al.*, 1992).

Hybridoma technology is largely restricted to making antibodies of rodent origin, and it is notoriously difficult to make human hybridomas (Sa'adu and Zumla, 1995). One of the advantages of the phage display approach is that a wide variety of sources can be used for the V region genes. These include B cells from immunised mice or humans (for example as a result of infection, prophylactic immunisation or autoimmune disease (Barbas *et al.*, 1991; Burton *et al.*, 1991; Zebedee *et al.*, 1992; Hexham *et al.*, 1994)) and also 'naive' libraries which are derived from humans that have not been deliberately immunised against any particular antigen (Marks *et al.*, 1991a; Gram *et al.*, 1992). In theory it is possible to generate a library from B cells from any species whose V regions can be isolated, and libraries have been made using chicken V regions (Davies *et al.*, 1995). In addition synthetic libraries are

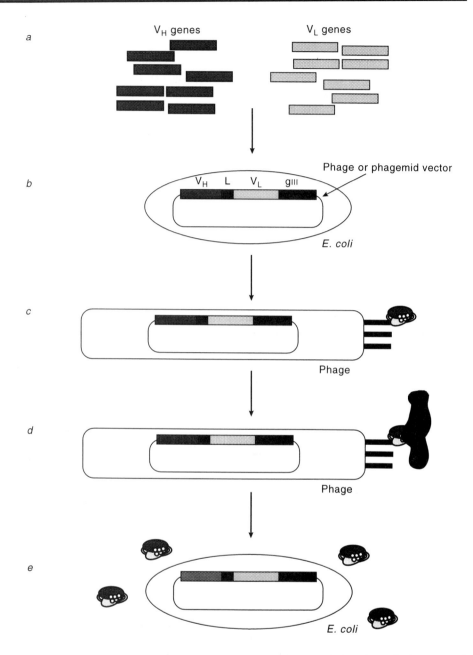

Figure 11 Isolation of novel antibodies using phage display technology. In the phage display approach the gene segments encoding the V_H and V_L domains are first isolated (*a*) using either PCR of cDNA, previously cloned V region segments or artificial sequences. These are cloned as a library in a phage or phagemid vector (*b*). This diagram illustrates an sFv consisting of a V_H domain followed by the linker peptide (L), the V_L domain and gene III (encoding pIII, in black). The library is then expressed as phage particles, with the sFv fused to the pIII minor coat protein (*c*). The number of sFv expressed on each phage will be dependent on whether a phage or phagemid vector is used, the nature of the helper phage and the efficiency with which the sFv is expressed. Only a single sFv is illustrated. Affinity techniques can then be used to isolate those phage that express the appropriate antibody specificity (*d*), thus isolating the genes encoding the sFv. Transfer of the gene constructs into bacteria allows expression of the isolated sFv (*e*).

being generated that consist of germ line variable region genes, together with artificial sequences corresponding to the CDR regions of the antibodies (Barbas *et al.*, 1992; Hoogenboom and Winter, 1992; Griffiths *et al.*, 1994; Nissim *et al.*, 1994). Attention has concentrated on the CDR3 regions, in particular of the heavy chain, as this is where the most diversity is in natural antibodies. The random sequences have been made of different lengths, mimicking the heterogeneity seen in the size of natural CDR3 regions.

A number of different constructs have been used in antibody phage display libraries. In addition to sFv, dsFv (Brinkmann *et al.*, 1995) Fab (Barbas *et al.*, 1991; Garrad *et al.*, 1991; Hoogenboom *et al.*, 1991; Kang *et al.*, 1991a) and artificial antigen-binding domain structures (Martin *et al.*, 1994; Ku and Schultz, 1995) constructs have been used, fused to both the pIII and also to the major coat protein, pVIII (Kang *et al.*, 1991a). The pVIII protein is expressed at many copies on the cell surface, and so fusion to this protein should provide an increased valency that may be useful in isolating low-affinity antibodies. However, in practice, this has not been widely adopted..

There has also been a move away from phage vectors, which can be difficult to manipulate, to phagemid vectors, which consist of plasmids containing the phage origin of replication (Hoogenboom *et al.*, 1991). Phagemids can be manipulated and propagated in a similar manner to plasmids, simplifying the generation of the library and the manipulation of the resulting antibodies. However, if the bacteria containing a phagemid are infected with helper phage that provide the necessary proteins for the replication and assembly of phage particles, then single-stranded DNA copies of the phagemids are made. The DNA is then packaged and assembled into phage particles which can be affinity-selected on antigen.

It is possible to use phage display libraries derived from immunised animals to derive high-affinity antibodies. However, the manufacture of a new library for each antigen is laborious and time consuming. This has led to the increased use of 'naive' or synthetic libraries, where one library can be used against a range of antigens. The major disadvantage of this approach is that the resulting antibodies are of low affinity. There have been several strategies to overcome this. One is to take the antibodies and mutate them, and then use affinity techniques to select variants with higher affinity. Several mutating strategies can be used, including error-prone PCR (Gram *et al.*, 1992; Hawkins *et al.*, 1992), 'spiked' PCR (Hermes *et al.*, 1989), passage through a mutating strain of bacteria (Schaaper, 1988), random mutagenesis of CDRs (Barbas *et al.*, 1994), and 'chain shuffling' in which one of the chains of the antibody is randomly changed, in order to find an improved combination with higher affinity (Clackson *et al.*, 1991; Kang *et al.*, 1991b; Marks *et al.*, 1992). These techniques are on the whole very successful, and can be used to increase the affinity of the antibody to the same order of magnitude as a good hybridoma antibody.

Mutagenesis, allied to selection techniques, can also be used to change the specificity of an antibody. Thus, chain shuffling has been used to convert an anti-lysozyme antibody to one with specificity for a T cell receptor (Ward, 1995). Additionally mutagenesis of CDR3 of the heavy chain has been used to change the specificity of an antibody from tetanus toxoid to fluorescein (Barbas *et al.*, 1992). The ability to alter the specificity of an antibody in this way may prove very important in immunoassay development, allowing the prevention or introduction of crossreactivity, for example to different isoenzymes.

An alternative strategy is to use the technology to isolate a high-affinity antibody directly, without the need for subsequent mutation. The major approach to this is to use enormous libraries, such that there is a very high probability of finding a high-affinity antibody of the desired specificity. These libraries are too large to make by conventional techniques, and so recombination strategies have been developed in which two libraries, one containing V_H and the other V_L regions, are combined using a *cre* recombinase system (Griffiths *et al.*, 1994). Libraries containing 6.5×10^{10} different antibodies have been reported. It is interesting to consider that the total number of B cells in a mouse at any one time is $<10^9$ (Picker and Siegelman, 1993), so the phage display library can offer a greater repertoire of antibodies to choose from than that found in a mouse. Using these libraries it has been possible to isolate high-affinity antibodies without the need to go through subsequent mutation and further selection (Griffiths *et al.*, 1994).

What are the advantages of phage display libraries? The four major advantages are:

1   it is possible to use antibodies derived from any species, not just rodents;

2   it is possible to isolate very rare antibodies;

3   it is possible to develop novel isolation techniques to obtain new specificities;

4   the antibodies have not undergone negative selection in an animal.

The use of species other than rodents has already been discussed. The ability to isolate rare antibodies is inherent in the affinity-selection method used. With a conventional-sized library (say 10^8 specificities) it is possible to contain the entire library in a few microlitres of buffer. Thus selection of antibodies from that library, by panning and passing down a column or fluid phase, allows one to select the desired antibody from 10^8 different clones. In hybridoma technology, by contrast, one has to screen individual wells following the fusion to determine if they make the desired specificity. In practice this restricts one to screening $<10^3$ different hybridomas. Therefore, if the specificity that one requires is rare, the chances of isolating it from a phage library are considerably higher than that from a conventional hybridoma system.

It is also possible to design selection techniques that allow isolation of particular specificities. For example, a library was made from the bone marrow of a patient infected with HIV-1 (Burton *et al.*, 1991). The resulting phage were panned on recombinant gp120 derived from the IIIB strain of HIV, which the patient had not been infected with. The result was the isolation of a crossreactive antibody that could block the binding of CD4 to the gp120 of several HIV strains (Burton *et al.*, 1991). One can also use antibodies against particular epitopes on the antigen either to block the epitope prior to panning, thus directing the specificity of the antibodies isolated from the library away from that particular epitope (Ditzel *et al.*, 1995), or specifically to elute phage binding to that epitope (Meulemans *et al.*, 1994). It may also be possible to set up negative selection techniques to remove unwanted specificities. In addition fluorescence-activated cell sorting (FACS) has been used to isolate phage binding to cell populations, using conventional antibodies to sort the cells (de-Kruif *et al.*, 1995).

Another important feature is that the antibodies displayed on the phage have not been negatively selected in an animal. As a result it is possible to isolate antibodies that one would not be able to obtain using conventional hybridoma technology. This might include antibodies against conserved epitopes and autoantibodies (Griffiths *et al.*, 1993, 1994; Nissim *et al.*, 1994). In addition antibodies have been made against molecules such as mammalian BiP (heavy chain binding protein) which cannot conventionally be generated as they are held up in the endoplasmic reticulum of B cells (Nissim *et al.*, 1994).

CONCLUSION

Antibody engineering has had a minimal impact on the development of immunoassays since the first edition of this book (1991). However, it is important to have an understanding of antibody engineering for several reasons. It is likely that engineered antibodies will be increasingly used in immunoassays, as their convenience and low cost make them more competitive. But perhaps most important is the possibility of using phage display technology to make a new generation of antibodies, with improved specificities and affinities. Hybridoma technology helped to provide a quantum leap in the development of immunoassays, by providing the means to make reproducibly large amounts of an antibody. The use of recombinant techniques, in particular phage display, to make novel specificities may offer a similar advance in the production of immunoassay reagents, by opening up the possibility of making antibodies directed against epitopes that, previously, we have not had access to.

REFERENCES

Adams, G. P., McCartney, J. E., Tai, M. S., *et al.* (1993) Highly specific *in vivo* tumor targeting by monovalent and divalent forms of 741F8 anti-c-*erb*B-2 single-chain Fv. *Cancer Res.* **53**, 4026–4034.

Ayala, M., Balint, R. F., Fernández-de-Coss'o, M. E. *et al.* (1995) Variable region sequence modulated periplasmic export of a single-chain Fv antibody fragment in *Escherichia coli*. *Biotechniques* **18**, 832–842.

Barbas, C. F. III, Bain, J. D., Hoekstra, D. M. *et al.* (1992) Semisynthetic combinatorial antibody libraries: A chemical solution to the diversity problem. *Proc. Natl Acad. Sci. USA* **89**, 4457–4461.

Barbas, C. F. III, Hu, D. Dunlop, N., *et al* (1994) *In vitro* evolution of a neutralising human antibody to human immunodeficiency virus type 1 to enhance affinity and broaden strain cross-reactivity. *Proc. Natl Acad. Sci. USA* **91**, 3809–3813.

Barbas, C. F., III, Kang, A. S., Lerner, R. A. *et al.* (1991) Assembly of combinatorial antibody libraries on phage surfaces: The gene III site. *Proc. Natl Acad. Sci. USA* **88**, 7978–7982.

Barclay, A. N., Birkeland, M. L., Brown, M. H., *et al.* (1993) *The Leukocyte Antigen Facts Book* (Academic Press, London).

Batra, J. K., Fitzgerald, D. J., Chaudhary, V. K. *et al.* (1991) Single-chain immunotoxins directed at the human transferrin receptor containing *Pseudomonas* exotoxin A or diphtheria toxin: anti-TFR(Fv)–PE40 and DT388–anti-TFR(Fv). *Mol. Cell. Biol.* **11**, 2200–2205.

Bei, R., Schlom, J. & Kashmiri, S. V. (1995) Baculovirus expression of a functional single-chain immunoglobulin and its IL-2 fusion protein. *J. Immunol. Meth.* **186**, 245–255.

Better, M., Chang, C. P., Robinson, R. R. & Horwitz, A. H. (1988) *Escherichia coli* secretion of an active chimeric antibody fragment. *Science* **240**, 1041–1043.

Bird, R. E., Hardman, K. D., Jacobson, J. W., *et al.* (1988) Single-chain antigen-binding proteins. *Science* **242**, 423–426.

Boleti, E., Deonarain, M., Spooner, R. A. *et al.* (1995) Construction, expression and characterisation of a single-chain anti-tumour antibody-IL-2 fusion protein. *Ann. Oncol.* 6, 945–947.

Bosslet, K., Czech, J., Lorenz, P. *et al.* (1992) Molecular and functional characterisation of a fusion protein suited for tumour specific prodrug activation. *Brit. J. Cancer* 65, 234–238.

Boulianne, G. L., Hozumi, N. & Shulman, M. J. (1984) Production of functional chimaeric mouse/human antibody. *Nature* 312, 643–646.

Brinkmann, U., Chowdhury, P. S., Roscoe, D. M. *et al.* (1995) Phage display of disulfide-stabilised Fv fragments. *J. Immunol. Meth.* 182, 41–50.

Brinkmann, U., Reiter, Y., Jung, S. H. *et al.* (1993) A recombinant immunotoxin containing a disulfide-stabilised Fv fragment. *Proc. Natl Acad. Sci. USA* 90, 7538–7542.

Burioni, R., Plaisant, P., Riccio, M. L., *et al.* (1995) Engineering human monoclonal antibody fragments: A recombinant enzyme-linked Fab. *Microbiologica* 18, 127–133.

Burton, D. R., Barbas, C. F. III, Persson, M. A. *et al.* (1991) A large array of human monoclonal antibodies to type 1 human immunodeficiency virus from combinatorial libraries of asymptomatic seropositive individuals. *Proc. Natl Acad. Sci. USA* 88, 10134–10137.

Capon, D. J., Chamow, S. M., Mordenti, J. *et al.* (1989) Designing CD4 immunoadhesins for AIDS therapy. *Nature* 337, 525–531.

Carter, P., Kelly, R. F., Rodrigues, M. L. *et al.* (1992) High level *Escherichia coli* expression and production of a bivalent humanised antibody fragment. *Bio/technology* 10, 163–167.

Casey, J. L., Keep, P. A., Chester, K. A. *et al.* (1995) Purification of bacterially expressed single chain Fv antibodies for clinical applications using metal chelate chromatography. *J. Immunol. Meth.* 179, 105–116.

Chaudhary, V. K., Queen, C., Junghans, R. P. *et al.* (1989) A recombinant immunotoxin consisting of two antibody variable domains fused to Pseudomonas exotoxin. *Nature* 339, 394–397.

Chothia, C., Lesk, A. M. & Gherardi, E. (1992) Structural repertoire of the human V_H segments. *J. Mol. Biol.* 227, 799–817.

Chothia, C., Lesk, A. M., Tramontano, A. *et al.* (1989) Conformations of immunoglobulin hypervariable regions. *Nature* 342, 877–883.

Clackson, T., Hoogenboom, H. R., Griffiths, A. D. *et al.* (1991) Making antibody fragments using phage display libraries. *Nature* 352, 624–628.

Cook, G. P. & Tomlinson, I. M. (1995) The human immunoglobulin V_H repertoire. *Immunol. Today* 16, 237–242.

Corr, M., Slanetz, A. E., Boyd, L. F. *et al.* (1994) T-cell receptor-MHC class I peptide interactions: Affinity, kinetics, and specificity. *Science* 265, 946–949.

Courtenay-Luck, N. S., Epenetos, A. A. & Sivolapenko, G. B. *et al.* (1988) Development of anti-idiotypic antibodies against tumour antigens and autoantigens in ovarian cancer patients treated intraperitoneally with mouse monoclonal antibodies. *Lancet* ii, 894–897.

Courtenay-Luck, N. S., Epenetos, A. A., Winearls, C. G. *et al.* (1987) Preexisting human anti-murine immunoglobulin reactivity due to polyclonal rheumatoid factors. *Cancer Res.* 47, 4520–4525.

Cumber, A. J., Ward, E. S. & Winter, G. *et al.* (1992) Comparitive stabilities *in vitro* and *in vivo* of a recombinant mouse antibody FvCys fragment and a bisFvCys conjugate. *J. Immunol.* 149, 120–126.

Das, C., Kulkarni, P. V., Constantinescu, A. *et al.* (1992) Recombinant antibody-metallothionein: Design and evaluation for radioimmunoimaging. *Proc. Natl Acad. Sci. USA* **89**, 9749–9753.

Davies, E. L., Smith, J. S., Birkett, C. R. *et al.* (1995) Selection of specific phage-display antibodies using libraries derived from chicken immunoglobulin genes. *J. Immunol Meth.* **186**, 125–135.

Davies, J. & Riechmann, L. (1994) 'Camelising' human antibody fragments: NMR studies on V_H domains. *FEBS Lett.* **339**, 285–290.

de-Kruif, J., Terstappen, L., Boel, E. *et al.* (1995) Rapid selection of cell subpopulation-specific human monoclonal antibodies from a synthetic phage antibody library. *Proc. Natl Acad. Sci. USA* **92**, 3938–3942.

Deng, S. J., MacKenzie, C. R., Sadowska, J. *et al.* (1994) Selection of antibody single-chain variable fragments with improved carbohydrate binding by phage display. *J. Biol. Chem.* **269**, 9533–9538.

Desplancq, D., King, D. J., Lawson, A. D. *et al.* (1994) Multimerization behaviour of single chain Fv variants for the tumour-binding antibody B72.3. *Protein Engng* **7**, 1027–1033.

Ditzel, H. J., Binley, J. M., Moore, J. P. *et al.* (1995) Neutralising recombinant human antibodies to a conformational V2- and CD4-binding site-sensitive epitope of HIV-1 gp120 isolated by using an epitope-masking procedure. *J. Immunol.* **154**, 893–906.

Dorai, H., McCartney, J. E., Hudziak, R. M., *et al.* (1994) Mammalian cell expression of single-chain Fv (sFv) antibody proteins and their C-terminal fusions with Interleukin-2 and other effector domains. *Bio/technology* **12**, 890–897.

Dübel, S., Breitling, F., Kontermann, R. *et al.* (1995) Bifunctional and multimeric complexes of streptavidin fused to single chain antibodies (scFv). *J. Immunol. Meth.* **178**, 201–209.

Dübel, S., Breitling, F., Seehaus, T. *et al.* (1992) Generation of a human IgM expression library in *E. coli. Meth. Mol. Cell. Biol.* **3**, 47–52.

Ducancel, F., Gillet, D., Carrier, A. *et al.* (1993) Recombinant colorimetric antibodies: Construction and characterisation of a bifunctional F(ab')2/alkaline phosphatase conjugate produced in *Escherichia coli. Biotechnology N. Y.* **11**, 601–605.

Duncan, A. R. & Winter, G. (1988) The binding site for C1q on IgG. *Nature* **332**, 738–740.

Duncan, A. R., Woof, J. M., Partridge, L. J. *et al.* (1988) Localisation of the binding site for the human high-affinity Fc receptor on IgG. *Nature* **332**, 563–564.

Eshhar, Z., Waks, T., Gross, G. *et al.* (1993) Specific activation and targeting of cytotoxic lymphocytes through chimeric single chains consisting of antibody-binding domains and the γ or ζ subunits of the immunoglobulin and T-cell receptors. *Proc. Natl Acad. Sci. USA* **90**, 720–724.

Foote, J. & Winter, G. (1992) Antibody framework residues affecting the conformation of the hypervariable loops. *J. Mol. Biol.* **224**, 487–499.

Gandecha, A. R, Owen, M. R., Cockburn, B. *et al.* (1992) Production and secretion of a bifunctional staphylococcal protein A:antiphytochrome single-chain Fv fusion protein in *Escherichia coli. Gene* **122**, 361–365.

Gandecha, A., Owen, M. R., Cockburn, W. *et al.* (1994) Antigen detection using recombinant, bifunctional single-chain Fv fusion proteins synthesised in *Escherichia coli. Protein Expr. Purif* **5**, 385–390.

Garrad, L. S., Yang, M., O'Connell, M. P. *et al.* (1991) F_{AB} assembly and enrichment in a monovalent phage display system. *Bio/technology* **9**, 1373–1377.

Gascoigne, N. R., Goodnow, C. C., Dudzik, K. I. *et al.* (1987) Secretion of a chimeric T-cell receptor-immunoglobulin protein. *Proc. Natl Acad. Sci. USA* **84**, 2936–2940.

Ge, L., Knappik, A., Pack, P. *et al.* (1995) Expressing antibodies in *Escherichia coli*. In: *Antibody Engineering: A Practical Approach* 2nd edn., (ed Borrebaeck, A. K.) pp. 229–266 (Oxford University Press, Oxford).

George, A. J. T. (1995) Bispecific antibodies in tumour therapy. *Tumor Targeting* **1**, 185–187.

George, A. J. T. & Epenetos, A. A. (1996) Advances in antibody engineering. *Expert Opinion on Therapeutic Patents* **6**, 441–456

George, A. J. T., Huston, J. S. & Haber, E. (1996) Exploring and exploiting the antibody and Ig superfamily combining Sites. *Nature Biotechnology* **14**, 584.

George, A. J. T., Jamar, F., Tai, M.-S. *et al.* (1995a) Radiometal labeling of recombinant proteins by a genetically engineered minimal chelation site: Technetium–99m coordination by single-chain Fv antibody fusion proteins through a C-terminal cysteinyl peptide. *Proc. Natl Acad. Sci. USA* **92**, 8358–8363.

George, A. J. T., Spooner, R. A. & Epenetos, A. A. (1994a) Applications of monoclonal antibodies in clinical oncology. *Immunol. Today* **15**, 559–561.

George, A. J. T., Titus, J. A., Jost, C. R. *et al.* (1994b) Redirection of T-cell-mediated cytotoxicity by a recombinant single-chain Fv molecule. *J. Immunol.* **152**, 1802–1811.

George, A. J. T., Titus, J. A., Jost, C. R. *et al.* (1995b) Redirection of cellular cytotoxicity; A two step approach using recombinant single-chain Fv molecules. *Cell Biophys.* **26**, 153–165.

Glockshuber, R., Malia, M., Pfitzinger, I. *et al.* (1990) A comparison of strategies to stabilise immunoglobulin Fv-fragments. *Biochemistry* **29**, 1362–1367.

Goshorn, S. C., Svensson, H. P., Kerr, D. E. *et al.* (1993) Genetic construction, expression, and characterisation of a single chain anti-carcinoma antibody fused to β-lactamase. *Cancer Res.* **53**, 2123–2127.

Gram, H., Marconi, L. A., Barbas, C. F., III *et al.* (1992) *In vitro* selection and affinity maturation of antibodies from a naive combinatorial immunoglobulin library. *Proc. Natl Acad. Sci. USA* **89**, 3576–3580.

Griffiths, A. D., Malmqvist, M., Marks, J. D. *et al.* (1993) Human anti-self antibodies with high specificity from phage display libraries. *EMBO J.* **12**, 725–734.

Griffiths, A. D., Williams, S. C., Hartley, O. *et al.* (1994) Isolation of high affinity human antibodies directly from large synthetic libraries. *EMBO J.* **13**, 3245–3260.

Gruber, M., Schodin, B. A., Wilson, E. R. *et al.* (1994) Efficient tumor cell lysis mediated by a bispecific single chain antibody expressed in *Escherichia coli*. *J. Immunol.* **152**, 5368–5374.

Güssow, D. & Seemann, G. (1991) Humanisation of monoclonal antibodies. *Methods. Enzymol.* **203**, 99–121.

Haber, E. & Richards, F. F. (1966) The specificity of antigenic recognition of antibody heavy chain. *Proc. R. Soc. Lond. B* **166**, 176–187.

Hale, G., Dyer, M. J., Clark, M. R. *et al.* (1988) Remission induction in non-Hodgkin lymphoma with reshaped human monoclonal antibody CAMPATH–1H. *Lancet* ii, 1394–1399.

Hamers-Casterman, C., Atarhouch, T., Muyldermans, S. *et al.* (1993) Naturally occurring antibodies devoid of light chains. *Nature* **363**, 446–448.

Hasesmann, C. A. & Capra, J. D. (1990) High-level production of a functional immunoglobulin heterodimer in a baculovirus expression system. *Proc. Natl Acad. Sci. USA* **87**, 3942–3946.

Hawkins, R. E., Russell, S. J. & Winter, G. (1992) Selection of phage antibodies by binding affinity: Mimicking affinity maturation. *J. Mol. Biol.* **226**, 889–896.

Hayden, M. S., Linsley, P. S., Gayle, M. A., *et al.* (1994) Single-chain mono- and bispecific antibody derivatives with novel biological properties and antitumour activity from a COS cell transient expression system. *Ther. Immunol.* **1**, 3–15.

Hermes, J. D., Parekh, S. M., Blacklow, S. C. *et al.* (1989) A reliable method for random mutatagenesis: The generation of mutant libraries using spiked oligodeoxyribonucleotide primers. *Gene* **84**, 143–151.

Hexham, J. M., Partridge, L. J., Furmaniak, J. *et al.* (1994) Cloning and characterisation of TPO autoantibodies using combinatorial phage display libraries. *Autoimmunity* **17**, 167–179.

Hiatt, A., Cafferkey, R. & Bowdish, K. (1989) Production of antibodies in transgenic plants. *Nature* **342**, 76–78.

Hilyard, K. L., Reyburn, H., Chung, S. *et al.* (1994) Binding of soluble natural ligands to a soluble human T-cell receptor fragment produced in *Escherichia coli. Proc. Natl Acad. Sci. USA* **91**, 9057–9061.

Hollinger, P., Prospero, T. & Winter, G. (1993) 'Diabodies': Small bivalent and bispecific antibody fragments. *Proc. Natl Acad. Sci. USA* **90**, 6444–6448.

Holvoet, P., Laroche, Y., Lijnen, *et al.* (1991) Characterisation of a chimeric plasminogen activator consisting of a single-chain Fv fragment derived from a fibrin fragment D-dimer-specific antibody and a truncated single-chain urokinase. *J. Biol. Chem.* **266**, 19717–19724.

Hoogenboom, H. R., Griffiths, A. D., Johnson, K. S. *et al.* (1991) Multi-subunit proteins on the surface of filamentous phage: Methodologies for displaying antibody (Fab) heavy and light chains. *Nucleic Acids Res.* **19**, 4133–4137.

Hoogenboom, H. R. & Winter, G. (1992) By-passing immunisation. Human antibodies from synthetic repertoires of germline V_H gene segments rearranged *in vitro. J. Mol. Biol.* **227**, 381–388.

Horwitz, A. H., Chang, C. P., Better, M. *et al.* (1988) Secretion of functional antibody and Fab fragment from yeast cells. *Proc. Natl Acad. Sci. USA* **85**, 8678–8682.

Huston, J. S., George, A. J. T., Adams, G. P. *et al.* (1996) Single-chain Fv radioimmuno-targeting. *Q. J. Nuclear Med.* (in the press).

Huston, J. S., George, A. J. T., Tai, M.-S. *et al.* (1995) Single-chain Fv design and production by preparative folding. In: *Antibody Engineering: A Practical Approach*, 2nd edn., (ed. Borrebaeck, C. A. K.) pp. 185–225 (Oxford University Press, Oxford).

Huston, J. S., Levinson, D., Mudgett-Hunter, M. *et al.* (1988) Protein engineering of antibody binding sites: Recovery of specific activity in an anti-digoxin single-chain Fv analogue produced in *Escherichia coli. Proc. Natl Acad. Sci. USA* **85**, 5879–5883.

Huston, J. S., McCartney, J., Tai, M. S. *et al.* (1993) Medical applications of single-chain antibodies. *Int. Rev. Immunol* **10**, 195–217.

Inbar, D., Hochman, J. & Givol, D. (1972) Localisation of antibody-combining sites within the variable portions of heavy and light chains. *Proc. Natl Acad. Sci. USA* **69**, 2659–2662.

Isaacs, J. D., Watts, R. A., Hazleman, B. L. *et al.* (1992) Humanised monoclonal antibody therapy for rheumatoid arthritis. *Lancet* **340**, 748–752.

Jones, P. T., Dear, P. H., Foote, J. *et al.* (1986) Replacing the complementarity-determining regions in a human antibody with those from a mouse. *Nature* **321**, 522–525.

Jost, C. R., Kurucz, I., Jacobus, C. M. *et al.* (1994) Mammalian expression and secretion of functional single-chain Fv molecules. *J. Biol. Chem.* **269**, 26267–26273.

Kabat, E. A., Wu, T. T., Perry, H. M. *et al.* (1991) *Sequences of Proteins of Immunological Interest* (US Department of Health and Human Services, Bethesda, MD).

Kang, A. S., Barbas, C. F., Janda, K. D. *et al.* (1991a) Linkage of recognition and replication functions by assembling combinatorial antibody Fab libraries along phage surfaces. *Proc. Natl Acad. Sci. USA* **88**, 4363–4766.

Kang, A. S., Jones, T. M. & Burton, D. R. (1991b) Antibody redesign by chain shuffling from random combinatorial immunoglobulin libraries. *Proc. Natl Acad. Sci. USA* **88**, 11120–11123.

Karawajew, L., Behrsing, O., Kaiser, G. *et al.* (1988) Production and ELISA application of bispecific monoclonal antibodies against fluorescein isothiocyanate (FITC) and horseradish peroxidase (HRP). *J. Immunol. Meth.* **111**, 95–99.

Keinänen, K. & Laukkanen, M. L. (1994) Biosynthetic lipid-tagging of antibodies. *FEBS Lett.* **346**, 123–126.

Khazaeli, M. B., Conry, R. M. & LoBuglio, A. F. (1994) Human immune response to monoclonal antibodies. *J. Immunother.* **15**, 42–52.

Kipriyanov, S. M., Dübel, S., Breitling, F. *et al.* (1994) Recombinant single-chain Fv fragments carrying C-terminal cysteine residues: Production of bivalent and biotinylated miniantibodies. *Mol. Immunol.* **31**, 1047–1058.

Knappik, A. & Plückthun, A. (1995) Engineered turns of a recombinant antibody improve its *in vivo* folding. *Protein Engng* **8**, 81–89.

Knight, K. L. (1992) Restricted V_H gene usage and generation of antibody diversity in rabbit. *Annu. Rev. Immunol.* **10**, 593–616.

Kohl, J., Ruker, F., Himmler, G. *et al.* (1991) Cloning and expression of an HIV-1 specific single-chain Fv region fused to *Escherichia coli* alkaline phosphatase. *Ann. N. Y. Acad Sci.* **646**, 106–114.

Kontsekova, E., Kolcunova, A. & Kontsek, P. (1992) Quadroma-secreted bi(interferon alpha 2–peroxidase) specific antibody suitable for one-step immunoassay. *Hybridoma* **11**, 461–468.

Kostelny, S. A., Cole, M. S. & Tso, J. Y. (1992) Formation of a bispecific antibody by the use of leucine zippers. *J. Immunol.* **148**, 1547–1553.

Ku, J. & Schultz, P. G. (1995) Alternate protein frameworks for molecular recognition. *Proc. Natl Acad. Sci. USA* **92**, 6552–6556.

Kurucz, I., Jost, C. R., George, A. J. T. *et al.* (1993) A bacterially expressed single-chain Fv construct from the 2B4 T-cell receptor. *Proc. Natl Acad. Sci. USA* **90**, 3830–3834.

Kurucz, I., Titus, J. A., Jost, C. R. *et al.* (1995) Retargeting of CTL by an efficiently refolded bispecific single-chain Fv dimer produced in bacteria. *J. Immunol.* **154**, 4576–4582.

Larrick, J. W. and Fry, K. E. (1991) PCR amplification of antibody genes. *Methods: A Companion to Meth. Enzymol.* **2**, 106–110.

Laukkanen, M. L., Orellana, A. & Keinänen, K. (1995) Use of genetically engineered lipid-tagged antibody to generate functional europium chelate-loaded liposomes: Application in fluoroimmunoassay. *J. Immunol. Meth.* **185**, 95–102.

Lilley, G. G., Dolezal, O., Hillyard, C. J. *et al.* (1994) Recombinant single-chain antibody peptide conjugates expressed in *Escherichia coli* for the rapid diagnosis of HIV. *J. Immunol. Meth.* **171**, 211–226.

Lin, A. Y., Devaux, B., Green, A. *et al.* (1990) Expression of T-cell antigen receptor heterodimers in a lipid-linked form. *Science* **249**, 677–679.

Mallender, W. D. & Voss, E. Jr (1994) Construction, expression, and activity of a bivalent bispecific single-chain antibody. *J. Biol. Chem.* **269**, 199–206.

Marks, J. D., Griffiths, A. D., Malmqvist, M. *et al.* (1992) By-passing immunisation: Building high affinity human antibodies by chain shuffling. *Bio/technology* **10**, 779–783.

Marks, J. D., Hoogenboom, H. R., Bonnert, T. P. *et al.* (1991a) By-passing Immunisation: Human antibodies from V-gene libraries displayed in phage. *J. Mol. Biol.* **222**, 581–597.

Marks, J. D., Ouwehand, W. H., Bye, J. M. *et al.* (1993) Human antibody fragments specific for human blood groups antigens from a phage display library. *Bio/technology* **11**, 1145–1149.

Marks, J. D., Tristem, M., Karpas, A. *et al.* (1991b) Oligonucleotide primers for polymerase chain reaction amplification of human immunoglobulin variable genes and design of family-specific oligonucleotide probes. *Euro. J. Immunol.* **21**, 985–991.

Martin, F., Toniatti, C., Salvati, A. *et al.* (1994) The affinity-selection of a minibody polypeptide inhibitor of human interleukin-6. *EMBO J.* **13**, 5303–5309.

Max, E. E. (1993) Immunoglobulins: molecular genetics. In: *Fundamental Immunology* 3rd edn (ed. Paul, W. E.) pp. 315–382 (Raven Press. New York).

McCafferty, J., Griffiths, A. D., Winter, G. *et al.* (1990) Phage antibodies: Filamentous phage displaying antibody variable domains. *Nature* **348**, 552–554.

Meulemans, E. V., Slobbe, R., Wasterval, P. *et al.* (1994) Selection of phage-displayed antibodies specific for a cytoskeletal antigen by competitive elution with a monoclonal antibody. *J. Mol. Biol.* **244**, 353–360.

Milstein, C. & Cuello, A. C. (1983) Hybrid hybridomas and their use in immunohistochemistry. *Nature* **305**, 537–540.

Model, P. & Russel, M. (1988) Filamentous bacteriophage. In: *The Bacteriophages*, Vol. 2 (ed. Calendar, R.) pp. 375–456 (Plenum Press, New York).

Morrison, S. L., Coloma, M. J., Espinoza, D. *et al* (1995) Vectors and approaches for the eukaryotic expression of antibodies and antibody fusion proteins. In: *Antibody Engineering: A Practical Approach*, 2nd edn (ed. Borrebaeck, C. A. K.) pp. 267–293 (Oxford University Press, Oxford).

Morrison, S. L., Johnson, M. J., Herzenberg, L. A. *et al.* (1984) Chimeric human antibody molecules: mouse antigen-binding domains with human constant region domains. *Proc. Natl Acad. Sci. USA* **81**, 6851–6855.

Neri, D., de Lalla, C., Petrul, H. *et al.* (1995) Calmodulin as a versatile tag for antibody fragments. *Bio/technology* **13**, 373–377.

Neri, D., Momo, M., Prospero, T. *et al.* (1995b) High-affinity antigen binding by chelating recombinant antibodies (CRAbs). *J. Mol. Biol.* **246**, 367–373.

Neuberger, M. S., Williams, G. T. & Fox, R. O. (1984) Recombinant antibodies possessing novel effector functions. *Nature* **312**, 604–608.

Neuberger, M. S., Williams, G. T., Mitchell, E. B. *et al.* (1985) A hapten-specific chimaeric IgE antibody with human physiological effector function. *Nature* **314**, 268–270.

Nicholls, P. J., Johnson, V. G., Andrew, S. M. *et al.* (1993a) Characterisation of single-chain antibody (sFv)-toxin fusion proteins produced *in vitro* in rabbit reticulocyte lysate. *J. Biol. Chem.* **268**, 5302–5308.

Nicholls, P. J., Johnson, V. G., Blanford, M. D. *et al.* (1993b) An improved method for generating single-chain antibodies from hybridomas. *J. Immunol. Meth.* **165**, 81–91.

Nissim, A., Hoogenboom, H. R., Tomlinson, I. *et al.* (1994) Antibody fragments from a 'single pot' phage display library as immunochemical reagents. *EMBO J.* **13**, 692–698.

Orlandi, R., Güssow, D. H., Jones, P. T. *et al.* (1989) Cloning immunoglobulin variable domains for expression by the polymerase chain reaction. *Proc. Natl Acad. Sci. USA* **86**, 3833–3837.

Pack, P. & Plückthun, A. (1992) Miniantibodies: Use of amphipathic helices to produce functional, flexibly linked dimeric FV fragments with high avidity in *Escherichia coli*. *Biochemistry* **31**, 1579–1584.

Padlan, E. A. (1991) A possible procedure for reducing the immunogenicity of antibody variable domains while preserving their ligand-binding properties. *Mol. Immunol.* **28**, 489–498.

Padlan, E. A. (1994) Anatomy of the antibody molecule. *Mol. Immunol.* **31**, 169–217.

Painter, R. G., Sage, H. J. & Tanford, C. (1972) Contributions of heavy and light chains of rabbit immunoglobulin G to antibody activity. I. Binding studies on isolated heavy and light chains. *Biochemistry* **11**, 1327–1337.

Pantoliano, M. W., Bird, R. E., Johnson, S. *et al.* (1991) Conformational stability, folding, and ligand-binding affinity of single-chain Fv immunoglobulin fragments expressed in *Escherichia coli*. *Biochemistry* **30**, 10117–10125.

Pedersen, J. T., Henry, A. H., Searle, S. J. *et al.* (1994) Comparison of surface accessible residues in human and murine immunoglobulin Fv domains. Implication for humanisation of murine antibodies. *J. Mol. Biol.* **235**, 959–973.

Pessi, A., Bianchi, E., Crameri, A. *et al.* (1993) A designed metal-binding protein with a novel fold. *Nature* **362**, 367–369.

Picker, L. J. & Siegelmann, M. H. (1993) Lymphoid tissues and organs. In: *Fundamental Immunology* 3rd edn (ed. Paul, W. E.) pp. 145–197 (Raven Press, New York).

Plückthun, A. (1990) Antibodies from *Escherichia coli*. *Nature* **347**, 497–498.

Poljak, R. J., Amzel, L. M., Avey, H. P. *et al.* (1973) Three-dimensional structure of the Fab' fragment of a human immunoglobulin at 2,8-Å resolution. *Proc. Natl Acad Sci USA* **70**, 3305–3310.

Ratcliffe, M. J. H. & Jacobsen, K. A. (1994) Rearrangement of immunoglobulin genes in chicken B cell development. *Semin. Immunol.* **6**, 175–184.

Reichmann, L., Clark, M., Waldmann, H. *et al.* (1988) Reshaping human antibodies for therapy. *Nature* **322**, 323–327.

Reiter, Y., Brinkmann, U., Jung, S. H. *et al.* (1994a) Improved binding and antitumor activity of a recombinant anti-erbB2 immunotoxin by disulfide stabilisation of the Fv fragment. *J. Biol. Chem.* **269**, 18327–18331.

Reiter, Y., Brinkmann, U., Kreitman, R. J. *et al.* (1994b) Stabilisation of the Fv fragments in recombinant immunotoxins by disulfide bonds engineered into conserved framework regions. *Biochemistry* **33**, 5451–5459.

Reiter, Y., Kurucz, I., Brinkmann, U. *et al.* (1995) Construction of a functional disulfide-stabilised TCR Fv indicates that antibody and TCR Fv frameworks are very similar in structure. *Immunity* **2**, 281–287.

Reiter, Y., Pai, L. H., Brinkmann, U. *et al.* (1994c) Antitumor activity and pharmacokinetics in mice of a recombinant immunotoxin containing a disulfide-stabilised Fv fragment. *Cancer Res.* **54**, 2714–2718.

Rodrigues, M. L., Presta, L. G., Kotts, C. E. *et al.* (1995) Development of a humanised disulfide-stabilised anti-p185HER2 Fv-β-lactamase fusion protein for activation of a cephalosporin doxorubicin prodrug. *Cancer Res.* **55**, 63–70.

Roguska, M. A., Pedersen, J. T., Keddy, C. A. *et al.* (1994) Humanisation of murine monoclonal antibodies through variable domain resurfacing. *Proc. Natl Acad. Sci. USA* **91**, 969–973.

Sa'adu, A. & Zumla, A. (1995) Human monoclonal antibodies: Production, use problems. In: *Monoclonal Antibodies. Production, Engineering and Clinical Application* (eds Ritter, M. A. & Ladyman, H. M.) pp. 85–120 (Cambridge University Press, Cambridge).

Sambrook, J., Fritsch, E. F. & Maniatis, T. (1989) *Molecular Cloning: A Laboratory Manual* (Cold Spring Harbor Laboratory Press. New York).

Saragovi, H. U., Fitzpatrick, D., Raktabutr, A. *et al.* (1991) Design and synthesis of a mimetic from an antibody complementarity-determining region. *Science* **253**, 792–795.

Sastry, L., Alting-Mees, M., Huse, W. D. *et al.* (1989) Cloning of the immunological repertoire in *Escherichia coli* for generation of monoclonal catalytic antibodies: Construction of a heavy chain variable region-specific cDNA library. *Proc. Natl Acad. Sci. USA* **86**, 5728–5732.

Savage, P., So, A., Spooner, R. A. *et al.* (1993) A recombinant single chain antibody interleukin-2 fusion protein. *Brit. J Cancer* **67**, 304–310.

Sawyer, J. R., Tucker, P. W. & Blattner, F. R. (1992) Metal-binding chimeric antibodies expressed in *Escherichia coli*. *Proc. Natl Acad. Sci. USA* **89**, 9754–9758.

Schaaper, R. M. (1988) Mechanisms of mutagenesis in the *Escherichia coli* mutator *mut D5*: Role of DNA mismatch repair. *Proc. Natl Acad. Sci. USA* **85**, 8126–8130.

Scott, J. K. & Smith, G. P. (1990) Searching for peptide ligands with an epitope library. *Science* **249**, 386–390.

Searle, S. J., Pederen, J. T., Henry, A. H. *et al.* (1995) Antibody structure and function. In: *Antibody Engineering: A Practical Approach* 2 edn. (ed. Borrebaeck, C. A. K.) pp. 3–51 (Oxford University Press, Oxford).

Skerra, A., Pfitzinger, I. & Plückthun, A. (1991) The functional expresssion of antibody Fv fragments in *Escherichia coli*: improved vectors and a generally applicable purification technique. *Bio/technology* **9**, 273–278.

Skerra, A. & Plückthun, A. (1988) Assembly of a functional immunoglobulin Fv fragment in *Escherichia coli*. *Science* **240**, 1038–1041.

Smith, G. P. (1985) Filamentous fusion phage: novel expression vectors that display cloned antigens on the virion surface. *Science* **228**, 1315–1317.

Spooner, R. A., Murray, S., Rowlinson-Busza, G. *et al.* (1994) Genetically engineered antibodies for diagnostic pathology. *Hum. Pathol.* **25**, 606–614.

Stanfield, R. L., Takimoto-Kamimura, M., Rini, J. M. *et al.* (1993) Major antigen-induced domain rearrangements in an antibody. *Structure* **1**, 83–93.

Tai, M. S., Mudgett-Hunter, M., Levinson, D. *et al.* (1990) A bifunctional fusion protein containing Fc-binding fragment B of staphylococcal protein A amino terminal to antidigoxin single-chain Fv. *Biochemistry* **29**, 8024–8030.

Tomlinson, I. M., Cox, J. P. L., Gherardi, E. *et al.* (1995) The structural repertoire of the human V_K domain. *EMBO J.* **14**, 4628–4638.

Tomlinson, I. M., Walter, G., Jones, P. T. *et al.* (1996a) The imprint of somatic hypermutation on the repertoire of human germline V genes. *J. Mol. Biol.* **256**, 813–817.

Tomlinson, I. M., Walter, G., Marks, J. D. *et al.* (1992) The repertoire of human germline V_H sequences reveals about fifty groups of V_H segments with different hypervariable loops. *J. Mol. Biol.* **227**, 776–798.

Tomlinson, I. M., Williams, S. J. C., Cox, J. P. L. *et al.* (1996b) *The V BASE Directory of Human V Gene Sequences.* (MRC Centre for Protein Engineering, Hills Road, Cambridge CB2 2QH, UK; http://www.mrc–cpe.cam.ac.uk/imt–doc/vbase–home–page.html).

Traunecker, A., Lanzavecchia, A. & Karjalainen, K. (1991) Bispecific single chain molecules (Janusins) target cytotoxic lymphocytes on HIV infected cells. *EMBO J.* **10**, 3655–3659.

Turner, D. J., Ritter, M. A. & George, A. J. T. (1996) Importance of the linker in expression of single-chain Fv antibody fragments: optimisation of peptide sequence using phage display technology. (Manuscript submitted for publication.)

Ward, E. S. (1995) V_H shuffling can be used to convert an Fv fragment of anti-hen egg lysozyme specificity to one that recognises a T-cell receptor V alpha. *Mol. Immunol.* **32**, 147–156.

Ward, E. S., Güssow, D., Griffiths, A. D. *et al.* (1989) Binding activity of a repertoire of single immunoglobulin variable domains secreted from *Esherichia coli. Nature* **341**, 544–546.

Ward, V. K., Schneider, P. G., Kreissig, S. B. *et al.* (1993) Cloning, sequencing and expression of the Fab fragment of a monoclonal antibody to the herbicide atrazine. *Protein Engng* **6**, 981–988.

Webber, K. O., Reiter, Y., Brinkmann, U. *et al.* (1995) Preparation and characterisation of a disulfide-stabilised Fv fragment of the anti-Tac antibody: comparison with its single-chain analog. *Mol. Immunol.* **32**, 249–258.

Weiss, E. & Orfanoudakis, G. (1994) Application of an alkaline phosphatase fusion protein system suitable for efficient screening and production of Fab-enzyme conjugates in *Escherichia coli. J. Biotechnol.* **33**, 43–53.

Wels, W., Harwerth, I.-M., Zwickl, M. *et al.* (1992) Construction, bacterial expression and characterisation of a bifunctional single-chain antibody-phosphatase fusion protein targeted to the human ERBB-2 receptor. *Bio/technology* **10**, 1128–1132.

Whitelam, G. C., Cockburn, W. & Owen, M. R. (1994) Antibody production in transgenic plants. *Biochem. Soc. Trans.* **22**, 940–944.

Whitlow, M., Bell, B. A., Feng, S. L. *et al.* (1993) An improved linker for single-chain Fv with reduced aggregation and enhanced proteolytic stability. *Protein Engng* **6**, 989–995.

Whitlow, M., Filpula, D., Rollence, M. L. *et al.* (1994) Multivalent Fvs: Characterisation of single-chain Fv oligomers and preparation of a bispecific Fv. *Protein Engng* **7**, 1017–1026.

Williams, W. V., Moss, D. A., Kieber-Emmons, T. *et al.* (1989) Development of biologically active peptides based on antibody structure. *Proc. Natl Acad. Sci. USA* **86**, 5537–5541.

Winter, G., Griffiths, A. D., Hawkins, R. E. *et al.* (1994) Making antibodies by phage display technology. *Annu. Rev. Immunol.* **12**, 433–455.

Winter, G. & Milstein, C. (1991) Man-made antibodies. *Nature* **349**, 293–299.

Wognum, A. W., Lansdorp, P. M., Eaves, A. C. *et al.* (1989) An enzyme-linked immunosorbent assay for erythropoietin using monoclonal antibodies, tetrameric immune complexes, and substrate amplification. *Blood* **74**, 622–628.

Wülfing, C. & Plückthun, A. (1994) Protein folding in the periplasm of *Escherichia coli*. *Mol. Microbiol.* **12**, 685–692.

Yang, W. P., Goldstein, J., Procyk, R. *et al.* (1994) Design and evaluation of a thrombin-activable plasminogen activator. *Biochemistry* **33**, 606–612.

Yoo, T. J., Roholt, O. A. & Pressman, D. (1967) Specific binding activity of isolated light chains of antibodies. *Science* **157**, 707–709.

Zebedee, S. L., Barbas, C. F., III, Hom, Y. L. *et al.* (1992) Human combinatorial antibody libraries to hepatitis B surface antigen. *Proc. Natl Acad. Sci. USA* **89**, 3175–3179.

Chapter 5

Reaction Kinetics

Robert Karlsson and Håkan Roos

INTRODUCTION

The wide repertoire of antibody specificities that can be generated by real and artificial immune systems provides a rich pool of potential reagents for diagnostic and therapeutic use. For each antibody, the antigen recognition properties, i.e. the kinetic and affinity properties, along with class and specificity, will determine its utility.

There are numerous techniques and methods used for the characterisation of antigen-antibody interactions (Phizicky and Fields, 1995). They can be subdivided into two categories, 'direct' and 'indirect'. With a direct technique the molecular interaction can be monitored without the use of labels, whereas for an indirect technique a label such as an enzyme or a fluorophore is needed for detection. A number of optical and gravimetric techniques (Ramsden, 1993; Ebara and Okahata, 1994) permit direct observation of binding events at sensor surfaces. When these detection techniques are combined with sophisticated surface chemistry and efficient sample handling they can be used for kinetic analysis (Karlsson *et al.*, 1991; Jönsson and Malmqvist, 1992). This is illustrated in Figure 1 where binding curves obtained with three different monoclonal antibodies (MAb) reacting with the same antigen are compared. The antibodies are immobilised to different sensor surfaces. A baseline level is recorded with buffer in contact with the surface. Antigen is introduced and reacts with immobilised antibody. After a few minutes the antigen is replaced by buffer and the stability of the antigen-antibody complex is studied in the absence of antigen. The amplitudes of the response curves are not directly comparable because different levels of antibodies were immobilised, but clearly these antibodies have very different kinetic properties. For instance, antigen does not appear to dissociate at all from MAb 1, whereas dissociation from MAb 3 is very rapid. In an immunoassay these antibodies would perform very differently and the key to their performance is to be found in their kinetic properties.

In this chapter we will briefly discuss how the knowledge of antigen-antibody kinetics can be used for immunoassay development, to address items such as selection of antibodies, sensitivity and robustness. We will outline how affinity and kinetic parameters can be determined and will focus on the use of optical sensors for this purpose.

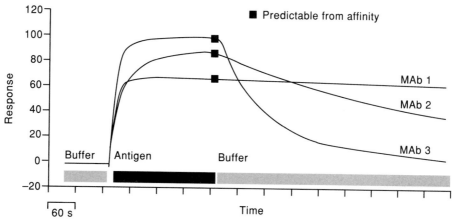

Figure 1 Response curves illustrating the interaction of p24 antigen (125 nM) with three different monoclonal antibodies (MAbs).

KINETIC ANALYSIS OF ANTIGEN-ANTIBODY INTERACTIONS AND IMPLICATIONS FOR IMMUNOASSAY DEVELOPMENT

When the affinity constant, K_a, for the reaction between antibody and antigen combining sites

$$Ab + Ag \Leftrightarrow AbAg$$

is known, it is in principle possible to predict the equilibrium concentration of the antigen-antibody complex for all combinations of total antibody and total antigen concentrations. Only the equilibrium state can be predicted (Figure 1) and the affinity in itself gives no information on how rapidly or how slowly the equilibrium is approached. This information can be obtained from an analysis of the kinetics of the antigen-antibody interaction. Rate constants, association rate (k_a) and dissociation rate (k_d) constants (known or assumed), can be used to predict the time course of an interaction. The value of such predictions for immunoassay development is illustrated in Figures 2 and 3. Figure 2 demonstrates the dose-response curve for antibodies with a moderate affinity of 5×10^8 l mol^{-1}. Three antibodies of this affinity but with different kinetic properties are considered. The rate constants assumed are typical for antigen-antibody interactions. The response range is 1,000 arbitrary units and the equilibrium responses are identical for all three antibodies. The cut-off level indicates the sensitivity of the assay, and is close to 20 pmol l^{-1}. The inserted binding curves illustrate the time needed to reach 98% of the steady-state level at an antigen concentration of 2 nmol l^{-1}. This value is reached in 8.3 minutes when MAb 1 is used but not until after 2.7 hours when MAb 3 is used. Thus if a rapid assay is considered, MAb 1 appears to be a suitable candidate.

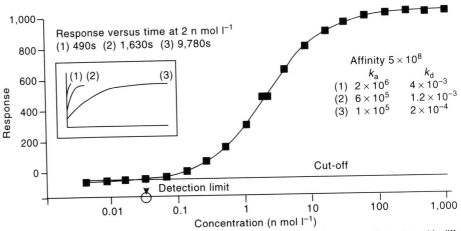

Figure 2 Calculated dose-response curves for three antibodies with the same affinity but with different kinetic properties. The binding curves in the insert demonstrate the time needed to reach the equilibrium level at the K_d concentration.

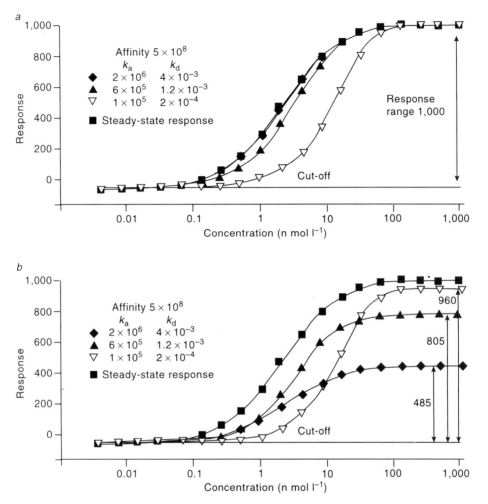

Figure 3 Calculated dose-response curves for three MAbs with the same affinity but different kinetic properties after *a*, 10-minutes incubation; *b*, 10-minutes incubation and a 3-minutes wash step.

Next (Figure 3a) the dose-response curves obtained after 10-minute incubation with antigen are compared. When MAb 1 is used the response curve is almost identical to the predicted affinity (infinite time) curve and the sensitivity is close to 30 pmol l^{-1}. The sensitivity is lower and approximately 60 pmol l^{-1} when MAb 2 is used but only about 250 pmol l^{-1} when MAb 3 is used. The response range for all three antibodies is still 1,000 arbitrary units. A wash step of 3 minutes is now included and the dose-response curves are recalculated (Figure 3b). Because of rapid dissociation of antigen the response range for MAb 1 is now only 485 arbitrary units. The sensitivity for this antibody is reduced to 70 pmol l^{-1}. For MAb 2 the response range is 805 arbitrary units but the sensitivity (70 pmol l^{-1}) has not been drastically impaired by the washing procedure. Finally, for MAb 3 the sensitivity and also the response range is almost unaffected by the washing procedure. Thus if antibody 1 is used in an assay, wash periods would have to be short and the assay would have to run under tight time control. This indicates that automation of the assay is required. Although antibody 3 would give a more robust assay, and automation would not be necessary, longer incubation times would be required for highest sensitivity. In reality many solid-phase assays are not performed in a kinetic mode; binding rates may instead be governed by the diffusion of analyte to the surface. As a consequence the difference in performance between these antibodies would be less pronounced but not insignificant.

These examples demonstrate the kind of information relevant to assay design that is obtained when the kinetic properties of antibodies are considered. Strengths and/or weaknesses in the assay procedure can be identified and the selection of antibodies is facilitated. The sensitivity and the robustness of the assay can be estimated; furthermore by considering the kinetics of crossreactivity the specificity may be improved, and by comparing the kinetics before and after a labelling procedure reagents may be optimised.

Classical Techniques for Kinetic and Affinity Analysis

Numerous techniques (chromatographic (Hummel and Dreyer, 1962; Chaiken *et al.*, 1992), sedimentation (Rivas and Minton, 1993), spectroscopic (Oberfelder and Lee, 1985; Ward, 1985)) exist for the study of protein-protein and protein-ligand interactions and many of them are used to estimate or determine binding constants (Phizicky and Fields, 1995). The basic issue in affinity and kinetic analysis is the measurement of some property related to the concentration, either of reactants or of the product(s) formed during the reaction. The change in concentration can then be related to the affinity or kinetic properties of the interacting system. The range of rate constants that can be measured in a kinetic assay is determined by the sensitivity and by the time-resolution of the assay. Similarly the range of affinity constants that can be experimentally resolved is determined by the sensitivity of the assay. When the separation of bound and free entities is a step in the analysis, the degree by which the separation procedure perturbs the equilibrium state will be important. Spectroscopic techniques and titration calorimetry (Wiseman *et al.*, 1989) are examples of direct nonseparation techniques, whereas ELISA is an indirect separation technique.

Spectroscopic Techniques can be used when the formation of the antigen-antibody complex can be linked to a change in the spectroscopic signal. Spectroscopic methods can be used both for affinity and kinetic analysis (Foote and Milstein, 1991). Often only the association rate constant and the affinity constant are measured.

For affinity measurements a normal spectrophotometer is sufficient, but for kinetic analysis a stopped-flow instrument is preferred. In such an instrument, antibody and antigen are precisely and rapidly mixed and transferred to the observation cell in a few milleseconds or less. The subsequent reaction can then be followed by absorbance or fluorescence spectrophotometry. In some cases the fluorescence spectrum of tryptophan residues can be used but it is also common to introduce a fluorescent label on either the antigen or the antibody. For low molecular-mass antigens fluorescence polarisation may be an alternative (Gaikwad *et al.*, 1993; Checovich *et al.*, 1995). These methods have the potential of providing both affinity and kinetic data sometimes without the need to label molecules and always without the need to separate bound and free species. The techniques are sensitive and both rapid interactions and high-affinity interactions can be investigated. Fluorescence methods are often the first choice when the kinetics of antigen-antibody interactions in solution are investigated (Goldberg, 1991). Some drawbacks are that the dissociation-rate constant can be difficult to measure, that labelling is often required and that the systems may have to be calibrated to determine conditions where the signal is proportional to a change in the concentration of the antigen-antibody complex.

Calorimetry is widely applicable in that the heat of the reaction is measured. This is proportional to the amount of complex formed. One interaction partner, the antibody or the antigen, is titrated with the other (titration calorimetry) and the heat generated in each titration step is measured. Both interaction partners have to be present in rather high ($>\mu$mol l^{-1}) concentrations. Typically a titration experiment can be performed in less than an hour. It allows the calculation of the number of binding sites, the affinity constant and changes in enthalpy and entropy (Wiseman *et al.*, 1989). One limitation is the sensitivity of the calorimeter, and with present instrumentation, affinities higher than 10^8 l mol^{-1} can normally not be resolved. Calorimetry is not used for kinetic analysis.

Enzyme-linked Immunosorbent Assay (ELISA) is perhaps the most frequent technique used for affinity analysis of antigen-antibody interactions. In particular the Friguet method (Friguet *et al.*, 1985) is useful. In this method antibody at fixed concentration is first incubated in solution with antigen at varying concentrations. When equilibrium is reached the solution is transferred to a microtitre plate coated with antigen. Here free antibody reacts with coated antigen. After washing, the antibody bound to the microtitre plate is detected by means of an enzyme-labelled secondary antibody. The advantages of this technique are that labelling procedures are avoided, that crude antibody preparations can be used and that the technique is sensitive, so that high-affinity interactions can be investigated. One drawback is that it sometimes may be difficult to setup the ELISA in such a way that the equilibrium obtained in solution is not shifted during the ELISA procedure (Seligman, 1994; Friguet *et al.*, 1995). ELISA is not suitable for kinetic analysis.

NEW OPTICAL TECHNIQUES FOR ANALYSIS OF BIOMOLECULAR INTERACTIONS

Whereas classical techniques measure interactions in solution, a new family of optical sensors allows direct detection of molecular interactions at a sensor surface. One interaction partner is attached to the surface and samples containing the other partner in solution are brought into contact with the surface.

Commercially available systems BIAcore from Pharmacia Biosensor, IAsys from Affinity Sensors and BIOS-1 from Artificial Sensing Instruments do this by detecting changes in refractive index close to the sensor surface. In each instance, the technology used to observe these changes is based on evanescent wave detection. However, the actual mode of detection and the design of the optical layers of the sensor surface differ. BIAcore systems are based on surface plasmon resonance (SPR) detection (Jönsson and Malmqvist, 1992). The surface consists of a thin gold film on a glass support (Löfås and Johnsson, 1990). IAsys uses a resonant mirror (RM) technique and the surface consists of a combination of high-and low-refractive index layers on a prism (Cush *et al.*, 1993). The BIOS-1 system makes use of waveguiding film materials (SiO_2–TiO_2) in combination with a diffraction grating on a glass or plastic support (Tiefenthaler, 1993). The basic versions of SPR and RM surfaces are coated with dextran films, of similar but not identical nature. These films provide a hydrophilic environment in which molecular interactions take place and facilitate covalent coupling of ligands to the sensor surface; other surface chemistries are also available. A hydrophobic surface intended for use in combination with lipid films is provided by BIAcore AB and an aminosilane surface is provided by Affinity Sensors. Both these surfaces are flat, lacking an extended dextran matrix.

In BIAcore the sample is brought into contact with the surface by means of a microfluidic system; the sample volume in direct contact with the surface is approximately 60 nl. Fresh sample is continuously pumped over the sensor surface using flow rates from 5 to 100 μl min^{-1}. A flow system is also used in the BIOS-1 system but here the flow cells are much larger (10–100 μl). In IAsys the sensor surface is integrated with a small cuvette (250 μl) and a stirring device provides efficient mixing.

The similarities and differences of these systems have been surveyed (Panayotou *et al.*, 1993b; Hodgson, 1994). In the context of biological chemistry, when the actual use of optical sensors is considered, most of the papers describe results obtained with the SPR sensor.

System properties
– the way to introduce sample
– dynamic range
– response/concentration and time unit
– noise
– drift
– automation

Surface properties
– stability of optical layers
– stability of chemical layers
– degree of nonspecific binding
– surface capacity
– possibilities for ligand immobilisation

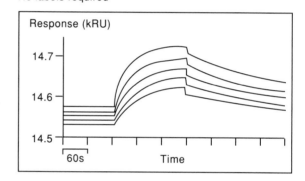

Analyte ranges from small molecules to cells
Direct interaction analysis
No labels required

Figure 4 Optical sensors: important system parameters and application areas. Biomolecular interaction analysis: identity binding sites (Bartley *et al.*, 1994); map binding sites (Fägerstam *et al.*, 1990; Nice *et al.*, 1993; Daiss and Scalice, 1994); building macromolecular complexes (Schuster *et al.*, 1993); perform enzyme reactions on surface complex (Schuster *et al.*, 1993; Nilsson *et al.*, 1994); measure concentration (Fägerstam *et al.*, 1992; Karlsson *et al.*, 1993); determine affinity (Cunningham and Wells, 1993; Karlsson, 1994; Karlsson and Ståhlberg, 1995; Morelock *et al.*, 1995); determine kinetic properties (Panayotou *et al.*, 1993a; Zeder-Lutz *et al.*, 1993; Fisher *et al.*, 1994; Van Cott *et al.*, 1994).

As illustrated in Figure 4 these sensor systems have the capability to provide direct interaction analysis data for a very wide range of biological systems. No labelling of analytes is required. Analytes range from whole cells (Watts *et al.*, 1994) to molecules with a molecular mass as low as a few hundred Da (Karlsson and Ståhlberg, 1995). The basic procedure for all types of interaction analysis is simple. The sensor surface is sequentially contacted with buffers, reagents and samples. The consequences of these actions are immediately displayed on a computer screen. The surface can in most cases be regenerated so that many cycles can be performed on one surface. The binding events studied may be interpreted in many different ways. The quality of binding data and the ease of obtaining them depends on the quality of the measuring system and especially on factors such as sensitivity, drift, surface stability, temperature stability and degree of automation.

BINDING EVENTS, 'BULK' EFFECTS AND MASS TRANSFER

Two factors that influence the shape of the binding curves are the 'bulk' effect and mass transfer. The 'bulk' effect is a consequence of the measuring technique, and mass transfer may determine the actual concentration of analyte close to the sensor surface. An understanding of both these phenomena is important for the correct interpretation of binding data.

Binding Events and 'Bulk' Effects

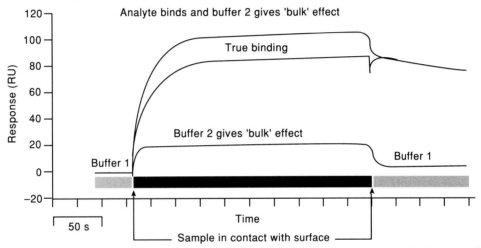

Figure 5 'Bulk' effects and binding events measured with SPR sensor. The 'true' binding curve is obtained after subtraction of the bulk effect.

The signal obtained from optical sensors is related to the refractive index in a small volume close to the sensor surface. As soon as the refractive index changes, a response is recorded. The bottom curve in Figure 5 demonstrates the bulk effect. When a new buffer is brought in contact with the sensor surface there is a rapid change in the signal and a new plateau level is reached; when the first buffer is again brought into contact with the surface the signal returns to the original baseline level. The bulk effect is thus only related to the difference in refractive index between the two buffers; it does not reflect a binding event. When a sample containing an analyte that reacts with the immobilised binding agent is introduced, the refractive index will also change as more mass becomes bound to the surface. The signal recorded in this case (top curve in Figure 5) will reflect both the binding event and the bulk effect. The 'true' binding curve is obtained after subtraction of the bulk effect. The response obtained is directly proportional to the mass of bound analyte (Stenberg *et al.*, 1991). In the absence of nonspecific binding and of bulk effect the response curve reflects the concentration of the complex between the analyte and the immobilised binding partner. It is important to discriminate between binding events and bulk effects. In particular the bulk effect should not be misinterpreted as a secondary binding event characterised by a rapid approach to steady state followed by rapid dissociation.

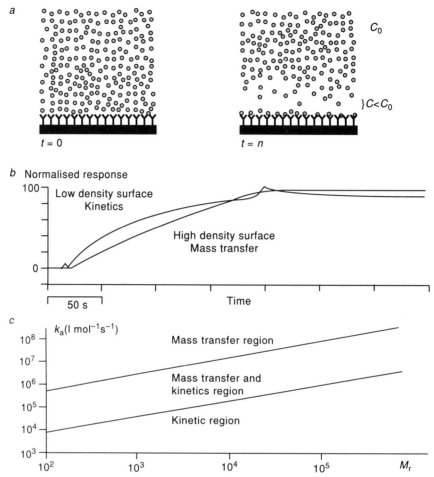

Figure 6 *a*, Binding of antigen to immobilised antibody lowers the concentration of antigen close to the surface; *b*, when antigen reacts with surfaces with different levels of immobilised antibody, the immobilisation level determines the shape of the binding curve and the information that can be obtained; *c*, the balance between mass transfer and kinetics for analytes of different molecular mass.

Reactions at Surfaces, Mass Transfer and Sample Depletion

Consider a binding agent immobilised on a surface. The corresponding binding partner, the analyte, is introduced at concentration C_0 and layered over the surface. The balance between how fast the analyte is consumed by the reaction and how efficient the analyte can be transported to the surface will determine the concentration of analyte close to the surface. If binding is rapid the concentration of analyte close to the surface, C_s, will drop, and C_s will become less than C_0 (Figure 6a). A concentration gradient effective over a certain distance will develop. Analyte is transported by diffusion into the region where $C < C_0$. The rate with which the analyte binds to the surface therefore reflects the diffusion of analyte molecules into the depleted region (Stenberg *et al.*, 1988). For kinetic analysis this situation is clearly unsatisfactory. The situation can be improved in different ways. The most efficient action is to decrease the number of molecules attached to the surface. With fewer binding agents immobilised, depletion will become less severe because fewer analyte molecules bind. Next we can shake or stir the solution or introduce the sample in a flow. These actions may be equally effective. They work by reducing the extension of the depleted layer so that diffusion occurs over shorter distances. When these actions are taken it is often possible to establish conditions where the difference between C_s and C_0 becomes insignificant. The kinetic properties of the reagents will then determine the binding rate (Sadana and Sii, 1992; Glaser, 1993; Karlsson *et al.*, 1994). Binding curves obtained on surfaces with high and low levels of immobilised binding agent are illustrated in Figure 6b; here the response values have been normalised in order to facilitate the comparison. At high levels of immobilisation mass transfer effects dominate. The binding rate is limited by diffusion and is almost constant during the injection of analyte. At low levels of immobilisation the binding curve is more curved and reflects the kinetics of the interaction; mass transfer effects are also visible after the injection when analyte dissociates in buffer flow. At high levels of immobilisation, dissociated molecules are more likely to rebind to the surface; the dissociation observed here is therefore slower than the dissociation observed from the surface with a low level of immobilised binding partner, where the analyte is transported out from the surface before it can rebind. Additional transfer effects on matrix surfaces have been suggested (Schuck, 1996). In practice, mass transfer effects are easy to detect since the binding rate will increase with increasing flow or stir rate.

In the BIAcore instrument, the range of association rate constants that can be determined under near optimal conditions (maximum response 100 resonance units (RU), flow rate 30 μl min^{-1}) is presented in Figure 6c; for low molecular weight analytes the range is narrower than for high molecular weight analytes. This is because detection is mass-sensitive. To detect the binding of a small molecule the level of immobilised binding agent cannot be reduced as much as for high molecular weight analytes; consequently mass transfer limitations become more severe. Figure 6c also demonstrates the balance between kinetics and mass transfer. For each type of analyte there is a kinetic region, a region where the binding is influenced both by mass transfer and by the kinetic properties, and a region where binding is determined almost exclusively by mass transfer. In the mid-region kinetic data may be obtained when weight transfer is considered in the evaluation procedure. Clearly, it will be difficult to obtain high quality kinetic data for many hapten-antibody interactions because these are often very rapid and involve low molecular weight analytes.

Although mass transfer effects should be reduced as far as possible for kinetic analysis they can be used to advantage for concentration analysis. When mass transfer effects dominate, the initial binding rate will only reflect the concentration of analyte, and it may be possible to discriminate affinity and concentration parameters (Karlsson *et al.*, 1993).

USE OF OPTICAL SENSORS FOR AFFINITY AND KINETIC ANALYSIS

Affinity Analysis

An equivalent to the Friguet assay is easy to set up. The antigen (or the antibody) is immobilised to the sensor surface and the solution where antibody and antigen are present at equilibrium is brought in contact with the surface. The use of real-time detection is now a clear advantage because initial binding rates can be used to determine the concentration of free antibody (or antigen). Independently of how the sample is introduced, reliable binding rates can be obtained in 10–20 s so the risk of perturbing the equilibrium in solution is reduced. When the sample is introduced in a flow the situation is even more favourable (Nieba *et al.*,

1996). When a flow rate of 10 μl min^{-1} is used in BIAcore, it takes only 0.4 s to exchange the entire sample volume over the sensor surface. New sample is continuously brought into contact with the surface and the total contact time can therefore be extended without affecting the equilibrium in solution. When the contact time is increased, lower concentrations can be determined; typically concentrations as low as 0.1 nmol l^{-1} can be accurately quantified in 5 minutes in a one-step assay. With this type of sensitivity, low concentrations of antibody can be used in the solution experiment, and nanomolar affinities can be determined (Karlsson, 1994). For affinities in the micromolar range, where steady-state levels are reached in a few minutes, the surface equilibrium values can be used to determine the concentration of free antibody or free antigen (Morelock *et al.*, 1995). This extends the use of the Friguet assay to low-affinity interactions.

Kinetic Analysis

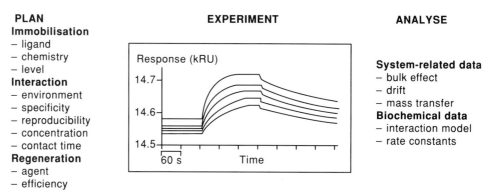

PLAN
Immobilisation
– ligand
– chemistry
– level
Interaction
– environment
– specificity
– reproducibility
– concentration
– contact time
Regeneration
– agent
– efficiency

EXPERIMENT

Response (kRU)

14.7

14.6

14.5

60 s   Time

ANALYSE

System-related data
– bulk effect
– drift
– mass transfer
Biochemical data
– interaction model
– rate constants

Figure 7 Three steps in kinetic analysis with optical sensors.

The steps in a kinetic experiment are outlined in Figure 7. A number of practical issues have to be considered in the planning phase, including into how much detail the interaction should be analysed.

For MAb selection, a presentation of data in overlay plots like Figure 1 is often sufficient. It is easy to identify antibodies that give rise to stable binding and a first impression of the speed of binding is obtained. Selected MAbs can later be characterised in more detail, for instance by using a concentration series of the antigen. Antigen-antibody interactions can be complex; an in-depth analysis of the interaction may include a further variation of ligand densities, interaction times and different environmental conditions (pH, ionic strength, temperature, additives). This type of experiment may help to differentiate antibodies, can be used to find optimal reaction conditions and may give clues to the actual reaction mechanism.

Immobilisation

Prior to the kinetic experiments it is important to decide which partner to immobilise. When quantitative data, i.e. the determination of apparent rate constants, is of interest, it is better to immobilise the antibody. Simple interaction models can then be assumed, at least when the antigen does not carry repeated epitopes. When the antigen is immobilised and intact anti-

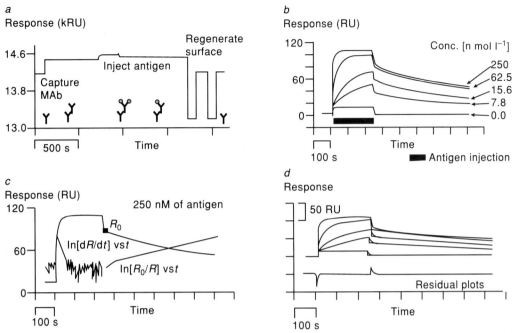

Figure 8 Kinetic analysis of MAb-antigen interactions and plots used in data analysis: *a*, the kinetic experiment; *b*, overlay plot of different antigen concentrations; *c*, data transformation to aid selection of interaction model; *d*, overlay plot of observed and calculated binding curves and residual plots.

body is used as analyte, the bivalent nature of IgG antibodies makes data analysis more difficult. The binding curves from such an experiment are easy to interpret in a qualitative manner (Karlsson *et al.*, 1995). However, the actual determination of rate constants using a bivalent interaction model (see model B in Figure 9) has, to our knowledge, not been reported. Immobilisation of the antigen should be considered when the antigen is a hapten or when the final immunoassay involves surface-bound antigen.

Different immobilisation chemistries can be used: amine coupling (Löfås *et al.*, 1993), coupling by thiol groups (Johnsson *et al.*, 1995), by oxidised sugar groups (Johnsson *et al.*, 1995) or by using streptavidin surfaces and biotinylated antibodies (Johnsson *et al.*, 1995). Amine coupling is straightforward and is the first choice. In cases where immobilisation through amine groups leads to inactivation of the antibody the alternatives should be investigated. Different immobilisation procedures can be used to identify suitable chemistry for the final immunoassay. For monoclonal antibody work it is convenient to immobilise a capturing antibody: for instance, a rabbit antibody directed to the Fc part of mouse antibody. This RAMFc antibody can then be used to capture mouse antibodies in an oriented way (Karlsson *et al.*, 1991) and furthermore monoclonal antibodies can be captured directly from culture media. Equally important is that the regeneration of the sensor surface can be standardised. There is no need to find suitable regeneration conditions for each and every antibody, only the RAMFc antibody surface has to be regenerated.

When Fab and ScFv fragments are used, new functional groups, for instance thiol groups or histidines (Gershon and Khilko, 1995), can be introduced and used for immobilisation or capture. In this case, as well as when other labels are introduced, it is important to keep the

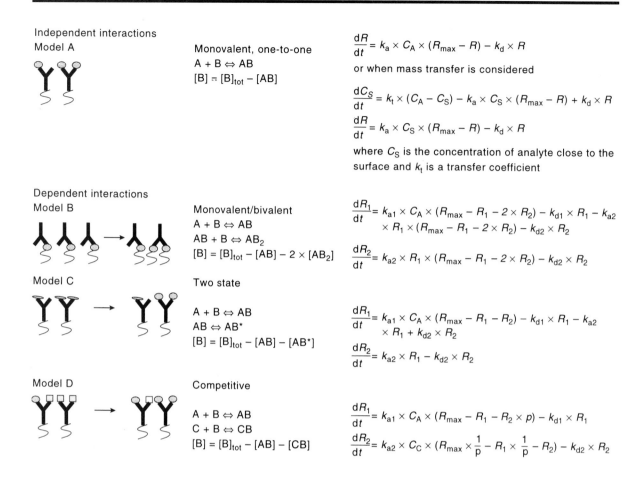

Independent interactions

Model A

Monovalent, one-to-one

A + B ⇔ AB

[B] = [B]$_{tot}$ − [AB]

$$\frac{dR}{dt} = k_a \times C_A \times (R_{max} - R) - k_d \times R$$

or when mass transfer is considered

$$\frac{dC_S}{dt} = k_t \times (C_A - C_S) - k_a \times C_S \times (R_{max} - R) + k_d \times R$$

$$\frac{dR}{dt} = k_a \times C_S \times (R_{max} - R) - k_d \times R$$

where C_S is the concentration of analyte close to the surface and k_t is a transfer coefficient

Dependent interactions

Model B

Monovalent/bivalent

A + B ⇔ AB

AB + B ⇔ AB$_2$

[B] = [B]$_{tot}$ − [AB] − 2 × [AB$_2$]

$$\frac{dR_1}{dt} = k_{a1} \times C_A \times (R_{max} - R_1 - 2 \times R_2) - k_{d1} \times R_1 - k_{a2} \times R_1 \times (R_{max} - R_1 - 2 \times R_2) - k_{d2} \times R_2$$

$$\frac{dR_2}{dt} = k_{a2} \times R_1 \times (R_{max} - R_1 - 2 \times R_2) - k_{d2} \times R_2$$

Model C

Two state

A + B ⇔ AB

AB ⇔ AB*

[B] = [B]$_{tot}$ − [AB] − [AB*]

$$\frac{dR_1}{dt} = k_{a1} \times C_A \times (R_{max} - R_1 - R_2) - k_{d1} \times R_1 - k_{a2} \times R_1 + k_{d2} \times R_2$$

$$\frac{dR_2}{dt} = k_{a2} \times R_1 - k_{d2} \times R_2$$

Model D

Competitive

A + B ⇔ AB

C + B ⇔ CB

[B] = [B]$_{tot}$ − [AB] − [CB]

$$\frac{dR_1}{dt} = k_{a1} \times C_A \times (R_{max} - R_1 - R_2 \times p) - k_{d1} \times R_1$$

$$\frac{dR_2}{dt} = k_{a2} \times C_C \times (R_{max} \times \frac{1}{p} - R_1 \times \frac{1}{p} - R_2) - k_{d2} \times R_2$$

Figure 9 Interaction models and differential rate equations. The differential rate equations listed in above are stated in response terms. R_1 and R_2 refer to the concentration of the molecular complexes formed; C_A is the concentration of the analyte; R_{max} is related to the total concentration of the immobilised partner (Karlsson *et al.*, 1991); $(R_{max} - R)$ reflects the concentration of the free binding sites of the immobilised partner; p is introduced as a normalising factor when analytes of different molecular mass compete for the binding site (Karlsson, 1994). This variable is introduced because the specific response of each component has to be considered.

degree of modification low. Preferably only one or two groups should be introduced in order to maintain the activity of the antibody (Johnsson *et al.*, 1995; Hemminki *et al.*, 1995).

The Kinetic Experiment

It is wise to use solution conditions (pH, ionic strength, temperature) that mimic the ones to be used in the final immunoassay. The buffer used to establish the baseline conditions and the solution in which the antigen is dissolved should be as closely matched as possible. This helps to minimise the bulk effect and to establish similar interaction conditions during and after the injection. Injection times from 2 to 5 minutes are suitable for initial experiments. An example is given in Figure 8a; here RAMFc has been immobilised to the sensor surface. MAb at 30 μg ml^{-1} is injected and captured by RAMFc. The stability of the RAMFc-MAb interaction is tested by introducing a wait period of 5 to 10 minutes before antigen is contacted with the surface. After the antigen injection the analysis cycle is finished by removing both MAb and antigen from the surface by injecting 0.1 mol l^{-1} hydrochloric acid. The entire analysis cycle can then be repeated. With a cycle time of 20 to 30 minutes, a large number of MAbs can be compared in a very short time using one antigen concentration. For more detailed analysis the antigen concentration is normally varied over one to two orders of magnitude.

DATA ANALYSIS

Inspection by Eye

Prior to data analysis it is useful to inspect the binding curves in an overlay plot (Figure 8b); here it is easy to see that there is a bulk effect, that the response is concentration-dependent and that interaction curves appear exponential. The binding curves for the two highest concentrations come very close immediately after the injection; the response levels obtained here are therefore close to the saturation level. The activity of the captured antibody can be estimated by comparing the level of captured MAb with the level of bound antigen at saturation (Karlsson *et al.*, 1993).

$$\text{The activity} = \frac{\text{Antigen level}}{M_w \text{ antigen}} * \frac{M_w \text{ antibody}}{\text{antibody level}} * \frac{1}{\text{antibody valency}}$$

M_w represents the molecular weight of antigen and antibody. Activities >0.9 are often obtained when RAMFc is used as capturing agent. When the antibody is immobilised directly the activity is often lower; low values may indicate that the antibody is partly inactivated or contaminated with inactive antibody. The number of available sites can possibly also be reduced by steric effects in the dextran matrix. This appears to be more pronounced with the RM surface where steric effects have been demonstrated even at low levels of immobilised antibody (2.5 ng mm^{-2}) (Edwards *et al.*, 1995). Similar experiments on the SPR surface have demonstrated a high and constant antibody activity at immobilisation levels as high as 15 ng mm^{-2} (Johnsson *et al.*, 1995). Values higher than unity may indicate nonspecific binding or aggregation of antigen molecules.

Finally (Figure 8b), by looking at the top and bottom curves it is evident that the plateau levels are very stable; the drift is negligible. This also confirms that the dissociation of MAb from the RAMFc surface is very small.

Selection of Interaction Model and Determination of Rate Constants

For the analysis of binding data the reaction mechanism and an appropriate interaction model (Hulme and Birdsall, 1992) must first be considered; some useful models are presented in Figure 9. The models describe the reaction with a number of parameters (a1, a2, a3...) such as time, the rate constants, the concentration of immobilised binding partner (the ligand), the concentration of analyte and the concentration of the analyte: ligand complex. More parameters are needed for complex models than for simple models; some of these parameters are known, some are measured and some are unknown.

The model is used to calculate a response curve as a function of these parameters, $R(t)_{\text{calc}}$ = $f(a1, a2, a3...)$. The aim of data analysis is to find values for the unknown parameters (the rate constants) so that the residual, i.e. the difference between measured and calculated response curves, becomes as small as possible. The parameter estimates must also be physically meaningful. In a perfect match between measured and calculated data the residual should only reflect the noise level of the instrumentation. This level is seldom if ever achieved for a complete set of data. Careful analysis of the residuals (Straume and Johnson, 1992) may reveal systematic trends. When factors linked to the instrumentation and to surface chemistry can be ruled out, remaining non random residuals may suggest that the model in use has to be modified. To verify this the experimental design often has to be improved.

When observed and calculated data are close, this is still not proof of the assumed reaction mechanism. It merely demonstrates that the chosen model is sufficient to describe the interaction data. The rate constants calculated are therefore apparent rate constants and should be reported as such.

One-to-one-Binding

The selection of an interaction model is obviously a critical issue. In a first attempt we may assume that antigen binding is monovalent and that binding to the antibody sites are independent of each other (model A in Figure 9). If this model is valid and data is transformed as illustrated in Figure 8c, the resulting plots should be linear. In Figure 8c the $\ln(dR/dt)$ versus t plot is linear at first but when steady state is approached the plot levels off. The nonlinear region reflects the noise level of the instrument and therefore it does not contradict the assumption that data may be analysed with the one-to-one model. The $\ln(R_0/R)$ versus t plot is also linear. Accordingly these transformations indicate that the one-to-one model may be valid. It is possible to use linear analysis and to obtain numerical values for the rate constants by analysing the linear parts of the transformed response curve as originally described (Karlsson *et al.*, 1991). There are several drawbacks with this approach. First, only a part of the data is analysed; second, the transformation of data may distort the error distribution (Leatherbarrow, 1990) and third, linear analysis is restricted to the one-to-one model and generally not applicable to more complex interaction models. Some of these drawbacks are evident from Figure 8c. In linear analysis the slope of the $\ln(dR/dt)$ plot is calculated. Here the linear part extends over approximately 100 seconds. The rest of the injection phase must be omitted from the analysis. The slope value would turn out completely wrong if the entire injection phase was used. By using nonlinear regression (Leatherbarrow, 1990; Duggleby, 1991; Johnson, 1992), i.e. by using nontransformed data and by calculating the best-fit curve rather than the best-fit line, (Marquardt, 1963) these shortcomings are avoided and the entire curve can be used for analysis. Nonlinear analysis of kinetic data can be used to various degrees of sophistication. The injection phase and the buffer flow phase can be analysed separately (O'Shannessy *et al.*, 1993) using the appropriate analytical equations. Simultaneous analysis, or global fitting of all data, not only from one binding curve but including all the curves in the experiment is more attractive (Fisher and Fivash, 1994; Morelock *et al.*, 1995; Morton *et al.*, 1995). In global analysis the residual is minimised for the entire data set and not only for one curve at a time. This gives more reliable results, and a practical aspect is that only one set of rate constants is calculated instead of one set for each curve. Figure 8d demonstrates the result from a global analysis of the data in Figure 8 using the one-to-one model. The bulk effect was modelled as an offset and the spikes in the residual plots reflect the few seconds over which the bulk effect is developed. The rate constants found were $k_a = 3.5 \times 10^5$ l mol^{-1}s^{-1} and $k_d = 1.2 \times 10^{-3}$ s^{-1}. The average difference between measured and calculated data points (excluding the spikes) was approximately 1% of the maximum response. The residual is rather small, 2 to 3 times the noise level. Clearly the calculated rate constants describe the interaction over a wide range of concentrations and also over a reasonable time frame.

More Complex Interactions

When complex interaction models are used, analytical solutions to the differential rate equations are often difficult if not impossible to find. By using numerical integration the response curves can easily be calculated and later analysed. For kinetic analysis a combination of numerical integration of differential rate equations with nonlinear analysis and global fitting appears to be a very powerful technique (Fisher and Fivash, 1994; Morton *et al.*, 1995). Numerical integration and global analysis require intensive calculation. Normally 5 to 10 curves with 1,000 data points in each curve can be analysed in less than 10 minutes on a reasonably fast personal computer.

In order to find experimental evidence for a more complex interaction model it is helpful to examine the $\ln(dR/dt)$ and $\ln(R_0/R)$ versus t plots. These plots are linear for a one-to-one binding event, and a deviation from linearity will easily be picked up by the eye. It can sometimes be explained by a drift in the signal, by nonspecific binding or by a mass transfer influence, but could also indicate that the interaction itself is more complex. There are now two alternatives. The first is to go ahead and analyse the data with the one-to-one model. The residuals will now be larger and not randomly distributed; the rate constants found may not describe the interaction in detail but the purpose of the investigation may still be fulfilled. The other alternative is to try to fit the data to other models. For instance, the immobilised ligand may be heterogeneous, leading to parallel interactions. These types of reactions are additive and can be analysed using the sum of two or more rate equations (model A in Figure 9). A change in conformation can lead to a gradual stabilisation of the antigen-antibody complex (model C in Figure 9). Alternatively the antigen could be present in different forms where both forms bind to the antibody in a competitive manner (model D in Figure 9). When there is a mass transfer limitation the one-to-one model can be corrected to account for this (Karlsson *et al.*, 1994). When a laminar-flow system is used, the set of differential equations in model A in Figure 9 describe the situation. When mass transfer limits the initial binding rate, the mass transfer coefficient, k_t, can be determined independently. The k_t is then found as the slope from a plot of initial binding rate versus analyte concentration.

The differential rate equations listed in Figure 9 are valid when the analyte concentration can be considered constant during the entire injection phase. Experimentally this is easily achieved in a flow system, but also in a cuvette system when the volume is large and only a fraction of the sample binds to the surface. Similarly the analyte concentration is assumed to be zero during the buffer phase after the injection. Again this assumption is valid in the flow-through system but it may not be valid in the cuvette system, because the released analyte accumulates in the cuvette. When the affinity is high, even a low concentration (0.1 nmol l^{-1}) of released antigen will be significant. An equation describing the increase in antigen concentration over time should then be included in the model.

Discriminating between Different Reaction Mechanisms

It is often possible to obtain good fits with several models when a limited set of experimental data is used. More experiments are normally needed in order to discriminate between different interaction mechanisms. A variation of ligand density or flow/stir rate is useful in identifying a mass transfer limitation. The addition of free ligand (the immobilised partner) to the buffer after the injection of analyte has been used to prevent rebinding of the analyte (Panayotou *et al.*, 1993); in the presence of free ligand the dissociation rate can be increased. Whether this procedure can be used to obtain dissociation data corresponding to the true dissociation rate constant or whether a more active displacement of analyte from the immobilised ligand is also involved has not been clarified. A variation of ligand density and of analyte concentration can demonstrate ligand or analyte heterogeneity. A variation of interaction time can reveal the existence of linked interactions and discriminate them from independent (parallel) interactions. When several mechanisms are considered, crucial experiments can be identified by simulating interaction curves using different models. When the simulation reveals significant differences the corresponding experiments are performed. It may thus be possible to discard one or several interaction mechanisms.

RATE CONSTANTS: EXPECTED AND MEASURED VALUES

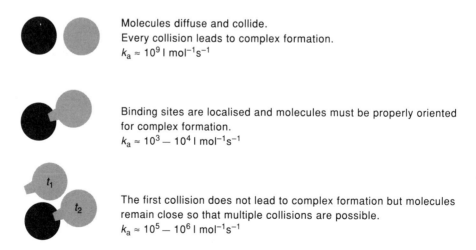

Molecules diffuse and collide.
Every collision leads to complex formation.
$k_a \approx 10^9$ l mol^{-1}s^{-1}

Binding sites are localised and molecules must be properly oriented for complex formation.
$k_a \approx 10^3 - 10^4$ l mol^{-1}s^{-1}

The first collision does not lead to complex formation but molecules remain close so that multiple collisions are possible.
$k_a \approx 10^5 - 10^6$ l mol^{-1}s^{-1}

Figure 10 Illustration of simplified collision theory for antigen-antibody interactions.

When two molecules interact in solution the collision frequency and the orientation of interaction sites may determine the reaction rate (Northrup and Erickson, 1992); this is illustrated in Figure 10. When the molecules are viewed as spheres and the entire surface area is reactive, so that every collision results in a binding event, the association rate constant would be high and approximately 1×10^9 l mol^{-1}s^{-1}. For protein-protein interactions this view is too simplified. The complementarity determining regions (CDRs) on the Fab fragment, the regions involved in antigen binding, have a surface area of approximately 2,800 Å^2 (Padlan, 1994). This area is only a fraction of the total surface area of the antibody. The CDRs differ in topography and may be characterised by depressions and protrusions sometimes containing pockets or clefts (Padlan, 1994). The structures of antigen-antibody complexes indicate that the antigen surface is complementary in shape. Structural analysis also demonstrates that the surface used in binding to antigen is smaller than the total CDR area (Padlan, 1994). The probability that a random encounter of two molecules would lead to a precise match of binding sites lowers the expected association rate constant to about 1×10^3 l mol^{-1}s^{-1} (Northrup and Erickson, 1992). This value is much smaller than measured values. Simulations using Brownian dynamics (Northrup and Erickson, 1992) suggest that molecules remain close to each other for a prolonged time, that reorientation is possible and that multiple collisions occur during this encounter period. This would give rise to association rate constants close to 1×10^6 l mol^{-1}s^{-1}. By including weak attractive forces, higher association rate constants could be expected. Lower association rate constants indicate a smaller effective binding surface or repulsive forces. Reported values for antigen-antibody interactions are often in the range from 10^5 to 10^6 l mol^{-1}s^{-1}. Such values suggest that the rate of complex formation is mainly controlled by the diffusion properties of antibody and antigen.

For haptens the association rate constants can be much higher because of more rapid diffusion and less dependence on orientation.

Conformational change (Stanfield and Wilson, 1994) and loss of water of hydration lead to an increased 'goodness-of-fit' (Van Oss, 1995) and improves the stability of the antibody and antigen complex. The contacts between paratope and epitope are mainly hydrophobic and electrostatic (Van Oss, 1995) but there appears to be no obvious correlation between the number of such contacts and antibody affinity (Webster *et al.*, 1994). Although a large number of contacts are formed between antibody and antigen, a single point mutation can lead to drastic changes in the affinity (Altschuh *et al.*, 1992; Kelley and O'Connell, 1993). The dissociation rate constant is usually more affected and can sometimes be reduced more than a 1,000-fold (Kelley and O'Connell, 1993). An amino acid exchange may also lead to an improvement in antibody affinity (Barbas III *et al.*, 1994). A biologically useful lower limit for the dissociation rate constant of 10^{-3} to 10^{-4} s^{-1}, corresponding to half-times ($\ln2/k_d$) of approximately 10 minutes to 2 hours, has been suggested (Foote and Eisen, 1995). In practice dissociation rate constants for antigen-antibody interactions ranging from 0.01 to 1×10^{-5}s^{-1} are frequently found.

Rate Constants for Immobilised Antibodies

The rate constants found for immobilised antibodies may differ from those found in solution. One reason for this is that the immobilisation itself may affect the activity, because it may involve the active site. When a capture reagent such as a RAMFc antibody is used, this risk is probably small. Another reason is that the diffusion properties are not the same for 'immobilised' antibodies as for antibodies in solution. For a reaction limited by diffusion both the association and the dissociation constants are proportional to the sum of the diffusion coefficients ($D_{Ab}+D_{Ag}$). When antibody is immobilised on a solid support we can assume that D_{Ab} drops to zero and that, disregarding other effects of the immobilisation, k_a and k_d will decrease by a factor of $D_{Ag}/(D_{Ab}+D_{Ag})$. D_{Ab} and D_{Ag} are the diffusion coefficients in solution. If the antibody has the smaller diffusion coefficient the decrease is never more than a factor of two. When the antibody is immobilised in a highly flexible matrix, such as the dextran matrix on SPR and RM sensor surfaces, D_{Ab} will in practice not be zero. For a reaction limited by diffusion we could still expect the rate constants determined with surface techniques to be somewhat lower than the rate constants determined in solution (Karlsson *et al.*, 1994).

Affinity constants obtained with BIAcore and with calorimetry are close (Ladbury *et al.*, 1995). Furthermore rate constants obtained in the lysozyme/anti-lysozyme system (Yeung *et al.*, 1995) support the hypothesis that rate constants obtained with optical sensor techniques do not differ widely from those obtained in solution.

CONCLUSIONS

Knowledge of the kinetic properties of antibodies is important for immunoassay design. Association rate constants are often limited by diffusion but still k_a values for a number of antibodies directed against the same antigen may differ by a factor of at least 10. The dissociation rate constant can vary considerably more, at least over four orders of magnitude. Selection of antibodies for immunoassay on kinetic grounds and a consideration of kinetic properties during immunoassay development may lead to more rapid, more sensitive, more specific and more robust assays.

With optical sensors the binding between antibody and antigen can be directly observed, no labelling is required, and furthermore, antibodies from culture media can be used directly. A kinetic assay can be set up in a few hours and a large number of antibodies may be analysed in a short time. For immunoassay purposes a direct comparison of binding curves in an overlay plot is often sufficient for the selection of suitable antibodies.

The effect of introducing labels on antibody or antigen can also be investigated. Quantitative analysis of binding curves allows the calculation of apparent rate constants. Optical sensors thus provide key kinetic information for developers of immunoassay.

REFERENCES

Altschuh, D., Dubs, M-C., Weiss, E. *et al.* (1992) Determination of kinetic constants for the interaction between a monoclonal antibody and peptides using surface plasmon resonance. *Biochemistry* **31**, 6298–6304.

Barbas C. F. III, Hu, D., Dunlop, N. *et al.* (1994) In vitro evolution of a neutralising human antibody to human immunodeficiency virus type 1 to enhance affinity and broaden cross-reactivity. *Proc. Natl Acad. Sci. USA* **91**, 3809–3813.

Bartley, T. D., Hunt, R. W., Welcher, A. A. *et al.* (1994) B61 is a ligand for the ECK receptor protein-tyrosine kinase. *Nature* **368**, 558–560.

Chaiken, I., Rosé, S. & Karlsson, R. (1992) Analysis of macromolecular interactions using immobilised ligands. *Anal. Biochem.* **201**, 197–210.

Checovich, W. J., Bolger, R. E. & Burke, T. (1995) Fluorescence polarisation: A new tool for cell and molecular biology. *Nature* **375**, 254–256.

Cunningham, B. C. & Wells, J. A. (1993) Comparison of a structural and functional epitope. *J. Molec. Biol.* **234**, 554–563.

Cush, R., Cronin, J. M., Stewart, W. J. *et al.* (1993) The resonant mirror: A novel optical biosensor for direct sensing of biomolecular interactions. Part I: Principle of operation and associated instrumentation. *Biosens. Bioelectron.* **8**, 347–354.

Daiss, J. L., & Scalice, E. R. (1994) Epitope mapping on BIAcore: Theoretical and Practical Considerations. *Methods: A Companion to Meth. Enzymol.*, **6**, 143–156.

Duggleby, R. G. (1991) Analysis of biochemical data by non-linear regression: Is it a waste of time? *Trends Biol. Sci.* **16**, 51–52.

Ebara, Y. & Okahata, Y. (1994) A kinetic study of concanavalin A binding to glycolipid monolayers by using a quartz-crystal microbalance. *J. Amer. Chem. Soc.* **116**, 11209–11212.

Edwards, P. R., Gill, A., Pollard-Knight, D. V. *et al.* (1995) Kinetics of protein-protein interactions at the surface of an optical biosensor. *Anal. Biochem.* **231**, 210–217.

Fågerstam, L., Frostell, Å., Karlsson, R. *et al.* (1990), Detection of antigen-antibody interactions by surface plasmon resonance. Application to epitope mapping. *J. Mol. Recognit.*, **3**, 208–214.

Fågerstam, L. G., Frostell-Karlsson, Å., Karlsson, R. *et al.* (1992), Biospecific interaction analysis using surface plasmon resonance detection applied to kinetic, binding site and concentration analysis. *J. Chromatogr.* **597**, 397–410.

Fisher, R. J. & Fivash, M. (1994) Surface plasmon resonance based methods for measuring the kinetics and binding affinities of biomolecular interactions. *Curr. Opin. Biotechnol.* **5**, 389–395.

Fisher, R. J., Fivash, M., Casas-Finet, J. *et al.* (1994) Real-time DNA binding measurements of the ETS1 recombinant proteins reveal significant kinetic differences between the p42 and p51 isoforms. *Protein Sci.* **3**, 257–266.

Foote, J. & Eisen, H. N. (1995) Kinetic and affinity limits on antibodies produced during immune responses. *Proc. Natl Acad. Sci. USA* **92**, 1254–1256.

Foote, J. & Milstein, C. (1991) Kinetic maturation of an immune response. *Nature* **352**, 530–532.

Friguet, B., Chafotte, A. F., Djavadi-Ohaniance, L. *et al.* (1985) Measurement of the true affinity constant in solution of antigen-antibody complexes by enzyme-linked immunosorbent assay. *J. Immunol. Meth.* **77**, 305–319.

Friguet, B., Chafotte, A. F., Djavadi-Ohaniance, L. *et al.* (1995) Under proper experimental conditions the solid-phase antigen does not disrupt the liquid phase equilibrium when measuring dissociation constants by competition ELISA. *J. Immunol. Meth.* **182**, 145–147.

Gaikwad, A., Gómez-Hens, A. & Pérez-Bendito, D. (1993) Use of stopped-flow fluorescence polarisation immunoassay in drug determinations. *Anal. Chim. Acta* **280**, 129–135.

Gershon, P. D. & Khilko, S. N. (1995) Stable chelating linkage for reversible immobilisation of oligohistidine tagged proteins in the BIAcore surface plasmon resonance detector. *J. Immunol. Meth.* **183**, 65–76.

Glaser, R. W. (1993) Antigen-antibody binding and mass transport by convection and diffusion to a surface: A two dimensional computer model of binding and dissociation kinetics. *Anal. Biochem.* **213**, 152–161.

Goldberg, M. E. (1991) Investigating protein conformation dynamics and folding with monoclonal antibodies. *Trends Biol. Sci.* **16**, 358–362.

Hemminki, A., Hoffrén, A. M., Takkinen, K. *et al.* (1995) Introduction of lysine residues on the light chain constant domain improves the labelling properties of a recombinant Fab fragment. *Protein Engng.* **8**, 185–191.

Hodgson, J. (1994) Light, Angles, Action. Instruments for label-free, real-time monitoring of intermolecular interactions. *Bio/technology* **12**, 31–35.

Hulme, E. C. & Birdsall, J. M. (1992) Strategy and tactics in receptor binding studies. In: *Receptor Ligand Interactions: A Practical Approach.* (ed. Hulme, E. C.) pp. 63–176 (Oxford University Press, Oxford).

Hummel, J. P. & Dreyer, W. J. (1962) Measurement of protein-protein binding phenomena by gel filtration. *Biochim. Biophys. Acta* **63**, 530–532.

Johnson, M. L. (1992) Why, when and how biochemists should use least squares. *Anal. Biochem.* **206**, 215–225.

Johnsson, B., Löfås, S., Lindquist, G. *et al.* (1995) Comparison of methods for immobilisation to carboxymethyl dextran sensor surfaces by analysis of the specific activity of monoclonal antibodies. *J. Molec. Recognit.* **8**, 125–131.

Jönsson, U. & Malmqvist, M. (1992) Real-time biospecific interaction analysis. The integration of surface plasmon resonance detection, general biospecific interface chemistry and microfluidics into one analytical system. *Adv. Biosens.*, **2**, 291–336.

Karlsson, R. (1994) Real time competitive kinetic analysis of interactions between low molecular weight ligands in solution and surface immobilised receptors. *Anal. Biochem.* **221**, 142–151.

Karlsson, R., Fägerstam, L., Nilshans, H. *et al.* (1993) Analysis of active antibody concentration. Separation of affinity and concentration parameters. *J. Immunol. Meth.* **166**, 75–84.

Karlsson, R., Michaelsson, A. & Mattson, L. (1991) Kinetic analysis of monoclonal antigen-antibody interactions with a new biosensor based analytical system. *J. Immunol. Meth.* **145**, 229–240.

Karlsson, R., Mo, J. A. & Holmdahl, R. (1995) Binding of autoreactive mouse anti-type II collagen antibodies derived from the primary and the secondary immune response to type II rat collagen investigated with biosensor technique. *J. Immunol. Meth.*, **188**, 63–71.

Karlsson, R., Roos, H., Fägerstam, L. *et al.* (1994) Kinetic and concentration analysis using BIA technology. *Methods: A Companion to Meth. Enzymol.* **6**, 99–110.

Karlsson, R. & Ståhlberg, R. (1995) Surface plasmon resonance detection and multi-spot sensing for direct monitoring of interactions involving low molecular weight analytes and for determination of low affinities. *Anal. Biochem.* **228**, 274–280.

Kelley, R. F. & O'Connell, M. P. (1993) Thermodynamic analysis of an antibody functional epitope. *Biochemistry*, **32**, 6828–6835.

Ladbury, J. E., Lemmon, M. A., Zhou, M. *et al.* (1995) Measurement of the binding of tyrosyl phosphopeptides to SH2 domains: A reappraisal. *Proc. Natl Acad. Sci. USA* **92**, 3199–3203.

Leatherbarrow, R. J. (1990) Using linear and non-linear regression to fit biochemical data. *Trends Biol. Sci.* **15**, 455–458.

Löfås, S. & Johnsson, B. (1990), A novel hydrogel matrix on gold surfaces in surface plasmon resonance sensors for fast and efficient covalent immobilisation of ligands. *J. Chem. Soc. Chem. Commun.* **21**, 1526–1528.

Löfås, S., Johnsson, B., Tegendahl, K. *et al.* (1993) Dextran modified gold surfaces for surface plasmon resonance sensors: Immunoreactivity of immobilised antibodies and antibody-surface interaction studies. *Colloids & Surfaces B: Biointerfaces* **1**, 83–89.

Marquardt, D. W. (1963) An algorithm for least squares estimation of non-linear parameters. *J. Soc. Indust. Appl. Math.* **11**, 431–441.

Morelock, M. M., Ingraham, R. H., Betageri, R. *et al.* (1995) Determination of receptor-ligand kinetics and equilibrium binding constants using surface plasmon resonance: Application to the lck SH2 domain and phosphotyrosyl peptides. *J. Med. Chem.* **38**, 1309–1318.

Morton, T. A., Myszka, D. G. & Chaiken, I. M. (1995) Interpreting complex binding kinetics from optical biosensors: A comparison of analysis by linearisation, the integrated rate equation and numerical integration. *Anal. Biochem.* **227**, 176–185.

Nice, E., Layton, J., Fabri, L. *et al.* (1993), Mapping of the antibody- and receptor-binding domains of granulocyte colony-stimulating factor using an optical biosensor. Comparison with enzyme-linked immunosorbent assay competition studies. *J. Chromatogr.* **646**, 159–168.

Nieba, L., Krebber, A. & Plückthun, A. (1996) Competition BIAcore for measuring true affinities: Large differences from values determined from binding kinetics. *Anal. Biochem.* **234**, 155–165.

Nilsson, P., Persson, B., Uhlén, M. *et al.* (1994) Real-time monitoring of DNA-manipulations using biosensor technology. *Anal. Biochem.* **224**, 400–408.

Northrup, S. H. & Erickson, H. P. (1992) Kinetics of protein-protein association explained by Brownian dynamics computer simulation. *Proc. Natl Acad. Sci. USA* **89**, 3338–3342.

O'Shannessy, D. J., Brigham-Burke, M., Soneson, K. K. *et al.* (1993) Determination of rate and equilibrium binding constants for macromolecular interactions using surface plasmon resonance: Use of non linear least squares analysis methods. *Anal. Biochem.* **212**, 457–468.

Oberfelder, R. W. & Lee, J. C. (1985), Measurement of ligand-protein interactions by electrophoretic and spectroscopic techniques. *Meth. Enzymol.* **117**, 381–399.

Padlan, E. A. (1994) Anatomy of the antibody molecule. *Molec. Immunol.* **31**, 169–217.

Panayotou, G., Gish, G., End, P. *et al.* (1993a) Interactions between SH2 domains and tyrosine-phosphorylated platelet derived growth factor β-receptor sequences: Analysis of kinetic parameters by a novel biosensor based approach. *Molec. Cell. Biol.* **13**, 3567–3576.

Panayotou, G., Waterfield, M. D. & End, P. (1993b) Riding the evanescent wave. *Curr. Biol.* **3**, 913–915.

Phizicky, E. M. & Fields, S. (1995), Protein-protein interactions: Methods for detection and analysis. *Microbiol. Rev.* **59**, 94–123.

Ramsden, J. J. (1993) Experimental methods for investigating protein adsorption kinetics at surfaces. *Quart. Rev. Biophys.* **27**, 41–105.

Rivas, G. & Minton, A. P. (1993), New developments in the study of biomolecular associations via sedimentation equilibrium. *Trends Biol. Sci.* **18**, 284–287.

Sadana, A. & Sii, D. (1992) The binding of antigen by immobilised antibody: Influence of a variable adsorption rate coefficient on external diffusion limited kinetics. *J. Colloid Interface Sci.* **151**, 166–177.

Schuck, P. (1996). Kinetics of ligand binding to receptor immobilised in a polymer matrix, as detected with an evauescent wave biosensor. I. A computer simulation of the influence of mass transport. *J. Biophys.* **70**, 1230–1249.

Schuster, S., Swanson, R., Alex, A. *et al.* (1993) Assembly and function of a quaternary signal transduction complex monitored by surface plasmon resonance. *Nature*, **365**, 343–347.

Seligman, S. J. (1994) Influence of solid-phase antigen in competition enzyme linked immunosorbent assays on calculated antigen-antibody dissociation constants. *J. Immunol. Meth.*, **168**, 101–110.

Stanfield, R. L. & Wilson, A. (1994) Antigen-induced conformational changes in antibodies: A problem for structural prediction and design. *Trends Biotechnol.* **12**, 275–279.

Stenberg, E., Persson, P., Roos, H. *et al.* (1991) Quantitative determination of surface concentration of protein with surface plasmon resonance using radiolabeled proteins. *J. Colloid Interface Sci.* **143**, 513–526.

Stenberg, M., Werthén, M., Theander, S. *et al.* (1988) A diffusion limited reaction theory for a microtiter plate assay. *J. Immunol. Meth.* **112**, 23–29.

Straume, M. & Johnson, M. L. (1992) Analysis of residuals: Criteria for determining goodness-of-fit. *Meth. Enzymol.* **210**, 87–105.

Tiefenthaler, K. (1993) Grating couplers as label-free biochemical waveguide sensors. *Biosens. Bioelectron.* **8**, xxxv–xxxvii.

Van Cott, T. C., Bethke, R. F., Polonis, V. P. *et al.* (1994) Dissociation rate of antibody –gp120 binding interactions is predictive of V3-mediated neutralisation of HIV-1. *J. Immunol.* **153**, 449–459.

Van Oss, C. J. (1995) Hydrophobic, hydrophilic and other interactions in epitope-paratope binding. *Molec. Immunol.* **32**, 192–211.

Ward, L. D. (1985) Measurement of ligand binding to proteins by fluorescence spectroscopy. *Meth. Enzymol.* **117**, 400–414.

Watts, H. J., Lowe, C. R. & Pollard-Knight, D. V. (1994) Optical biosensor for monitoring microbial cells. *Anal. Chem.* **66**, 2465–2470.

Webster, D. M., Henry, A. H. & Rees A. R. (1994) Antigen-antibody interactions. *Curr. Opin. Struct. Biol.* **4**, 123–129.

Wiseman, T., Williston, S., Brandts, J. F. *et al.* (1989) Rapid measurement of binding constants and heats of binding using a new titration calorimeter. *Anal. Biochem.* **179**, 131–137.

Yeung, D., Gill, A., Maule, C. H. *et al.* (1995) Detection and quantification of biomolecular interactions with optical biosensors. *Trends Anal. Chem.* **14**, 49–56.

Zeder-Lutz, G., Wenger, R., Van Regenmortel, M. H. V. *et al.* (1993) Interaction of cyclosporin A with an Fab fragment or cyclophilin-affinity measurements and time-dependent changes in binding. *FEBS Lett.* **326**, 153–157.

Chapter 6

Assessment and Selection of Antibodies

David J. Newman and Christopher P. Price

INTRODUCTION

Preceding chapters discuss the molecular interactions that define the specificity and affinity of the binding interaction between epitope and paratope (Chapter 2) and the importance of measuring that affinity (Chapter 5). Other chapters discuss the production of specific high-affinity immunoreagents including the production of both polyclonal and monoclonal antibodies (Chapter 3), the design of recombinant antibodies (Chapter 4) and the preparation of synthetic binding agents (antibody mimics) (Chapter 7). All these chapters cover various aspects of selection and characterisation of binding agents of a certain specificity and affinity but here we will attempt to integrate all of this to give an overview of the assessment of binding agents with regards to their use in different assay formats. We will also include, for completeness, comparisons with alternative binding agents such as receptors, lectins and other alternatives to antibodies. The requirements of immunosensor technologies are in general similar to those for more conventional immunoassays and for the purposes of this discussion they will be treated as such unless there is a particular reason not to.

The absolute cost of an antibody will be a combination of the difficulty of initial development and the scale and ease of production. Commercial sources of monoclonal antibodies, lectins and protein A/G can all be expensive, costing hundreds of pounds per milligram. These costs can apparently be reduced by 'in-house' production but usually only if the true labour costs are defrayed or if there is the possibility for the generation of patent and licensing royalties from unique antibodies, particularly those produced by hybridoma or recombinant antibody technologies. Most diagnostic applications now use monoclonal antibodies where the advantages of continual production of a defined specificity are of considerable value and the availability of large-scale *in vitro* cell culture systems producing many grams makes the process viable.

With some immunosensor systems, regeneration of the antibody or binding agent is possible, which could provide an economic advantage for such a system; however, this puts stringent demands on the stability of the antibody under the regeneration conditions. Furthermore the use of very high-affinity binding agents, e.g. streptavidin, could be problematic because of the need for strong denaturing conditions to disrupt the binding interaction.

Development of immunoassay technologies for commercial exploitation requires a close eye on the patent literature. With regard to antibody selection the most crowded area is in immunogen design where there are a whole host of protected conjugation techniques, linker sequences and even peptide sequences (Dorman, 1977; Dean, 1986). With regard to selection of the type of antibody, there are licensing restrictions on the use of paired monoclonal antibodies in 'sandwich' assays (Ekins, 1989; Greene and Duft, 1990). The latter has resulted in significant royalties to the company owning the patent and in several approaches to circumvent the patent. These issues mainly relate to the cost of assembling the final assay reagents but need to be considered at the outset of the selection procedure.

Strategy

Selection of an antibody should be considered with regard to different levels of need: clinical, economical and operational. An assay has to meet the required clinical sensitivity and specificity but at a reasonable cost, both in terms of reagents and the complexity (time/difficulty) required to complete the analysis. The clinical need may be relatively easy to meet but combining this with the need for ever-faster delivery of results requires higher affinity constants and therefore more careful selection.

In selecting an antibody there are four main characteristics to consider in connection with the final assay performance: specificity, sensitivity, reaction time and stability. Achieving the desired specificity, sensitivity and reaction time is dependent upon the affinity constant of the antibody and its inherent paratopic conformation. Although different antibodies may show greater thermal stability, enabling higher temperatures to be used, overall stability will probably be dependent mostly upon the solid phase to which the antibody is conjugated. If regeneration of the surface is required, as can be the case in some types of immunosensor, then stability of the antibody to pH changes and other denaturing or dissociative conditions becomes even more important. In the main the initial selection of an antibody is dependent upon assessment of affinity constant (K_a) and demonstration of a lack of cross reactivity to a panel of potential interfering molecules, selected on the basis of structural similarity and clinical importance.

The most important aspect of the selection of an antibody or a binding agent is that the selection process should use a procedure that reflects, as nearly as possible, the final assay format. This may, however, mean that derivatives or conjugates of a range of reagents need to be prepared and this can be expensive and time-consuming; therefore a certain amount of preliminary screening is usually necessary. Thus measurement of antibody affinity as described in Chapter 5 allows a minimal K_a for a particular detection limit to be selected. The minimum affinity that will be required for a particular analytical task will depend upon the design of the analytical system and upon the concentration of the ligand to be measured; in the latter case the K_a will need to be at least the same order of magnitude as the molarity of the ligand of interest, particularly in limited-reagent assays where the affinity constant of the antibody is the major determinant of assay sensitivity (see Chapter 9) (Berzofsky *et al.*, 1989). At concentrations of analyte much below $1/K_a$ most of the antibody binding sites are unoccupied, thus competition between labelled and unlabelled analyte will be less effective; reducing the number of antibody binding sites will help but is limited by the inability to detect ever decreasing amounts of antibody:antigen complex.but see the later discussion in Chapter 24 on radiometric or ambient analyte assays for other advantages of this approach. For excess-reagent systems the affinity constant is less important to overall assay sensitivity, and specific activity of the label and the nonspecific binding are the predominant factors; in this case the higher the affinity constant, the less antibody will be required to achieve equilibrium in a given time. However, in general it can be assumed that the higher the affinity constant the more sensitive the resultant assay will be in a given time, as the antibody:antigen complex will be formed faster and will be more resistant to dissociation during the wash steps that will be required to reduce the nonspecific binding. The use of two antibodies in a sandwich format further complicates kinetic considerations as cooperativity can occur, with the binding of one antibody to the antigen either increasing or decreasing the affinity of binding to the second antibody (Johne *et al.*, 1995). This requires careful consideration about which antibody to use as the label and which as the capture and can only be investigated using the final assay format.

Characterisation of specificity starts with epitope mapping, enabling a minimum level of crossreactivity and specificity to be chosen. The difficulties arise when enzyme conjugation or solid-phase derivatisation is carried out; these processes can introduce structural alterations that can influence both affinity and specificity. A particular solid-phase format may require extensive washing conditions, or a particular antigen may require a particular anticoagulant for sample preservation; these requirements may place certain demands on the binding reagent's characteristics, e.g. dissociation constant, k_d. These issues have been covered in a number of other reviews including (Day, 1990; Multiple Authors, 1993; Newman *et al.*, 1997).

AFFINITY

The affinity of a bimolecular interaction is dependent not only on the intrinsic reaction but also on the reaction conditions under which it is measured e.g. pH, temperature. The rate of attainment of equilibrium will be similarly influenced by the law of mass action, i.e. predominantly by the concentration of the reactants and the volume used for the reaction. Thus if an antibody is immobilised onto a microtitre plate the limited surface area and relatively large reaction volume will significantly reduce the rate of attainment of equilibrium. Furthermore this ignores the potentially damaging effects of adsorbing the antibody to the plastic surface, which could alter the equilibrium position that was ultimately obtained by changing the intrinsic K_a of the reaction (Olsen *et al.*, 1989; Spitznagel and Clark, 1993; Karlsson *et al.*, 1994). Thus, knowing the kinetic rate constants for an interaction under one set of conditions may not be an accurate predictor of performance in an immunoassay under very different reaction conditions, particularly solid-phase immobilisation (Johne *et al.*, 1995; Newman and Price, 1996). An excellent example of this was described by Johne *et al.* (1995) where the relative affinity and specificity of antigen capture by antibodies to myoglobin, selected by BIAcore analysis, were altered by whether they were used as label or capture antibody (Johne *et al.*, 1995). It is thus important that the technique used to characterise the kinetics uses the immunoreagents in as close a condition to their final intended usage as possible.

Techniques for Measuring Affinity Constants

Techniques for the measurement of the affinity constants for bimolecular interactions have been discussed in Chapter 5. Suffice to say that the method of choice at present would be the use of a surface-effect optical sensor system using real-time analysis. If this is not available then the more traditional equilibrium techniques using enzyme-linked immunoassay (ELISA) or radioimmunoassay (RIA) can still be used to provide useful information; one helpful review is that of Friguet *et al.* (1985). In general the techniques are quite simple but certain pieces of detailed information, e.g. specific activity of the label, nonspecific binding, etc., are required if an accurate assessment is to be made. Experimental data is analysed using the Langmuir isotherm or its derivative, the better-known Scatchard equation (1949):

$$\text{Langmuir:} \quad \frac{1}{b} = \frac{1}{Ab_t \, [Ag] \, K_a} + \frac{1}{Ab_t} \qquad \text{Plot:} \quad \frac{1}{b} \quad \text{versus} \quad \frac{1}{[Ag]}$$

$$\text{Scatchard:} \quad \frac{b}{[Ag]} = nK_a - b \, K_a \qquad \text{Plot:} \quad \frac{b}{[Ag]} \quad \text{versus} \quad b$$

where b = moles of antigen bound, $[Ag]$ = moles of free antigen, n = valency of antibody, K_a = equilibrium constant and Ab_t = total number of binding sites. Figure 1 gives representations of the expected plots for a monoclonal and a polyclonal antibody. The single class of binding

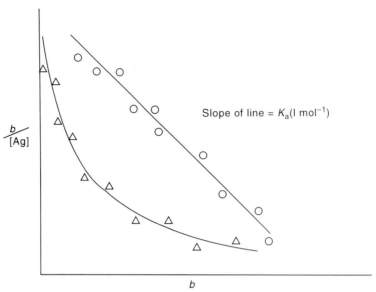

Figure 1 Scatchard plots for monoclonal (circles) and polyclonal (triangles) antibodies. b = bound antigen concentration and [Ag] = free (unbound) antigen concentration.

site of the monoclonal antibody gives a linear plot, the slope of which is K_a and the complex curvilinear plot of the polyclonal antibody shows the range of affinities that are present within it.

Accurate assessment of the distribution and amount of free and bound antigen is very important, including accurate values of the amount of labelled molecules and the nonspecific binding contribution. It is also essential that the separation technique used should not disturb the primary antigen-antibody interaction. A competitive labelled antigen approach is usual, using an amount of antibody that will bind approximately 30–50% of the total labelled antigen added (Berzofsky *et al.*, 1989, and *see* Chapter 9). A standard curve, in at least triplicate, with at least 10 points over a wide concentration range is set up and allowed to reach equilibrium (this can take several days). The complexity of the experimental detail is one reason why differing assessments of the K_a of an antibody are produced by workers using slightly different protocols. For screening purposes, however, a completely accurate assessment of the K_a of different antibodies is probably not needed; using a fixed protocol the different antibodies screened can be ranked for relative affinity.

The association reaction is often diffusion limited and the major determinant of K_a is the k_d and not k_a, and it is with k_d that most variation is seen (Berzofsky *et al.*, 1989, and *see* Chapter 5). If an antibody is intended for use in an assay format where stringent washing is necessary then a slow k_d should be looked for because a fast dissociation rate would mean that significant amounts of the antigen-antibody complex would dissociate during the washing steps. The half-life ($t_{1/2}$) of the complex is $0.7/k_d$, with the range of k_d found being approximately 10^4 to 10^{-6} per second; this represents half-lives from microseconds to several days.

As indicated in Chapter 5 a high K_a reaction can be achieved in a number of ways and measurement of the component kinetic rate constants can be useful in identifying such important characteristics. Indeed this has been one of the major benefits of the optical sensor systems that are becoming so established as tools for automated ranking and absolute measurement of the kinetic rate constants of a wide range of bimolecular interactions (*see* Chapter 5). The limitation of these technologies lies with their lack of resemblance to many of the immunoassay formats that are in commercial use, so any measurement needs to be carefully interpreted with this limitation in mind as discussed above (Johne *et al.*, 1995). However, experience has shown that a knowledge of these important defining characteristics of an interaction does provide useful pointers in antibody selection but what they cannot do is replace experimental verification in the final assay format.

SPECIFICITY

For a measurement to be termed specific it is necessary to define the molecular or biological characteristic that a system should exclusively recognise. This can be a particular molecular mass, molecular charge or shape, epitope or a particular chemical or biological activity. In some cases a less 'specific' antibody may be required, for instance if it is necessary to monitor the metabolites of, for example, a drug as well as the parent molecule if they retain biological activity. The ability to recognise the selected molecular characteristic will be in part determined by the antibody and partly by the detection technology used. The specificity of the antibody can be characterised and one with the desired behaviour selected; although affinity and specificity are intimately linked (the paratope binding affinity is highest for a particular epitope, but it may recognise a small range of similar epitopes with reduced affinity) they need to be investigated separately.

Specificity can be measured in two ways: first by demonstrating a lack of crossreaction, that is, no measurable binding of molecules other than the one of first choice (the classical crossreaction study using similar molecular structures looking for whether they will bind to the selected antibody); second by demonstrating a lack of interference by other molecules in the binding of the primary reactant (whether competing molecular structures can cause a change in the measured response for the specific molecule).

Crossreactivity is best assessed using epitope mapping for large molecular mass antigens (see next section) but useful information can be generated by performing serial dilutions of a potential interferent in parallel with similar dilutions of the specific antigen. The relative degree (%) of interference can then be calculated; this approach is also the only practical way of assessing antibodies for haptens. A similar study can be performed looking at the change in response caused by a range of interferent concentrations to a fixed concentration of the specific antigen. These approaches are illustrated in Figure 2 and, as can be seen, an antibody may not crossreact with a molecule but if that molecule is present in significant amounts it may interfere with the binding of the specific antigen with its antibody.

When assessing antibody specificity it is important to use the final assay format because conjugation to labels or to solid phases can cause conformational changes in the immunoglobulin structure that could alter specificity as well as affinity.

Epitope Mapping

Epitope mapping is the assessment of a panel of antibodies to determine which structural region of the antigen each individual antibody recognises; this enables complementary pairs of antibodies to be recognised so that they can be selected for use in sandwich immunoassays of

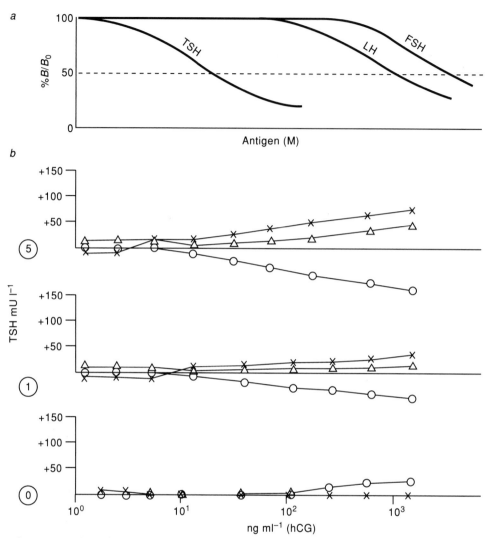

Figure 2 *a*, Assessment of crossreactions of luteinising hormone (LH) and follicle-stimulating hormone (FSH) with a polyclonal, antiserum for thyroid-stimulating hormone (TSH). Dotted line represents 50% displacement. *b*, Interference in a TSH immunoradiometric assay, using a common capture antibody and three different labelled antibodies. In the absence of TSH (0) only one of the labelled antibodies gives any evidence of interference from hCG. In the presence of TSH (1 and 5 mU l⁻¹) all three antibodies show some interference, but not all in the same direction.

enhanced specificity. This has traditionally been carried out using solid-phase ELISA techniques, e.g. Figure 3, but, as discussed above, the introduction of automated optical immunosensor systems has revolutionised the mapping of large arrays of monoclonal antibodies.

Essentially either the antigen of interest is conjugated to the sensor surface or an anti species antibody or protein A/G surface is prepared (in this case the antibodies under investigation are captured and the antigen binding is monitored in a second reaction). Then different antibodies are allowed to react with the surface with and without the other antibodies in the panel; with a sequential analysis of the type illustrated in Figure 4 the pattern of interactions can be elucidated and the antibodies grouped into different epitopic groups.

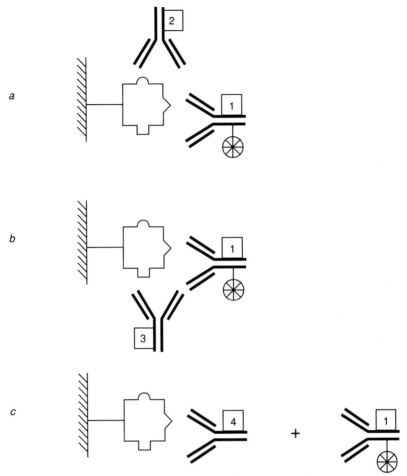

Figure 3 Epitope mapping. One monoclonal antibody is labelled, the competing antibodies (in excess) are added to microtitre plate wells coated with antigen and, after incubation and washing, the labelled antibody is added. In *a* and *b*, antibodies 2 and 3 recognise different epitopes to antibody 1 but in *c*, antibody 4 recognises the same epitope as antibody 1. By examining all the pairs, epitope complementarity can be established and if the sequences recognised by one or more of the antibodies are known then further characterisation is possible.

For some analytes more detailed analysis may be necessary, for instance if there are different isoforms of the molecule found in the biological fluid of interest, e.g. alkaline phosphatase (bone versus liver). This may require Western blotting of serum samples or measurement of chromatographic fractions; these techniques may, however, introduce some alteration to the structure of the antigen, causing a difference in binding with the antibody compared with the molecule in free solution. The final proof of specificity may have to be a clinical study using the final assay format.

Combining automated epitopic mapping and kinetic rate constant ranking enables rapid and more complete analysis of hybridomas at an earlier stage than in the usual screening cycle. Peptide series in which sequential mutations are introduced can be readily investigated for differences in binding affinity and specificity, by binding one sequence to the sensor surface and looking at competition for binding with the antibody.

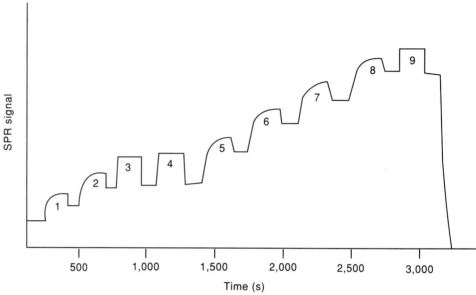

Figure 4 In this example, nine different antibodies to the same antigen are passed sequentially over the sensor surface upon which the antigen is immobilised. If the antibodies recognise distinct epitopes then they will be able to bind concurrently, e.g. antibodies 1, 2 and 5–8. If an antibody recognises an overlapping or similar epitope then it will not be able to bind concurrently, e.g. antibodies 3, 4 and 9. By altering the order of addition a complete map of the different antibody specificities can be obtained.

SELECTION OF A BIOAFFINITY MOLECULE

The primary characteristic of a bioaffinity molecule is that it should be specific for the desired molecular characteristic or biological function, and the characterisation of the specificity and affinity of the antibody has been described in the previous section. It should be borne in mind that absolute specificity is not always required. It can be beneficial to have an antibody that recognises a group of metabolites as well as the parent compound. Having obtained the desired specificity and affinity there are several other characteristics that can help in the selection of the most appropriate agent for use in a particular system: stability, tolerance to pH changes, purity, cost of production and coupling chemistry (Table 1). The strategy for selection of the appropriate bioaffinity molecule remains the same as that described for antibodies.

Polyclonal versus Monoclonal Antibodies

Polyclonal antibodies are easier and simpler to produce than monoclonal antibodies and in general it is easier to produce high-affinity polyclonal antibodies (Albert, 1984). Monoclonal antibodies require considerable initial investment in time and equipment but offer the ultimate advantage of providing the continuous production of a defined reagent, once they have been identified. They can also be produced using partially purified immunogens, whereas polyclo-

---

Assay detection limit and working range

    Absolute: measurement, assay requirements, washing effects

    System reaction conditions

    Introduction of labelled molecule

    Conjugation to a solid phase

    Single or multiple use

Assay specificity

    Absolute: crossreactivity and interference; assay requirements; nonspecific effects

    Receptor versus immunological agent

    System reaction conditions

    Introduction of labelled molecule

    Conjugation to a solid phase

    Single or multiple use

Costs

    Patents on immunogens

    Patents on type and combinations of antibodies

    Costs of production

    Single or multiple use

Table 1 Selection characteristics.

nal antibody production requires the use of highly purified antigens. Monoclonal antibodies, by definition, are more specific than polyclonal antibodies. However, this unique specificity can occasionally complicate matters. The unique epitope recognised by one antibody could have a different half-life to that of another epitope on the same specific antigen that is recognised by another monoclonal antibody. The absolute specificity of monoclonal antibodies has allowed the quantification of different forms of human chorionic gonadotrophin (hCG): β-sub-unit, intact molecule and different cleaved forms (Stenman, 1993). Some workers have suggested that the best interim arrangement is to develop defined polyclonal antibodies using mixtures of monoclonal antibodies, thus recognising all the circulating isoforms until their unique biological roles and clinical utility can be determined.

As mentioned above, most of the very high-affinity antibodies that have been produced have been polyclonal. This situation is changing with improved fusion and selection protocols for monoclonal antibodies. The development of heterohybridomas using spleen cells from species such as sheep, which are known to produce higher-affinity antibodies than mice, may become increasingly common. This is, however, of most importance to limited-reagent assays for certain haptens, e.g. thyroxine and triiodothyronine, that have proved difficult to raise even high-affinity polyclonal antibodies against. With regard to excess reagent assays monoclonal antibodies are much to be preferred to polyclonal because of their defined specificity and high purity. It is mainly with agglutination assays that polyclonal antibodies still have the advantage but even here there is an increasing use of mixtures of monoclonal antibodies.

Specific Recognition Using Nonimmunological Recognition

Lectins

Lectins are a class of carbohydrate-binding proteins of nonimmune origin that agglutinate cells or precipitate polysaccharides and exhibit antibody-like sugar-binding specificity (Liener *et al.*, 1986). Lectins have been used extensively in the study of blood group antigens and other cellular interactions but have as yet received little use as recognition molecules in immunoassays and immunosensors, one exception being the measurement of the bone isoform of alkaline phosphatase (Rosalki and Foo, 1984).

Receptors

For certain drugs it can be very important to identify pharmacologically active structures, i.e. for their ability to bind to a particular receptor. Receptors are proteins, which usually consist of one or more sub-units and, although varying significantly in molecular mass, generally have a relative molecular mass of 100,000 or larger. There has been for example much discussion of the use of digoxin receptors as a specific binding agent (Soldin, 1992); another example is the use of cyclophilin for the measurement of cyclosporin (Soldin *et al.*, 1993). With the use of molecular biology techniques these receptors can be cloned for large-scale production, which can overcome some of the difficulties of obtaining large-scale reliable sources of receptor proteins.

Interference

Immunoassays using intact immunoglobulins can be prone to interferences that are unrelated to the specificity of the antigen binding site, for instance binding of rheumatoid factors and complement proteins to the Fc portion (Chambers *et al.*, 1987). Removal of the Fc portion leaving an $F(ab)_2$ or Fab fragment can prevent this type of interference. These antibody fragments are generated by proteolytic cleavage (papain) of the intact antibody and chromatographic purification of the cleaved products (Lamoyi and Nisonoff, 1983; Rousseaux *et al.*, 1983). This process requires careful optimisation to ensure a high yield of pure antibody fragment and adds significantly to the cost of the final antibody reagent; thus clear evidence of an interference with a particular antibody is needed before such a procedure should be considered. Not all assays that use intact immunoglobulins are prone to these interferences and there is some evidence that this may be due to the reaction conditions selected; furthermore there is the possibility of using sulphydryl reagents such as dithiothreitol to eliminate the interference at a more reasonable cost (Eng and Person, 1981).

Other interferences include human anti-mouse antibody (HAMA) and other human anti-animal species antibodies which can cause nonspecific binding of antibodies used in immunoassays. These can generally be blocked by addition of nonimmune immunoglobulin from the species in which the primary antibodies were prepared (Howanitz *et al.*, 1982).

Purity

In the case of polyclonal antibodies it is better that either an immunoglobulin fraction or an affinity-purified preparation is used. In the case of monoclonal antibodies, antibody fragments and sFvs (single-chain antibodies), chromatographically pure preparations should be made; for lectins and proteins A and G the commercial sources should already be pure, but there are always possibilities of batch-to-batch variations. A further alternative is to use purified second-antibody systems to capture the primary antibody. When an impure bioaffinity molecule is all that is available, e.g. for measuring an antibody concentration in a human serum sample, then it can be more appropriate to couple the ligand of interest to a surface. However, the coupling of a ligand will be much more idiosyncratic than binding an antibody, because of the much wider range of molecular structures, and can increase the possibility of nonspecific binding reactions.

STABILITY

Any alteration to the structure of the binding molecule will at least potentially alter the inherent kinetics of its interaction with a ligand (Olsen *et al.*, 1989; Spitznagel and Clark, 1993; Karlsson *et al.*, 1994). Adsorption to plastic can deform the protein; conjugation to an enzyme, fluorophore, isotope etc. can also cause the same effect either as a result of the size of the attached molecules or as a consequence of the conjugation reaction itself. Some immunoglobulin species may also be more prone to deformation and already weakened structures such as antibody fragments (as a result of exposure to enzymic digestion) may also be more compromised.

Immunoglobulin molecules are generally very robust and when conjugated to solid phases retain their immunological activity for several years (Butler, 1991; Thakkar *et al.*, 1991). Peptides can also be more stable conjugated to a solid phase than in free solution. The long-term stability of lectins on a solid phase is also likely to be good although there is little actual data; the least stable of the bioaffinity agents discussed are likely to be the receptor molecules, and their actual stability will be an individual characteristic. This can also be true for monoclonal antibodies, and the stability of these pure proteins needs to be individually determined.

The coupling of proteins to a solid phase *per se* has been shown to enhance the stability of a wide range of proteins (Butler, 1991; Thakkar *et al.*, 1991); the difficulties lie not with the storage of the coupled proteins but in their ability to retain their activity in multiple-use immunosensor systems when regeneration cycles are required. The primary determinant of the stability of the antibody under regeneration conditions will be the care with which these conditions have been optimised. Information on the likely stability of different antibody molecules to regeneration can often be obtained from publications concerning their use in affinity chromatography systems. Thus stability is inherently interlinked with tolerance to pH as modulation of pH is one of the most important dissociation factors. The coupling of enzymes and immunoglobulins to solid phases has been shown to enhance their tolerance to pH to include short exposure to pHs between 1 and 13 (Monsan and Combes, 1988). The pH range used can be reduced by inclusion of chaotropic agents such as acetonitrile (Hodginkson and Lowry, 1982) and the use of high ionic strength and detergents (Fulop *et al.*, 1993). These factors can be important for optimising regeneration conditions for multiple-use immunosensors.

Coupling Technique

The technique used to couple an antibody can have a profound effect on its utility (Al-Abdullah *et al.*, 1989; O'Shanessy *et al.*, 1992; Davies *et al.*, 1995; Hidalgo-Alvarez and Galisteo-Gonzalez, 1995). Most workers would agree that a covalent coupling technique is required for immobilisation to the surface and there is a wide range available (*see* Chapter 8). These can be complemented by techniques that enable spacers of various length to be introduced; the general aim of these techniques is to ensure a stable conjugation with an appropriate orientation of the molecules to enable fully functional interactions. These all require the molecule to be conjugated to have a suitable active residue for conjugation, most commonly a free amino group but carboxyl, aldehyde and sulphydryl groups can also be used. The different conjugation techniques use a range of pHs and reagents and these can have a profound effect upon the activity and stability of the conjugated antibody. If an appropriate orientation or activity cannot be obtained using direct coupling techniques then an indirect one such as second-antibody, protein A/G or biotin-streptavidin should be used. Further possibilities of protecting or stabilising unstable macromolecules include adding the antigen/ligand to the antibody to form a more stable complex which can then be conjugated to the solid phase, and the ligand removed.

CONCLUSIONS

Determination of an antibody's inherent affinity and specificity can be a useful pointer to selection of the reagent with the desired characteristics. The possibilities of real-time kinetic rate analysis and automated epitope mapping has resulted in the use of the BIACore™ and IA-Sys™ to characterise and select antibody combinations for use in other immunological systems. However, selection is a process with many stages and no final choice can be made until the prime candidates have been compared in the final assay format. Experience of multiple assay developments within different companies and research groups can give rise to a knowledge base concerning particular system-dependent characteristics of antibodies. This will obviously help in the designing of system-dependent approaches to selection. In general, however, selection of the best antibody or other binding agent is an iterative process requiring experience and a fundamental understanding of the intermolecular interaction involved and the system within which it is to be measured.

REFERENCES

Al-Abdulla, I. H., Mellor, G. W., Childerstone, M. S. & Smith, D. S. (1989) Comparison of three different activation methods for coupling antibodies to magnetisable cellulose particles *J. Immunol. Meth.* **122**, 253–258.

Albert, W. H. W. (1984) Monoclonal antibodies: Advantages and disadvantages in production of a test system. In: *New Technologies in Clinical Laboratory Science* (ed. Shinton, N. K.) pp. 83–96.

Berzofsky, J. A., Epstein, S. L. & Berkower, I. J. (1989) Antigen-antibody interactions and monoclonal antibodies. In: *Fundamental Immunology* 2nd edn (ed. Paul, W. E.) pp. 315–356, (Raven Press, New York).

Butler, J. E. (1991) The behaviour of antigens and antibodies immobilised on a solid phase. In: *Structure of Antigens* Vol I (ed. Van Regenmortel, M. H. V) pp. 209–260 (CRC Press New York).

Chambers, R. E., Whicher, J. T., Perry, D. E. *et al.* (1987) Overestimation of immunoglobulins in the presence of rheumatoid factor by kinetic immunonephelometry. *Ann. Clin. Biochem.* **24**, 520–524.

Davies, J., Dawkes, A. C., Haymes, A. G. *et al.* (1995) Scanning tunnelling microscopy and dynamic angle studies of the effects of partial denaturation on immunoassay solid phase antibody. *J. Immunol. Meth.* **186**, 111–123.

Day, E. D. (1990) Specificity and complementarity. In: *Advanced Immunochemistry* 2nd Edn, pp. 281–293 (Wiley-Liss, New York).

Dean, K. K. (1986) Immunoassay for non-enzymatically glucosylated proteins and protein fragments: an index of glycaemia. *US Patent* No. 4,629,692.

Dorman, L. (1977) Method for forming an amide bond between a latex and protein. *US Patent* No. 4,045,384.

Ekins, R. P. (1989) A shadow over immunoassay. *Nature* **340**, 256–258.

Eng, R. H. K. & Person, A. (1981) Serum cryptococcal antigen determination in the presence of rheumatoid factor. *J. Clin. Microbiol.* **14**, 700–702.

Friguet, B., Chafotte, A. F., Djavadi-Ohaniance, L. *et al.* (1985) Measurement of the true affinity constant in solution of antigen/antibody complexes by enzyme-linked immunosorbent assay. *J. Immunol. Meth.* **77**, 305–319.

Fulop, M. J., Webber, T. & Manchee, R. J. (1993) Use of a zwitterionic detergent for the restoration of the antibody binding capacity of immunoblotted *Francisella tubarensis* lipopolysaccharide. *Anal. Biochem.* **203**, 141–145.

Greene, H. E. & Duft, B. J. (1990) Disputes over monoclonal antibodies. *Nature* **347**, 117–118.

Hidalgo-Alvarez, R. & Galisteo-Gonzalez, F. (1995) The adsorption characteristics of immunoglobulins. *Hetero. Chem. Rev.* **2**, 249–268.

Hodgkinson, S. C. & Lowry, P. J. (1982) Selective elution of immunoadsorbed anti- (human prolactin) immunoglobulins with enhanced immunochemical properties. *Biochem. J.* **205**, 535–541.

Howanitz, P. J., Howanitz, J. H., Lamberson, H. V. *et al.* (1982) Incidence and mechanism of spurious increases in serum thyrotropin. *Clin. Chem.* **28**, 427–431.

Johne, B., Hansen, K., Mork, E. *et al.* (1995) Colloidal gold conjugated monoclonal antibodies, studied in the BIAcore biosensor and in the Nycocard immunoassay format. *J. Immunol. Meth.* **183**, 167–174.

Karlsson, R., Roos, H., Fägerstam, L. *et al.* (1994) Kinetic and concentration analysis using BIA technology. *Methods: A Companion to Meth. Enzymol.* **6**, 99–110.

Lamoyi, E. & Nisonoff, A. (1983) Preparation of F(ab)$_2$ fragments from mouse IgG of various subclasses. *J. Immunol. Meth.* **56**, 235–243.

Liener, I. E., Sharon, N. & Goldstein, I. J. (eds) (1986) *The Lectins, Properties, Functions, and Applications in Biology and Medicine* (Academic Press, New York).

Monsan, P. & Combes, D. (1988) Enzyme stabilisation by immobilisation. *Meth. Enzymol.* **137**, 584–598.

Multiple Authors (1993) Antibodies. In: *Methods of Immunological Analysis* Vol. 2 (eds Albert W. H. and Staines N. A.) pp. 147–427 (VCH, Basel).

Newman, D. J. & Price, C. P. (1996) Molecular mechanisms in immunoassay for drugs. *Ther. Drug Monit.* 18, 493–497.

Newman, D. J., Olabiran, Y. & Price, C. P. (1997) Bioaffinity agents for sensing systems. In: *Handbook of Biosensors and Electronic Noses: Medicine, Food, and the Environment* (ed. Kress-Rogers, E.) pp. 59–89 (CRC Press, Boca Raton, USA).

O'Shannessy, D. J., Brigham-Burke, M. & Peck, K. (1992) Immobilisation chemistries suitable for use in the BIAcore surface plasmon resonance detector. *Anal. Biochem.* 205, 132–136.

Olsen, W. C., Spitznagel, T. M. & Yarmush, M. L. (1989) Dissociation kinetics of antigen-antibody interactions: Studies on a panel of anti-albumin monoclonal antibodies. *Molec. Immunol.* 26, 129–136.

Rosalki, S. B. & Foo, A. Y. (1984) Two new methods for separating and quantifying bone and liver alkaline phosphatase isoenzymes in plasma. *Clin. Chem.* 30, 1182–1186.

Rousseaux, J, Rousseaux-Provost, R. & Bazin, H. (1983) Optimal conditions for the preparation of Fab and F(ab)$_2$ fragments from monoclonal IgG of different rat IgG subclasses. *J. Immunol. Meth.* 64, 141–146.

Scatchard, G. (1949) The attraction of proteins for small molecules and ions. *Ann. NY Acad. Sci. USA* 51, 660–672.

Soldin, S. J. (1992) Drug receptor assays: Quo vadis? *Ann. Clin. Biochem.* 29, 132–136.

Soldin, S. J., Murthy, J. N., Donnelly, J. G. *et al.* (1993) Immunophilin receptors for immunosuppressive drugs. *Ther. Drug Monit.* 15, 468–471.

Spitznagel, T. M. & Clark, D. S. (1993) Surface density and orientation effects on immobilised antibodies and antibody fragments. *Biotechnology.* 11, 825–829.

Stenman, U. H., Bidart, J. M., Birken, S. *et al.* (1993) Standardization of protein immunoprocedures – choriogonadotropin (CG). *Scand. J. Clin. Lab. Invest.* 51 (**suppl.** 205), 42–78.

Thakkar, H., Davey, C. L., Medcalf, E. A. *et al.* (1991) Stabilisation of turbidimetric immunoassay by covalent coupling of antibody to latex particles. *Clin. Chem.* 37, 1248–1251.

Chapter 7

Nonbiological Alternatives to Antibodies in Immunoassay

Lars I. Andersson and Klaus Mosbach

INTRODUCTION

The performance of an immunoassay or related technique critically depends on the properties of the ligand-binding species. Several types of binding molecule are available, but specific antibodies are the most familiar and the production of antibodies and their use in immunoassays form the focus of this book. Less widely used are assays based on naturally occurring circulating binding molecules (referred to as competitive protein-binding assays) or cellular receptors (receptor assays) (Barnett and Nahorski, 1983; Crevat-Pisano *et al.*, 1986; Ferkany, 1987; Iisalo *et al.*, 1988). For a given biologically active substance there exists a receptor site with which the substance must interact in order to evoke a response. The availability of a large number of endogenous compounds and receptor-active drugs labelled to a high specific activity allows the use of many such receptors in assay applications using membrane preparations obtained from biological tissue. The availability of an increasing number of cloned receptor preparations with much higher specific binding activity increases the utility of receptor assay technology.

The principal design of a receptor assay is analogous to the conceptually identical competitive immunoassay. The analyte ligand and a labelled specific ligand are presented to a restricted number of receptor sites. As the two ligands compete for binding to the same sites, the amount of labelled ligand bound to the receptors is quantitatively related to the amount of analyte present in the incubation medium. Some examples of substances measured by labelled receptor assay include anticholinergic drugs (Iisalo *et al.*, 1988), opiates (Levi *et al.*, 1987; Alburges *et al.*, 1991), β-blocking agents (Phan *et al.*, 1991), benzodiazepines (Bruhwyler and Hassoun, 1993), neuroleptic drugs (Rao, 1986), 1,25-dihydroxyvitamin D (Watanabe *et al.*, 1994), immunosuppressants (Murthy *et al.*, 1992), inositol phosphates (Bredt *et al.*, 1989), calcium channel antagonists (Quennedey *et al.*, 1989), leukotrienes (Kohi *et al.*, 1988; Simmet and Luck, 1988) and steroid drugs (Arts and Van den Berg, 1989; Soldin *et al.*, 1992).

The radioreceptor assays are experimentally simple and rapid and are sensitive and reliable. Their major limitation, which paradoxically is one of their benefits, is lack of specificity: any substance having an affinity for the receptor will displace the specifically bound radioligand. Hence the receptor assay determines the parent compound and active metabolites in proportion to their affinity for the specific receptor (Crevat-Pisano *et al.*, 1986; Iisalo *et al.*, 1988). This lack of specificity can be useful in applications such as the detection of previously unknown metabolites (Levi *et al.*, 1987), the measurement of total activity including active metabolites (Murthy *et al.*, 1992; Soldin *et al.*, 1992; Bruhwlyer and Hassoun, 1993) and the screening of drugs of abuse (Arts and Van den Berg, 1989; Alburges *et al.*, 1991). In the latter case, positive samples can subsequently be analysed with more sophisticated methods for confirmation of the identity of the compounds present.

Although animals can make antibodies against virtually any foreign chemical group (aided by the plethora of biotechnological and genetic methods available today), the availability of synthetically derived binding entities with predetermined specificities may create new opportunities for immunoassay technology. In applications such as on-line combination with chromatographic separation techniques and laboratory automation, among others, compatibility of the binding species with organic solvents and the ability to withstand thermal and mechanical stress are desirable properties. For many drug substances and other biologically active compounds of low molecular mass, their chromatographic separation from the other sample components is often affected by the use of eluents composed of organic solvents. The use of immunoassay for detecting and quantifying the eluted analyte peak provides the chromatographic separation system with excellent sensitivity. But such a combination requires antibodies resistant to organic solvent if the overall analysis scheme is to be run on-line. Stability of reagents is critical for automated analytical systems run outside the controlled laboratory environment, e.g. in production facilities. Several nonbiological binding systems can be envisaged, such as molecules designed and synthesised with the desired binding properties and synthetic polymers made by molecular imprinting techniques (Mosbach, 1992).

MOLECULAR IMPRINTING

Molecular imprinting (Wulff, 1986; Mallik *et al.*, 1994; Mosbach, 1994; Shea, 1994; Mosbach and Ramström, 1996) provides a means for the preparation of synthetic polymers with predetermined specificity. The polymerisation of monomers around a template species gives rise to imprints (actually 'cavities' or 'clefts') complementary to these template molecules in the resultant polymer. These imprints can be looked upon as synthetically derived counterparts to the antigen-combining sites of antibodies. To extend the analogy even further, in common with the immunogen-antibody relationship, the choice of imprint species determines the specificity of the respective polymer preparation.

Benefits

Provides a means for development of assays based both on organic solvent and on aqueous buffer.

Simple preparation: molecular imprinting of haptenic compounds is possible without prior chemical conjugation.

High tolerance to mechanical and thermal stress.

Excellent storage stability: ambient temperature and humidity is not problematic.

Nonbiological origin may lead to reduction in the number of laboratory animals used.

Limitations

Young technology: further research focusing on the analytical performance is desirable.

Table 1 Some characteristics of molecularly imprinted polymer (MIP)-derived antibody mimics.

Some features of the molecularly imprinted polymer (MIP)-based approach are summarised in Table 1. The high mechanical, thermal and solvent stability are characteristic of the polymer systems used. MIPs can be packed into high-performance liquid chromatography (HPLC) columns and used as specific chromatographic sorbents, demonstrating their resistance to high pressure and organic solvents. The column is packed using pressures of up to 35×10^6 Pa (350 bars) and such MIP columns have been used up to at least 100 times during a 9-month period with specificity maintained (Anderson *et al.*, 1994). The MIPs are compatible with autoclave conditions (120 °C, 20 min) and are unaffected by acid and base treatment (Kriz and Mosbach, 1995). The stability of the imprinted polymers is demonstrated further by their ability to be stored in the dry state at ambient temperatures for several years without detectable loss of recognition capabilities (Andersson *et al.*, 1994). In situations where it is desirable to bring the assay system out to the users in the field (e.g. in illegal drug control programmes) such technical features may be important decision criteria in the assay implementation.

Antibody preparation against low molecular mass compounds, i.e. haptens, necessitates conjugation of the hapten to a carrier protein (which may be difficult) before injection into the animal. Conjugation often changes the structural properties of the antigen exposed to the immune system and the antibodies elicited may be directed against a structure subtly different to the intended one. MIP preparation avoids the need for derivatisation of haptenic antigens as long as the hapten is soluble in the polymerisation mixture. For such antigens, molecular imprinting is increasingly becoming a viable alternative, especially when the antibody response is poor using traditional methods. In some instances, the absence of a requirement for derivatisation may result in superior specificity of the artificial system. Hence the imprint-derived antibody mimics may complement biological antibodies. Molecular imprinting is a simple and cheap experiment that can be performed in any reasonably equipped laboratory. How MIP preparation on an industrial scale will compare technically and economically with antibody production remains to be seen. Using laboratory equipment, molecular imprinting is, however, possible on a semi-industrial scale, with preparations of up to 250 g having been made (Andersson *et al.*, 1994). For an optimised assay system the amount of polymer used per individual assay is about 50 μg (Andersson, 1996), and hence such a batch size is sufficient for up to 5 million assays. On this scale the key consideration of MIP synthesis is the availability of the imprint species in sufficient quantity. The cost of the imprint species is, however, a minor issue because the production cost is split over a high number of analyses. A point worth mentioning is that MIP preparation does not involve the use of any material of biological origin, which may have good implications for the long-term availability of material with consistent quality. Provided the quality of the chemicals used is controlled, a MIP preparation can be reproduced with each batch having properties almost identical to those of the previous one. In our experience, the batch-to-batch variation of parameters, such as avidity, binding site density and specificity, have in most instances been small and could be considered negligible (Andersson, L. I., unpublished results). In those few cases for which variable results have been obtained, these have been due to variable quality of the imprint species.

Emerging antibody technologies, such as the use of naive libraries and antibody engineering (Borrebaeck, 1995), have many of the advantages described above for MIPs. These include the availability of antibodies against non-immunogenic substances, long-term production of antibodies of consistent quality, scale-up possibilities and predictable specificity pattern. Antibody technology is the alternative for the majority of antigens, such as biological macromolecules, whereas molecular imprinting is used for haptenic substances that can be dissolved together with the monomers in an organic solvent. For substances with limited water solubility and in situations where mechanical and chemical tolerance are desirable properties, MIPs may be a superior alternative. At present, MIPs are tools for the research scientist rather than the routine analyst although the increasing number of publications suggest that this may change in the not too distant future. Although early attempts in this field were of limited success, in recent years selective ligand-binding systems, not only examples mimicking those seen in biology but also quite novel ligand-receptor recognition systems, have been developed. Antibody-like affinities and selectivities are now becoming achievable with molecularly imprinted systems.

PREPARATION OF MOLECULAR IMPRINTS

As indicated above, MIP preparation involves the polymerisation of functional monomers in the presence of an imprint species (Figure 1). The monomers used are capable of engaging in reversible noncovalent (Andersson *et al.*, 1994, 1995b; Mosbach, 1994), reversible covalent (Wulff, 1986; Shea, 1994) or metal ion mediated (Mallik *et al.*, 1994) interactions with specific functionalities present in the imprint molecule. More specifically, the types of noncovalent interactions used are the very same as those involved in the antigen-antibody binding, namely hydrogen and ionic bonds, hydrophobic interactions, etc. During the polymerisation process the functional monomers become spatially fixed, via their interaction with the imprint species, in the polymer network. The end result is the formation of 'cavities' or 'clefts' with complementary shape and chemical functionality to the imprint molecule (Figure 1). Removal of the imprint species exposes these 'stamped memories' which later enable the polymer to re-bind the imprint molecule selectively from a mixture of closely related compounds.

Of the molecular imprinting approaches available, the noncovalent strategy (Andersson *et al.*, 1994, 1995b; Mosbach, 1994) is easier to use than its covalent (Wulff, 1986; Shea, 1994) counterpart. The imprint molecule is simply allowed to prearrange with the monomers in solution before initiation of the polymerisation (Figure 1), rather than requiring pre-derivatisation with functional monomers. Furthermore, a higher number of compounds are amenable to noncovalent imprinting and the final imprinted material is more versatile, at least for the type of application focused upon here (Andersson *et al.*, 1995b).

So far, bulk polymerisation, followed by grinding and particle sizing, has generally been the most often used technique for imprinted polymer preparation (Andersson *et al.*, 1994; Mosbach, 1994). More recently a technique has been developed leading to molecularly imprinted beaded polymers (Mayes and Mosbach, 1996). The imprint compound is dissolved in an organic solvent and mixed with the crosslinking monomer and one or more functional monomers. For maximal efficiency of imprint formation, at least for the type of polymers discussed here, the polymerisation reaction should take place in a solvent as apolar as possible without compromising solubility of the imprint species (Andersson *et al.*, 1994). This is to ensure maximal strength of the noncovalent interactions, such as hydrogen and ionic bonds. Following addition of azobis-nitrile initiators, the polymerisation is conducted either by elevating the temperature or by irradiation with UV light. To preserve the integrity of the imprints in the resultant MIP a very highly crosslinked polymer network is required. Ethylene glycol dimethacrylate is the most extensively used crosslinking monomer because of its mechanical and thermal stability, ease of removal of imprint molecule and the high selectivities that have been observed. Recently, some interesting more highly methacrylate-substituted crosslinkers have come into use in noncovalent imprinting applications and show promising properties (Kempe and Mosbach, 1995). Several functional monomers carrying chemical functionalities suitable for interacting noncovalently with the imprint molecule have been employed in MIP preparation. Methacrylic acid and vinyl-pyridine, in particular, have proved to be versatile in most situations. Combinations of these monomers can sometimes yield superior results (Ramström *et al.*, 1993). Generally, those monomers having methacrylate, acrylate or vinylic type polymerisable functionalities are compatible with the crosslinking strategies discussed here.

Although sometimes overlooked, the removal of the imprint species from the resultant polymer is critically important because a more thorough extraction yields a superior material where more of the high-avidity sites are free. Complete extraction requires extensive washing using solvents with strong elution power, such as aqueous ethanol containing acid or base.

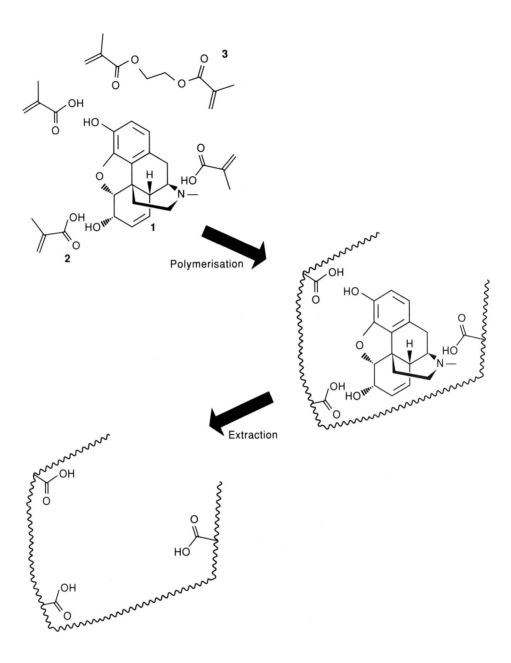

Figure 1 Scheme for the preparation of molecular imprints against morphine (1) using methacrylic acid (2) as the functional monomer and ethylene dimethacrylate (3) as the crosslinking monomer. In a typical preparation (Andersson *et al.*, 1995a) morphine-free base and 2,2'-azobis-(2-methylpropionitrile) (initiator of the polymerisation reaction) were dissolved in acetonitrile together with methacrylic acid and ethylene dimethacrylate. The mixture was sparged with nitrogen and polymerised at 60 °C for 16 h. The bulk polymer was ground to particles <25 μm and fines were removed by repeated sedimentation from ethanol for the extraction step. The particles were carefully washed with large amounts of ammonium acetate dissolved in a mixture of ethanol/acetic acid/water (2/1/1, *v/v/v*) followed by acetic acid in ethanol (1/3, *v/v*) and then by methanol. Finally, the particles were dried under vacuum and stored at ambient temperature until use. Reprinted with permission from *Nature* (1993) 361, 645–647. Copyright 1993 Macmillan Magazines Limited.

Intermittent acid and base washings may be beneficial. The prepared material can be stored in the dry state at ambient temperatures before use.

Safety precautions should be taken during the preparation of the polymerisation mixture and the grinding and extraction of the polymer. These steps should be performed in a fume cupboard because they involve the handling of organic solvents and monomers.

IMPRINTED POLYMER-BASED ASSAYS

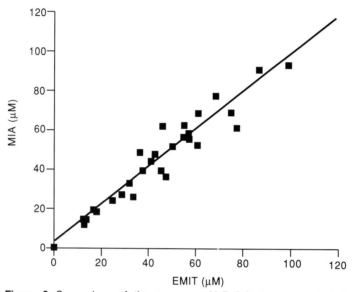

Figure 2 Comparison of the enzyme-multiplied immunoassay technique (EMIT) and MIP-based competitive binding assay (MIA) for determination of serum concentrations of theophylline in patient samples (Vlatakis *et al.*, 1993). Before the actual MIA assay, performed using an organic solvent, the analyte was extracted from serum. The sample was acidified with an equal volume of HCl and extracted with dichloromethane/isopropanolol (4/1, *v/v*). The organic layer was evaporated at 40 °C under a stream of nitrogen and redissolved in acetonitrile/acetic acid (99/1, *v/v*) containing [3H]theophylline. Antitheophylline polymer, suspended in the incubation solvent by vigorous stirring, was added and the mixture was incubated at room temperature. Bound and free radioligand were separated by centrifugation and the radioactivity in the supernatant was measured by liquid scintillation counting. Reprinted with permission from *Nature* (1993) 361, 645–647. Copyright 1993 Macmillan Magazines Limited.

In 1993 it was demonstrated that imprinted polymers can indeed be substituted for antibodies in immunoassay protocols (Vlatakis *et al.*, 1993). In this first study, molecular imprints against theophylline and diazepam were used in a competitive radioligand-binding assay for the determination of these drugs in human serum. The assay was given the acronym MIA for molecularly imprinted sorbent assay. Both drugs could be determined in clinically significant concentrations with an accuracy comparable to that obtained using a traditional immunoassay technique. Specifically, the calibration graphs of the assays for theophylline and diazepam were in the ranges 14–224 µmol l^{-1} and 0.44–28 µmol l^{-1} with detection limits of 3.5 µmol l^{-1} and 0.2 µmol l^{-1}, respectively, which in both cases are satisfactory for therapeutic monitoring of the drugs. Before the actual assay, performed under optimised incubation con-

Analyte	Imprint species	Medium	Detection limit	Reference
S-Propranolol	S-Propranolol	Buffer	6 nmol l^{-1}	Andersson (1996)
		Solvent	5.5 nmol l^{-1}	
Theophylline	Theophylline	Solvent	3.5 µmol l^{-1}	Vlatakis et al. (1993)
Benzodiazepines	Diazepam	Solvent	0.2 µmol l^{-1}	Vlatakis et al. (1993)
Morphine	Morphine	Buffer	0.22–0.79 µmol l^{-1}	Andersson et al. (1995a)
		Solvent	0.15 µmol l^{-1}	
Enkephalins	[Leu^5]-enkephalin anilide	Solvent		Andersson et al. (1995a)
Atrazine	Atrazine	Solvent	0.25 µmol l^{-1}	Siemann et al. (1995)
Atrazine	Atrazine	Solvent	4.6 µmol l^{-1}	Muldoon and Stanker (1995)

Table 2 Analytes that have been the focus for ligand-binding studies using MIPs.

ditions using organic solvents, the analyte is extracted from the serum using standard protocols derived from the corresponding high-performance liquid chromotography (HPLC) assay methods (see legend to Figure 2). Briefly, an organic solvent, such as heptane, diethyl ether, methylene chloride, etc., is added to the aqueous phase (in this instance the serum sample). The aqueous phase is adjusted to acidic, basic or neutral pH depending on which pH is most favourable for a quantitative extraction of the particular analyte into the organic phase. A comparison of the results obtained using a commercial immunoassay technique and the MIA competitive binding assay for the determination of theophylline in patient samples showed excellent correlation between the two methods (Figure 2). Since this first demonstration several further studies have been presented (Table 2), which have focused on improving the assay sensitivity and extending the assay to aqueous conditions.

Some of the more recently developed analyte MIP systems may be used equally well using an organic solvent or an aqueous buffer. This was demonstrated for morphine and enkephalin MIPs (Anderson et al., 1995a) and studied in detail using S-propranolol MIPs (Andersson, 1996) (Table 2). For the S-propranolol MIPs, an assay based on an aqueous buffer showed high substrate selectivity for propranolol in the presence of structurally similar β-blockers. The corresponding assay using toluene as the solvent showed excellent enantio-selectivity, the crossreactivity of the R-enantiomer being only 1%. These different selectivity profiles are due to a different balance between hydrophobic and polar interactions in toluene and water: polar interactions, such as hydrogen bonds, are strong in apolar solvents and hydrophobic interactions are strong in water. These achievements have extended molecular recognition by MIPs to aqueous buffers, adding flexibility to the development of the assay method. For example, in many environmental and bioanalytical methods a solvent extraction step is included in the sample work-up process. In such situations a MIP-based assay can be performed directly after the extraction, thus eliminating the need for evaporation of the solvent and reconstitution of the analyte in the assay buffer. Furthermore, some analytes are very poorly soluble in water, causing adsorption problems. Some attempts to use organic solvents with antibodies to such analytes have been described (Russell et al., 1989; Stöcklein et al., 1990; Weetall, 1991; Matsuura et al., 1993). The use of MIPs may enable extension of immunoassay technology to new analytical contexts and substances insoluble in water.

The low sensitivities of the early MIP-based assays have increasingly been improved by refinements of the MIP preparation and optimisation of the rebinding conditions (Andersson, 1996; Table 2).Because of the binding site heterogeneity, the apparent affinity (and hence the sensitivity) of the assay system is partly determined by the concentrations of polymer and labelled compound in the incubation mixture. At low polymer and radioligand concentrations, only the high-affinity sites are able to bind the radioligand and in the competitive assay the displacement events occur predominantly at these saturated high-affinity sites. Furthermore, under these conditions the nonspecific binding can be eliminated. Limits of determination as low as 6 nmol l^{-1} have been obtained (Andersson, 1996). Another one to two orders of magnitude improvement in detection limits may be achievable with the present detection system, which uses tritium-labelled tracers. Further increases in sensitivity may be obtainable with the use of other labelling techniques and detection systems, such as those based on recording fluorescence and enzymatic reactions. Future design of MIP-based assays is, however, open to speculation at this stage. The fact that the MIPs are insoluble polymer particles suggests that they might be used in assay formats such as particle counting assay and agglutination. Another area is that of biosensors where a biomolecule, such as an antibody or enzyme, is used in conjunction with an electronic transducer. Such sensory devices interact specifically with an analyte and provide a signal which may be monitored externally. Again, the greater inherent physical and chemical stability of MIPs make them suited to this role. The use of MIPs with field-effect type sensors (Hedborg *et al.*, 1993), amperometric sensors (Piletsky *et al.*, 1994; Kriz and Mosbach, 1995) and optic sensors (Kriz *et al.*, 1995) for substrate-selective determinations has been described.

Like polyclonal antibodies, the polymers contain a heterogeneous population of binding sites with a range of affinities for the imprint molecule. Thus, multiple equilibrium dissociation constants (K_D), varying from high to low affinity, are obtained on analysis of binding data. Apparent K_D values down to 10^{-9} mol l^{-1} have been obtained, which compare favourably with the 10^{-6}–10^{-14} mol l^{-1} range typical for antibodies. To obtain MIPs showing high avidity at least two issues need special attention. First, the imprint molecules must be removed quantitatively from the polymer and also from the very high-affinity sites. The use of a very thorough extraction protocol (as described above) improves assay sensitivity (Andersson, L. I., unpublished results). Second, the inherent affinity of the MIP needs to be increased through the preparation of imprints with a more precise complementarity to the imprint molecule. The noncovalent interactions that are used for imprinting are highly dependent on the medium used for polymerisation, which should be performed at low temperatures using a solvent as apolar as possible (see above). Further improvements are likely to follow the ongoing developments of the various imprinting technologies (Wulff, 1986; Mallik *et al.*, 1994; Mosbach, 1994; Shea, 1994). The combination of covalent imprinting with noncovalent rebinding may improve the homogeneity of the imprint population (Whitcombe *et al.*, 1995).

Both the theophylline and diazepam MIA methods described above show crossreactivity profiles for the major drug metabolites and structurally related drugs similar to the profiles obtained using commercial immunoassays based on biological antibodies. Anti-theophylline MIPs, for example, showed excellent selectivity for theophylline (1,3-dimethylxanthine) in the presence of the structurally related compound caffeine (1,3,7-trimethylxanthine) (Table 3). Despite their close resemblance (they differ by only one methyl group), caffeine showed less than 1% crossreactivity. More recently, some systems, such as morphine (Andersson *et al.*, 1995a) and *S*-propranolol (Andersson, 1996) MIPs, have been found to demonstrate selectivity profiles equal to or superior to those reported for biologically prepared antibodies. This is because MIP preparation avoids the need for derivatisation of haptenic antigens. Codeine,

Competitive ligand	Crossreaction (%)	
	MIP	Antibody
Theophylline (1,3-dimethylxanthine)	100	100
3-Methylxanthine	7	2
Caffeine (1,3,7-trimethylxanthine)	<1	<1
Theobromine (3,7-dimethylxanthine)	<1	<1
Xanthine	<1	<1
Hypoxanthine	<1	<1
Uric acid	<1	<1

Table 3 Selectivity profiles for theophylline assays based on MIPs and antibodies (Vlatakis *et al.*, 1993). Reprinted with permission from *Nature* (1993) 361, 645–647. Copyright 1993 Macmillan Magazines Limited.

which has a very closely related structure to morphine, interferes less with morphine binding to the imprinted polymers than with its binding to most of the anti-morphine antibodies reported so far. This finding is significant because codeine is a notoriously difficult crossreactant for biological anti-morphine antibodies. The use of a MIP-based *S*-propranolol assay can give enantio-selectivity that is superior to any of the corresponding biological antibodies reported so far (see above).

SUMMARY AND CONCLUSION

Molecular imprinting complements antibody technology in the context of assay development for low molecular mass compounds, i.e. haptens. In this area, molecular imprinting provides a tool by which recognition sites of predetermined specificity can be made for compounds of a diverse array of chemical classes. The imprinted polymers are resistant to harsh conditions, such as organic solvents, which most imprint-analyte binding experiments have, in fact, used so far. In the longer term, the organic solvent and mechanical stress tolerance of imprinted systems may allow the implementation of analytical methods combining immunoassay technology with chromatography, solid-phase extraction, liquid-liquid extraction, etc. Future research in this field is warranted, is expected to be rewarding, and should include the introduction of nonradioactive detection systems with a concomitant improvement in assay sensitivity.

REFERENCES

Alburges, M. E., Hanson, G. R., Gibb, J. W. *et al.* (1991) Fentanyl receptor assay. Development of a radioreceptor assay for analysis of fentanyl and fentanyl analogs in urine. *J. Anal. Toxicol.* 15 , 311–318.

Andersson, L. I. (1996) Application of molecular imprinting to the development of aqueous buffer and organic solvent based radioligand binding assays for (s)-propranolol. *Anal. Chem.* **68**, 111–117.

Andersson, L. I., Müller, R., Vlatakis, G. *et al.* (1995a) Mimics of the binding sites of opioid receptors obtained by molecular imprinting of enkephalin and morphine. *Proc. Natl Acad. Sci. USA* **92**, 4788–4792.

Andersson, L. I., Nicholls, I. A. & Mosbach, K. (1994) Molecular imprinting: A versatile technique for the preparation of separations materials of predetermined selectivity. In: *Highly Selective Separations in Biotechnology* (ed. Street, G.) pp. 206–224 (Blackie, Glasgow).

Andersson, L. I., Nicholls, I. A. & Mosbach, K. (1995b) Antibody mimics obtained by non-covalent molecular imprinting. In: *Immunoanalysis of Agrochemicals: Emerging Technologies* (eds Nelson, J. O., Karu, A. E. & Wong, R. B.) ACS Symposium Series 586 pp. 89–96 (American Chemical Society, Washington DC).

Arts, C. J. M. & Van den Berg, H. (1989) Multi-residue screening of bovine urine on xenobiotic oestrogens with an oestrogen radioreceptor assay. *J. Chromatogr.* **489**, 225–234.

Barnett, D. B. & Nahorski, S. R. (1983) Drug assay in plasma by radioreceptor techniques. *Trends Pharmacol. Sci.* **4**, 407–409.

Borrebaeck, C. A. K. (ed.) (1995) *Antibody Engineering* 2nd edn (Oxford University Press, New York).

Bredt, D. S., Mourey, R. J. & Snyder, S. H. (1989) A simple, sensitive and specific radioreceptor assay for inositol 1,4,5-triphosphate in biological tissues. *Biochem. Biophys. Res. Commun.* **159**, 976–982.

Bruhwyler, J. & Hassoun, A. (1993) Potential use of radioreceptor assay for the determination of benzodiazepine compounds in serum. *J. Anal. Toxicol.*, **17**, 403–407.

Crevat-Pisano, P., Hariton, C., Rolland, P. H. *et al.* (1986) Fundamental aspects of radioreceptor assays. *J. Pharm. Biomed. Anal.* **4**, 697–716.

Ferkany, J. M. (1987) The radioreceptor assay: A simple, sensitive and rapid analytical procedure. *Life Sci.* **41**, 881–884.

Hedborg, E., Winquist, F., Lundström, I. *et al.* (1993) Some studies on molecularly imprinted polymer membranes in combination with field effect devices. *Sens. Actuators* A37-38, 796–799.

Iisalo, E., Kaila, T. & Laurén, L. (1988) Radioreceptor assay of anticholinergic drugs. *Ann. Clin. Res.* **20**, 367–372.

Kempe, M. & Mosbach, K. (1995) Receptor binding mimetics: A novel molecularly imprinted polymer. *Tetrahedron Lett.* **36**, 3563–3566.

Kohi, F., Agrawal, D. K., Cheng, J. B. *et al.* (1988) The development of a sensitive and specific radioreceptor assay for leukotriene B_4. *Life Sci.* **42**, 2241–2248.

Kriz, D. & Mosbach, K. (1995) Competitive amperometric morphine sensor based on an agarose immobilised molecularly imprinted polymer. *Anal. Chim. Acta* 300, 71–75.

Kriz, D., Ramström, O., Svensson, A. *et al.* (1995) Introducing biomimetic sensors based on molecularly imprinted polymers as recognition elements. *Anal. Chem.* 67, 2142–2144.

Levi, V., Scott, J. C., White, P. F. *et al.* (1987) Improved radioreceptor assay of opiate narcotics in human serum: Application to fentanyl and morphine metabolism. *Pharm. Res.* **4**, 46–49.

Mallik, S., Plunkett, S. D., Dhal, P. K. *et al.* (1994) Towards materials for the specific recognition and separation of proteins. *New J. Chem.* **18**, 299–304.

Matsuura, S., Hamano, Y., Kita, H. *et al.* (1993) Preparation of mouse monoclonal antibodies to okadaic acid and their binding activity in organic solvents. *J. Biochem.* **114**, 273–278.

Mayes, A. & Mosbach, K. (1996) Molecularly imprinted beaded polymers and stabilised polymerisation of the same in perfluorocarbon liquids. PCT/US 96/06972.

Mosbach, K. (1992) Preparation of synthetic enzymes and synthetic antibodies and use of the thus prepared enzymes and antibodies. *US Patent* 5.110.833.

Mosbach, K. (1994) Molecular imprinting. *Trends Biochem. Sci.* **19**, 9–14.

Mosbach, K. & Ramström, O. (1996) The emerging technique of molecular imprinting and its future impact on biotechnology. *Bio/technology* **14**, 163–170.

Muldoon, M. T. & Stanker, L. H. (1995) Polymer synthesis and characterisation of a molecularly imprinted sorbent assay for atrazine. *J. Agric. Food Chem.* **43**, 1424–1427.

Murthy, J. N., Chen, Y., Warty, V. S. *et al.* (1992) Radioreceptor assay for quantifying FK-506 immunosuppressant in whole blood. *Clin. Chem.* **38**, 1307–1310.

Phan, T.-M. M., Nguyen, K. P. V., Giacomini, J. C. *et al.* (1991) Ophthalmic beta-blockers: Determination of plasma and aqueous humor levels by a radioreceptor assay following multiple doses. *J. Ocular Pharmacol.* **7**, 243–252.

Piletsky, S. A., Parhometz, Y. P., Lavryk, N. V. *et al.* (1994) Sensors for low-weight organic molecules based on molecular imprinting technique. *Sens. Actuators* B **18-19**, 629–631.

Quennedey, M-C., Ehrhardt, J-D., Welsch, M. *et al.* (1989) Improved radioreceptor assay for the determination of plasma levels of dihydropyridine calcium channel blockers in humans. *Ther. Drug Monitor.* **11**, 598–606.

Ramström, O., Andersson, L. I. & Mosbach, K. (1993) Recognition sites incorporating both pyridinyl and carboxy functionalities prepared by molecular imprinting. *J. Org. Chem.* **58**, 7562–7564.

Rao, M. L. (1986) Modification of the radioreceptor assay technique for estimation of serum neuroleptic drug levels leads to improved precision and sensitivity. *Psychopharmacology* **90**, 548–553.

Russell, A. J., Trudel, L. J., Skipper, P. L. *et al.* (1989) Antigen-antibody binding in organic solvents. *Biochem. Biophys. Res. Commun.* **158**, 80–85.

Shea, K. J. (1994) Molecular imprinting of synthetic network polymers: The *de novo* synthesis of macromolecular binding and catalytic sites. *Trends Polym. Sci.* **2**, 166–173.

Siemann, M., Andersson, L. I. & Mosbach, K. (1996) Antibody-like selective recognition of the herbicide atrazine in noncovalent molecularly imprinted polymers. *J. Agric. Food Chem.* **44**, 141–145.

Simmet, T. & Luck, W. (1988) Radioreceptor assay for leukotriene B_4. Use for determination of leukotriene B_4 formation by whole human blood. *Eicosanoids* **1**, 107–110.

Soldin, S. J., Rifai, N., Palaszynski, E. W. *et al.* (1992) Development of a radioreceptor assay to measure glucocorticoids. *Ther. Drug. Monitor.* **14**, 164–168.

Stöcklein, W., Gebbert, A. & Schmid, R. D. (1990) Binding of triazine herbicides to antibodies in anhydrous organic solvents. *Anal. Lett.* **23**, 1465–1476.

Vlatakis, G., Andersson, L. I., Müller, R. *et al.* (1993) Drug assay using antibody mimics made by molecular imprinting. *Nature* **361**, 645–647.

Watanabe, Y., Kubota, T., Suzumura, E. *et al.* (1994) 1,25-Dihydroxyvitamin D radioreceptor assay using bovine mammary gland receptor and non-high performance liquid chromatographic purification. *Clin. Chim. Acta* **225**, 187–194.

Weetall, H. H. (1991) Antibodies in water immiscible solvents. Immobilised antibodies in hexane. *J. Immunol. Meth.* **136**, 139–142.

Whitcombe, M. J., Rodriguez, M. E., Villar, P. *et al.* (1995) A new method for the introduction of recognition site functionality into polymers prepared by molecular imprinting: Synthesis and characterisation of polymeric receptors for cholesterol. *J. Am. Chem. Soc.* **117**, 7105–7111.

Wulff, G. (1986) Molecular recognition in polymers prepared by imprinting with templates. In: *Polymeric Reagents and Catalysts* (ed. Ford, W. T.) ACS Symposium Series vol. 308, pp. 186–230 (American Chemical Society, Washington DC).

Chapter 8

Separation Techniques

David J. Newman and Christopher P. Price

INTRODUCTION

All heterogeneous immunoassays require a procedure to separate the bound labelled ligand from the free. There have been several reviews focusing on this important aspect of immunoassay, notably Ratcliffe (1974), a multiauthor section in the book edited by Hunter and Corrie (1983) and more recently by Gosling (1990) and Masseyeff *et al.* (1993). Gosling reviewed the changing usage of the different approaches to separation; during the 1980s the use of solid-phase techniques increased from 40% to nearly 70% of new immunoassays and the majority of these (nearly 70%) were based on microtitre plates (Gosling, 1990). In the 1990s automated immunoassay systems have provided an increasing amount of new assay development and most of these use solid-phase technologies but relatively few are based on microtitre plates. Here we will summarise the salient features that are expected of a separation technique and, with passing reference to historical approaches, focus on those in current use with concluding comments on some future possibilities.

REQUIREMENTS OF A SEPARATION TECHNIQUE

An ideal separation technique will ensure complete separation of free and bound labelled antibody or antigen, without modulation of the primary antigen-antibody reaction and while remaining indifferent to the composition of the reaction matrix. If separation is incomplete, misclassification errors arise that result in assay bias and, if there is a lack of robustness, there will be an increase in assay imprecision. Such a lack of 'efficiency' in a separation technique can be due to physical trapping of the free ligand, adsorption of the free ligand to the assay tube, impurities in the labelled ligand or simply to a failure to remove all the supernatant liquid. The conventional measure of this 'efficiency' is the assay nonspecific binding.

If the separation technique interferes with the primary antigen-antibody reaction, and this can be by changing the rate of attainment of equilibrium or the equilibrium position reached, then a bias will be introduced that may also be variable (e.g. dependent on reaction time) and thereby increase imprecision. As immunoassays are performed in a variety of biological matrices e.g. whole blood, serum, plasma, urine, faeces, CSF, etc., a separation technique should be robust to the influence of 'matrix' effects.

In addition to the above fundamental attributes any separation system must also be practical (i.e. simple, quick and cheap), preferably be readily automated and be applicable to a wide range of analytes.

HETEROGENEOUS IMMUNOASSAY

Heterogeneous versus Homogeneous

The lack of a separation step is the mark of a homogeneous assay and this can be advantageous in terms of the speed and convenience of an assay. However, the inclusion of such a separation step provides the opportunity for introducing a wash step, which has many advantages for improving assay detection limits by removing interferents that can compromise the detection system and particularly reducing nonspecific binding, which is critical to overall performance of noncompetitive assays. Thus, although homogeneous assays have proved extremely useful for analytes in the micromolar concentration range and above, it is the heterogeneous systems that have demonstrated the sensitivity to measure analytes such as thyroid stimulating hormone (thyrotropin, TSH) in the pico to femtomolar concentration range.

Limited-reagent versus Excess-reagent Assays

As is discussed by Ekins in Chapter 9, and by other authors in this volume, it is the excess-reagent (or noncompetitive) assay systems that are the most influenced in their performance by nonspecific binding.

By contrast the performance of limited-reagent (or competitive) assays is determined more by the equilibrium constant of the reagent antibody. Thus the precision and detection limit of exces-reagent assays is significantly improved by the ability to wash the immunoaggregate; the development of these systems has thus been associated with the development of solid-phase separation technologies, which began in the early 1960s (Wide and Porath, 1966; Miles and Hales, 1968).

CLASSIFICATION OF SEPARATION TECHNIQUES

Separation systems can be classified as shown in Table 1 and represent a chronicle of assay development and increasing sophistication. The first separation procedures in immunoassay

Principle	Examples
Physicochemical characteristics of antibody or antigen	Electrophoresis: charge Chromatography: molecular size
Adsorption	Coated charcoal: binds free fraction Ion-exchange resins: charge Hydroxyapatite: charge
Fractional precipitation	Ethanol (usually at −20 °C) Polyethylene glycol, PEG (at around 200 g l⁻¹) Cross-linked dextran (at around 200 g l⁻¹) Ammonium or sodium sulphate (at around 200 g l⁻¹ or greater)

Immunological
  i) liquid phase
  ii) solid phase
	Anti-species secondary antiserum (± PEG)
	Primary antibody: particles, membranes, tubes, microtitre plates, paddles, etc.
	Secondary antibody: particles, membranes, tubes, microtitre plates, paddles, etc. anti-FITC–FITC

Non-immunological	Universal capture: protein A/G, streptavidin/biotin, lectins

Table 1 Classification of separation techniques.

were performed using the physicochemical differences between the immunoglobulin and the antigen. This approach, if size-related, was limited to assays for smaller molecules, e.g. haptens. Chromatography (thin-layer chromatography (TLC) initially) and electrophoresis gave high nonspecific binding, in the region of 20% or more of the total activity and were time-consuming and slow. These techniques were superseded by the dextran-coated charcoal and fractional precipitation approaches which were widely used in the 1970s and even the early 1980s. Although they were more practicable they still gave unacceptably high nonspecific binding in the range of 10–20%, required the use of a refrigerated centrifuge and, in the case of dextran-charcoal, could significantly interfere with the primary antigen-antibody reaction. Although the fractional precipitation techniques enhanced the molecular size range for analytes that could be measured, these techniques all suffered from an essential lack of specificity for the antibody. Their major advantage, and the reason that they survived so long, was that they used cheap reagents.

The introduction of secondary anti-species antisera was a major advance in finally introducing specificity for the essential component of the immunoassay reaction (Utiger *et al.*, 1962), bringing nonspecific binding down to the 5–10% region. The second antibody acted to increase the size of the immune complex to enable easier separation by direct centrifugation. The essential immunological specificity of this interaction also ensured that there was no interference with the primary antigen-antibody reaction. The downside was that they were relatively expensive and time-consuming, requiring overnight reactions and refrigerated centrifuges. This resulted in the development of a more economical approach to the use of secondary antibodies by combining them with a low concentration of polyethylene glycol (PEG, 40 g l^{-1}), thus reducing antisera usage, reaction time and the need for a refrigerated centrifuge, and further reducing the nonspecific binding to the region of 2% (Edwards, 1983b). This review will focus on the continuing development of immunologically based separation systems, which are now almost exclusively used with the primary antibody conjugated directly or indirectly to a solid phase.

IMMUNOLOGICAL SEPARATION SYSTEMS

Anti-species second antibodies became available in the late 1970s and early 1980s, and they are now widely available as both poly- and monoclonal antibodies. The ability to couple secondary antibodies (and more recently the primary antibody) to a solid phase has led to immunological separation systems being almost exclusively used in modern heterogeneous immunoassays. In an extension to the immunological specificities of primary and secondary antibodies there is now the potential to use the bacterial protein A or protein G, both having specific binding sites for the Fc region of immunoglobulins; lectins and the streptavidin-biotin reaction are other examples of separation systems of excellent specificity (Oliver *et al.*, 1982; Newman *et al.*, 1989).

The use of liquid-phase second-antibody systems, as described above, has the disadvantage of requiring relatively large amounts of antibody, long reaction times and the use of a refrigerated centrifuge. Using a liquid-phase system also has the disadvantage that washing of the precipitate requires great care. The development of particulate and subsequently tube and microtitre plate solid phases has enabled frequent washing ultimately without the requirement for a centrifuge and has reduced nonspecific binding to a fraction of 1%.

Size	Examples	Advantages	Disadvantages
Small particle (<20 μm)	Latex Microcrystalline-cellulose Fine porous glass Some magnetic particles Liposomes Starburst™ dendrimers	Dispensing as for liquids Agitation not required High antibody-binding capacity	Centrifugation required (unless used with a membrane capture) Long magnetic precipitation
Medium particle (<1mm)	Sepharose beads Sephacryl beads Sephadex beads	Centrifugation not required Short magnetic separation	Agitation required Slower reaction kinetics than above Moderate antibody-binding capacity
Single particle (>1mm)	Polystyrene Nylon	Centrifugation not required Agitation not required	Some variability in antibody coupling Lower antibody-binding capacity Difficulty in dispensing Poor reaction kinetics
Fibres	Membranes Glass fibre, nylon, silicone rubber	Centrifugation not required Agitation not required No dispensing of reagent Simple to use	Medium antibody binding capacity can be fast reaction kinetics
Solid surface	Coated tubes Dipsticks Microtitre plates	Centrifugation not required Agitation rare No dispensing of reagent Simple to use	Variability in antibody coupling Lowest antibody-binding capacity Slowest reaction kinetics

Table 2 Solid-phase supports for use as separation systems in immunoassay.

Solid-phase Immunological Separation Systems

An enormous range of solid-phase supports is now available, ranging from microparticulate to microtitre plates and membranes (Table 2). The relatively slow introduction of these techniques – they were known in the early 1960s (Catt and Tregear, 1967) but were not in widespread use until the 1980s – was due to difficulties in producing reliable coating/coupling procedures to link the antibodies to the solid phase. This was particularly a problem with tube and plate supports and as a result particulate solid phases were the first to receive widespread acceptance because their large surface area enabled more reproducible reaction conditions (Axon *et al.*, 1967; Bolton and Hunter, 1973; Chapman *et al.*, 1983; Douglas and Montieth, 1994).

Indirect

Immobilised capture agent	Ligand
Protein A	Fc of IgG, mouse IgG_{2A}, IgG_{2b}, IgG_3
Protein G	Fc of IgG, mouse IgG_1, IgG_{2A}, IgG_{2b}, IgG_3, IgG_4
Anti-species antibody	Primary antibody species of immunoglobulin
Streptavidin	Biotinylated antibody/antigen
Anti-DNP antibody	DNP-conjugated antibody/antigen
Anti-FITC antibody	FITC-conjugated antibody/antigen

Direct

Surface residue	Ligand active group	Conjugation chemistry
–COOH	$-NH_2$	Carbodiimide
$-NH_2$	$-NH_2$	Glutaraldehye
–OH	$-NH_2$	Cyanogen bromide
$-CONH_2$	$-NH_2$	Hydrazide
$-CONHNH_2$	–CHO	Hydrazine
–*N*-oxysuccinimide	$-NH_2$	Succinimide
–Maleimide	–SH	Maleimide
–Hydrazide	Periodate activated Carbohydrate	
Heterobifunctional agents	Various	Various

Table 3 Immobilisation techniques.

Coupling of Antigen/antibody to a Solid Phase

It should be remembered from the outset that it is possible to couple both the antibody and the antigen to a solid phase and both approaches have been used in heterogeneous immunoassays (Table 3). Proteins form the majority of molecules that will be conjugated to a solid-phase surface and can be either passively adsorbed or covalently coupled. For haptens, either small peptides or drugs, indirect conjugation via a linker or carrier protein will often be necessary and this will require covalent coupling techniques. Whole serum can be used as a source of antibody for conjugation but it is likely that the use of either an immunoglobulin G (IgG) fraction or even an affinity-purified antibody will result in better performance and a more reproducible product.

Adsorption. This is a process that is primarily dependent upon the p*I* of the protein and the nature of the surface (Horbett, 1992; Hidalgo-Alvarez and Galisteo-Gonzalez, 1995). Adsorption can also be a competitive process and displacement of an adsorbed protein by a serum protein such as albumin that occurs in relatively high concentrations may cause analytical difficulties (Elgersma *et al.*, 1992a, b). Other difficulties associated with adsorption are that first, although it is quite a high-affinity process, the use of detergents in washing solutions could at least potentially cause elution of protein; second, there is little control over the adsorption process and it is therefore impossible to control the orientation of the adsorbed protein and it is possible that this results in less immunoactive material on the surface (Spitznagel and Clark, 1993; Davies *et al.*, 1995). The denaturation effects of protein adsorption to polystyrene has even been put to use in the development of an immunoassay for glycated haemoglobin (Engbaek *et al.*, 1989). Thus in general the use of covalent coupling chemistries is to be preferred (Wood and Gadow, 1983).

Covalent Coupling. A wide range of coupling technologies has been used ranging from simple noncovalent adsorption to a plethora of covalent coupling methodologies (Table 3)(Axon *et al.*, 1967; Engvall and Perlmann, 1971; Bolton and Hunter, 1973; Chapman *et al.*, 1983; Wood and Gadow, 1983; Kemeny and Challacombe, 1988; Al-Abdulla *et al.*, 1989; O'Shannessy *et al.*, 1992; Veilleux and Duran, 1996). They range from the use of toxic agents, such as cyanogen bromide (Axon *et al.*, 1967), which require the appropriate facilities and experience to use, to less toxic agents, which enable smaller laboratories to prepare their own reagents with ease (Engvall and Perlmann, 1971; Chapman *et al.*, 1983; Wood and Gadow, 1983; Kemeny and Challacombe, 1988; Al-Abdulla *et al.*, 1989; O'Shannessy *et al.*, 1992; Veilleux and Duran, 1996). Whole antiserum, IgG preparations, affinity-purified antibodies, ascites fluid and antibody fragments have all been successfully coated onto solid-phase supports. Monoclonal antibodies tend to be more variable in the reaction conditions required than are polyclonal antisera, but their ready availability in large quantities makes their use much more attractive.

One aspect of coupling immunoreagents to solid phases is that their stability is enhanced. Thus latex particle-coupled antibody is stable for over a year stored as a liquid reagent (Thakkar *et al.*, 1991) and if solid phases are dried and stored desiccated the antibody is stable almost indefinitely (Voller *et al.*, 1979). Noncovalently bound antibody is less resistant to desorption than covalently bound but care is required in the selection of a benign coupling technique that does not damage the antibody in its own right (Wood and Gadow, 1983).

Primary versus Secondary Antibody versus Antigen

The advantages of coupling a secondary antibody to a solid phase are: no effect on the kinetics of the primary antigen-antibody reaction; applicability to a wide range of assays; and efficient use of primary antibody (Table 3). If the primary antibody is coupled to a solid phase this restricts the movement of the antibody and can considerably slow the rate of reaction with the antigen; also the solid phase is only suited for one assay (Nygren and Stenberg, 1989). The coupling process, whether covalent or noncovalent, will result in partial denaturation of the antibody molecule and it has been shown that the affinity constant of an antibody may change on coupling to a solid phase (Stenberg and Nygren, 1988). This loss of affinity/avidity can thus result in an increased usage of precious primary antibodies; this limited the usage of primary antibody solid phases until the advent of monoclonal antibodies rendered this a financial rather than a volume consideration. The continuing dilemma with solid-phase technologies is choosing between high antibody binding capacity and low nonspecific binding, because in general there is an inverse relationship between the two as the larger the surface area the greater the chance of nonspecific intereactions.

Antigen-antibody Kinetics at a Solid-phase Surface

The physical coupling of an antibody restricts its movement and the degree to which this influences the reaction kinetics depends upon the nature of the solid-phase surface and on the surface area of coupled antibody in relation to the volume and concentration of the other immunoreactants. As mentioned above, the intrinsic antigen-antibody reaction rates are lower for surface reactions than in free solution; the forward rate constant is reduced, but so is the reverse, and often to a greater extent, which can result in an overall increase in the equilibrium constant (Stenberg and Nygren, 1988; Nygren and Stenberg, 1989). However, because of the essentially irreversible nature of this binding interaction, the surface antigen/antibody can be considered multivalent, thus significantly increasing chances of reassociation; overall reaction rates can also become limited by the rate of diffusion of the solution-phase component as the surface concentrations become depleted.

The significance of diffusion effects will depend upon the geometry of the solid-phase surface, the intrinsic reaction rate and the surface concentration of antigen/antibody. The geometry is determined by particle size/surface area and the surface concentration by the choice of surface and coupling technique, with the intrinsic reaction rate determined by the choice of antibody. Diffusion effects are considered to be limiting only when the particle size of the solid phase exceeds 40 µm; that in general means large balls, paddles, tubes and microtitre plates. Membranes can be used to actively concentrate immunoreactants, increasing reaction rates (as described in Chapter 21) because of the large surface areas formed by the vast numbers of individual fibres. Microtitre plates will in general provide more favourable reaction kinetics than tubes as the local concentration of immunoreactants can be higher than in the larger volumes used in tube assays; however, overall microparticulate solid phases offer the fastest reaction kinetics because of their large surface area.

Antigen-coated solid phases can also be used; again care is required with larger protein molecules, and even some smaller peptides, as the partial denaturation that will occur on coupling to the solid phase will alter the expression of epitopes. Antigen-coated matrices have often been used in limited-reagent systems and as such are most appropriate to the measurement of small molecules, e.g. haptens. However, the recent development of anti-idiotypic antibodies has now enabled the development of excess-reagent systems for these same small molecules (Barnard and Kohen, 1990).

Universal Binding Agents

The main use of universal binding agents is in indirect coupling techniques (Table 3), enabling a standardised surface to be produced for use in a number of different applications (Voller *et al.*, 1979). Second, the use of a binding protein that is specific for a particular part of a bioaffinity agent, such as the Fc region of an immunoglobulin in the case of the bacterial, proteins A and G can result in a more favourable orientation of the bioaffinity molecule than direct coupling would allow.

Proteins A and G

Bacterial proteins with nonimmune binding specificities for the Fc portion of immunoglobulins have been found on the surface of a variety of *Streptococcus* and *Staphylococcus* species. Proteins A and G are examples of this type of bioaffinity agent (Boyle, 1990a). Protein A is a component of the cell wall of *Staphylococcus aureus*. It has a relative molecular mass of 42,000 and six independent binding sites for the Fc region of immunoglobulins from most mammalian species. Some binding to the Fab region also occurs, resulting in binding of IgA, M and E; the specificity of binding is enhanced by careful selection of the reaction conditions used for binding, particularly the pH.

Protein A is the prototype IgG-binding protein and has been used extensively for many immunochemical procedures, although the major use has been purification of IgG (Boyle, 1990b). Protein A reagents are extremely versatile: they can be used as secondary reagents for primary antibodies of different species, and may be radiolabelled, or fluorochrome or enzyme-conjugated. Protein G (Langone, 1978), a cell surface protein of group G *streptococci* is of the type III Fc receptor-binding proteins and binds to immunoglobulins by a similar manner to that of protein A, but its binding profile differs from that of protein A depending on the species origin of the immunoglobulin. However, neither have been extensively used in immunoassay or immunosensor systems and their potential may have been restricted by their relatively high price. Multiple use of a common surface is probably the only cost-effective means of using these reagents. The other difficulty lies with their specificity: the use of serum would be impracticable because of the binding of human immunoglobulins to protein A or G; this could give rise to a limited binding capacity for the specific immune complex and to increased nonspecific interactions.

Avidin-Biotin

The avidin-biotin system has been widely used in biology and is particularly attractive as a sandwich system used in conjunction with antibodies (Cruss, 1986). Avidin is a tetrameric protein with essentially identical subunits, each of relative molecular mass 15,000, found in egg white and with extremely high affinity (10^{-15} l mol^{-1}) for the water-soluble vitamin B$_6$, biotin (Bayer and Wilcheck, 1978). Biotin is relatively polar and can be coupled to antibodies under very mild conditions with little disruption to their structure. Avidin, coupled to fluorochromes, enzymes and other molecules may then be used as a stable high-affinity detection system. Both avidin and biotin are readily available commercially at little cost. The disadvantage of the system is the extremely basic nature of avidin (pI = 10.5) and thus it may bind nonspecifically by electrostatic forces.

Streptavidin, a binding protein isolated from *Streptomyces*, is an alternative to avidin. It has four identical chains, but amino acid analysis and comparison to avidin shows that strepavidin has only half the number of basic amino acids and therefore it would be expected to have a much less basic isoelectric point and correspondingly less nonspecific binding (Green, 1975). The streptavidin-biotin system can also be used as an enhancement technique as four biotin molecules can in theory be bound by each streptavidin molecule. Streptavidin-biotin in particular has found significant usage in immunoassay applications allowing liquid-phase reactions followed by rapid separation using a universal separation system with obvious cost benefits.

WASHING, NONSPECIFIC BINDING AND MATRIX EFFECTS

During the development of an immunoassay the optimisation of the reaction and washing buffers is of prime concern in reducing nonspecific binding and the influence of the biological

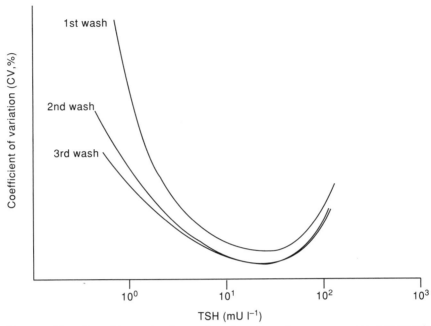

Figure 1 The effect of increasing the number of washing steps on an excess reagent assay precision profile.

matrix (Wood, 1991). The inclusion of buffer salts, chaotropes, proteins, e.g. BSA, and detergents such as Tween 20 is usual in the development of most immunoassays.

Most pertinent to this discussion is the effect of the buffer used in the washing step. In Figure 1 the effect of repeated washing on the precision profile for a TSH immunoradiometric assay (IRMA) is shown (a further example is given in Chapter 9, Figure 14). This demonstrates the improvement in detection limit and working range that wash steps can introduce, brought about essentially by reducing the nonspecific binding. The physical flushing that introducing a wash buffer produces is only one component of this effect. The inclusion of the same or similar agents as mentioned above for the reaction buffer, is also important. Washing removes entrapped label, reduces adsorption of label to surfaces and aids removal of the reaction supernatant. There is even recent evidence that wash steps can improve assay specificity (Self *et al.*, 1996). When using manual assays there was the choice as to whether to aspirate or decant the supernatant; despite early doubts concerning the reliability of decanting this is now the preferred technique, not only on the grounds of convenience but also of improved assay precision (Edwards, 1983a).

The manner in which the wash buffer is applied will vary depending upon the solid-phase matrix used. Particles, beads and microtitre plates can be washed actively but in general membranes will be washed by capillary flow or 'radial partition'. When the flow rate is slow, as in the latter case, the use of detergents and proteins in the wash fluid are even more important in reducing nonspecific binding.

Washing and separation steps have been automated in a variety of systems, e.g. microtitre plates (various commercial plate washers), membranes (Abbott Laboratories ImX®, Behring Opus-PB®), magnetic particles (Boehringer Mannheim, Elecys; Serono-Baker, SRI®; Tosoh, AIA 600®; Bayer, Immuno-1®; and the Corning ACS:180) and coated tubes (Boehringer, ES-600® and the Becton-Dickinson, Affinity®). The automation of these vital parts of a heterogeneous immunoassay has been among the most important developments in automating immunoassay (Wright and Hunter, 1983; Ehrhardt *et al.*, 1988) (see Chapter 13 for further discussion).

Mixing

The efficiency of washing as well as the overall rate of reaction can be profoundly influenced by the efficiency of the mixing approach used. The simplest form of mixing is to use the force of fluid dispensing; however, more efficient mixing can be provided by ultrasonic horns (Chen *et al.*, 1984) and in the case of magnetic particles by applying pulsed magnetic fields (Loebel, 1991); the DPC Immulite®; uses an ingenious form of centrifugal washing and mixing (Babson, 1991). All of these are likely to be more efficient at washing than the use of capillary flow and nonturbulent flow through systems that form the bulk of immunosensor technologies.

PARTICULATE SOLID PHASES

Particulate solid phases can be roughly divided into two types: nonmagnetic and magnetic.

Nonmagnetic Particulate Matrices

Nonmagnetic particulate matrices include latex, glass, Sepharose™, Sephadex™, Sephacryl™, nylon particles and beads. The choice between them is based on the relative coupling capacities of the different plastics and the size and density of the particles. The agaroses, e.g. Sephadex, and celluloses have higher antibody-binding capacities than polystyrene, nylon or glass although the absolute capacity per gram of particles will clearly depend upon the surface area available, i.e. on the size of the individual particles. On the basis of size, smaller polystyrene and glass particles can be more easily made. The choice of appropriate size will, as mentioned previously, depend upon the ease of use and reaction kinetics that are required (*see* Table 2). Examples of nonmagnetic particle systems in widespread use are the single, large (0.5 cm) nylon beads used in the kits from the Nichols Institute and in the Olympus automated immunoassay analyser, the Sucrosep separation system used in the Boots-Celltech range of assays and the microcrystalline cellulose system described by Chapman *et al.* (1983). The Sucrosep system used Sepharose beads in combination with a sucrose 'wash' solution, which prevented the need for a centrifugation step; this procedure was extremely efficient as a separation system (nonspecific binding <0.1%) but cumbersome to handle (Wright and Hunter, 1983).

There are several examples of particles used in combination with other matrices. These include the Abbott ImX, which uses primary antibody-coated latex particles to perform the primary antigen-antibody reaction and captures these particles on a glass-fibre membrane for separation and washing (Fiore *et al.*, 1988). Another combination approach is the use of antigen-coated particles as an affinity column, which acts both as a separation system and as part of the primary antigen-antibody reaction. Affinity column-mediated immunoassay (ACMIA) requires careful control of the elution step and as such is best performed in an automated fashion as exemplified by Freytag *et al.* (1984). A further example of an automated particle heterogeneous immunoassay was the use of the Centria® centrifugal analyser, which was used to automate a centrifugal separation step (Mériadec *et al.*, 1979).

Particle-based separation systems have been used with both hapten and protein assays and with all detection systems so far described for heterogeneous immunoassays.

Magnetic or Magnetisable Matrices

Magnetic or magnetisable particles have long been the favourite means for immunoassayists to avoid the use of a centrifugation based separation system (Hersh and Yaverbaum, 1975; Forrest and Rattle, 1983). The use of magnetic supports in immunoassay dates back to the early 1970s. The advantages of a magnetic particle are a high surface area, rapid analyte capture and properties that lead to efficient separation and washing. The most commonly used magnetic particle has been that made from paramagnetic ferrous oxide (Robinson *et al.*, 1973) and described by Forrest and Landon and used by Serono, Corning and other commercial companies (Forrest, 1977; Nargessi *et al.*, 1978; Milne *et al.*, 1988; Harmer and Samuel, 1989). The ferrous oxide is incorporated into a cellulose matrix, to which the antibody is coupled, to provide a stable reagent with low nonspecific binding. This was extended to develop a magnetisable charcoal reagent by co-trapping charcoal and ferrous oxide in a polyacrylamide gel. This approach considerably enhanced the use of charcoal as a separation matrix for hapten assays, in that it removed the centrifugation step but also in that there was less effect on the primary antigen-antibody reaction (Al-Dujaili *et al.*, 1979).

The ferrous oxide has proved superior to other magnetic components mainly because of its small particle size (10–20 nm) combined with a good magnetic response; the size is, however, increased dramatically during entrapment in the cellulose, the final particle size being determined by milling (1–3 μm). There have been relatively few advances in magnetic particle technology apart from the introduction of chromium dioxide particles in 1987 (Birkmeyer *et al.*, 1987). Deriving from audio-tape technologies, CrO_2 was suggested to offer less residual magnetism than ferrous oxide particles, i.e. offering better resuspension kinetics, and low nonspecific binding was achievable without incorporation into a polymer matrix, which thus allowed an overall smaller particle size of <5 μm without milling (Birkmeyer *et al.*, 1987). The low nonspecific binding characteristics of these particles are such that they have recently been used in a nonmagnetic ACMIA format in a whole-blood assay for cyclosporin (Hansen *et al.*, 1990). Other more recent advances include the development of ferrofluids, which are particles <50 nm in size that are almost as easy to handle as liquids (Weetall and Gaigalas, 1992).

The first magnetic particle assays used either batch processing in magnetic racks (e.g. Ciba-Corning) or automation in continuous flow systems. Automation has included unit-dose systems, such as the Serono-Baker SRI and the Tosoh AIA-600, as well as the Bayer Immuno-1 format multidose system. Magnetic particles have been used as secondary antibody separation systems and coupled to primary antibodies, in assays for haptens and proteins using a range of detection systems from isotopes, enzymes and fluorophores to chemiluminescence (ACS:180 from Ciba-Corning).

SOLID SURFACE MATRICES

The choice of a macro-solid phase is in general determined by a desire to simplify an assay protocol as much as possible. The choice of which plastic support to select is determined by the antibody-binding characteristics provided and the desired reaction kinetics. Macro-solid phases come in several formats described below.

Fibres (Membranes)

Two types of fibre have been used in immunoassays: first, cellulose or nitrocellulose, e.g. filter paper, and second, glass-fibre; both are used as part of larger membranous supports. The use of fibrous membranes provides a high surface area with high antibody-binding capacity. Direct coupling to cellulose is simple and has been mentioned above; coupling to glass-fibre is also simple and reproducible.

Cellulose membranes have been used in a wide variety of systems using a variety of washing protocols. The Dade Stratus® uses radial partition to wash an antibody-coated central portion of a glass-fibre membrane (Giegel *et al.*, 1982) (*see* also Chapter 22). The Hybritech ICON® uses monoclonal antibodies coupled to a cellulose matrix washed by the flow that is encouraged by an adsorbent layer below the membrane (Valkirs and Barton, 1985); a similar approach is found in the Behring-Syva Opus system (*see* also Chapter 21). Monoclonal antibodies have also been coupled to cellulose membranes in the Clearblue One Step™ (May, 1994), nitrocellulose in the FIAX® system (Wang *et al.*, 1980) and cellulose again in the immunochromatography systems (Zuk *et al.*, 1985) (*see* also Chapter 21).

Nitrocellulose membranes are commonly used in western blotting and this approach is extended to the so-called dot-ELISAs. These have been mainly limited to infectious disease assays so far but offer great potential for providing a simple multianalyte approach by immobilising several antibody 'spots' on a single strip of membrane (Pappas, 1988).

Coated Tubes

Coated tubes are one of the lowest-capacity solid phases used in immunoassay, although one of the earliest to be exploited (Catt and Tregear, 1967). Along with large single beads and microtitre plates their effective use is critically dependent upon the reproducibility of coupling of the antibody to each tube. Difficulties in achieving this led to very high rejection rates of batches of tubes in order to ensure satisfactory precision in the final assay. Coated-tube systems are in commercial use and have been automated by a number of manufacturers especially Boehringer in their ES series (Chan *et al.*, 1987). The low capacity of the solid phase can produce extremely low nonspecific binding, values of less than 0.01% are achievable although these are not routinely available because coated-tube enzyme-labelled systems rarely use 'total' tubes, which are needed to assess nonspecific binding.

Analogous to the use of coated tubes is the use of 'dip-sticks', which have not been widely used but are best suited to qualitative or semiquantitative assays and offer extremely simple protocols (Kemeny and Challacombe, 1988; Rasmussen 1988).

Microtitre Plates

Microtitre plates are probably the most popular solid phase in use at the present time despite the fact that they also have the lowest antibody-binding capacity. Plates are available in a range of plastics treated in a variety of ways (Kemeny and Challacombe, 1988; Rasmussen, 1988; Douglas and Monteith, 1994). The use of polystyrene plates that have been irradiated has been recommended by several authors (Kemeny and Challacombe, 1988; Rasmussen, 1988), with the capacity of the plates further enhanced by drying the antibody onto the plate. The standard format is the 96-well plate but strips and even individual wells are available. Although microtitre plates have been used with radiolabels (by cutting up the plates) they are most commonly used with nonisotopic systems using enzyme, chemiluminescent and fluorescent labels. The widespread application of microtitre plates required the development of suitable plate-based detection systems and it was delays in the development of these instruments that held back their introduction. One great advantage of microtitre plates that was immediately apparent to the immunoassayist was that less labelling of the tube/plate was required, reducing a very tedious and labour-intensive activity.

Difficulties with the plate format have included drift across the plate due to pipetting delays and temperature gradients across the plates due to their thermal insulating qualities. Batch-to-batch difficulties in preparation are also a problem and careful attention to quality control is required by commercial plate manufacturers. Because of the low capacity of the solid phase, reaction kinetics have been improved by incubating at elevated temperatures (37 °C) and using continuous vibration. Combinations of these approaches have resulted in extremely sensitive assays for proteins in only a few hours, e.g. the enzyme-amplified TSH assay using a kinetic plate reader (Clark and Price, 1986). The microtitre plate format does not lend itself to complete automation but there have been significant advances in work simplification that have resulted in partial automation, e.g. the Amerlite automated system (Johnson & Johnson) and the Auto-Delfia (Wallac).

CONCLUSIONS

A wide variety of solid-phase immunological separation systems has been developed and highly sensitive assays using a variety of detection systems have been achieved. Because of the use of washing techniques it is probably fair to say that it is the detection systems that limit the sensitivity of the assays (both excess and limited reagent) and not the capacity of the solid phase. The solid phase can, however, dictate the flexibility in the delivery system and the antibody binding capacity and reaction kinetics. The introduction of Starburst™ dendrimers (Dade International) and the magnetic particle system for the Boehringer Mannheim Elecys offer some interesting possibilities (Blackburn *et al.*, 1991; Singh *et al.*, 1994, 1996; Hoyle *et al.*, 1996).

FUTURE PROSPECTS

There are further advances in heterogeneous immunoassay that now extend to dry-film technologies (Hiratsuka *et al.*, 1982). The development of 'ambient analyte' assays (*see*

Chapter 9) offers a challenge to the traditional separation between heterogeneous and homogeneous immunoassays; although requiring solid-phase technology, it is inappropriate to consider its use as that of a separation system (*see* Chapter 9). A similar position applies to the surface-effect immunoassay techniques such as surface plasmon resonance and ellipsometry where the reaction is monitored 'through' the solid-phase matrix to which the immunoreactant is coupled and thus the 'solid phase' is an integral part of the measuring system (*see* Chapter 21). The future of immunoassay may thus not include separation as we know it, incorporating nanotechnology with vanishingly small reaction volumes and operator-transparent heterogeneous immunoassays (Kricka and Wilding, 1996).

REFERENCES

Al-Abdulla, I. H., Mellor, G. W., Childerstone, M. S. *et al.* (1989) Comparison of three different activation methods for coupling antibodies to magnetisable cellulose particles. *J. Immunol. Meth.* **122**, 253–258.

Al-Dujaili, E. A. S., Forrest, G. C., Edwards, C. R. W. *et al.* (1979) Evaluation and application of magnetizable charcoal for separation in radioimmunoassays. *Clin. Chem.* **25**, 1402–1405.

Axon, R., Porath, J. & Ernback, S. (1967) Chemical coupling of peptides and proteins to polysaccharides by means of cyanogen bromide. *Nature* **214**, 1302–1304.

Babson, A. L. (1991) The Cirrus Immulite™ Automated Immunoassay Analyser. *J. Clin. Immunoassay* **14**, 94–102.

Barnard, G. & Kohen, F. (1990) Idiometric assay: Non competitive immunoassay for small molecules typified by the measurement of estradiol in serum. *Clin. Chem.* **36**, 1945–1950.

Bayer, E. A. & Wilcheck, M. (1978) The avidin-biotin complex as a tool in molecular biology. *Trends Biochem. Sci.* **3**, N257–259.

Birkmeyer, R. C., Diaco, R., Hutson, D. K. *et al.* (1987) Application of novel chromium dioxide magnetic particles to immunoassay development. *Clin. Chem.* **33**, 1543–1547.

Blackburn, G. F., Shah, H. P., Kenten, J. H. *et al.* (1991) Electrochemiluminescence detection for the development of immunoassays and DNA probe assays for clinical diagnostics. *Clin. Chem.* **37**, 1534–1539.

Bolton, A. E. & Hunter, W. M. (1973) The use of antisera covalently coupled to agarose, cellulose and Sephadex in radioimmunoassays for proteins and haptens. *Biochim. Biophys. Acta.* **329**, 318–330.

Boyle, M. D. P. (ed.) (1990a) *Bacterial Immunoglobulin-Binding Proteins* Vol I: *Microbiology, Chemistry and Biology* (Academic Press, New York).

Boyle, M. D. P. (ed.) (1990b) *Bacterial Immunoglobulin-Binding Proteins* Vol II: *Applications in Immunotechnology.* (Academic Press, New York).

Catt, K. & Tregear, C. W. (1967) Solid-phase radioimmunoassay in antibody coated tubes. *Science.* **158**, 1570–1572.

Chan, D. W., Waldron, C., Bill, M. J. & Drew, H. (1987) The performance of a totally automated enzyme immunoassay system (ES 600). *Clin. Chem.* **33**, 947 [Abstract].

Chapman, R. S., Sutherland, R. M. & Ratcliffe, J. G. (1983) Application of 1,1'-carbonyldiimidazole as a rapid practical method for the production of solid-phase immunoassay reagents. In: *Immunoassays for Clinical Chemistry* 2nd ed. (eds Hunter, W. M. & Corrie, J. E. T.) pp. 178–190 (Churchill-Livingstone, Edinburgh).

Chen, R., Weng, L., Sizto, N. C. *et al.* (1984) Ultrasound accelerated immunoassay as exemplified by enzyme immunoassay of chorionic gonadotrophin. *Clin. Chem.* **30**, 1446–1451.

Clark, P. M. S. & Price, C. P. (1986) Enzyme amplified immunoassays: a new ultrasensitive assay of thyrotropin evaluated. *Clin. Chem.* **32**, 88–92.

Cruss, B. (1986) Structure of the IgG-binding regions of streptococcal protein G. *EMBO. J.* **5**, 1567–1575.

Davies, J., Dawkes, A. C., Haymes, A. G. *et al.* (1995) Scanning tunnelling microscopy and dynamic angle studies of the effects of partial denaturation on immunoassay solid phase antibody. *J. Immunol. Meth.* **186**, 111–123.

Douglas, A. S. & Monteith, C. A. (1994) Improvements to immunoassays by use of covalent binding assay plates. *Clin. Chem.* **40**, 1833–1837.

Edwards, R. (1983a) Discussion: Separation techniques. In: *Immunoassays for Clinical Chemistry* 2nd edn (eds Hunter, W. M. & Corrie, J. E. T.) p. 191 (Churchill-Livingstone, Edinburgh).

Edwards, R. (1983b) The development and use of a PEG assisted second-antibody as a separation technique in RIA. In: *Immunoassays for Clinical Chemistry* 2nd edn (eds Hunter, W. M. & Corrie, J. E. T.), pp. 139–146 (Churchill-Livingstone, Edinburgh).

Ehrhardt, V., Neumeier, D. & Meyer, H. D. (1988) Mechanization of heterogeneous immunoassays. *J. Clin. Immunoassay.* **11**, 74–80.

Elgersma, A. V., Zsom, R. L. J., Lykelma, J. *et al.* (1992a) Adsorption competition between albumin and monoclonal immuno-gamma-globulins on polystyrene latices. *J. Coll. Inter. Sci.* **152**, 410–428.

Elgersma, A. V., Zsom, R. L. J., Lykelma, J. *et al.* (1992b) Kinetics of single and competitive protein adsorption studied by reflectometry and streaming potential. *Coll. Surfaces* **65**, 17–28.

Engbaek, F., Christensen, S. E. & Jespersen, B. (1989) Enzyme immunoassay of haemoglobin A_{1c}: Analytical characteristics and clinical performance for patients with diabetes mellitus, with and without uremia. *Clin. Chem.* **35**, 93–97.

Engvall, E. & Perlmann, P. (1971) Enzyme-linked immunosorbent assay (ELISA): quantitative assay of IgG. *Immunochemistry* **8**, 871–874.

Fiore, M., Mitchell, J., Doan, T. *et al.* (1988) The Abbott ImX™ automated benchtop immunochemistry analyzer system. *Clin. Chem.* **34**, 1726–1732.

Forrest, G. C. (1977) Development and application of a fully automated continuous flow radioimmunoassay system. *Ann. Clin. Biochem.* **14**, 1–11.

Forrest, G. C. & Rattle, S. J. (1983) Magnetic particle radioimmunoassay. In: *Immunoassays for Clinical Chemistry* 2nd ed. (eds Hunter, W. M. & Corrie, J. E. T.), pp. 147–162 (Churchill-Livingstone, Edinburgh).

Freytag, J. W., Dickinson, J. C. & Tseng, S. Y. (1984) A high sensitivity affinity-column-mediated immunometric assay as exemplified by digoxin. *Clin. Chem.* **30**, 417–420.

Giegel, J. L., Brotherton, M. M., Cronin, P. *et al.* (1982) Radial partition immunoassay. *Clin. Chem.* **28**, 1894–1898.

Gosling, J. P. (1990) A decade of development in immunoassay methodology. *Clin. Chem.* **36**, 1408–1427.

Green, N. M. (1975) Avidin. *Adv. Prot. Chem.* **29**, 85–133.

Hansen, J. B., Lay, H. P., Janes, C. J. *et al.* (1990) A rapid and specific assay for cyclosporin on the DuPont aca discrete clinical analyser, performed directly on whole blood. *Transpl. Proc.* **22**, 1189–1192.

Harmer, I. J. & Samuel, D. (1989) The FITC-anti-FITC system is a sensitive alternative to biotin-streptavidin in ELISA. *J. Immunol. Meth.* **122**, 115–121.

Hersh, L. S. & Yaverbaum, S. (1975) Magnetic solid phase radioimmunoassay. *Clin. Chim. Acta.* **63**, 69–72.

Hidalgo-Alvarez, R. & Galisteo-Gonzalez, F. (1995) The adsorption characteristics of immunoglobulins. *Hetero. Chem. Rev.* **2**, 249–268.

Hiratsuka, N., Mihara, Y. & Miyazako, T. (1982) Method for immunological assay using multilayer analysis sheet. *U. S. Patent.* No 4,337,065.

Horbett, T. A. (1992) Adsorption of proteins and peptides at interfaces. In: *Stability of Protein Pharmacueticals, Part A: Chemical and Physical Pathways of Protein Degradation* (eds Ahern, T. A. & Manning, M. C.) pp. 195–214 (Plenum Press, New York).

Hoyle, N. R., Eckert, B. & Kraiss, S. (1996) Electrochemiluminescence: Leading edge technology for automated analyte detection. *Clin. Chem* **42**, 1576–1578.

Hunter, W. M. & Corrie, J. E. T. (eds) (1983) *Immunoassays for Clinical Chemistry* 2nd ed (Churchill-Livingstone, Edinburgh).

Kemeny, D. M. & Challacombe, S. J. (1988) Microtitre plates and other solid-phase supports. In: *ELISA and other Solid Phase Immunoassays: Theoretical and Practical Aspects* (eds Kemeny, D. J. & Challacombe, S. J.) pp. 31–56 (John Wiley and Sons, Chichester).

Kricka, L. J. & Wilding P. (1996) Micromechanics and nanotechnology. In: *Clinical Automation, Robotics and Optimisation* (eds Kost, G. J. & Welsh, J.) pp. 45–77 (John Wiley and Sons, New York).

Langone, J. L. (1978) [125]I Protein A: A tracer for general use in immunoassay. *J. Immunol. Meth.* **24**, 269–285.

Loebel, J. E. (1991) TOSOH AIA-1200/AIA-600 automated immunoassay analysers. *J. Clin. Immunoassay* **14**, 94–102.

Masseyeff, R. F., Delaage, M., Barbet, J. *et al.* (1993) Separation (distribution) methods In: *Methods of Immunological Analysis vol.1* (eds Masseyeff, R. F., Albert, W. H. & Staines, N. A.) pp. 475–533 (VCH, Basel).

May, K. (1994) Unipath Clearblue One Step[TM], Clearplan One Step[TM] and Clearview[TM]. In: The Immunoassay Handbook. (ed. Wild, D.) pp. 233–235 (Macmillan Press, London).

Mériadec, B., Jolu, J.-P. & Henry, R. (1979) A new and universal separation system technique for the 'Centria' automated radioimmunoassay system. *Clin. Chem.* **25**, 1596–1599.

Miles, L. E. M. & Hales, C. N. (1968) Labelled antibodies and immunological assay systems. *Nature* **219**, 186–189.

Milne, C. N., Pritchard, G. J., Allen, G. J. *et al.* (1988) Automation of enzyme immunoassays for hormones. *J. Endocr.* **119**, (suppl. 89) [Abstract].

Nargessi, R. D., Landon, J., Pourfarzaneh, M. *et al.* (1978) Solid phase fluoroimmunoassay of human albumin in biological fluids. *Clin. Chim. Acta* **89**, 455–460.

Newman, D. J., Medcalf, E. A., Gorman, E. G. *et al.* (1989) A novel solid phase enzyme-immunoassay for beta-2-microglobulin. *Biologie Prospective. Comptes Rendus du 7° Colloque de Ponte-à-Mousson.* (eds Galteau, M.-M., Siest, G. & Henny, J.) pp. 119–122 (John Libbey, Eurotext).

Nygren, H. & Stenberg, A. M. (1989) Immunochemistry at interfaces. *Immunology* **66**, 321–327.

O'Shannessy, D. J., Brigham-Burke, M. & Peck, K. (1992) Immobilisation chemistries suitable for use in the BIACore surface plasmon resonance detector. *Anal. Biochem.* **205**, 132–136.

Oliver, J. R., Hakendorf, P., Zeegers, P. *et al.* (1982) A proposed simple method for detection and measurement of antibodies to insulin in serum by use of staphylococcus aureus containing protein A. *Clin. Chem.* **28**, 121–123.

Pappas, M. G. (1988) Dot enzyme-linked immunosorbent assays. In: *Complementary Immunoassays* (ed. Collins, W. P.) pp. 113–134 (John Wiley and Sons, Chichester).

Rasmussen, S. E. (1988) Solid phases and chemistries. In: *Complementary Immunoassays.* (ed. Collins, W. P.) pp. 43–55 (John Wiley and Sons, Chichester).

Ratcliffe, J. G. (1974) Separation techniques in saturation analysis. *Brit. Med. Bull.* **30**, 32–37.

Robinson, P. J., Dunhill, P. & Lilly, M. D. (1973) The properties of magnetic supports in relation to immobilized enzyme reagents. *Biotech. Bioeng.* **15**, 603–606.

Self, C. H., Dessi, J. L. & Winger, L. A. (1996) Ultraspecific immunoassays for small molecules: role of wash steps and multiple binding formats. *Clin. Chem.* **42**, 1527–1531.

Singh, P., Moll III, F., Lin, S. H. *et al.* (1994) Starburst™ dendrimers: Enhanced performance and flexibility for immunoassays. *Clin Chem.* **40**, 1845–1849.

Singh, P., Moll III, F., Lin, S. H. *et al.* (1996) Starburst™ dendrimers: a novel matrix for multifunctional reagents in immunoassays. *Clin. Chem.* **42**, 1567–1569.

Spitznagel, T. M. & Clark, D. S. (1993) Surface density and orientation effects on immobilised antibodies and antibody fragments. *Biotechnology* **11**, 825–829.

Stenberg, M. & Nygren, H. (1988) Kinetics of antigen antibody reactions at solid-liquid interfaces. *J. Immunol. Meth.* **113**, 3–15.

Thakkar, H., Davey, C. L., Medcalf, E. A. *et al.* (1991) Stabilisation of turbidimetric immunoassay by covalent coupling of antibody to latex particles. *Clin. Chem.* **37**, 1248–1251.

Utiger, R. D., Parker, M. L. & Daughaday, W. H. (1962) Studies on human growth hormone. I:A radioimmunoassay for human growth hormone. *J. Clin. Invest.* **41**, 254–261.

Valkirs, G. E. & Barton, R. (1985) ImmunoConcentration®- a new format for solid-phase immunoassays. *Clin. Chem.* **31**, 1427–1431.

Veilleux, J. K. & Duran, L. W. (1996) Covalent immobilisation of bio-molecules to preactivated surfaces. *IVD Tech.* **2**, 26–31.

Voller, A., Bidwell, D. E. & Bartlett, A. (1979) *The Enzyme-linked Immunosorbent Assay (ELISA)* (Dynatech Europe, UK).

Wang, R., Merrill, B. & Maggio, E. T. (1980) A simplified solid phase immunofluorescence assay for measurement of serum immunoglobulins. *Clin. Chim. Acta* **102**, 169–177.

Weetall, H. H. & Gaigalas, A. K. (1992) Studies on antigen-antibody reactions using light scattering from antigen coated colloidal particles. *Anal. Lett* **25**, 1039–1053.

Wide, L. & Porath, J. (1966) Radioimmunoassays of proteins with the use of Sephadex coupled antibodies. *Biochim. Biophys. Acta.* **130**, 257–262.

Wood, W. (1991) Matrix effects in immunoassays. *Scand. J. Clin. Lab. Invest.* **51** (suppl. 205), 105–112.

Wood, W. G. & Gadow, A. (1983) Immobilisation of antibodies and antigens on macro solid phases: A comparison between adsorptive and covalent binding. Part 1 of a critical study of macro solid phases for use in immunoassay systems. *J. Clin. Chem. Clin. Biochem.* **21**, 789–797.

Wright, J. F. & Hunter, W. M. (1983) The sucrose layering separation: A non-centrifugation system. In: *Immunoassays for Clinical Chemistry* (eds Hunter, W. M. & Corrie, J. E. T.) 2nd ed., pp. 170–177 (Churchill-Livingstone, Edinburgh).

Zuk, R. F., Ginsberg, V. K., Houts, T. *et al.* (1985) Enzyme immunochromatography: A quantitative immunoassay requiring no instrumentation. *Clin. Chem.* **31**, 1144–1150.

Chapter 9

Immunoassay Design and Optimisation

Roger P. Ekins

INTRODUCTION

Immunoassay methods based on radioisotopic labels have played a major role in medicine during the past three-and-a-half decades. Their importance derives from the 'structural specificity' of antigen-antibody reactions and the 'detectability' of isotopically labelled reagents, the latter permitting observation of the binding reactions between exceedingly low reactant concentrations. These attributes have endowed radioimmunoassay (RIA) and immunoradiometric assay (IRMA) methods with unique specificity and sensitivity characteristics, largely accounting for their ubiquitous use in modern medicine and biology. More recently, interest has focused on non-isotopic techniques based on identical principles, albeit differing in the marker used to label the reactant (antibody or antigen) whose distribution between reacted ('bound') and unreacted ('free') moieties constitutes the immunoassay 'response'.

The reasons underlying this recent development are diverse. They embrace various environmental, legal, economic and practical considerations, such as the limited shelf life of isotopically labelled reagents, the problems of radioactive waste disposal, the cost and complexity of radioisotope counting equipment, the demand for simple diagnostic kits for home use etc., most of which are primarily of social or logistic significance. Other reasons are more fundamental, relating to the development of methodologies addressing analytical objectives unattainable by conventional isotopic techniques. Such prospective methodologies include transducer based 'immunosensors' for directly measuring analyte concentrations in biological and other fluids, and the 'multianalyte' immunoassay systems – briefly described in Chapter 24 – currently under investigation in the author's laboratory. The development of methods displaying improved performance compared with isotopically based techniques – in particular, greater sensitivity – also falls under this heading. The feasibility of this particular aim follows from the theoretical demonstration that, in certain assay designs, the specific activities of radioisotopes such as ^{125}I constitute a major limitation on sensitivity, implying that nonisotopic labels of higher specific activity offer the means of developing 'ultrasensitive' methods (Ekins, 1977).

A requirement for highly sensitive assay techniques capable of measuring very low concentrations of hormones and other such substances in biological fluids provided the principal initial stimulus for the development of RIA and other 'protein-binding' methods in the late 1950s and early 1960s. Moreover, the crucial need to identify assay conditions yielding maximal assay sensitivity (e.g. the physicochemical properties and optimal concentrations of the reagents used) underlay the independent construction of mathematical theories of 'ligand assay' design by both Yalow and Berson (1968) and me (1968) in the course of the original development of these techniques. Indeed, as discussed below, the description 'competitive assay' commonly applied to certain immunoassay (and other analogous ligand assay) methods does not represent a particular analytical concept, but merely reflects the finding that, in certain immunoassay designs, the attainment of maximal sensitivity demands the use of a relatively low antibody concentration (labelled and unlabelled forms of the analyte therefore being perceived as 'competing' for the limited number of antibody binding sites present). Further improvement in sensitivity (leading, *inter alia*, to further reductions in assay performance times) remains a prime (though not the sole) objective of methodological development in this field, despite the fact that many biologically important substances (such as drugs) that are conveniently measurable by immunoassay circulate at high concentration, and extreme sensitivity as such is of less importance in these cases.

In view of the crucial importance of assay sensitivity, it is perhaps surprising that the concept of sensitivity itself has, in the past, been widely misunderstood in this and other areas of science, and has therefore constituted the source of intense controversy relating to immunoassay design. Although confusion relating to the concept has now apparently been largely eliminated – at least amongst clinical chemists – certain mythologies remain as a legacy of past misunderstandings in this area. It is therefore important first to clarify the concept of 'sensitivity' and other terms descriptive of assay performance prior to discussion of the basic principles of immunoassay design.

TERMS DESCRIPTIVE OF ASSAY PERFORMANCE

Basic Concepts

The objective of all immunoassay procedures – as of other analytical methods – is to derive an estimate of the measured quantity as close as possible to the true or correct value, i.e. one that is devoid of error. In common usage, such a measurement is described as 'accurate', but unfortunately the meaning of this term has been distorted by clinical chemists and others (see below), and its use in the present context is therefore better avoided (Youden and Steiner, 1975). Meanwhile errors of measurement may conveniently be divided into two classes: (1) systematic errors, which consistently deflect all repeated measurements of the same quantity from the true value, thus constituting the source of assay bias, and (2) random errors, which affect individual measurements inconsistently and cause a scatter of results about some average value, generally termed imprecision (or precision).

There is, however, no hard and fast distinction between bias and imprecision; the classification of an error as systematic or random depends on the viewpoint from which the error is perceived. For example, replicate measurements (within an assay batch) of an analyte concentration in a test sample may be subject to a systematic error characteristic of the particular batch (due, for example, to error in the standards), implying that the mean result will be biased. If the measurements are subsequently repeated, the second batch may be subject to a systematic error of different magnitude, implying that the second mean result will be biased to a different extent. Further determinations will yield a succession of (randomly) biased mean results. Thus the overall scatter of individual results on the same sample as determined in the different batches (described as inter-assay, or inter-batch, imprecision) reflects both intra-assay (or 'intra-batch') imprecision and the variable bias characterising individual batches. For these reasons, inter-batch imprecision can never be less, and is almost invariably somewhat greater, than intra-batch imprecision (assuming the latter does not vary significantly between batches). It is nevertheless not unusual to see inter-assay coefficient of variation (CV) values reported in the literature that are less than intra-assay values. This is generally because inter-assay CVs have been calculated using the means of intra-assay replicate (e.g. duplicate, triplicate) determinations. The resulting estimate of inter-assay precision is therefore partially dependent on the particular habits of the analyst, and is a potentially misleading indicator of assay performance.

Precision and the Precision Profile

Although, as discussed below, precision – like sensitivity – has been defined in diverse ways, it is now generally accepted as relating to the reproducibility of replicate determinations, either within an assay batch, or between batches, laboratories, or methods, the scatter of such determinations being usually represented by their standard deviation (SD) or CV. This has led to an insistence by some authors on use of the word 'imprecision', on the syntactical grounds that the larger the SD or CV, the greater the imprecision. However, the concept of precision should not be confused with the particular parameter by which it is represented, and the term 'precision' will therefore be generally used in this chapter without, it is hoped, ambiguity or semantic contradiction. (Strict adherence to such rules would require replacement of 'sensitivity' by 'insensitivity' when referring to an assay system's ability to measure low analytic concentrations, since this is generally numerically represented by the lower limit of detection of the system or a closely related parameter.)

The precision of an analyte concentration measurement varies depending on whether replicate determinations are performed in the same sample or in different samples in the same batch, in different batches, in different laboratories, or using different assay methods. In short, a 'hierarchy' of precision values exists for any specified analyte concentration, each successive 'tier' encompassing a wider range of sources of random error. Clearly the precision estimate used to assess the significance of experimental results must correspond to the conditions of the study and the use to which the results are to be put. For example, when comparing the effect on serum insulin of the ingestion of a chocolate bar, it is desirable to measure all samples from the subject in the same batch, and to assess the statistical significance of differences in insulin concentration by reference to the intra-sample, intra-assay precision of the method. However, when monitoring a subject over the course of a year, serum samples are likely to be assayed in different batches, and intra-sample inter-assay (or 'inter-batch') precision thus constitutes the relevant parameter in assessing the statistical significance of any concentration changes observed.

A second general observation is that precision varies with analyte concentration, this variation being represented by the assay precision profile (Ekins, 1976) (Figure 1). Clearly the profile can be represented in as many ways as precision itself, for example, in terms of SD or CV. Analogously there exists a hierarchy of profiles – intra-assay, inter-assay, etc. – corresponding to the different circumstances in which precision may be assessed (Ekins, 1983b). However, for present purposes it is sufficient to consider only the intra-sample, intra-assay precision profile (on which assay design is increasingly commonly based).

The precision with which any two analyte concentrations are respectively determined defines the degree of confidence with which they can be said to differ. Because in most assay systems the SD of analyte measurements varies slowly with analyte concentration (Fig 1a), the SD of any specified 'basal' concentration essentially governs – to a close approximation – the minimum detectable difference (MDD) from it. For example, if the SD of serum thyroxine estimates at the 100 ng ml^{-1} level is 10 ng ml^{-1}, a measurement of 110 ng ml^{-1} implies an 84.1% probability (note that a one-tail statistical test is appropriate) that the sample actually contains a concentration >100ng ml $^{-1}$. Likewise a result of 120 ng ml^{-1} implies a 97.7% probability that the level exceeds 100 ng ml^{-1}. The MDD from 100 ng ml^{-1} can thus be said to be 10 or 20 ng ml^{-1} (or whatever), depending on the confidence level attaching to the claim. In short, the MDD from any specified analyte concentration constitutes an alternative representation of the latter's precision of measurement.

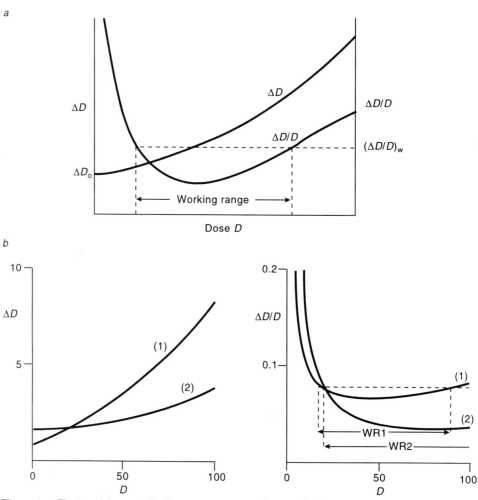

Figure 1 *a*, The 'precision profile' of an assay portrays the error in the dose estimate as a function of dose. The error may be represented, *inter alia*, by the absolute error (ΔD; e.g. SD of D) or the relative error ($\Delta D/D$; e.g. CV of D). ΔD_0, the error in the measurement of zero dose, represents the sensitivity of the assay. The working range may be defined as the range of dose estimates within which $\Delta D/D$ is less than a value $(\Delta D/D)$w acceptable to the investigator. *b*. The more sensitive of the two assays (assay 1) intercepts the ΔD axis at a lower value. Assay (2) is more precise at higher dose values, and has a much wider working range.

Concepts of Assay Sensitivity

The Lower Limit of Detection

A special case of the concepts discussed above is the MDD from a baseline analyte concentration of zero (or zero 'dose') which is primarily determined by the precision of the zero-dose estimate. This quantity is generally referred to as the 'minimum detectable dose', 'lower limit of detection', or 'detection limit' of the assay, and is indicative of the assay system's ability to determine analyte concentrations close to zero, i.e. its 'sensitivity'.

Certain authors have described statistically rigorous methods of calculation of the detection limit, taking into consideration such factors as the number of replicates, the required confidence level, the use of a one-tail test of significance, etc. (Rodbard 1978). Nevertheless, although examination of the immunoassay literature reveals that detection limits have often, in practice, been incorrectly determined, it is questionable whether the limit, even when correctly calculated in the manner described by Rodbard (1978), provides the most useful indicator of assay sensitivity. For example, it is evident that, if samples are measured in quadruplicate the means of the estimates are twice as precise as individual estimates, implying in turn that, other factors being equal, the formally calculated minimum detectable dose is halved. An assay based on quadruplicates might therefore be claimed to be twice as sensitive as one relying on singleton estimates, albeit the difference would not, of course, reflect superior assay performance, but merely the greater number of replicate determinations relied on by the analyst. But it is clearly misleading, when comparing the sensitivities of different assay methods, to use a parameter that encompasses factors (such as the number of replicates) that are not truly indicative of the performance characteristics of the assay system itself.

A second criticism of the detection limit (calculated formally as recommended by Rodbard (1978)) as a measure of sensitivity is that it constitutes no more than an unnecessarily complex representation of assay precision at dose levels close to zero. For both these reasons, my view is that the sensitivity of any assay system is most simply, logically and satisfactorily represented by the precision (i.e. standard deviation) of the zero-dose measurement, thus avoiding all unnecessary statistical complications involved in the calculation of the formal detection limit. The SD of the zero-dose measurement provides a clear and unambiguous indication of the lowest concentration levels that can be measured with acceptable precision with the system. For example, if the SD of zero-concentration measurements is 10 pg ml^{-1}, it may be legitimately inferred that (singleton) estimates of concentrations close to zero are characterised by random errors of the same order, and that the measurement of a concentration of about 100 pg ml^{-1} would thus be likely to possess a CV of approximately 10%. Such an assay would clearly be more sensitive than one characterised by a zero-dose SD of 10 ng ml^{-1}, which would be incapable of yielding precise measurements in the sub-nanogram per millilitre range. Assay sensitivity can, in short, be unambiguously represented by the zero-dose intercept of the (SD) precision profile (Figure 1a), the more sensitive of two assays being that yielding greater precision of (i.e. a lower SD in) the zero-dose estimate (Figure 1b).

Just as in the general case, there clearly exist 'intra-sample, intra-assay', 'inter-sample, intra-assay', 'intra-sample, inter-assay' precisions of the zero-dose measurement. In other words, an assay system displays a hierarchy of sensitivities. For example, if replicate measurements of a sample containing zero analyte are made within the same immunoassay run or batch, the SD of the estimates is likely to be less than if different samples, each known to contain no analyte, are examined in a similar fashion (Albano *et al.*, 1972). This difference arises because variations in sample viscosity, etc. (which give rise, in many immunoassays, to variable matrix effects) constitute an additional source of random error or variance. Thus inter-sample, intra-assay sensitivity is likely to be less than intra-sample, intra-assay sensitivity, although the latter is generally quoted in the published literature.

Regrettably no convention exists regarding the calculation and representation of assay sensitivities, and the claim that the sensitivity of a method is, for example, 10 pg ml^{-1} does not guarantee that it is superior to another supposedly possessing a sensitivity of 20 pg ml^{-1}. Fortunately, although differences in calculation methods complicate comparison of published assay techniques, this problem is of lesser importance in the context of assay design, i.e. in the identification of conditions yielding maximal sensitivity. In these circumstances, apparent sensitivity improvements deriving from changes in design are likely to be real, assuming that the assayist uses the same method of calculation throughout.

Attention should also be drawn in this context to another term that has recently appeared in the immunoassay literature: that is 'functional sensitivity'. This refers to the analyte concentration measured with an inter-assay precision (CV) of 20%. Essentially this parameter represents the lower limit of (a particular definition of) the assay working range, and represents a reasonable and useful concept, notwithstanding the differences in the manner in which analysts estimate interassay precision (see above), and the entirely arbitrary nature of the 20% cut-off. Furthermore it would seem preferable, to avoid further confusion, to distinguish the concept of sensitivity (i.e. the ability of an assay to detect an analyte concentration differing from zero) from that of the assay working range (the range of analyte concentrations that are measured with a precision appropriate to the particular needs of the analyst). In many cases (such as the detection of viral antigens in blood), the sensitivity of the assay (as represented by its lower limit of detection) is the parameter of special importance to the analyst, the working range (however defined) being essentially irrelevant.

The Slope of the Dose-Response Curve

An important corollary of these ideas is that the sensitivity of an assay methodology or design cannot be assessed unless errors in the zero-dose measurement are specifically estimated. This constitutes the crucial distinction between the statistical concept of sensitivity discussed above and the 'response curve slope' definition relied on by Yalow and Berson (1970) Berson and Yalow (1973) in their classic publications relating to immunoassay design. This fundamental difference underlay the controversies that centred on this topic during the mid-1960s to mid-1970s (see, for example, Ekins, 1968, Borth, 1970, Ekins *et al.*, 1970), controversies that have never been fully resolved and the effects of which have persisted to the present time. Thus many workers in the field continue to refer to 'sensitive curves', or to the 'sensitive part of the dose-response curve', and to use other similar expressions reflecting the identification of the response curve slope with sensitivity. Indeed certain official bodies continue formally to define the sensitivity of an analytical system or instrument in this manner, even if this definition has frequently been criticised as both illogical and unworkable (e.g. Jones, 1959), and leads to many absurdities. (For example, a recent publication, *International Vocabulary of Basic and General Terms in Metrology* (1993), prepared by a working group of experts appointed by the International Bureau of Weights and Measures (BIPM), the International Electrotechnical Commission (IEC), the International Federation of Clinical Chemistry (IFCC), the International Organisation for Standardisation (ISO), the International Union of Pure and Applied Chemistry (IUPAC), the International Union of Pure and Applied Physics (IUPAP) and the International Organisation of Legal Metrology (OIMI) reverts to a definition of sensitivity in terms of the slope of the dose-response curve.)

Confusion and disagreement on this issue have seriously influenced immunoassay development and indeed persist; the contrasting implications of these two concepts of sensitivity (Figure 2) should therefore be briefly illustrated. Figure 3a shows theoretical (labelled analyte) immunoassay dose-response curves relating analyte concentration ([A]) to the response variable fraction bound (B), calculated for different antibody concentrations ([Ab]). (The calculations are based on equations deriving from the mass action laws, assumed to govern antigen-antibody reactions.) It is visually apparent (and algebraically demonstrable) that the slope at zero dose ($dB/d[A]_0$) is maximal when $[Ab] = 0.5/K$ where K is the equilibrium constant, under which conditions the zero-dose response (B_0) = 0.33. This observation underlay Berson

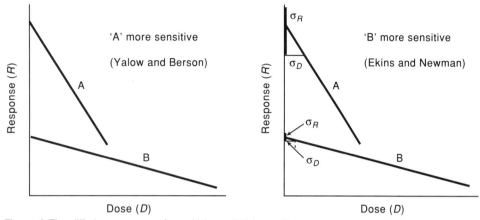

Figure 2 The differing concepts of sensitivity underlying radioimmunoassay design theories developed by Yalow and Berson (Ekins, 1968, 1983; Borth, 1970; Rodbard, 1978) and Ekins and Newman (Ekins, 1968, 1974; Ekins *et al.* 1968, 1970; Ekins and Newman, 1970). Yalow and Berson define assay A as the more sensitive because it yields a response curve of greater slope. Ekins *et al.* define assay B as more sensitive because the imprecision of measurement zero dose (σ_D) is less.

and Yalow's claim (Yalow and Berson, 1968, 1970; Berson and Yalow, 1973) that maximal RIA sensitivity is achieved using an antibody concentration resulting in 33.3 % binding of labelled antigen at zero dose: a dictum which remains a cornerstone of current immunoassay design practice.

Its fallacious nature is immediately revealed, however, simply by plotting identical data in other coordinate frames. For example, Figure 3b illustrates plots of $1/B$ against [A], the resulting curves progressively increasing in slope as [Ab] approaches zero, as is also the case when the response is expressed as B/B_0 (Figure 3c). Likewise, assuming the assayists choose to measure both free and bound labelled analyte fractions (as many workers in this field have done in the past), they will reach totally contradictory conclusions regarding the effects on assay sensitivity of a change in [Ab] depending on whether they plot response curves in terms of the free to bound ratio (F/B) or the bound to free ratio (B/F). Differences in slope are less conspicuous when data are plotted in terms of logit B/B_0 against log [A], but maximal slope is again observed as [Ab] tends to 0. In short, the antibody concentration yielding maximal slope is entirely dependent on the coordinate frame used to plot the response curve, illustrating the absurdity of regarding the slope as a valid indicator of assay sensitivity.

Defending their approach, Berson and Yalow argued that 'if the experimental error (in the response measurement) is unchanged, increasing the sharpness of the dose-response curve results in a reduction in minimal detectable quantity' (Berson and Yalow, 1973), illustrating this claim by an example involving the assumption that the statistical error (i.e. the CV) in the measurement of the response remained unchanged at 10%. (Elsewhere (Yalow, 1970) these authors defended the latter assumption by suggesting it was their common practice to count all radioactive samples for an equal number of counts, thus ensuring constancy of CV in regard to the counting component of the error in the response.) But the only circumstance in which the slope $dB/d[A]_0$ is a valid indicator of the detection limit arises when the standard deviation of B (not the CV) is constant, irrespective of the value of B. Thus even if the CV of B were constant, this would not lead to the conclusion that the detection limit is minimised (i.e. that assay sensitivity is maximised) when an antibody concentration of $0.5/K$ is selected;

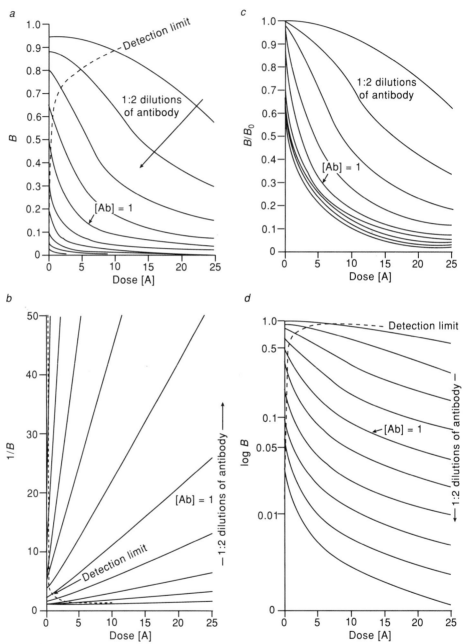

Figure 3 Typical RIA dose response curves plotted in terms of: *a*, fraction (or percentage) labelled analyte bound (*B*) versus analyte concentration [A]; *a*, b versus [A]; *b*, 1/*B* vs [A]; *c*, *B/B₀* versus [A]; *d*, log *B* versus [A]. All concentrations are expressed in terms of 1/*K*. The assay detection limit (based on the assumption of a 10% error in the measurement of the response at zero dose) is defined by the point of intersection of the response curve with the dotted line. Note that, irrespective of the manner in which the response curve is plotted, maximal sensitivity (minimal detection limit) is observed as the antibody concentration approaches zero.

indeed it is readily demonstrable that, in such circumstances, the value of [Ab] yielding maximal sensitivity is 0 (Figures 3a-d).

Although Berson and Yalow's justification for equating $dB/d[A]_0$ with the detection limit is clearly fallacious, such considerations reveal the implicit assumption underlying the common identification of the slope of the response curve with sensitivity, i.e. that the SD in the response variable (or response metameter) remains unchanged, irrespective of the latter's value and of any alteration in assay design. (When assay data conform to this condition, they are said to be 'homoscedastic'. 'Heteroscedasticity' implies nonuniformity of response variance, this being a common feature of immunoassay methods, irrespective of the response metameter used to plot assay results.) But even if this assumption were fortuitously true in the case of an individual assay using a particular response variable (e.g. fraction or per cent bound (B)), it would be false were results plotted in terms of some other variable (e.g. B/B_0 or logit B/B_0). In practice it is seldom, if ever, possible to identify an assay response variable for which the SD remains constant regardless of changes in assay design, implying that the slope of the response curve at zero dose would constitute a valid indicator of the assay detection limit.

Disagreement regarding the concept of assay sensitivity has inevitably led to dispute regarding optimal immunoassay design. Similar disagreements have also centred on precision, even though this attracted less attention than the conflicting definitions of sensitivity. Berson and Yalow defined precision as $dB/(d[A]/[A])$ (i.e. $dB/d\log[A]$), and identified the conditions under which this quantity (i.e. the slope of the B versus log dose-response curve) is maximal (Yalow and Berson, 1970; Berson and Yalow, 1973). As with these authors' concept of sensitivity, this definition disregards errors in the measurement of the assay response, and is therefore unrelated to the statistical concept of precision discussed above and accepted throughout all fields of analysis (Youden and Steiner, 1975).

To summarise, it is evident that untenable concepts of both sensitivity and precision underlie the theory of immunoassay design developed by Berson and Yalow, though conclusions deriving from it have profoundly influenced the immunoassay protocols adopted by many investigators and manufacturers and still do so. Examination of past debate and publications in this area thus reveals myths, preconceptions and prejudices have constituted a significant impediment to the development of new assay methods, such as 'ultrasensitive assays' in the mid-to-late 1970s, and the miniaturised array-based technology now under collaborative development by the author (*see* Chapter 24).

Bias and Accuracy

The concept of bias – the systematic error arising in a measurement – is both well understood and uncontroversial, and little needs to be added to the brief description of the meaning of this term given earlier in this chapter. Though the concept itself is straightforward, assessment of bias is difficult, because it presupposes knowledge of the true analyte concentrations against which measured values must be compared. In the case of certain analytes, the existence of a reference method – supposedly capable of yielding true values – may make such comparison possible, at least in principle. However, for many analytes (e.g. glycoprotein hormones such as thyroid-stimulating hormone (TSH), follicle-stimulating hormone (FSH), erythropoietin, etc.), true values for their concentrations in body fluids neither exist nor are reference methods available. Such analytes comprise a mixture of isohormonal forms, each differing in structure and biological activity. It is impossible to measure the concentration of

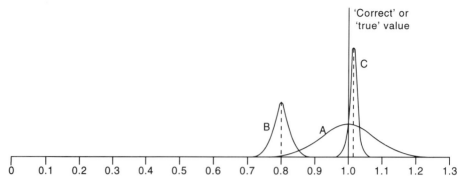

Figure 4 Distribution of assay results yielded by three (hypothetical) immunoassay kits with respect to a true analyte concentration of 1.0 (arbitrary units). Kit A is unbiased, but imprecise. Kit B is both biased and relatively imprecise. Kit C is extremely precise but slightly biased. Kit A is defined as the most accurate (IFCC definition (Büttner *et al.*, 1979)), albeit results yielded by Kit C are (on average) closer to the true value.

such a mixture meaningfully, and the concept of bias is therefore equally meaningless under these circumstances (*see* Ekins, 1991). In these circumstances assay bias is neither a valid concept, nor can it be measured in practice.

Another issue relating to assay bias is its identification, by certain official bodies, with the concept of accuracy (Büttner *et al.*, 1979). Although it is arguable that an organisation is free to define the meaning of words in whichever way it wishes, problems are likely to arise if the definition conflicts with the word's common meaning, or leads to absurdities of the kind that arise if 'sensitivity' is defined as the slope of the dose-response curve. Thus the identification of accuracy with bias, although not as serious in its consequences, can lead to nonsensical and contradictory conclusions: for example, the proposition that the majority of results yielded by the less accurate of two assay methods may in fact be closer to correct values (*see* Figure 4).

The Assay 'Working Range'

The 'working range' of an assay is that range of analyte concentrations over which measurements are of a precision sufficient for the particular needs of the assayist. Because this depends on the particular use to which assay results are put, the working range reflects a subjective judgement, though this does not imply that the judgement should be arbitrary and without scientific basis. In particular, proper assessment of the working range requires statistical information of the kind embodied in the precision profile. For example, if the assayist is willing to accept results for which the CV is less than 10%, a horizontal line drawn across the CV profile at this level (Figure 1) defines the range. Nevertheless, it is perhaps regrettable that no convention exists defining a standard CV value enabling the working ranges of different assay procedures to be compared, especially as such information is frequently of greater importance than knowledge of assay sensitivity, and the experimental steps required to maximise the range are therefore equally deserving of attention.

BASIC PRINCIPLES OF IMMUNOASSAY AND OTHER 'BINDING ASSAYS'

General Concepts

The terms 'binding assay' or 'protein binding assay' are generally applied to the broad category of techniques based on observation of the binding reaction between the analyte and a 'specific' protein (or mixture of proteins), i.e. one which essentially reacts only with the analyte. Antibodies – the reagent basis of immunoassays – constitute a class of binding proteins of special value in this context, since antibodies specific to most substances of biological interest can be readily prepared (if necessary in virtually pure form) by appropriate immunisation and selection procedures. But other classes of proteins have been used in a similar manner; likewise oligonucleotide probes have come into increasing use in assay techniques identical in principle to immunoassay and other protein binding assays.

It is inappropriate to review the history of these methods in detail in this chapter; however, it is relevant to identify certain conceptual milestones in their development, particularly those relating to assay design. Immunoassay was a well established technique by the early 1950s, but Berson and Yalow are generally credited with first recognising, in 1959, the possibility of assaying antigens such as insulin using a small amount of specific antibody and radiolabelled antigen as a marker of unlabelled antigen present in the system (Yalow and Berson, 1959). Termed radioimmunoassay (RIA), the analytical approach underlying this and other analogous binding assay techniques, and their physicochemical basis, had also been independently recognised by me in 1954, although experimental studies relating to its exploitation (in assays for thyroxine and, coincidentally, insulin) were delayed (through lack of funds) until 1957. As indicated earlier, the methodology has subsequently been frequently portrayed in terms of a 'competition' of labelled and unlabelled analyte molecules for a restricted number of protein binding sites. Such assays are consequently often referred to as 'competitive', albeit controversially: the term competitive was explicitly excluded from the title *Steroid Assay by Protein Binding*, one of a series of the Research Methods in Reproductive Endocrinology published by the Karolinska Institute and WHO (*see* Borth, 1970), on the grounds that, in many such assays, the labelled hormone is chemically identical to the unlabelled material, and no 'competition' (in the sense in which this term is conventionally used in biochemistry) is involved. But although it constitutes a simple and readily understandable representation of their mode of operation, this concept misrepresents the more fundamental principles by which these assays are governed (*see* below).

The next major advance in binding assay methodology was the development by Wide in Sweden (1967), and shortly after by Miles and Hales in the UK (1968a), of labelled antibody methods of immunoassay. When the label is a radioisotope, such techniques are generally referred to as immunoradiometric assays (IRMA) to distinguish them from conventional RIA, although this convention is not invariably adhered to. These methods represent an extension of the labelled reagent assay methods (relying on radiolabelled organic compounds such as ^{131}I-*p*-iodosulphonyl chloride, ^{3}H-acetic anhydride and other similar reagents) previously developed during the early 1950s by Keston *et al.* (1946), Avivi *et al.* (1954) and others for the measurement of amino acids, steroid and thyroid hormones, etc. A particular form of labelled antibody method introduced by Wide (1971) relied on 'immunoextraction' of the analyte by a second, unlabelled antibody coupled to a solid support (sometimes referred to as the capture antibody), leading to the description 'two-site' or 'sandwich' assay. Clearly a reliance on two antibodies recognising different antigenic sites (epitopes) on the analyte molecule decreases the chance of interference by other similar molecules, and sandwich methods are therefore generally more specific than simple single-site assays of either labelled antibody or labelled analyte format. Nevertheless the use of an antibody to isolate the analyte from a complex mixture constitutes a particular (albeit elegant) form of extraction/purification procedure, and does not differ in principle from other techniques used to achieve the same objective.

Although radiolabelled antibody methods were claimed originally (Miles and Hales, 1968b) to be more sensitive than methods (such as conventional RIA) based on the use of radiolabelled analyte, these claims were supported by neither rigorous theoretical analysis nor persuasive experimental evidence, and for some time remained controversial. Further doubt on their validity was cast by the publication by Rodbard and Weiss (1973) of a detailed theoretical analysis demonstrating both labelled analyte and labelled antibody methods to possess essentially equal sensitivities. (These authors suggested that IRMA methods might be more sensitive for the assay of small polypeptides in which radioiodine incorporation into the antigen molecule was restricted; conversely they would be less sensitive for the measurement of antigens of high molecular mass.) Nevertheless the (erroneous) belief that IRMA methods in particular, and labelled antibody methods in general, are – by virtue of the labelling of the antibody – intrinsically more sensitive than the corresponding labelled analyte methods has gained wide acceptance among clinical chemists.

Discussion of this issue is complicated by the frequent description of the labelled antibody approach as 'noncompetitive'. Given the grounds that led to the use of the term competitive to describe methods relying on labelled antigens, it is arguable that the description of labelled antibody methods as noncompetitive is justified, because the latter clearly do not involve 'competition' between labelled and unlabelled forms of the analyte. However, this simple distinction between competitive and noncompetitive methods has (*inter alia*) been undermined by the application of the term 'competitive' to certain labelled antibody assays, such as CELIA (competitive enzyme-linked immunoassay) (Yorde *et al.*, 1976). Depending on the manner in which such assay are performed, certain assays of this type also require, in practice, relatively small amounts of antibody to achieve maximal sensitivity, thus apparently justifying their description as competitive.

In the following section, I examine the fundamental distinction between these two immunoassay designs.

'Competitive' and 'Noncompetitive' Immunoassays

The perception that immunoassays are distinguished not only by which component of the system (antibody or analyte) is labelled, but also – and more importantly – by considerable differences in design (primarily by differences in the optimal concentration of antibody used) represents a significant advance in the understanding of immunoassay methodology (*see also* Chapter 9). To clarify the situation, I suggested (1977) the terms 'excess-reagent' and 'limited-reagent' methods to describe immunoassays which, for reasons discussed below, require optimal antibody concentrations tending to infinity and zero, respectively, to achieve maximal sensitivity. These terms broadly correspond to the more recent meanings placed upon the descriptions noncompetitive and competitive as implied in the acronym 'CELIA', and for the remainder of this chapter the terms may be regarded as essentially synonymous, despite a possibility of confusion.

It must again be emphasised that the distinction between excess-reagent (noncompetitive) and limited-reagent (competitive) assays does not coincide with the distinction between labelled antibody and labelled analyte methods; the particular component that is labelled constitutes a technical feature of little direct relevance to such aspects of assay performance as sensitivity, precision and specificity. The failure to recognise this point led to the debate in the early 1970s (referred to above) regarding the relative sensitivities of labelled antibody and labelled analyte methods; indeed the classification of assays on the basis of which reagent is labelled has continued to obscure the true reasons why certain immunoassay designs are potentially capable of yielding higher sensitivity than others. This point – and the fundamental difference between noncompetitive and competitive methods – may be more readily understood if the principles of immunoassay are portrayed somewhat differently from the way in which they are generally represented.

The 'Antibody Occupancy Principle'

When a 'sensor' antibody is introduced into an analyte-containing medium, antibody binding sites are occupied by analyte molecules to a fractional extent that reflects both the equilibrium constant governing the binding reaction, and the final free analyte concentration present in the mixture. This proposition stems immediately from the mass action law, which can be written as:

$$\frac{[AbAg]}{[fAg]} = K[fAg] \tag{1}$$

or fractional occupancy of antibody binding sites (i.e. [AbAg]/[total Ab])

$$= \frac{K[fAg]}{1 + K[fAg]} \tag{2}$$

where [AbAg], [fAb] and [fAg] represent the concentrations (at equilibrium) of bound antibody, free antibody and free antigen (analyte), respectively, and K is the equilibrium constant. The final free analyte concentration is generally dependent on both total analyte and antibody concentrations; however, when [total Ab] approximates to $0.05/K$ or less, free and total analyte concentrations do not differ significantly. Assays based on this concept have been termed 'ambient analyte immunoassays' (Ekins, 1983a); the fractional occupancy of the antibody being independent of both sample volume and antibody concentration.

All immunoassays essentially depend upon measurement of the 'fractional occupancy' of the sensor antibody following its reaction with analyte (*see* Figure 5). (N.b. this may erroneously suggest that the reaction between analyte and antibody must be allowed to reach completion before further binding reactions (requiring addition, for example, of labelled reagents) are initiated for the purpose of estimating antibody occupancy. The mode of operation of immunoassays is represented in this way solely to convey their underlying conceptual basis; in practice, the various binding reactions involved are often allowed to proceed simultaneously.)

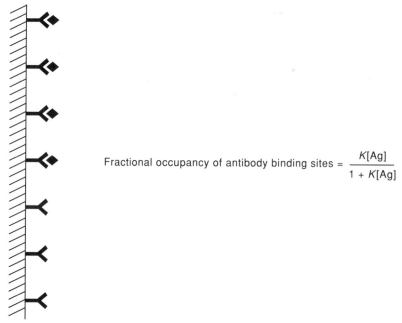

Fractional occupancy of antibody binding sites $= \dfrac{K[Ag]}{1 + K[Ag]}$

Figure 5 The antibody binding site occupancy principle of immunoassay. All immunoassays implicitly rely on the measurement of (fractional) binding site occupancy by the analyte.

Techniques relying on the measurement of residual, unoccupied antibody binding sites (from which antibody occupancy is implicitly deduced by subtraction) require – for the attainment of maximal sensitivity – the use of sensor-antibody concentrations tending to zero, and may thus be termed competitive. Conversely, techniques in which occupied sites are directly measured generally permit (but do not always require) the use of relatively high sensor-antibody concentrations and may be described as noncompetitive.

This difference in assay design reflects the proposition that, to maximise the precision of the measurement, it is generally undesirable to determine a small quantity by estimating the difference between two large quantities. Thus when an immunoassay relies on observation of unoccupied binding sites, the amount of antibody must be small to minimise error in the (indirect) estimate of occupied sites. Conversely, when occupied sites are measured directly, considerable advantage may derive from using relatively large amounts of sensor antibody in the system.

These concepts are illustrated in Figure 6 which portrays the basic immunoassay formats currently in common use. Conventional RIA and other similar labelled analyte techniques rely on measurement of unoccupied binding sites; this is generally effected by back-titration (either simultaneous or sequential) using labelled analyte, but anti-idiotypic antibody (reactive only with unoccupied sites on the sensor antibody) may in principle be used for the same purpose. Meanwhile, single-site and two-site labelled antibody methods are best considered separately. In the case of single-site assays, the labelled antibody itself constitutes the sensor antibody which, following reaction with analyte, may be separated into occupied and unoccupied fractions using, for example, an immunosorbent (comprising antigen, antigen analogue or anti-idiotypic antibody linked to a solid support). If, following separation, the signal emitted by labelled antibody bound to analyte (i.e. the occupied fraction) is measured directly, the assay

A Noncompetitive immunoassay   Ab → ∞ for maximum sensitivity

Measurement of occupied sites

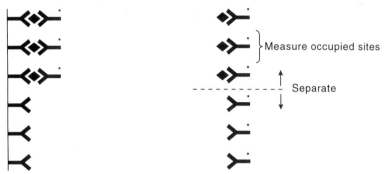

Two-site labelled antibody assay   Single-site labelled antibody assay

B Competitive immunoassay   Ab → 0 for maximum sensitivity

Measurement of unoccupied sites

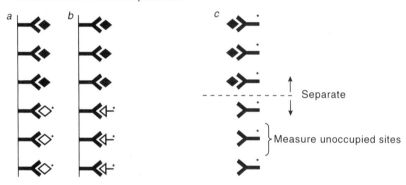

Single-site labelled antibody assay

Key

◇˙   Labelled antigen

⊰⊢˙   Labelled anti-idiotypic antibody

⊱—˙   Labelled antibody

◆   Analyte

Figure 6 Basic competitive and noncompetitive immunoassay designs. The distinction between noncompetitive (*a*) and competitive immunoassays (*b*) reflects the way in which antibody binding site occupancy is observed. Labelled antibody methods are noncompetitive if occupied sites of the (labelled) antibody are directly measured, but are competitive (*Bc*) when unoccupied sites are measured. Labelled antigen (*Ba*) or labelled anti-idiotypic antibody methods (*Bb*) rely on measurement of sites unoccupied by analyte, and are therefore invariably of competitive design.

can be classed as 'noncompetitive'. Conversely, if labelled antibody unbound to analyte (i.e. that attached to the immunosorbant) is measured, then the assay is 'competitive'. This is the approach adopted in the CELIA enzyme-labelled antibody methods.

Two-site sandwich assays are clearly more complex because they rely on two antibodies and can be considered from two points of view. As with single-site assays, the labelled antibody can be regarded as the sensor antibody, the solid-phase antibody (i.e. capture antibody) merely providing a means of separating occupied from unoccupied labelled antibody binding sites. Viewed from this standpoint, it is clear that if labelled antibody remaining attached (via analyte) to the capture antibody is directly measured (as is customary), the assay can be described as noncompetitive. But if unoccupied labelled antibody remaining in solution is measured, the assay should be classed as competitive. Conversely the solid-phase antibody can be viewed as the sensor antibody, with the labelled antibody enabling occupied sensor-antibody binding sites to be distinguished. Seen in this light, two-site assays must always be classed as noncompetitive.

The paradox that certain two-site assay designs may be described as both competitive and noncompetitive (depending on the viewpoint from which they are considered) highlights a potential source of confusion underlying the classification of assays in this manner. It reflects the possibility of constructing assays relying on the measurement of occupied binding sites on one antibody, and unoccupied sites on the other (implying, *inter alia*, differing optimal amounts of the two antibodies in the system). Fortunately, current sandwich assays invariably depend, in practice, on the observation of labelled antibody attached, via analyte, to the solid-phase capture antibody (implying that occupied sites of both antibodies are directly measured), so that confusion on these grounds is unlikely to arise.

However, other assay formats have been described (Ekins, 1993) that rely on the determination of both occupied and unoccupied binding sites on a capture antibody, and which are therefore of both noncompetitive and competitive design. Such an approach (described in greater detail in Chapter 24) is advantageous in certain circumstances by extending the assay working range. It therefore seems inevitable that the terms noncompetitive and competitive assay will be ultimately replaced by an improved terminology that more exactly relates to the fundamental concepts underlying the different ways in which antibody occupancy is determined.

As a further illustration of the above concepts, the design of true immunosensors should be briefly considered. Such devices (currently under development by several manufacturers) rely on a transduction mechanism (e.g. surface plasmon resonance) to signal analyte occupancy of antibody sites situated on the sensor surface. They can likewise be classed as competitive and noncompetitive, depending on whether the signal generated is maximal when sensor-antibody binding sites are fully unoccupied or fully occupied, respectively (*see* Figure 7). As in the case of conventional immunoassays, these alternative approaches to the measurement of antibody occupancy have important statistical consequences, which are likely, in turn, to affect sensor design and performance.

Such considerations emphasise that the differences in design distinguishing so-called competitive and noncompetitive methods are unrelated to which component (if any) of the reaction system is labelled. Also these terms do not enshrine different analytical principles, but merely reflect alternative approaches to the determination of antibody binding site occupancy, leading to differences in the optimal antibody concentration required to minimise the effects of random errors arising in the determination. Indeed, if occupancy measurements were error-free, no antibody concentration would be optimal, and the distinction between competitive and noncompetitive assays would effectively disappear. It should also be emphasised that, although optimal sensor-antibody concentrations tend to zero and infinity for competitive and noncompetitive respectively, this is true only when separation of reaction products is 'perfect'. When separation is incomplete, giving rise to significant misclassification of (for example) free

Noncompetitive immunosensor　　　　　Competitive immunosensor

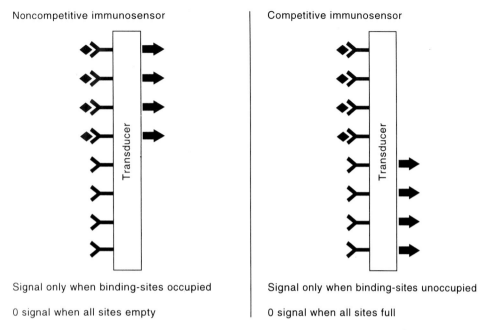

Signal only when binding-sites occupied　　Signal only when binding-sites unoccupied

0 signal when all sites empty　　　　　0 signal when all sites full

Figure 7 Noncompetitive and competitive immunosensors. A signal may be generated either when antibody binding sites are occupied (noncompetitive sensor) or unoccupied (competitive sensor).

labelled antigen as bound and vice versa, optimal antibody concentrations depart from these extremes and tend to converge.

In practice, competitive and noncompetitive immunoassays can be shown to differ significantly in many of their performance characteristics, including their potential sensitivities, in consequence of the differences in the optimal sensor-antibody concentration on which – given efficient separation methods – they are likely to rely. For example, an important theoretical prediction is that only by adoption of a noncompetitive approach and labels of higher specific activity than those of the commonly used isotopes can the sensitivities of isotopically based immunoassay methods be surpassed (see below). Competitive and noncompetitive methods also differ in the times required to attain (approximate) thermodynamic equilibrium in the system, noncompetitive methods generally requiring shorter incubation times. These issues are addressed in greater detail in the next section.

IMMUNOSSAY OPTIMISATION

General Concepts

Assay design constitutes the choosing of reagents and a protocol whereby the central objective of the assay, i.e. the most accurate measurement of analyte concentrations in test samples in the shortest reasonable time, is achieved. (The term 'accuracy' is used here in its original English and Latin sense i.e. that measurements should be carried out 'with care', implying that they are subject to minimal error). Assay design and optimisation are essentially synonymous terms, albeit assayists tend to use the term 'optimisation' when referring to measures taken to make best use of a given set of reagents within the constraints of an overall assay design. Immunoassay design in the widest sense clearly embraces, *inter alia*, selection of antibody (or antibodies) with appropriate specificity and affinity characteristics, and the choice of label, separation method (to isolate reaction products), data analysis procedure, etc. Detailed consideration of all such factors clearly lies beyond the scope of a single chapter, and this section is intended to address only the general principles underlying activities of this kind.

Aside from identifying an antibody, or antibodies, displaying high 'structural specificity', minimisation of assay bias requires that all samples in the assay system, i.e. unknowns, standards and QC samples, should be as alike in general composition as possible, and are subjected to identical treatments. For example, when assaying serum, standards should generally be made up in analyte-free serum deriving from the same animal species as test samples. Likewise, in the case of protein and polypeptide analytes, 'reference preparations' used to make up standards should ideally derive from the same animal species as the analyte itself. Unfortunately, many analytes (such as the glycoprotein hormones) do not comprise single substances, but mixtures of substances of closely related molecular structure. In these circumstances it is impossible to ensure that the spectrum of molecules in the standards recognised by a given antibody is identical to that in the test samples (which may itself vary from one sample to another). Results from different laboratories are therefore almost certain to differ, i.e. they will be biased with respect to each other, though no individual methodology can be claimed to be correct. Other important factors include the timing of the steps involved in the assay procedure (differences in incubation times between standards and unknowns sometimes leading, for example, to progressive biasing effects generally referred to as assay 'drift'), and the method adopted for computation of assay results, because significant bias can be caused by inappropriate curve-fitting procedures embodied in computer programs. These and other similar issues are addressed in detail elsewhere in this volume (Chapters 10, 11, 12).

Minimisation of the Biasing Effects of Crossreacting Substances

A particular source of bias arising in the case of individual samples is the presence of 'crossreacting' substances that simulate the analyte in its reaction with antibody. The extent to which such substances distort assay results depends in part on their relative antibody-binding affinity, and in part on the assay design. Regrettably, the observation that the potency of a cross-reacting substance relative to the analyte is not a constant has been obscured by the common practice of reporting the relative amounts of crossreactant and analyte that reduce the zero-dose response (e.g. B_0) by 50% (Abraham, 1969), this quantity sometimes being referred to as the 'coefficient of cross reactivity' (CR_{50}). However, for several reasons, the value of this coefficient may substantially misrepresent the biasing effect of the crossreactant in the system. For example, considering the simplest case of a conventional RIA relying on a monoclonal antibody the antibody reacting with the analyte, both labelled and unlabelled, with an affinity represented by K_a and with a crossreactant with an affinity represented by K_{CR}, it may be shown that, assuming equilibrium, the relative potency (RP) of analyte and crossreactant is given by (Ekins, 1974)

$$RP = (F \times K_a/K_{CR}) + B \tag{3}$$

where F and B are the free and bound labelled analyte fractions, respectively.

This equation implies that the relative potency of the crossreactant varies as a function of assay response (*see also* Rodbard and Lewald, 1970). For example, if the analyte binds to antibody with an affinity 100–fold greater than that of the crossreactant, then the analyte will display a 50.5-fold greater potency when 50% of the labelled material is antibody-bound, increasing to a 100-fold greater potency when 0% is bound. This implies a doubling in relative potency over the entire span of the dose-response curve, assuming this extends from 50% binding of label at zero dose to 0% at infinite dose.

The change in relative potency illustrated in this example reflects a more fundamental phenomenon, i.e. that the relative potencies of two different antigens competing for antibody binding site occupancy depend on the relative concentrations of antibody and antigens in the system. Thus all antigens react with antibody with equal potency in the presence of an infinitely large excess of antibody. This conclusion is illustrated by equation (3), from which it is apparent that when $B = 1$, the relative potency of two cross-reacting antigens is also unity, i.e. they are equipotent (assuming $K_{CR} \neq 0$).

Similar considerations reveal that, in a labelled antibody method, the relative potency of two antigens reacting with the same (labelled) antibody binding site is given by:

$$RP = \frac{([fAb] + 1/K_{CR})}{([fAb] + 1/K_a)} \tag{4}$$

where $[fAb]$ = the free (labelled) antibody concentration.

Thus, when $[fAb]$ is very large compared, in both cases, with $1/K$, both target analyte and crossreactant become equipotent. Conversely when $[fAb] \to 0$, RP approximates K_a/K_{CR}.

The situation is clearly more complex if the assay relies on a mixture of antibodies, some reactive with the analyte, some with the crossreactant, and some with both. In these circumstances computer methods are required to predict the biasing effects of crossreactants on assay results. However, probably the most important point emerging from these considerations is that adoption of a single-site noncompetitive assay design (relying on a relatively large amount of antibody to maximise assay sensitivity) is also likely to lead to a concomitant increase in the relative potency of any crossreactants present in the system, i.e. to a loss in assay specificity. Such a loss of specificity may be obviated by the use of two-site sandwich assay designs; however, caution is clearly required in the case of analytes (such as steroid hormones) which are too small to bind simultaneously to two antibodies directed against different regions of the molecule.

Minimisation of Random Errors

Random errors arising in a typical immunoassay procedure can be conveniently categorised under two headings: 'experimental' (or manipulation) errors, and 'signal measurement' errors. Minimisation of both of these types of error (i.e. maximisation of assay precision and sensitivity) needs, *inter alia*, great care with regard to pipetting and other reagent manipulation steps, certain of which – such as the addition of antibody and labelled antigen in a conventional 'competitive' assay – are of crucial importance in this context.

In methodologies in which 'signal measurement' involves photon counting – for example, assays relying on the use of radioisotopic or fluorescent labels – sufficient 'counts' must be accumulated to ensure the statistical counting error is small relative to the 'manipulation' errors arising in the procedure. The SD of a total accumulated count of 10,000 photons is 100, implying a CV in the measured count rate of 1%. Counting the sample ten times longer would yield a total count of 100,000 ± 316, i.e. a CV in the measured count rate of about 0.3%. Considerable care is required to reduce the statistical sum of manipulation errors to 1% or less, so that little increase in overall precision can generally be expected from counting samples for a longer time than is necessary to accumulate a total of 10,000 counts. The overall error in the response measurement is therefore likely, at best, to be approximately 1.5%, and (in my experience) only laboratory personnel of exceptional skill (or very well designed automatic instruments) can consistently surpass this level of precision.

Error in measurement of the assay response clearly leads to a corresponding error in the analyte concentration (or 'dose') estimate. A fundamental objective of assay optimisation is to ensure that error in the response causes minimal error in the dose measurement. This objective can be addressed theoretically and/or empirically, as discussed in greater detail in the following sections. (In practice many assayists have not adopted a logical approach to assay design, and have been guided by a blend of intuition and arbitrary rules of thumb. This has been the source of many of the myths that continue to exist in the field.)

Theoretical Approach to Immunoassay Optimisation

Theoretical studies of immunoassay performance are primarily of value in clarifying the broad principles governing immunoassay design, and identifying the key parameters that determine the sensitivity and precision of alternative assay procedures. For example, early mathematical models revealed that the sensitivity of a 'labelled analyte' immunoassay is critically dependent on the equilibrium (or affinity) constant of the antibody used. (Although a definition of sensitivity as $dB/d[A]$ is unsustainable, certain of the conclusions to which it leads are fortuitously correct. Although this provides the immunoassay design theory based on the definition with a semblance of validity, other conclusions to which it leads are demonstrably false.) The same conclusion has subsequently been shown to apply to labelled antibody techniques whether 'competitive' or 'noncompetitive' in format, albeit higher sensitivity is likely to be obtained when a given antibody is used in a noncompetitive mode (see below). Such theoretical analysis has, in my experience, been of value, not only in suggesting how best to perform a particular assay, but in pointing the way to new methodologies, the emergence of which might have been considerably delayed using a purely empirical approach.

Theoretical studies of immunoassay optimisation essentially rely on the combination of two models: (1) a physicochemical model descriptive of the binding reactions between antibody, analyte and, when appropriate, labelled analyte, and (2) an error model representing the random errors incurred in the measurement of the assay response. In the case of the physicochemical model, it is generally assumed that the reactions involved are governed by the mass action laws, and that only a single 'species' of antibody is implicated in the binding reaction in the case of 'single-site' assays, or two antibodies directed against different antigenic sites (epitopes) on the analyte molecule in the case of two-site assays. The construction of an error model is, in general, considerably more difficult, ideally entailing assessment of the variability of every individual step in an assay protocol. The two models can, in combination, provide the basis of computer programs, enabling such questions as the effect of increasing the amount of antibody in the system, either on assay sensitivity or on the precision of measurement of any defined 'target' analyte concentration, to be addressed. Moreover, using hill-climbing techniques, the optimal combination of reagents required to yield measurements of maximal precision over any defined range of analyte concentrations can be determined. Computer models of this kind (of varying degrees of complexity) have been developed by me and by others (e.g. Rodbard *et al.*, 1978).

Although of considerable value in assay development, such computer models have not found widespread application, perhaps due, in part, to the fact that they have not been widely distributed. Moreover, many experimentalists are reluctant to dissect their assay systems in order to identify and assess the magnitudes of all individual sources of error, preferring a more empirical approach of the kind described below.

Somewhat simpler theoretical models have also been devised that rely on broad assumptions regarding the overall magnitude and variation of the error in the response variable, albeit they do not identify individual sources of error. Such models are of less value in the establishment of individual assay protocols, but nevertheless yield useful general insights into assay design and optimisation. Theoretical studies that my colleagues and I have done will be used to illustrate this point. Figure 8 shows relationships between assay sensitivity (expressed in terms of molecules per ml) and antibody affinity in an optimised competitive (labelled analyte) assay assuming (1) use of a label of infinite specific activity (i.e. that no statistical error arises in the measurement of the label), and (2) use of ^{125}I as a label, samples being counted for a 'reasonable' counting time of the order of 2 minutes. The theoretically-optimal reagent concentrations on which the calculations represented in this figure rely were deduced from equations described in Ekins *et al.*, 1968 and Ekins and Newman, 1970 and were based on the further assumptions (3) that the antibody-bound labelled analyte fraction was counted, and (4) that the (relative) 'experimental error' component in the measurement of the bound fraction (σ_B/B) (i.e. the total error arising from pipetting of sample and reagents, separation of reaction products and other manipulations, but excluding the counting, or 'signal measurement', error) was 1%. Given these assumptions, it may be readily shown that the maximal (or 'potential') sensitivity attainable in such an assay (i.e. using a label of infinite specific activity) is given by σ_B/Kb where K is the affinity constant of the antibody. (For example, if the affinity constant is 10^{12} l mol^{-1}, and σ_B/B is 0.01 (i.e. 1%), maximal assay sensitivity is 10^{-14} mol l^{-1}, or about 6 x 10^6 molecules per ml). The additional 'signal measurement error' arising in consequence of counting radioactive samples for a finite time implies a loss of assay sensitivity, as shown by the upper curves in the figure. However, it is also apparent that the resulting sensitivity loss is relatively small for antibodies of affinities less than about 10^{12} l mol^{-1}, and is negligible for antibodies with affinities less than about 10^{11} l mol^{-1}. In other words, provided the assayist is prepared to accept individual sample counting times in the order of 2 to 3 minutes, little is gained in regard to sensitivity improvement by using alternative labels displaying higher specific activities than ^{125}I. However, similar considerations suggest that radioisotopic labels (such as ^3H) of much lower specific activity than ^{125}I may

Competitive immunoassay

Noncompetitive immunoassay

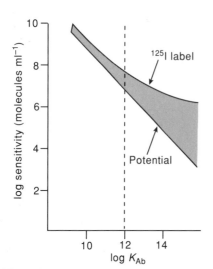
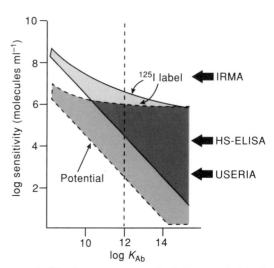

Figure 8 Theoretically predicted sensitivities of competitive and noncompetitive immunoassay methods (represented by the SD of zero analyte measurements, expressed as molecules per ml) plotted as a function of antibody affinity (K). (Note: in the case of noncompetitive sandwich assays, the antibody affinity referred to is that of the labelled antibody.) In the case of competitive assays, calculations are based on the assumption that the experimental error (CV) incurred in the measurement of the assay response (e.g. fraction of labelled antigen bound) is 1%. The potential sensitivity curve assumes the use of a label of infinite specific activity, implying that the error is the measurement of the label *per se* is zero. The ^{125}I label curve indicates the loss in sensitivity arising from the statistical error incurred in counting ^{125}I disintegrations for a reasonable (albeit finite) counting time. Note that, using antibodies with an affinity $< 10^{-12}$ l mol^{-1} (the maximum achieved in practice), little increase in sensitivity can be achieved by using labels of higher specific activity than ^{125}I. In the case of noncompetitive assays, the potential sensitivity curves shown relate to values of nonspecific binding of labelled antibody of 1% (upper curves) and 0.01% (lower curves), and reveal the improvement in potential sensitivity by minimising nonspecific binding. The corresponding ^{125}I label curves demonstrate the much greater loss in sensitivity (as compared with that potentially attainable) resulting from the use of a radioisotopic marker, and the special advantages of nonisotopic labels of higher specific activity in noncompetitive assay designs (particularly if nonspecific binding is reduced to 0.1% or less). Arrows indicate assay sensitivities reported for noncompetitive immunoassays based on ^{125}I (IRMA), and enzymes relying on fluorogenic (HS-ELISA) and radioactive (USERIA) substrates. The conclusions deriving from this figure underlie my original collaborative development (Marshall *et al.*, 1981) of time-resolved fluoroimmunoassay (DELFIA).

significantly limit the sensitivities of assays (such as steroid assays) in which they are used, notwithstanding the use of comparatively long sample counting times.

Other conclusions stemming from such analysis are the importance both of minimising 'manipulation' errors, and of using antibodies of high binding affinity. For example, an increase in σ_B/B to 3% implies an approximate threefold loss in sensitivity, notwithstanding the fact that an assay reoptimised in response to the deterioration in operator skill that these figures imply would use less antibody and labelled analyte, thereby partially offsetting the latter's effects. But the most important conclusion emerging from the analysis is the near-impossibility, in practice, of achieving immunoassay sensitivities better than about 10^7 molecules per ml using a competitive approach, irrespective of the nature of the label used, assuming an upper limit to antibody binding affinities in the order of 10^{12} l mol^{-1}.

The results of an analogous analysis of the sensitivity limitations applying to noncompetitive (two-site) assays (Jackson *et al.*, 1983) are also illustrated in Figure 8. Two sets of curves are portrayed in this figure, corresponding to the assumptions of 1% and 0.01% nonspecific binding of labelled antibody to the capture-antibody substrate. Such analysis likewise yields important broad conclusions relevant to assay design; for example, the crucial importance of reducing nonspecific binding to an absolute minimum. Furthermore, assuming nonspecific binding is reduced to about 0.01%, it is evident that the sensitivity achievable using an antibody of affinity 10^8 l mol^{-1} in an optimised noncompetitive assay design, can be just as high as using an antibody of 10^{12} l mol^{-1} in a competitive method. The analysis also predicts that, given a nonspecific binding value of this order, assay sensitivities higher by some four orders of magnitude are potentially achievable using a particular antibody in a noncompetitive assay as compared with its use in a competitive system. However, the sensitivities potentially attainable with high-affinity antibodies ($K>$ about 10^{10} l mol^{-1}) are beyond the reach of radioisotopically based methods, which (because of the relatively low specific activities of isotopes such as ^{125}I) are limited in practice to sensitivities of the order of 10^6–10^7 molecules per ml and above. In short, although under certain circumstances noncompetitive IRMA methods are likely to prove somewhat more sensitive than corresponding RIA techniques (assuming the use of the same antibody), the potential advantages (with regard to sensitivity) of the noncompetitive approach can only be realised using nonisotopic labels of much higher specific activity than ^{125}I. The superiority of such labels is most apparent when they are combined with high-affinity antibodies, although Figure 8 demonstrates that, even using antibodies with affinities of about 10^8–10^9 l mol^{-1} nonisotopic labels may yield significant sensitivity improvement.

These theoretical conclusions (together with the development by Köhler and Milstein (1975) of methods of *in vitro* monoclonal antibody production) was the basis of my decision (in about 1976) to initiate collaborative development (together with LKB/Wallac) of the time-resolved fluorometric immunoassay methodology now known as DELFIA (Marshall *et al.*, 1981; Soini and Lövgren, 1987). The same approach has since been adopted by other manufacturers using a variety of high specific activity labels, as indicated in Table 1. A more detailed review of such labels has been published by Kricka (1993).

Specific activity of ^{125}I	One detectable event per 7.5×10^6 labelled molecules
Specific activity of enzyme label	Determined by the enzyme 'amplification factor' and detectability of reaction product
Specific activity of chemiluminescent label	One detectable event per labelled molecule
Specific activity of fluorescent label	Many detectable events per labelled molecule

Table 1 General indication of relative activities of commonly used labels.

Although the attainment of high sensitivity is clearly an important general objective of immunoassay optimisation and development, high sensitivity is of limited value in many analytical applications, the sensitivities of current technologies being adequate for all practical purposes. However, circumstances clearly exist in which the development of 'ultrasensitive' immunoassay methods (a term generally applied to methods of higher sensitivity than conventional RIA) is essential. Such methods have already proved clinically useful for the measurement of certain hormones such as TSH (Spencer, 1989), but are also potentially of great importance for the detection of, for example, viral and tumour antigens in biological fluids. However, high specific activity labels also offer other potential benefits in the present context. For example, they permit faster throughput of samples in signal measuring equipment; they also facilitate 'miniaturisation' of immunoassay methodology, and thus the development of multianalyte immunoassay methods of the kind briefly described in Chapter 24.

Experimental Approach to Immunoassay Optimisation

Particular attention has been focused above on the use of theoretical models to design assays of maximal sensitivity, albeit such models can also be used more generally to define conditions yielding maximal precision of target-analyte concentrations other than zero. Maximising assay sensitivity is equivalent to maximising the precision with which the system measures a target analyte concentration of zero (cf. definition of sensitivity). In practice, however, most investigators have used more empirical methods of assay optimisation, albeit relying in part on the theoretical concepts discussed above. Regrettably pragmatic approaches have sometimes led to the elevation of simple rules of thumb to the status of scientific law, obscuring fundamental concepts of assay design, and significantly impeding progress towards improved assay methodologies.

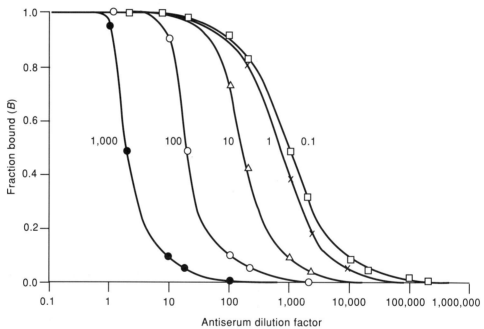

Figure 9 Theoretical antibody dilution curves using different labelled antigen concentrations typical of those obtained in practice (see, for example Hunter, 1983). The antiserum dilution factor of 1 shown corresponds to an antibody concentration on $1/K$; antigen concentrations are likewise expressed in units of $1/K$.

The validity of this assertion may be illustrated by a consideration of common methods whereby the optimal antibody concentration for use in a conventional RIA is selected. One typical approach has been discussed in some detail by Hunter (1983), and may be summarised as follows. Assuming the availability of a high-affinity antibody, and a reliable separation procedure, an experiment may be conducted in which different antibody concentrations are allowed to react (to equilibrium) with different concentrations of labelled antigen.

From such experiments, a set of dilution curves of the kind shown in Figure 9 can be drawn (confirming the predictions of the mass action laws). Hunter has suggested that, in the light of such information, a labelled antigen concentration of 0.01 ng ml^{-1} (in his particular example) would be initially chosen, and dose-response relationships established (in a further series of experiments), again using different antibody concentrations, albeit over a narrower range, and encompassing values for B_0 (the binding of labelled antigen in the absence of unlabelled antigen) of about 65% and below. Hunter claims (correctly) that the response curves deriving from this second series of experiments would be likely to be closely similar (i.e. superimposable) when normalised, i.e. when plotted in terms of B/B_0 (the curves nevertheless becoming progressively less steep using the higher antibody concentrations (see Figure 3c). He further asserts (but without providing evidence) that the correct antibody concentration is that resulting in the highest value of B_0 while also yielding a normalised response curve essentially superimposable with others in the set. Assuming use of a high-quality tracer, Hunter claims that this value of B_0 generally approximates to 65%.

Other authors have adopted closely comparable strategies in choosing supposedly optimal antibody concentrations, arriving at broadly similar conclusions. For example, as indicated earlier, Berson and Yalow – in order to maximise the slope of the B versus analyte concentration response curve – selected concentrations yielding B_0 values of either 50% or 33% (their conclusions changing during the 1960s). Most conventional immunoassay kits conform to these precepts.

Assays so constructed are likely to yield adequate sensitivity and an acceptable working range, and it is probably for this reason that the approach to assay design they embody has endured for so long, and is so widely accepted. However, it relies essentially on semi-intuitive judgements based primarily on the appearance of response curves plotted in particular coordinate frames, and disregards the errors incurred in measurement of the response variable (and the effect thereupon of changes in antibody concentration), without consideration of which genuine assay optimisation is impossible. In other words, empirical assay design rules of this nature have been formulated entirely without regard to the effect of changes in antibody concentration on assay sensitivity or precision, and thus lack any valid scientific basis.

What, then, is a more logical, rigorous and statistically sound experimental approach to the selection of the optimal antibody concentration for use in a conventional labelled-antigen immunoassay? To simplify discussion of this issue, we assume that the basic objective is to maximise assay sensitivity, and that the lowest usable concentration of labelled antigen (commensurate with the need to register a measurable signal (i.e. count-rate) for bound fractions down to, e.g., 1% binding of label) has been ascertained. It is also assumed, as above, that a reliable separation system is available, and that the assay system (conveniently) relies on measurement of the bound antigen fraction only. An experiment can be performed (similar to that described above) in which labelled antigen is incubated (1) alone with a series of antibody dilutions, and (2) with the same set of dilutions but together with a small increment of unlabelled antigen ($[\Delta Ag]$), sufficient in magnitude to cause a significant displacement of the resulting antibody dilution curve as shown in Figure 10. A further crucial feature of the experiment is that each point on each of the antibody dilution curves is determined at least in duplicate, and preferably using 5–10 replicates, implying that the entire study requires the use of, say, 100 incubation tubes (or more) in total. The experiment thus yields not only the two dilution curves shown in Figure 10, but, equally importantly, an estimate of the standard deviation of the response at each measured point along the curves. However, because the number of replicate estimations at each point is limited (thereby causing SD estimates to be statistically unreliable) it is useful to plot the measured SD values as a function of the re-

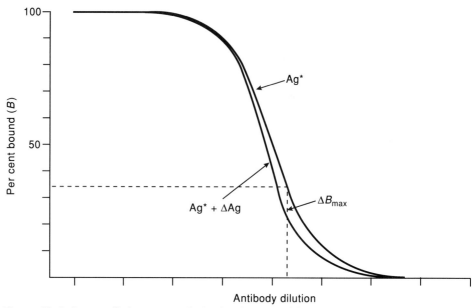

Figure 10 Antiserum dilution curves obtained using trace labelled antigen only (Ag*) and labelled antigen together with a small increment of unlabelled antigen (Ag*+ΔAg). Note that the maximal difference in the fraction of antigen bound (ΔB_{max}) is observed when Ag* is 33% bound.

sponse variable (B), permitting the fitting of a further curve – representing the response error relationship (RER) – through the points (*see* Figure 11).

Turning again to the dilution curves, it is also evident that the vertical distance between them varies as a function of antibody concentration. This difference, representing the change in the bound labelled antigen fraction (ΔB) caused by the increment in antigen concentration ($[\Delta Ag]$), may likewise be plotted (Figure 12) as a function of the corresponding value of B_0 (i.e. the value of B when only labelled antigen is present), again reducing the effects of experimental errors on the individual measurements of ΔB.

We now have two curves: one relating the SD in the measurement of B (i.e. σ_B) to B; the other the reduction in B (ΔB), caused by the presence of $[\Delta Ag]$ in the system, also as a function of B. We are thus able to calculate the quotient $\sigma_B/\Delta B$ as a function of B. This quotient represents the estimated precision of measurement of zero dose (i.e. assay sensitivity corresponding to all values of B_0, and implicitly to all antibody dilutions. It may likewise be plotted, either as a function of B or of antibody dilution (Figure 13), its minimum value corresponding to the conditions yielding maximal assay sensitivity.

This example has been described in some detail in order to illustrate a logical and scientifically sound approach to the choice of the antibody concentration yielding maximal assay sensitivity. Analogous procedures can readily be devised to establish the values of other key parameters, for example, the optimal labelled antigen concentration, the optimal amount of adsorbent to separate bound and free antigen fractions, etc. Moreover, the same approach can be used to establish optimal conditions yielding maximal precision of measurement of any target-analyte concentration (representative of the range of concentrations of interest to the analyst). For example, the antibody concentration maximising the precision of measurement of a target concentration ($[A_t]$) can be identified essentially as described above, but including

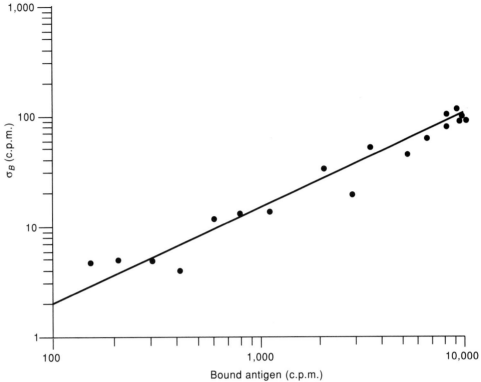

Figure 11 Curve representing the response error relationship (RER), i.e. the standard deviation in bound counts per min (σ_B) plotted as a function of bound counts per min (c. p. m.).

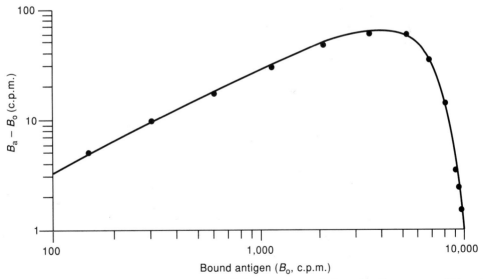

Figure 12 Curve representing the difference (ΔB) in counts per min bound in the presence (B_a) and absence (B_o) of the antigen increment ΔA.

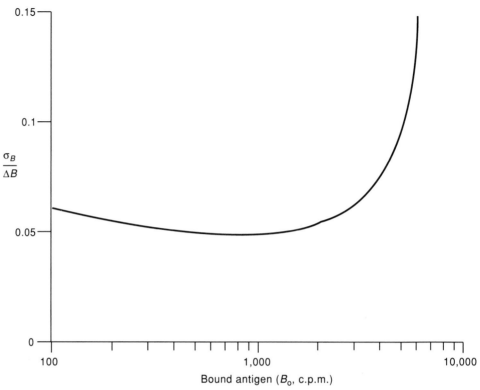

Figure 13 Curve representing the quotient $\sigma_B/\Delta B$ plotted as a function of bound counts per min. The value of the response variable B_0 (bound counts per min) at which $\sigma_B/\Delta B$ is minimal (i.e. about 1,000 counts per min) indicates the antibody dilution at which the SD in the zero-dose measurement ((σ_A), given by $\Delta A\sigma_B/\Delta B$) is minimal, i.e. sensitivity is maximal.

unlabelled analyte concentrations of $[A_t]$ and $[A_t] + [\Delta A]$ (together with labelled analyte) in the incubation tubes containing the selected range of antibody dilutions.

The distinguishing feature of this approach is that it relates to the valid, statistically based, concepts of assay sensitivity and precision now generally accepted in the field. In certain circumstances it will fortuitously yield assay designs coinciding broadly to those suggested by empirical methods. In others, it will yield quite different values of key parameters. For example, it reveals that, if care is taken to minimise nonspecific binding of labelled antigen to a solid-phase antibody support (such as cellulose or Sephadex), the antibody concentration yielding maximal sensitivity is likely to be considerably less than commonly used, implying that B_0 values may be as low as 3–4% or less as demonstrated by Wide (1978). This reduction is accompanied by an improvement in assay sensitivity over that obtained using antibody concentrations as recommended by Hunter and others. Indeed, the essential reason for the long survival of the myth that concentrations yielding B_0 values of about 50% are optimal is that such concentrations are appropriate to assay systems in which the misclassification of free labelled antigen activity as bound (commonly referred to as nonspecific binding) is high (i.e. in the order of 5–10%). This justification for the use of relatively high antibody concentrations is, of course, logical in such circumstances; it is, however, entirely unrelated to specious arguments based on consideration of the slopes of dose-response curves, and is therefore no longer valid when better methods of reagent separation are used.

A consequence of the faulty reasoning underlying Hunter's optimisation procedure summarised above has been that many assays (and assay kits) have, in practice, been constructed suboptimally, causing them to be of lower sensitivity and precision than would otherwise have been the case. However, in many situations, suboptimal assay design is likely to be of relatively little practical significance. More importantly, a reliance on empirical, often invalid, rules of immunoassay design rather than on a rational approach based on sound statistical concepts has tended to delay the development of improved methodologies. For example, the notion that maximal RIA sensitivity is obtained using antibody concentrations of $0.5/K$ for many years effectively deflected attention from the great importance of minimising non-specific binding of labelled antigen, and the considerable improvements in working range (and assay sensitivity) that flow from such action. Unsound assay design concepts likewise obscured the basis of the ultrasensitive immunoassay methods now in common use, and impeded the development of miniaturised immunoassay methodologies of the kind discussed in Chapter 24.

Fortunately, however, the importance of error analysis in the assessment of assay performance, and hence in assay design, is becoming widely recognised, one example being the increasing use of the precision profile in this context by many immunoassay kit manufacturers and others.

The Precision Profile

The assay precision profile – a term coined by me some 20 years ago (Ekins, 1976) – has already been briefly discussed in this chapter. It represents a simple concept applicable to all measurement systems used in science, but only in recent years has its importance in regard to immunoassay design become more generally recognised. A simple description of the basic derivation of the intra-assay profile is given in Ekins (1983), and other authors have incorporated more sophisticated methods of calculation into widely-available computer programs (e.g. Raab, 1983). Essentially all calculation methods rely on combining information regarding the dose-response relationship for all values of dose (that is, expressed in pictorial terms, the slope of the dose-response curve at all points along its length) with information regarding the random error incurred in the measurement of the response for all values of the response variable (as represented by the RER, see above). Computer methods of calculation rely on simple mathematical expressions representing each of these relationships, which are used to derive the precision profile from an appropriate set of assay data.

An example of the use of the profile in optimising assay performance was given in Ekins (1983), and may be summarised here. It relates to a simple decision – typical of many made by the practising immunoassayist – regarding the extent to which solid-phase antibody precipitates (e.g. antibody-coated cellulose) should be washed. Figure 14 shows a hypothetical set of precision profiles (albeit one reflecting practical experience) based on data generated in experiments in which precipitates are repeatedly washed. The profiles show that, following one wash, sensitivity is improved and the working range is increased. Further improvements in sensitivity and working range occur with further washings, but these benefits are likely to diminish progressively and to be eventually replaced by a deterioration in assay performance as precipitates are (variably) washed out of incubation tubes. Clearly only by statistical analysis of the results of such experiments can a rational decision on the extent to which precipitates should be washed (or analogous questions of this kind) be reached.

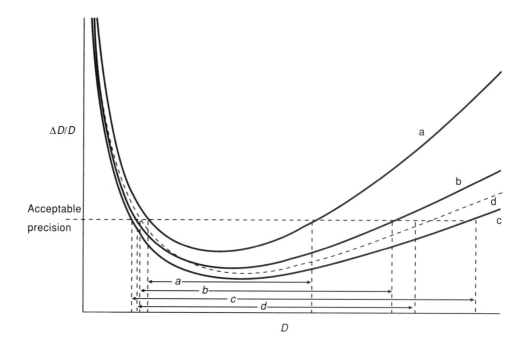

Figure 14 Precision profiles reflecting the effects of repeated washing of solid-phase (e.g. microcrystalline cellulose) antibody precipitates. Curves a, b and c reflect the progressive improvements in precision and working range resulting from repeated washings (curve a being yielded by the least washed precipitate). Curve d reflects the loss in precision and working range that may ultimately arise in consequence of loss of precipitate from the incubation tube. Although the curves are diagrammatic, they represent practical experience with a variety of reagent separation procedures, including those relying on the use of charcoal, second antibody, etc. and a variety of solid-phase antibody techniques.

It must be emphasised, however, that the precision profile (being invariably based on limited data) is itself subject to error. In other words, an error envelope surrounds the profile analogous to that which surrounds an immunoassay response curve. For these reasons, it is important to bear in mind, when relying on the profile to monitor changes in performance caused by changes in assay design, that large amounts of data are required to confer a reasonable degree of reliability on the profile's shape and position. For example, in observing the effects on assay performance of changes in antibody concentration, I have typically used a minimum of about 100 sample tubes (including standards and unknowns) for each concentration examined in order to establish the optimal value.

The necessity for large amounts of data to reach valid conclusions regarding the effects of changes in assay design clearly constitutes a major practical obstacle to the use of the profile in this context. However, as has repeatedly been emphasised in this chapter, past failure by workers in the field to recognise that the relative merits of different immunoassay procedures can be correctly assessed only by statistical analysis of effects on assay performance (as represented by the precision profile) constitutes the underlying cause of many of the myths that have accumulated in this area.

SUMMARY AND CONCLUSION

The primary objective of immunoassay design is to maximise the accuracy of (i.e. to minimise the error) in the measurement of analyte concentrations in a specified range, albeit bearing in mind the costs involved, and the use for which the measurements are intended. In short, whether the analyst relies on an experimental or theoretical approach (or a combination of both), the effect of any alterations in assay protocol on measurement errors constitutes a key issue, implying a requirement for detailed statistical analysis to ascertain the effects on assay precision and bias resulting from changes in design. Regrettably, because of past confusion regarding the concepts of precision, sensitivity, accuracy, etc. and the relatively large amounts of data required to evaluate these parameters when correctly defined, such analysis has not generally been performed, practitioners reaching superficial conclusions based primarily on the appearance of dose-response curves. In consequence, a number of erroneous concepts have become incorporated within currently accepted rules of immunoassay design. This point has been illustrated by consideration of the correct choice, in a so-called 'competitive assay' of the antibody concentration that yields maximal sensitivity (or, more generally, maximal precision of measurement of any target analyte concentration), but the same statistical approach should ideally be used in addressing, in a scientifically sound and rational manner, all decisions relating to immunoassay design. Failure to adopt such an approach has not only had the effect of creating myths in this field, but has delayed the emergence of new methodologies that conflict with widely accepted assay design concepts.

REFERENCES

Abraham, G. E. (1969) Solid-phase radioimmunoassay of estradiol-17 beta. *J. Clin. Endo.* **29**, 866–870.

Albano, J. D. M., Ekins, R. P., Maritz, G. *et al.* (1972) A sensitive, precise radioimmunoassay of serum insulin relying on charcoal separation of bound and free hormone moieties. *Acta. Endocrin.* **70**, 487–509.

Avivi, P., Simpson, S. A., Tait, J. F. *et al.* (1954) The use of ^{3}H and ^{14}C labelled acetic anhydride as analytical reagents in microbiochemistry. In: *Radioisotope Conference, 1954* (eds Johnston, J. E., Faires, R. A. & Millett, R. J.) pp. 313–323 (Butterworths, London).

Berson, S. A. & Yalow, R. S. (1973) Measurement of hormones: Radioimmunoassay. In: *Methods in Investigative and Diagnostic Endocrinology*, Vol. 2A. (eds Berson, S. A. & Yalow, R. S.) pp. 84–135 (North Holland/Elsevier, Amsterdam).

Borth, R. (1970) Discussion. In: *Steroid Assay by Protein Binding. Karolinska Symposia on Research Methods in Reproductive Endocrinology* (eds Diczfalusy, E. & Diczfalusy, A.) pp. 30–36 (WHO/Karolinska Institute, Stockholm).

Büttner, J., Borth, R., Boutwell, J. H. *et al.* (1979) IFCC: Approved recommendation on quality control in clinical chemistry. Part 1. General principles and terminology. *Clin. Chim. Acta.* **98**, 129F–143F.

Ekins, R. P. (1968) Limitations of specific activity. In: *Protein and Polypeptide Hormones Part 3 (Discussions)* (ed. Margoulies, M.) pp. 612–616 (Excerpta Medica, Amsterdam); Concentrations of tracer and antiserum, time and temperature of incubation, volume of incubation. ibid. 672–682.

Ekins, R. P. (1974) Basic principles and theory. *Brit. Med. Bull.* **30/1**, 3–11.

Ekins, R. P. (1976) General principles in hormone assay. In: *Hormone Assays and their Clinical Application* 4th edn (eds Loraine, J. A. & Bell, I.) pp. 1–72 (Churchill Livingstone, Edinburgh).

Ekins, R. P. (1977) The future development of immunoassay. In: *Radioimmunoassay and Related Procedures in Medicine* Vol. 1. pp. 241–268, (International Atomic Energy Agency Vienna, Vienna).

Ekins, R. P. (1983a) Measurement of analyte concentration. *British Patent* No. 8224600.

Ekins, R. P. (1983b) The precision profile: its use in assay design, assessment and quality control. In: *Immunoassays for Clinical Chemistry* (eds Hunter, W. M. & Corrie, J. E. T.) pp. 76–105 (Churchill Livingstone, Edinburgh).

Ekins, R. P. (1991) Immunoassay standardisation. *Scan. J. Clin. Lab. Invest.* **51** (Suppl. 205), 33–46.

Ekins, R. P. (1993) Back titration assay using two different markers. *British Patent No.* 9326451.3

Ekins, R. P. & Newman, B. (1970) Theoretical aspects of saturation analysis. In: *Steroid Assay by Protein Binding. Karolinska Symposia on Research Methods in Reproductive Endocrinology* (eds Diczfalusy, E. & Diczfalusy, A.) pp. 11–30 (WHO/Karolinska Institute, Stockholm).

Ekins, R. P., Newman, B. & O'Riordan, J. L. H. (1968) Theoretical aspects of 'saturation' and radioimmunoassay. In: *Radioisotopes in Medicine: in vitro Studies* (eds Hayes, R. L., Goswitz, F. A. & Murphy, B. E. P.) pp. 59–100 (US Atomic Energy Commission, Oak Ridge, Tennessee).

Ekins, R. P., Newman, B. & O'Riordan, J. L. H. (1970) Competitive protein-binding assays. Discussion. In: *Statistics in Endocrinology* (eds McArthur, J. W & Colton, T.) pp. 379–392 (MIT Press, Cambridge, MA).

Hunter, W. M. (1983) Optimisation of RIA: some simple guidelines. In: *Immunoassays for Clinical Chemistry* (eds Hunter, W. M. & Corrie, J. E. T.) pp. 69–75 (Churchill Livingstone, Edinburgh).

International Vocabulary of Basic and General Terms in Metrology (1993) ISBN 92–67–01075.

Jackson, T. M., Marshall, N. J. & Ekins, R. P. (1983) Optimisation of immunoradiometric assays. In: *Immunoassays for Clinical Chemistry* (eds Hunter, W. M. & Corrie, J. E. T.) pp. 557–575 (Churchill Livingstone, Edinburgh).

Jones, R. C. (1959) Phenomenological description of the response and detecting ability of radiation detectors. *Proc. Inst. Radio. Eng.* **47**, 1495–1502.

Keston, A. S., Udenfriend, S. & Cannan, S. (1946) Micro-analysis of mixtures (amino acids) in the form of isotopic derivatives. *J. Am. Chem. Soc.* **68**, 1390.

Köhler, G. & Milstein, C. (1975) Continuous culture of fused cells secreting specific antibody of predefined specificity. *Nature* **256**, 495–497.

Kricka, L. J. (1993) Trends in immunoassay technologies. *J. Clin. Immunoassay* **16**, 267–271.

Marshall, N. J., Dakubu, S., Jackson, T. & Ekins, R. P. (1981) Pulsed light, time resolved fluoroimmunoassay. In: *Monoclonal Antibodies and Developments in Immunoassay* (eds Albertini, A. & Ekins, R. P.) pp. 101–108 (Elsevier/North Holland, Amsterdam).

Miles, L. E. H. & Hales, C. N. (1968a) Labelled antibodies and immunological assay systems. *Nature* **219**, 186–189.

Miles, L. E. H. & Hales, C. N. (1968b) An immunoradiometric assay of insulin In: *Protein and Polypeptide Hormones Part 1* (ed. Margoulies, M.) pp. 61–70 (Excerpta Medica, Amsterdam).

Raab, G. (1983) Validity tests in the statistical analysis of immunoassay data. In: *Immunoassays for Clinical Chemistry* (eds Hunter, W M. & Corrie, J. E. T.) pp. 614–623 (Churchill Livingstone, Edinburgh).

Rodbard, D. (1978) Statistical estimation of the minimal detectable concentration ('sensitivity') for radioligand assays. *Anal. Biochem.* 90, 1–12.

Rodbard, D. & Lewald, J. E. (1970) Computer analysis of radioligand assay and radioimmunoassay data. In: *Steroid Assay by Protein Binding. Karolinska Symposia on Research Methods in Reproductive Endocrinology* (eds Diczfalusy, E. & Diczfalusy, A.) pp. 79–98 (WHO/Karolinska Institute, Stockholm).

Rodbard, D. & Weiss, G. H. (1973) Mathematical theory of immunometric (labelled antibody) assay. *Anal. Biochem.* 52, 10–44.

Rodbard, D., Munson, P. J. & De Lean, A. (1978) Improved curve-fitting, parallelism testing, characterisation of sensitivity and specificity, validation, and optimisation for radioligand assays. In: *Radioimmunoassay and Related Procedures in Medicine 1977* Vol. 1 pp. 469–503 (International Atomic Energy Agency Vienna, Vienna).

Soini, E. & Lövgren, T. (1987) Time-resolved fluorescence of lanthanide probes and applications in biotechnology. *CRC Crit. Rev. Anal. Chem.* 18, 105–154.

Spencer, C. A. (1989) Thyroid profiling for the 90's: Free T4 estimate or sensitive TSH measurement. *J. Clin. Immunoassay* 12, 82–89.

Wide, L. (1971) Solid-phase antigen-antibody systems. In: *Radioimmunoassay Methods* (eds Kirkham, K. E. and Hunter, W. M.) pp. 405–412 (Churchill Livingstone, Edinburgh).

Wide, L. (1978) Solid-phase radioimmunoassays. In: *Radioimmunoassay and Related Procedures in Medicine 1977* Vol. l pp. 143–153 (International Atomic Energy Agency Vienna, Vienna).

Wide, L., Bennich, H. & Johansson, S. G. O. (1967) Diagnosis of allergy by an in-vitro test for allergen antibodies. *Lancet* ii, 1105–1107.

Yalow, R. S. (1970) Competitive protein-binding assays. Discussion. In: *Statistics in Endocrinology* (eds McArthur, J. W. & Colton, T.) pp. 379–392 (MIT Press, Cambridge, MA).

Yalow, R. S. & Berson, S. A. (1959) Assay of plasma insulin in human subjects by immunological methods. *Nature* 184, 1648–1649.

Yalow, R. S. & Berson, S. A. (1968) General principles of radioimmunoassay. In: *Radioisotopes in Medicine: in vitro Studies* (eds Hayes, R. L., Goswitz, F. A. & Murphy, B. E. P.) pp. 7–39 (US Atomic Energy Commission, Oak Ridge, Tennessee).

Yalow, R. S. & Berson, S. A. (1970) Radioimmunoassays. In: *Statistics in Endocrinology.* (eds McArthur, J. W & Colton, T.) pp. 327–344, (MIT Press, Cambridge, MA).

Yorde, D. E., Sasse, E. A., Wang, T. Y. *et al.* (1976) Competitive enzyme-linked immunoassay with use of soluble enzyme antibody immune complexes for labelling. 1. Measurement of human choriogomadotrophin. *Clin. Chem.* 22, 1372–1377.

Youden, W. J. & Steiner, E. H. (1975) *Statistical Manual of the Association of Official Analytical Chemists* (Association of Official Analytical Chemists, Washington DC).

207

Chapter 10

Quality Assurance

John Seth

INTRODUCTION

Laboratory data are widely used in health care, environmental monitoring, industry and research, and laboratories are increasingly required to demonstrate that their output meets defined quality standards. In health care, quality standards may be defined in government legislation (e.g. the US Clinical Laboratory Improvement Amendments of 1988 (CLIA-88)), or by the relevant professions (e.g. the clinical laboratory accreditation scheme operated in the UK by Clinical Pathology Accreditation, UK, Ltd). Quality assurance describes all activities undertaken by a laboratory to ensure that its work meets defined quality standards. The principles of quality assurance are common to all measurements in laboratory medicine, and are well described in standard textbooks (Westgard, 1994), but immunoassays present some special requirements that have been recently described (Jeffcoate, 1981; Franzini *et al.*, 1991). This chapter describes the principles and practice of quality assurance with particular reference to the internal quality control and external quality assessment of immunoassays in the clinical laboratory. Many points will, however, be equally relevant to other laboratory settings.

DEFINITIONS

The following definitions, based on International Union of Pure and Applied Chemistry (IUPAC) guidelines (Thompson and Wood, 1993) and World Health Organization (WHO) reports (WHO, 1981) are used in this chapter:

Quality assurance (QA) All those planned and systematic actions necessary to provide adequate confidence that a product or service will satisfy given requirements for quality.

Internal quality control (IQC) The set of procedures undertaken by the staff of a laboratory for continuously assessing laboratory work and the emergent results, in order to decide whether they are reliable enough to be released, either in support of clinical decision making or for epidemiological or research purposes.

External quality assessment (EQA) The set of procedures operated by an external agency for objectively comparing a laboratory's results with an agreed target. It provides a retrospective assessment of performance, and is not used to decide on acceptability of results in real time. Where EQA is used to assess laboratory performance for licensing or accreditation purposes, it is often described as proficiency testing. In the older literature EQA was often described as external quality control.

Accuracy Closeness of agreement between the result of a measurement and the true value of the measurand.

Bias Difference between the expectation of the test results and an accepted reference value.

Precision Closeness of agreement between independent test results obtained under prescribed conditions.

Repeatability conditions Conditions where independent test results are obtained with the same method on identical test items in the same laboratory by the same operator using the same equipment within short intervals of time.

Run (analytical run) Set of measurements obtained under repeatability conditions. (Under CLIA-88 regulations, a run cannot be for more than 24 h).

QUALITY ASSURANCE

Clinical laboratory investigations comprise a complex series of steps (Figure 1) that can be broadly grouped as specimen collection, laboratory processing, and reporting and interpretation. IQC covers only the analytical steps in the sequence, while EQA monitors the analytical steps plus a wider range of laboratory activities, such as reliability of specimen handling in reception. EQA can also monitor reporting and interpretation of results. QA covers a still wider range of activities, most importantly the specimen collection, reporting and interpretation

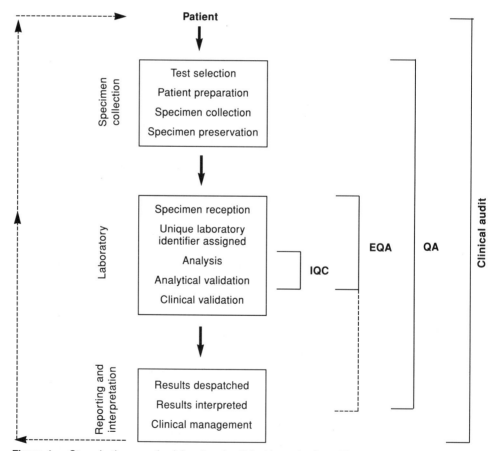

Figure 1   Steps in the use of a laboratory in clinical investigations. The steps monitored by internal quality control (IQC), external quality assessment (EQA), quality assurance (QA) and clinical audit are shown.

stages. Although these stages are often not under direct control of the laboratory, the laboratory has a responsibility to provide its users with clear advice on correct use of the laboratory services and, where appropriate, interpretation of the results. These aspects of QA are particularly relevant to the use of immunoassays for hormones, tumour markers and drugs, where considerations of patient preparation (e.g. fasting, possible interfering medication), time of specimen collection (e.g. time of day or month), and specimen stability (e.g. hormone degradation during specimen transit) are of equal importance to analytical factors in ensuring reliability of the result. A laboratory handbook that clearly and concisely summarises investigative protocols is invaluable for both laboratory staff and users, although this will need to be supplemented by continuing education of users. QA should also assess turnaround times, and the completeness and clarity of laboratory reports.

QA of laboratory work has an important, although often understated, role in ensuring quality of patient care, the latter being the subject of a still wider range of standard setting and monitoring activities falling under the umbrella of clinical audit.

INTERNAL QUALITY CONTROL

The purpose of IQC is to ensure that the analytical process meets predefined criteria with respect to bias and precision. Three broad areas of activity need to be considered: (1) preanalytical quality control; (2) statistical quality control; and (3) review of quality control. The principles of these activities are summarised in Table 1, and are discussed below.

Preanalytical quality control

- Laboratory facilities and equipment adequate for assays to be performed competently and safely.
- Reagent preparation and method design optimised.
- Method protocols adhered to.
- Staff appropriately trained.

Statistical quality control

- IQC specimens (e.g. serum pools) should have identical properties to the test specimens in the assay.
- Baseline assay performance (precision and bias) estimated under stable assay conditions.
- IQC specimens processed identically to test specimens through the entire assay procedure.
- IQC results simply and clearly presented.
- There should be defined criteria for run rejection (e.g. control rules).
- The IQC plan should take account of the quality goals.

Review of quality control

- IQC failures explored in a constructive manner and remedial action taken.
- IQC and other data (e.g. EQA) reviewed regularly to search for trends in performance.

Table 1 Principles of IQC.

Preanalytical Quality Control

Laboratory Facilities and Equipment

Adequate laboratory space, lighting and heating are prerequisites for analysts to perform skilled work. Equipment should be appropriate for the task and properly maintained, e.g. pipettes capable of adequate accuracy and precision. For radioimmunoassay, special attention to cleanliness and calibration of gamma counters is needed, and calibrator sets are available for this purpose. Nonisotopic methods are increasingly used and care is required to avoid environmental contaminants, e.g. dust and fluorophores or quenching agents. Where automated analysers are used diligent adherence to analyser maintenance schedules is vitally important. These procedures are analyser specific but, in general, obvious problem areas such as probes, wash-stations and priming before running must receive careful attention. Some of the more mundane tasks, unless self-monitored by the analyser or recorded on a maintenance chart, may be overlooked. Changes in output because of lack of maintenance of the optical system or overheating due to failure to clean air filters can also cause deterioration and IQC failure.

Method Design and Protocols

Methods and reagents should be optimised so that minor changes in conditions have minimum effect on performance. The precision of any quantitative measurement is the square root of the sum of the variances of the component steps (Eurachem Working Group, 1995):

$$(SD) = \sqrt{SD_a^2 + SD_b^2 + SD_c^2 + \ldots\ldots}$$

where SD_a, SD_b, SD_c are the standard deviations of steps a, b, c and so on (e.g. pipetting, washing, absorbance measurement); i.e., attempts to improve assay precision must focus first on the steps that are least precise. There should be written 'standard operating procedures' for reagent preparation, assay procedure and instrument operation, and more importantly these should be adhered to. Assay procedure should not be modified without verifying that performance is not adversely affected, and laboratory accreditation agencies will usually require documentary evidence of this.

Staff Training

Manual immunoassays are among the more technically demanding of laboratory methods, and can be vulnerable to changes in performance depending on the analyst. Training of staff is vitally important therefore, and it is desirable that changes of analyst with staff rotation are kept to a minimum (e.g. 3-monthly) in line with the overall training programme. Immunoassay automation has the benefit of permitting greater flexibility in staff deployment, but does not obviate the need for adequate training in analyser operation and maintenance. Training should be the responsibility of a named person and not delegated to successive operators, which might risk undesirable changes from recommended practice becoming established.

- Matrix identical to test specimens in assay.
- Analyte concentrations close to decision levels of test.
- Stable (before and after reconstitution if lyophilised).
- Free from infectious hazards (negative for hepatitis B, hepatitis C and HIV antigens).
- Target value preassigned, or determined in-house.
- Large volume of single batch available.
- Economical.

Table 2 Desirable properties of IQC specimens.

Statistical Quality Control

Choice of IQC Material

The desirable properties of IQC specimens are summarised in Table 2, although rarely are all the listed requirements met.

Several types of material may be used to assess precision and accuracy, and their roles are complementary rather than mutually exclusive alternatives.

Stable test material, e.g. pooled serum. For monitoring precision, a homogeneous supply of the test material is required, divided into aliquots in sufficient quantity for use over a period of several months. A human serum matrix is a prerequisite for clinical immunoassays of serum analytes. Possible sources of IQC serum are: (1) unwanted serum from blood donations; and (2) commercially available lyophilised sera. Pooling of residues from patient specimens routinely received in the laboratory is not recommended owing to the risk of infection and the cost and inconvenience of virological screening. Note that not all commercially available IQC sera are negative for hepatitis C antigen.

Because of the wide concentration ranges covered by most immunoassays, it is accepted practice to use IQC specimens covering the low, medium and high concentration ranges. Whichever source of IQC material is used, this may require analyte stripping and addition to achieve low and high levels, respectively, challenging the first of the requirements in Table 2. The analyte concentration in the control specimens may be assigned in-house as the mean result determined in not less than 15 assay runs when the analysis is in control or, in the case of commercial QC specimens, it may be preassigned by the supplier. Note that preassigned targets in immunoassay often vary according to the method used, and are of limited value in assessing accuracy. It will usually be necessary to determine target values locally.

Lyophilised commercial IQC sera do not always behave identically to patient sera, perhaps reflecting the presence of different molecular forms of the analyte, or alterations in the properties of the serum protein matrix. Use of lyophilised sera also introduces the potential for errors in reconstitution. Liquid IQC sera should be stored at $-80\,^{\circ}$C to minimise degradation, and not $-20\,^{\circ}$C which under working conditions will give temperatures near the eutectic point of serum, where protein breakdown may occur.

Certified reference materials (CRM). A CRM is a material in which the analyte is certified to have a concentration within stated confidence limits, determined by a reference method, i.e. one that has negligible inaccuracy in relation to its precision. The purpose of CRM is for the occasional assessment of accuracy, by providing traceability of results to a reference method value (RMV). CRM for a limited range of analytes, e.g. serum proteins, alphafetoprotein, apolipoprotein, thyroglobulin, thyroxine, cortisol and progesterone, are available through the European Commission (Joint Research Centre, Institute for Reference Materials and Measurements (IRMM), Retieseweg B-2440, GEEL, Belgium).

Other types of specimen occasionally used in IQC. In view of the limited availability of CRM, other IQC materials are often used in the assessment of accuracy. Recovery specimens can be prepared by adding known quantities of the calibrant to analyte-free serum, taking care to use independently prepared solutions of the calibrant for assay calibration and preparation of the recovery specimens. External quality assessment scheme specimens with a target assigned as the consensus mean may also provide an indication of accuracy, and are discussed more fully later in this chapter. Blank specimens prepared by physicochemical removal of the analyte (e.g. charcoal absorption), or pharmacological suppression in donor subjects may be helpful in assessing background interference as a cause of inaccuracy.

Assessment of Baseline Assay Performance

	Precision	Bias
Within-run	Within-sample, within-run CV (precision profile)	Mean difference between results on IQC pool in a run and target value
Between-run	Within-sample, between-run CV of IQC pools across runs	Mean difference between results on IQC pool across several runs and target value

Table 3 Basic IQC performance statistics and their derivation.

Table 3 summarises a basic approach to the estimation of within- and between-run precision and accuracy. These performance statistics should be made at an early stage in method development or evaluation under 'optimal conditions', in order to define criteria for acceptance or rejection of runs as part of the IQC programme.

Precision. Within-run precision is best estimated from replicated estimates on test specimens in the form of a precision profile, showing the plot of coefficient of variation (CV) against concentration. The calculation and use of the precision profile is discussed elsewhere in this book (*see* Chapter 9) and many software packages for processing immunoassay data compute and plot a precision profile. In IQC the profile is particularly valuable in comparing the effects of changes in assay conditions on precision, and in determining the working range of the assay, defined for example as the concentration range within which the precision is less than 10% CV.

Between-run precision can also be estimated from results on test specimens, replicated across runs to give a between-assay precision profile, as outlined above. However, for IQC purposes between-run precision is best estimated as the standard deviation of IQC pool results, across at least 15 assay runs. It is the between-run SD that is used to plot the control limits on IQC charts. IQC performance statistics are calculated as follows, where x_i is the control result in each of n runs:

$$\text{Mean } (\bar{x}) = \frac{\sum\limits_{i=1}^{n} x_i}{n}$$

$$\text{Standard deviation (SD)} = \sqrt{\frac{n\sum\limits_{i=1}^{n} x_i^2 - \left(\sum\limits_{i=1}^{n} x_i\right)^2}{n(n-1)}}$$

$$\text{Coefficient of variation (CV)} = \frac{SD}{\bar{x}} \times 100\%$$

Bias. Within-run bias is indicated by a consistent deviation of pool results from target, and reflects a systematic error affecting that run due, for example, to miscalibration, high background etc. Bias persisting across runs indicates a more fundamental problem due to, for example, deterioration of reagents or calibrators. Bias is calculated as follows, where x_w is the mean of IQC results within a run, x_b is the mean across runs, and x_t is the target previously determined for the same IQC material:

$$\text{Bias within run} = \frac{(\bar{x}_w - x_t) \times 100\%}{x_t}$$

$$\text{Bias across runs} = \frac{(\bar{x}_b - x_t) \times 100\%}{x_t}$$

Inclusion of IQC Specimens in Assay Run

A key assumption is that the IQC results will reflect the quality of the test results in the assay run. IQC specimens should therefore be inserted in random positions in the run, and must be taken through all steps (e.g. including any extraction or chromatography steps) of the assay procedure. Failure to observe these points will result in underestimation of errors. Under routine conditions, a basic approach would be to include in each run IQC pools at three concentrations to assess precision and shifts in accuracy. For troubleshooting and to investigate suspected shifts in accuracy, CRM, EQA or recovery specimens should be included.

Control Charts

IQC data are intended to control the assay process in real time and presentation should be clear and straightforward. Recording the IQC results in tabular or spreadsheet form, together with details of assay run (date, reagent and calibrator batches, analyst name) is a basic minimum. However, graphical presentation in the form of a Levey-Jennings chart (also known as Shewhart chart) can be helpful. Details of the design and use of these charts have been described in standard texts (Westgard, 1994) but the principles are shown in Figure 2. Under stable conditions, not more than 1 in 20 IQC results should exceed the 2 SD limits, and not more than 3 in 1,000 should exceed the 3 SD limits. The chart shows stable assay conditions up to run 6, followed by persistent negative bias up to run 12, followed by correction of the bias but poor precision from run 13.

217

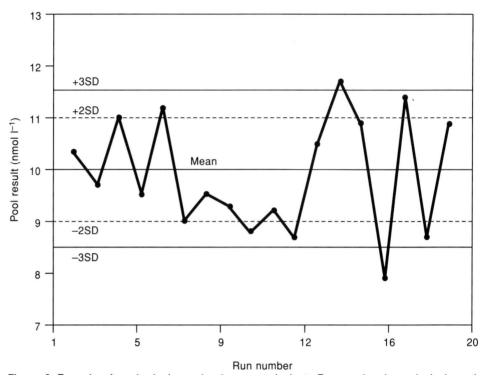

Figure 2 Example of a simple Levey-Jennings control chart. Run number is marked along the horizontal axis, and pool results are on the vertical axis. The horizontal lines drawn from the vertical axis indicate the pool mean, the 'warning' limits (±2 SD), and the 'action' limits (±3 SD) where SD is the between-run precision. See text for details of bias and precision changes, and run rejections.

Control charts for immunoassay. Immunoassays present particular features that often make it necessary to modify the general approach to chart plotting described above. An example of a Levey-Jennings chart for a testosterone radioimmunoassay (RIA) is shown in Figure 3, which illustrates the following points.

1 Immunoassays often cover a wide working range, with several 'clinical decision' levels. It is usually necessary therefore to include several IQC pools of different concentration in each run. A separate chart will be needed for each pool.

2 In scaling the y-axis, it is preferable to use relative error (e.g. percentage deviation of pool result from mean) rather than absolute error (e.g. SD in concentration units). This is because the SD increases markedly with concentration, resulting in widely differing scales for the different pools. Each pool mean is accordingly set at zero, the mean in concentration units being marked on this line.

3 Control lines are marked on the charts at ±1 CV, ±2 CV, and ± 3 CV around the zero line. In the charts in Figure 3 for the testosterone RIA with a between-run CV of 6% for all three pools, the lines are drawn at ±6%, ±12% and ± 18%.

Software packages for processing immunoassay data often provide facilities for plotting Levey-Jennings charts.

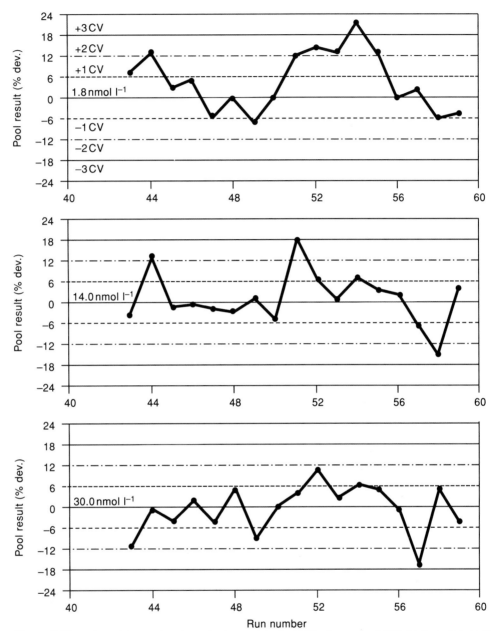

Figure 3 Examples of Levey-Jennings charts used in the IQC of a manual RIA for testosterone in serum. Note that, in order to achieve similar scales for different pools, the *y*-axes are plotted in terms of relative error (percentage deviation of pool result from mean), with pool concentration marked on the zero line. The control lines are also marked in units of relative error (coefficient of variation, CV) rather than absolute error (SD).

Interpretation of IQC Results

The principle of interpretation is to detect significant changes in bias and precision while not rejecting runs under 'in-control' conditions (false rejection). In a simple IQC procedure using one control specimen per run (Figure 2), an out-of-control condition is signalled if any of the following occur (Thompson and Wood, 1993).

1   The IQC result falls outside the action limits.

2   The current IQC result and the previous run IQC result lie between the warning and action limits.

3   Nine successive IQC results fall on the same side of the mean line.

Criteria (1) and (2) will detect changes in precision and bias, whereas (3) will be more effective in detecting a persistent change in bias. In the example shown (Figure 2), runs 14 and 16 would be rejected (criterion 1), as would run 18 (criterion 2).

Limitations of the above simple approach are that the power of the rules to detect errors are not explicitly defined, and when several IQC specimens are included in each run, and some are 'in control' and others are out of control, IQC results can be difficult to interpret. In addition the control criteria are defined simply in terms of the established performance of the method, without reference to the quality requirements of the user of the laboratory data.

Control Rules

These limitations can be overcome by use of the approach developed by Westgard and co-workers (Westgard *et al.*, 1981), which is based on computer simulation techniques to estimate the probability for detecting stated sizes of systematic error (bias), and random error (precision) using different numbers of control observations and different rejection criteria, or control rules. Figures 4a and b show power function graphs for the control rules listed in the right-hand panels, the rules being abbreviated as follows.

1_{3s} Reject when one control measurement exceeds ± 3 SD control limits.

2 of 3_{2s} Reject when any two of three consecutive control measurements exceed the same $+ 2$ SD or -2 SD control limits.

R_{4s} Reject when one control measurement exceeds the $+2$ SD control limit, and another exceeds the -2 SD control limit.

3_{1s} Reject when three consecutive control observations exceed the same $+1$ SD or -1 SD control limit.

6_x Reject when six consecutive control measurements fall on the same side of the mean.

Where combinations of the above rules are used in a 'multirule' approach (e.g. $1_{3s}/2$ of $3_{2s}/R_{4s}/3_{1s}$) the run is judged out of control when any one of the rules is broken.

Figure 4a shows that the probability of detecting a systematic error of 2 SD (e.g. 10% shift in bias in an assay with a between-run precision of 5%) would be only 0.15 using the 1_{3s} rule with one control sample per run, but this could be improved to about 0.4 using 3 pools per run, and further improved to 0.55 using a multirule approach. Use of rules more sensitive to bias (e.g. 3_{1s}, 6_x, over 2 runs) greatly improves detection to 0.94. The probability for false rejection is shown by the intercept on the y-axis, and remains acceptable at 0.04.

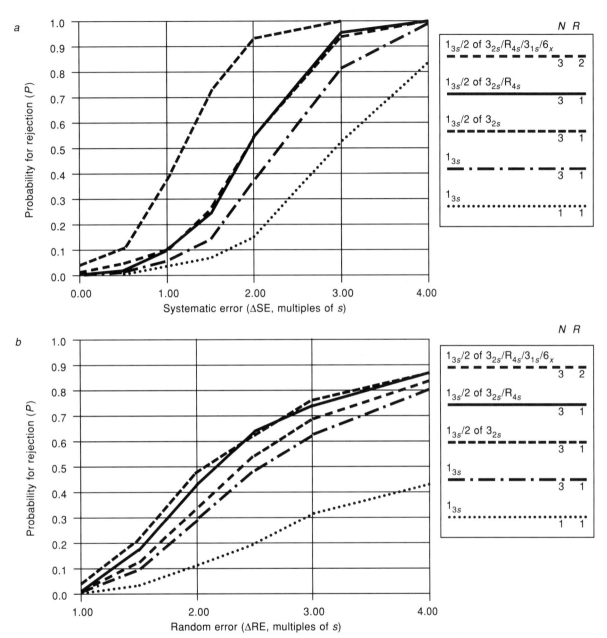

Figure 4 Examples of 'power function graphs' illustrating the effect of varying the number of IQC results and rejection criteria (control rules) on the probability of detection of systematic error, panel *a*, and random error, panel *b*. The errors are expressed as multiples of the between-run standard deviation (s). The key to the graph lines, are shown in the right panel. *N*, number of control observations per run; *R*, number of runs. See text for key to control rules. Figures plotted using the 'QC Validator, version 1.1' software package (Westgard Quality Corporation, 112 Shore Road, PO Box 2026, Ogonquit, ME 03907, USA).

Figure 4*b* shows that the probability of detecting a doubling in imprecision (e.g. 10% CV in an assay normally with a CV of 5%) is not better than 0.5 using the control strategies shown, illustrating that shifts in bias are often more reliably detected than changes in precision.

Planning IQC Strategy to Achieve Quality Goals

The IQC planning process developed by Westgard and co-workers (Westgard and Weibe, 1991), uses the above concepts to select the control strategy required to achieve a specified level of performance. The level of performance is defined in terms of the total allowable error and may be based on analytical requirements (e.g. performance criteria in an EQA scheme), or user requirements (e.g. clinically significant change in results). Owing to the difficulty in quantifying the latter for all clinical applications, analytical requirements are most commonly used. In principle, the steps in the planning process are as follows.

1   Determine the quality requirement as total allowable error, e.g. target value ± 3 SD in an EQA scheme, or target value $\pm$ stated per cent.

2   Determine the between-run precision (SD) and bias of the assay. Bias is calculated as per cent deviation from a reference method target, or other valid target in an EQA scheme.

3   Calculate the critical-size errors that must be detected using the formulae:

$$\Delta SE_{crit} = [(TE - bias_{meas})/s_{meas}] - 1.65$$

$$\Delta RE_{crit} = (TE - bias_{meas})/1.65 s_{meas}$$

where ΔSE_{crit} and ΔRE_{crit} are the critical-size systematic and random errors, TE is the total allowable error, $bias_{meas}$ and s_{meas} are the assay bias and precision (CV) under stable conditions, and 1.65 is the statistical z-value which allows for a 5% error rate before the process is stopped.

4   From power function graphs select the number of control observations and control rules to give probabilities of error detection and of false rejection at the critical-size error of about 0.9 and less than 0.05, respectively.

5   Review the IQC strategy as required in relation to changes in quality requirements, and changes in method performance.

The above steps are easily performed using the QC Validator software (see Figure 4 legend for details). Quality requirements (analytical or clinical) are entered, together with details of assay bias and precision. The power of alternative combinations of number of IQC observations and control rules to detect significant errors can be explored, and a rational IQC strategy selected.

This approach to planning IQC offers several advantages.

1   The quality requirement, i.e. size of errors to be detected, is an explicit part of the IQC plan.

2   The probability of detection of significant errors is approximately known.

3   The size of the analytical errors in relation to quality requirements highlights aspects of the process that most need attention. Where the critical error is large (measurement error small in relation to allowable error) a minimum of IQC samples with a simple control

rule and wide limits (e.g. 1_{3s}) might be adequate. When the critical error is small (measurement error large in relation to allowable error), a more demanding IQC plan and efforts to reduce analytical errors are indicated.

4   Where IQC results fail control rule criteria, the rule failed can indicate the type of error (bias or precision) occurring.

Application of Statistical IQC Principles in Immunoassay

The above principles are applicable to all quantitative tests but some additional considerations arise in their application to immunoasay. These considerations differ between manual immunoassays run in batch mode and automated assays in which tests are done sequentially.

Manual Immunoassay

An example of IQC planning for the serum testosterone RIA shown in Figure 3 is illustrated below. The steps were performed using the QC Validator software package (see Figure 4 legend for details)

1   The quality requirement for serum testosterone in females was taken as target $\pm$ 25% at a level of 3.0 nmol l^{-1} (the upper limit of normal in females).

2   Between-run precision using commercial IQC pools over 15 runs under stable conditions was previously estimated as 6% CV over the concentration range 2.0–30.0 nmol l^{-1}. Bias was assumed to be zero, on the basis of satisfactory performance in an EQA scheme.

3   Critical-size systematic error was calculated to be 2.52 SD, and critical-size random error was calculated to be 2.53 SD.

4   Power function graphs for 3 IQC specimens per run were plotted and the critical-error lines marked (Figure 5a and b). Optimum detection of systematic and random errors (0.86 and 0.65, respectively, with 0.02 false rejections) is given by the $1_{3s}/2$ of $3_{2s}/R_{4s}/3_{1s}$ multirule. Note that a 1_{2s} rule gives higher error detection but an unacceptably high rate of false rejection.

5   Application of the multirule to the testosterone RIA data indicated IQC failure of 4 runs as summarised in Table 4.

Assumptions in the approach that might not always be valid in manual immunoassay are that the errors affect all IQC samples equally. This may not be the case where there is concentration-dependent bias (due to, for example, incorrect points on a calibration curve, or high background interference) or there are differences in the incubation conditions across the assay run (due to, for example, nonuniformity of temperature or shaking conditions across microtitre plates or tube racks). Clearly, such errors will require remedial action, but in controlling immediate release of results, a judgement may need to be made as to whether only part of the run needs to be repeated. The judgement should take into account the size of the IQC error, and the likely effect of the error on the interpretation of the result. The need for flexibility in applying rejection criteria to immunoassay has been stressed elsewhere (Jeffcoate, 1981). A theoretically sound and practically acceptable approach to IQC in immunoassay

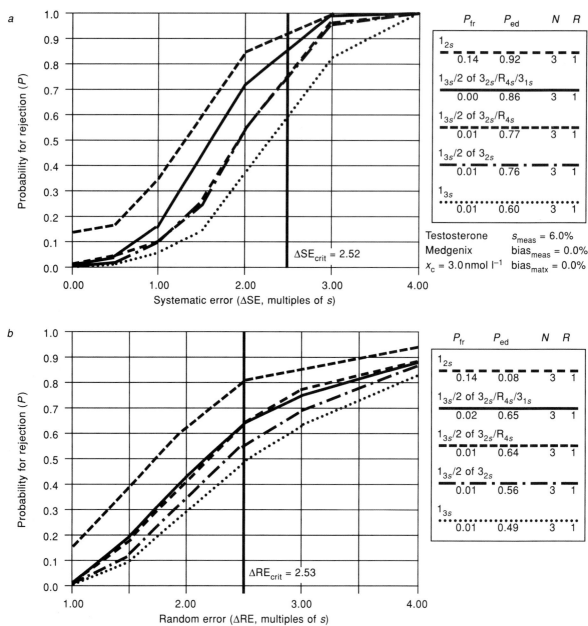

Figure 5 Critical error graphs for testosterone RIA, showing probability of detection of critical systematic error ΔSE_{crit}, panel *a* and critical random error ΔRE_{crit}, panel *b*, to achieve a quality goal of target ±25%. P_{fr} and P_{ed} are probability of false rejection, and probability of error-detection, respectively. The unbroken line shows the control rule selected. Figures plotted using QC Validator software (see Figure 4 for details).

would be to use appropriate control rules, with some latitude in interpretation depending on specific circumstances.

Run No.	Rule failed	IQC specimen
44	2 of 3_{2s}	Low, medium
51	1_{3s}	Medium
52	3_{1s}	Low, medium, high
54	1_{3s}	Low

Table 4 Application of the $1_{3s}/2$ of $3_{2s}/R_{4s}/3_{1s}$ multirule to the testosterone RIA IQC data shown in Figure 3.

Automated Immunoassay Analysers

Automated immunoassays generally present different requirements to those of manual batch assays.

(1) Calibration is performed relatively infrequently on many automated systems, with sample results being calculated from stored calibration curve parameters, unlike batch assays, where calibrators are included in every run. This economy of calibration is made possible by the stability of the analytical process, but implies that errors of bias are most likely to occur after the instrument has been idle, or maintenance work has been done. Where IQC results fall outside limits at analyser start-up, a one- or two-point recalibration may be done to adjust the calibration curve parameters. An IQC plan with high error detection at start-up is therefore advisable (*see* Chapter 12).

(2) In many automated systems, tests are performed sequentially during the working day, whereas in batch analysis tests (unknowns and IQC) are run simultaneously. Consequently, in batch analysis all IQC results are available at the time of reporting, maximising the power of the QC rules. This is not practicable with automated sequential analysers unless IQC validation of results is delayed until the end of the working day. Unlike batch mode, run acceptance should be confirmed before the unknowns have been analysed. This again implies the need for an IQC plan with high error detection at start-up. From this point on IQC specimens can be randomly placed throughout the day, culminating in one IQC specimen before close-down at the end of the day.

The reagent and consumables costs of IQC on automated systems are relatively high, and the IQC plan must be carefully defined to balance effectiveness and economy. In order to comply with regulatory requirements, laboratories should as a minimum follow manufacturers' recommended IQC protocols. However, the IQC planning approach of Westgard and colleagues (Westgard and Wiebe, 1991) provides a more objective approach. Application of this process to several immunoassays (Mugan *et al.*, 1994) run on automated equipment (Abbott IMx®) led to the conclusions that CLIA or College of American Pathologists (CAP) performance criteria could be met by a two-stage IQC process, using a 1_{3s} or $1_{2.5s}$ rule with $N=6$ at weekly instrument start-up when measurement instability might be greatest, and $N=2$–3 for daily monitoring.

The availability of analysers with on-board data processing facilities to store user-defined control rules and alert the operator to failures will simplify the routine application of this approach.

Other Strategies in IQC

Other techniques in IQC may be used, although these are usually in addition to rather than as an alternative to the above use of stable control material.

Cumulative Sum (CUSUM) Chart

Cumulative sum (CUSUM) charts can be helpful in identifying trends in performance. The chart is prepared using IQC specimen results as in the Levey-Jennings chart. Run number is plotted on the *x*-axis, but the *y*-axis now shows the cumulated sum of the difference between the observed result and the target value of the IQC specimen, i.e. if the differences between the IQC results and the target in runs 1, 2 and 3 were 10, −8 and 12 concentration units, respectively, the plotted CUSUM values would be 10, 2 and 14. A horizontal line is drawn at the mid-point of the *y*-axis at CUSUM=0, and for an assay under in-control conditions, the CUSUM plot would follow, with minor positive and negative deviations, the zero line. IQC results falling persistently on one side of the mean will cause the CUSUM plot to slope away from the zero line. A persistent positive or negative CUSUM slope therefore indicates assay bias. Difficulties with CUSUM charts are that the target value must be assigned with care to avoid a sloping plot under in-control conditions, and determination of a significant change in slope can be somewhat subjective. A simple, more objective approach is to scale the chart so that the distance between two runs on the *x*-axis equals twice the between-run SD on the *y*-axis. A 45° slope then represents a bias of 2 SD.

Repeat Analytical Controls (RAC)

Some of the limitations associated with pools can be overcome by the repeat analysis of 1 to 3 selected patient specimens from the previous assay run. Repeat analytical controls (RAC) and IQC provide complementary information: RAC reflect performance on authentic patient specimens over a wide concentration range, and can detect errors in specimen identification, whereas pools reflect performance with specimens that have often been modified (addition or removal of analyte) at a few concentrations that become well known to the analyst. RAC do not, however, provide an indication of long-term assay stability. Between-run precision can be estimated as:

$$SD = \sqrt{\frac{\sum d^2}{2N}}$$

where *d* is the difference between repeat observations, and *N* is number of repeated specimens.

Patient Data

The mean or median of results on patient specimens within an assay run, calculated after trimming to remove low and high values, has been used as an additional control parameter in general clinical biochemistry. The technique is not widely used as it cannot detect imprecision and it has poor sensitivity to bias changes relative to the use of stable IQC material. However, it may have a value in certain circumstances in immunoassay, e.g. in maternal serum screening programmes for Down's syndrome and neural tube defects, where continuous monitoring of patient medians for serum alphafetoprotein, chorionic gonadotrophin and other analytes can provide information on assay stability and confirmation of the validity of the parameters for risk calculation.

Assay Parameters

IQC results on test material indicate the quality of the entire assay procedure, but it may also be helpful to record key parameters of assay performance. These include the background and maximum signals (absorbance, radioactivity, luminescence etc.), the calibration curve parameters (slope, intercept), and scatter of the calibrator points about the calculated curve. Inspection of these parameters, together with records of reagent or kit batch number, can assist in determining the cause of trends and failures in IQC results.

Review of Quality Control Data

The daily quality control procedures are the responsibility of the analyst but, depending on circumstances, it is often beneficial to have a second person involved in data interpretation. There is evidence (Seth and Hanning, 1988) that among laboratories performing manual RIAs for growth hormone, laboratories in which the IQC data were validated by a second person performed better than those in which only the analyst did the IQC checking. It must, however, be emphasised that IQC is a collaborative activity involving all staff: attempts to operate IQC as a 'policing' regime are not likely to be successful. Where a run fails to meet quality criteria, the reasons should be explored in a constructive, noncritical manner. Often a lesson will be learnt that benefits future practice.

In addition to the use of IQC data for daily control, the accumulated data should be periodically reviewed to monitor longer-term trends in performance. EQA data should be simultaneously reviewed and interpreted in relation to IQC performance. Gradual shifts in bias and/or precision may be identified. Such reviews are best undertaken at regular, e.g. monthly, meetings of all staff involved in providing the service. Audit of pre- and postanalytical errors can also be reviewed at such meetings, providing a forum for continuous and comprehensive audit of the laboratory service.

Troubleshooting

It is difficult to generalise about the causes of IQC failure, as these depend on the type of immunoassay. However, a guide to which features of an assay to examine in the event of IQC failure is summarised in Table 5.

Limitations of IQC

IQC ensures that assay runs conform to defined quality standards; it cannot ensure that errors

Assay stage	Bias	Precision
Set up	• Incorrect or degraded calibrant • Incorrect calibrant matrix • Delay between set up of calibrants and test samples	• Imprecise pipetting of samples and reagents • Reagents not mixed • Temperature gradients
Separation of free and bound label	• Separation reagents not optimised	• Inadequate washing • Inadvertent loss of solid phase
Signal detection	• High background signal	• Nonequivalence of detectors (especially multihead gamma counters) • Contaminants on reaction tubes or detectors • Environmental contaminants (especially fluorescence, chemiluminescence)
Data processing	• Incorrect curve fit model • Incorrect calibrant conversion factor (mass to IU)	

Table 5 Some causes of errors in bias and precision in IQC of immunoassays.

do not occur with individual test specimens. Table 6 summarises some of the errors that might go undetected.

The prevalence of such errors will depend on individual laboratory circumstances but in general clinical chemistry an annual error rate of 0.1% of requests has been reported from two departments (Lapworth and Teal, 1994). Errors were approximately equally divided between the preanalytical, analytical and postanalytical stages. Specific sources of error will be analyte-dependent, e.g. specimen degradation will be important in the immunoassay of unstable hormones, whereas dilution errors, high-dose hook effects, and interference from human anti-mouse antibodies are likely to be important in tumour marker immunoassays.

IQC can detect shifts in bias with time, but in order to assess bias in relation to independent target values, analysis of CRM or EQA specimens is required. The uses of EQA in QA are discussed in the following section.

Preanalytical	Analytical	Postanalytical
• Incorrect specimen identity	• Insufficient sample due to pipette/probe blockage	• Incorrect results transcription
• Specimen degraded on storage	• Incorrect reagent addition	
• Incorrect type of specimen tube	• Interferences in test specimen, e.g. heterophilic antibodies, lipaemia	
	• High-dose hook effect Incorrect / missing dilution factor	

Table 6 Errors in immunoanalysis that may not be detected by IQC.

EXTERNAL QUALITY ASSESSMENT

While IQC ensures the consistency of quality within the laboratory, EQA provides data that retrospectively compare laboratory performance with an external and objective standard. Conventionally, an EQA organising centre distributes identical samples of test material to participant laboratories. The laboratory results are reported to the EQA centre for statistical analysis, which then returns an EQA report describing each participant's performance in relation to an agreed target. EQA has therefore a complementary role to IQC in quality assurance.

EQA schemes operate in all major laboratory disciplines in health care, and vary in their approach. Some are primarily educational with voluntary participation, whereas others, often with compulsory participation, set mandatory performance standards which laboratories must achieve in order to practice. EQA schemes may be provided commercially, or on behalf of professional associations.

The EQA of immunoassays has developed along the principles established for general clinical chemistry (Westgard, 1994) but present some additional problems arising from the use of biological reagents to measure complex analytes. Several EQA schemes have recently been reviewed (Franzini *et al.*, 1991).

Principles of EQA

The principles of EQA are common to the EQA of any analyte, and are summarised in Table 7. The features outlined are also those that participating laboratories should seek in selecting an EQA scheme.

Scheme Design

Regular and frequent sample distribution is essential if statistically valid data are to be obtained in a realistic time-frame. The external quality assessment scheme (EQAS) centre should also return reports promptly to participants if the results are to be of other than historical interest. The methods used by participants must be correctly identified, including any modifications made, if valid conclusions are to be drawn on method-group performance. The need for all participants to report in common units will be obvious. For hapten immunoassays there are relatively few difficulties provided that mass or molar units are specified. For peptides, international units (IU) of the current WHO standard are strongly preferred. Difficulties can arise, however, where methods are calibrated in mass units of other standard preparations, necessitating the use of conversion factors. There is good evidence that use of a common standard can dramatically improve between-laboratory agreement (Franzini *et al.*, 1991). This should encourage laboratories to report all results in terms of common units, although selective conversion of EQA results without converting patients' results does occur, hindering progress towards harmonisation of results, and introducing the potential for errors. As in IQC, EQA samples should be handled identically to samples routinely received. Preferential treatment of EQA samples can improve the laboratory's apparent, if not actual, performance. This does, however, diminish the value of EQA to the QA activities of the laboratory.

Scheme design
- Frequent sample distribution to provide practically relevant and statistically valid data.
- Rapid return of EQA reports to participants.
- Accurate documentation of methods used.
- Common units for reporting results.
- EQA samples assayed by participants in exactly the same way as routine specimens.
- Reports clear and concise.

Sample material distributed
- Properties identical to patient samples in all assay systems.
- Analyte concentrations appropriate to clinical use of test.
- Stable under conditions of sample distribution.
- Present no avoidable infectious hazard.

Definition of target values
- Reference method values provided where possible.
- Validate accuracy and stability of consensus mean targets.

Assessment of performance
- Appropriate statistics used.
- Overall, method-group and individual laboratory performances estimated.
- Gross errors (outliers) highlighted.
- Other aspects of performance (e.g. test interferences, interpretation) assessed where appropriate

---

Table 7 Principles of EQA.

Sample Material Distributed

The requirements of samples for distribution through EQAS (Table 7) are similar to those for IQC samples (Table 2). These are demanding requirements to meet, but their importance cannot be overstated as sample suitability is often questioned in response to evidence of poor laboratory or method performance.

Identity of behaviour between EQA samples and those routinely received (e.g. patients' samples) can be difficult to ensure. The use of pooled sera can obscure differences in bias that might be revealed by use of serum from individual patients (Bacon *et al.*, 1983). In addition, serum pools containing pure exogenous analyte can reveal a different pattern of performance compared to pools containing the endogenous form. For several peptide hormones and tumour markers, between-laboratory scatter is greater with specimens containing endogenous in contrast to exogenous (e.g. pure standard) analyte. This probably reflects greater molecular heterogeneity in samples containing endogenous hormone, and the differing specificity of immunoassays for these substances.

The analyte concentrations in the EQA samples must be appropriate for the major application of the assay. A laboratory performing maternal serum alphafetoprotein and chorionic gonadotrophin assays for screening for Down's Syndrome will require samples at concentrations around the cutoffs for recommending further action; samples covering the wider concentration range found in using these assays as tumour markers would be less helpful. For some analytes where the clinical application includes identification of suppressed levels (e.g. thyroid-stimulating hormone (thyrotrophin; TSH) and other anterior pituitary hormones), zero-analyte samples should also be distributed from time to time. These can be prepared by a variety of methods, e.g. by collection of sera after pharmacological or physiological suppression of hormone production in normal volunteers, or by removal of endogenous analyte from normal serum, using resin, charcoal or immunoaffinity stripping.

Sample stability is a major concern, as degradation of the analyte or matrix will affect immunoassay results. Many EQA schemes use lyophilised samples, but this can induce changes in the matrix of serum samples and consequent differences in behaviour between the lyophilised EQA sera and the test sera. In addition, reconstitution errors may occur. Liquid specimens avoid some of these difficulties, but they can only be used where rapid specimen delivery can be guaranteed. Liquid specimens should contain a bacteriostat, although evidence that this does not interfere in the immunoassays is essential. In the United Kingdom National External Quality Assessment Schemes (UK NEQAS), 0.05% azide is suitable for use with many immunoassays, but interferes in some assays using horseradish peroxidase labels, and for these assays 1% kathon® (Rohm and Hass (UK) Ltd, Lennig House, 2 Masons Avenue, Croydon, UK) is preferred.

Definition of Target Values

The target value is the analyte concentration in the sample against which performance is assessed, and it may be defined on the basis of one of the following.

1   *Reference method value (RMV)*: This is the preferred target if EQA is to promote the use of accurate methods, but in practice such targets have limited application in immunoassay owing to the lack of reference methods for other than a few analytes. They have been most widely used for steroid assays, where isotope dilution-mass spectrometry methods are available. Replication of RMVs in more than one centre is essential and considerable financial and experimental resources are needed to sustain this approach.

2   *All-laboratory consensus mean*: The mean (or median) of results from all laboratories is applicable to a wide range of analytes, is easily calculated and, provided that there are sufficient participating laboratories (at least 15), is statistically reasonably robust. The stability of the estimates of mean and overall scatter can be improved by excluding 'outlier' values, which is best done by the trimming technique described by Healy (1979).

3   *Method or grouped method means*: This is analogous to the all-laboratory consensus mean but includes users of only a single method, or a group of closely related methods. Caution is required in the use of single-method means; although this might assist comparison of laboratory performance with that of its peers, poor performance of the method will be obscured. In addition, the estimate of the mean will be less reliable when there are few laboratories using the method. A grouped-method target, calculated by combining results from several closely related methods, may be appropriate where methods for the same analyte fall into groups that differ according to the measurement

principle used, e.g. chorionic gonadotrophin methods measuring either the intact hormone plus its β-subunit, or the intact hormone only.

4   *Value defined by preparative procedure*: This can be appropriate where an adequate supply of the pure analyte is available and can be accurately weighed to make up the specimen, e.g. in EQA of a drug immunoassay. However, such specimens will not reflect the effect of metabolites in endogenous specimens.

5   *Mean of reference laboratory group*: The mean of results reported by a group of laboratories selected as 'centres of excellence' has been used to supply target values. Although the approach may be useful for newly developed assays performed in a few laboratories, it has found little place in established, large-scale schemes.

Validation of Target Values

In practice, the majority of EQA schemes use all-laboratory consensus means, grouped-method or single-method means as targets. Whichever of these is used, it is important to demonstrate that the targets meet minimum criteria of validity, which are stability between repeat distributions of the same pool, and accuracy. These are important criteria if EQA schemes are to guide users towards accuracy rather than towards the more limited goal of simply achieving between-laboratory agreement.

Stability of the target values is relatively easy to demonstrate, but accuracy presents both conceptual and practical problems. For some relatively simple analytes, e.g. steroids, it may be possible to demonstrate agreement between a consensus mean and the RMV (Middle and Singh, 1995). For more complex analytes, e.g. protein hormones and tumour markers that exhibit molecular heterogeneity, the concept of accuracy is difficult to apply. However, it should be possible to demonstrate agreement between the calculated and observed target values of sera to which known amounts of standard have been added (Table 8). Although this cannot demonstrate accuracy with patients' sera, distortion of the consensus mean by incorrectly calibrated methods can be identified, and the confidence of participants in the utility of the scheme increased.

The data in Table 8 illustrate several points. First, targets for some analytes such as free hormones are not easily validated either by RMV or recovery methods. Second, recovery is difficult to estimate when there is no suitable international standard and the analyte is unstable (e.g. parathyroid hormone and adrenocorticotrophic hormone). Finally, the reproducibility of the all-laboratory mean can be relatively poor in small schemes where several different methods are used (e.g. peptide hormones).

Assessment of Performance

Many EQA schemes provide data describing all-laboratory, method-group and laboratory performance. The details of how this is done differ between schemes, e.g. choice of target, use of log-transformation, methods of outlier rejection, etc. The underlying statistical concepts are, however, similar and are shown in Figure 6.

Analyte	N labs	ALTM Recovery (%)	Stability (%)	Between-lab agreement (%)
Thyroid hormones				
TSH	337	97	1.6	12
Total thyroxine	132	93	0.9	8
Total triiodothyronine	113	101	1.2	12
Free thyroxine	260	ND	1.0	17
Free triiodothyronine	169	ND	2.9	23
Protein hormones				
Growth hormone	77	93	0.5	20
Follicle-stimulating hormone	240	104	0.5	15
Luteinising hormone	240	111	0.7	22
Prolactin	240	114	0.5	20
Peptide hormones				
Parathyroid hormone	74	70	2.9	20
Adrenocorticotrophic hormone	29	55	2.4	35
Calcitonin	12	107	11.9	20
Tumour markers				
Alphafetoprotein	83	102	0.4	10
Chorionic gonadotrophin (total)	95	100	1.7	20
Chorionic gonadotrophin (intact)	24	100	0.8	20
Carcinoembryonic antigen	87	92	1.5	25
Steroids				
Cortisol	237	102	1.0	12
Oestradiol	159	74	2.0	20
Progesterone	193	84	1.0	15
Testosterone (female)	112	98	2.5	25
Testosterone (male)	11	89	2.0	12

Table 8 Validity of the target values (all-laboratory trimmed mean, ALTM) in the UK National External Quality Assessment Schemes (UK NEQAS), 1995. *N* labs is the number of participating laboratories. The ALTM recovery (%) is the agreement between the calculated and found value of the ALTM on adding pure analyte or WHO standard to serum. (ND, not determined). Stability is the mean CV (%) of the ALTM on repeat distributions of EQA samples. The between-laboratory agreement is the approximate overall spread of results (CV or GCV, %) across all laboratories.

Overall Performance

The all-laboratory mean (x_0) and scatter (SD_0) of results provides a measure of the 'state of the art' for measurement of the analyte. The closeness of the overall mean to an RMV (where

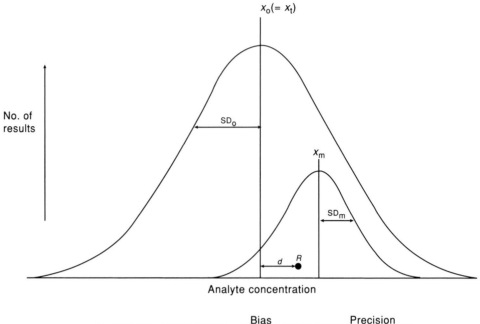

Figure 6 Principles of assessing overall, method and laboratory performance in EQA. The overall distribution of results, mean x_o, standard deviation SD_o, reflects the between- and within- method scatter of results on a single sample. The distribution of results among users of a single method M are shown by x_m and SD_m. In the absence of a RMV to define the target (x_t), x_o or in some schemes x_m is used as the target. R is the result from a laboratory using method M. R has a positive deviation (d) from target x_o, but a negative deviation from target x_m. See text for explanation of table.

	Bias	Precision
All laboratory	$(x_o - x_t) \times 100/x_t$	SD_o
Method	$(x_m - x_t) \times 100/x_t$	SD_m
Laboratory	mean $(d \times 100/x_t)$	$SD_d \times 100/x_t$

available), or to a recovery-validated target can indicate the accuracy of methods in use. Where an RMV is unavailable, as is the usual case, the overall mean is often used as the target, i.e. $x_o = x_t$. The scatter (SD_o) of the overall distribution reflects the closeness of agreement between methods and laboratories. The limits of the overall distribution ($x_o \pm 3\ SD_o$) may be used to define the criteria for acceptable performance in some proficiency-testing schemes.

Overall between-laboratory agreement for a wide range of immunoassays in the UK NE-QAS is summarised in Table 8. Several points are illustrated: agreement is not as good at low concentrations (e.g. female compared to male testosterone), and for technically demanding analytes (e.g. adrenocorticotrophic hormone). Agreement is relatively good for high concentration, relatively simple analytes (e.g. total thyroxine, alphafetoprotein). Trends towards improved overall agreement for several analytes have been shown in different national EQA schemes since the 1980s (Franzini *et al.*, 1991). Methodological advances have undoubtedly contributed to this, although the contribution of EQA activity *per se* is less easily determined.

Method Performance

EQA provides a powerful tool for assessing method performance. Provided that the method has a sufficient number of users (approximately 10), and that the target value can be validated as above, the relative deviation of the method mean from target $((x_m-x_t) \times 100/x_t)$ and the within-method, between-laboratory scatter of results (SD_m) indicate the method bias and between-laboratory precision. Pooling of these statistics across several samples is required to give robust estimates of method performance. These data are of unique value because they describe the performance of the methods under routine conditions and in many laboratories.

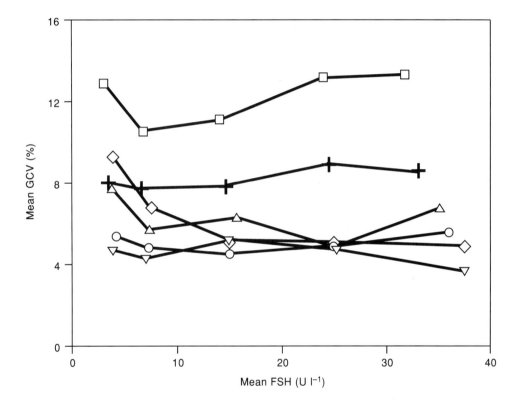

Figure 7 Within-method, between-laboratory precision profiles for serum follicle-stimulating hormone (FSH) methods in the UK NEQAS, 1995. Square symbols, manual RIA method; other symbols, automated nonisotopic methods. GCV is the geometric coefficient of variation, calculated from log-transformed results.

Data illustrating how EQA can compare and evaluate methods are shown in Figures 7 and 8. The precision profiles (Figure 7) show that automated nonisotopic methods for follicle-stimulating hormone (FSH) give better between-laboratory agreement than manual RIA, but that there are differences in precision among the automated methods, which might indicate differences in the robustness of assay chemistries and/or instrumentation.

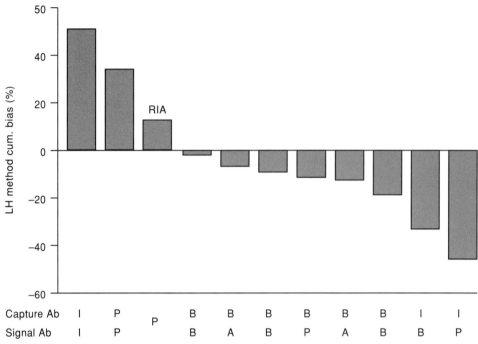

Figure 8 Bias of methods to the all-laboratory consensus mean in the UK NEQAS for luteinising hormone (LH), 1995. Antibody (Ab) specificity (data provided by manufacturers) is indicated as I, anti-intact; B, anti-beta chain; A, anti-alpha chain; P, polyclonal.

The bar chart (Figure 8) shows the wide spread of bias among methods for luteinising hormone (LH). The causes of bias are complex but the figure shows that antibody specificity is important, with methods using the more specific anti-intact antibodies tending to give negative bias to the all-laboratory trimmed mean (ALTM), and methods using less specific polyclonal antibodies giving high bias. The lack of complete correspondence between method bias and antibody specificity indicates that other factors (e.g. accuracy of calibration, nonspecific interference) also contribute to method bias.

Other aspects of method performance can also be assessed through EQA, although this will usually require the distribution of nonroutine, experimental samples. For example, in the UK NEQAS for thyroid hormones (Mackenzie, 1995), differences in the sensitivity of TSH methods have been revealed by distributing serum from triiodothyronine-suppressed subjects, providing a valuable guide as to which methods are likely to be most discriminating in the investigation of suspected hyperthyroidism. In the UK NEQAS for peptide hormones and tumour markers, some methods have been shown to be vulnerable to interference from human anti-mouse antibodies (Ellis *et al.*, 1996), an important cause of potentially serious clinical error. Differences in method specificity can also be demonstrated by distribution of specimens containing potential crossreactants. Experimental samples that probe these additional aspects of method performance need only be distributed occasionally, but can be of great educational value to laboratory users and manufacturers of *in vitro* diagnostic (IVD) products.

A role for EQA in the surveillance of IVD products in use has been proposed (Commission of the European Communities, 1995). Such a role requires firm evidence that the samples are appropriate, and that the target values are valid, as discussed above.

EQA ideally provides independent estimates of laboratory bias and precision, which complement estimates of these performance parameters obtained through IQC. The approaches to estimation of these parameters differ between EQA and IQC, because in EQA the estimates are made across samples whereas in IQC they are made within sample.

Bias. This is ideally determined against an RMV target, although in practice a consensus mean is usually used. As discussed above, the target value should have some proof of validity (stability and quantitative recovery of standard) if laboratories are to have confidence in the EQA data. Many EQA schemes provide reports describing the bias on each (e.g. monthly) specimen distribution, together with an 'end-of-term' (e.g. six-monthly) report. The former indicates the relative deviation of laboratory results from target ($d \times 100/x_o$, Figure 6) at the time the EQA specimens were assayed, in a single assay run. The latter six-month or cumulative bias (mean $(d \times 100)/x_t$) gives an estimate of long-term performance on many, e.g. 12–30 EQA specimens, depending on scheme design. It is important to appreciate that pooling of results across specimens to estimate bias in this way is vulnerable to concentration-dependent bias, which is a feature of many immunoassays. In addition, the type of specimen (e.g. whether it contains endogenous, or purified exogenous analyte) can affect assay bias. Estimates of laboratory bias in EQA often depend therefore on the concentration range and type of sample included in the assessment 'window'.

Precision. Changes in assay precision are less easily detected in EQA schemes than changes in bias. This is in part a consequence of the concepts shown in the 'power function' graphs in IQC (Figure 4), together with the relatively low frequency of control observations made in EQA. EQA schemes adopt either of two alternative approaches to estimating laboratory precision: (1) distribution of duplicate samples, and estimation of precision as the SD of duplicates (e.g. as described above for RAC); and (2) distribution of nonreplicated samples, and estimation of the scatter of relative deviations (SD of $d \times 100/x_o$, Figure 6) from target. Whichever approach is used, it will be appreciated that the same reservations attached to pooling data across samples to estimate bias also apply to the pooling of data to estimate precision.

Gross errors. Gross errors, or laboratory blunders (Table 7), may be detected in EQA schemes. They may be defined as results outside specified limits (e.g. $x_o \pm 3$ SD_o of the all-laboratory distribution). It is preferable to exclude these from the calculations of laboratory precision and bias, so as to give a more reliable estimate of the underlying assay performance, but the numbers of blunders occuring in the laboratory must be recorded.

Interpretation of results. EQA scheme participants can be asked to interpret their results in the context of clinical information on a real or fictional patient. Such exercises need careful planning if they are to be realistic, unambiguous and sufficiently challenging, but performed occasionally they can add interest and educational value (Sturgeon, 1996).

Surveys of laboratory practice. EQA provides an effective audit tool to assess laboratory practice. Differences in normal ranges, even among laboratories using the same methods, can be shown (Sturgeon, 1996) as can changes in methods used, and test profiles offered (e.g. for thyroid function tests). By making this information available to participants, EQA can be a medium for encouraging best laboratory practice.

	UK NEQAS for AFP, CEA and hCG.	Laboratory:
	Distribution: 98 Date: 9-Apr-96	Page 4 of 5
	Analyte: A.F.P. (kU/L BS 72/227)	

Pool (exclusion) [Type]	Distribution 93 17-Oct-95 result **target** % bias	Distribution 94 14-Nov-95 result **target** % bias	Distribution 95 12-Dec-95 result **target** % bias	Distribution 96 6-Feb-96 result **target** % bias	Distribution 97 5-Mar-96 result **target** % bias	Distribution 98 9-Apr-96 result **target** % bias
(T316)			(2.6) **2.7** (−1.8)			
(T317)				(3.9) **3.5**(+11.7)		
T318				8.8 **8.4** +4.7	7.3 **8.5** −14.1	
T314	12.0 **12.2** −1.7					
T319					12.4 **13.6** −9.2	13.6 **13.4** +1.3
T281			15.9 **15.9** −0.1			
T327					15.0 **16.0** −6.0	
T307		15.7 **16.3** −3.5			14.8 **16.4** −9.7	
T326					15.0 **17.2** −12.8	
T315		17.7 **18.4** −3.9				
T324				23.4 **18.8** +24.6		
T302			19.0 **19.4** −2.1	23.5 **19.6** +20.0		
T320						19.3 **19.4** −0.4
T312	22.4 **22.5** −0.7					
T300		23.5 **23.9** −1.8	23.6 **24.0** −1.5			
T330						28.5 **28.2** +1.1
T313	53.1 **53.5** −0.8					
T331						70.2 **70.4** −0.4
T285			72.7 **73.7** −1.4			
T288		78.1 **85.1** −8.2				
T304	98.4 **100.2** −1.8	87.7 **99.6** −12.0				
T323				180.0 **143.6** +25.3		
T329						194.7 **191.1** +1.9
T303	256.0 **238.8** +7.2					

method mean bias	Development +0.4	Development −5.9	Development −1.3	Development +18.7	Development −10.4	Development +0.7
BIAS	−3.0	−3.6	−2.6	+ 0.0	−2.5	−1.4
VAR	5.4	4.7	3.9	6.4	9.1	7.7

Figure 9 Table from a personalised laboratory report in the UK NEQAS for alphafetoprotein (AFP), summarising laboratory's performance over a six-month period. The distribution date is shown across the columns and pool identity is shown ranked by increasing concentration down the rows. The figures within each column show the laboratory's result, the target, and percentage deviation of the result from target.

Presentation of Results

EQA reports should present overall, method and individual laboratory performance in a clear and concise format. The use of simple scoring systems that combine bias and precision errors into a single performance parameter (Whitehead, 1977) may have a value in permitting rapid screening of EQA data on several analytes to detect problem areas requiring closer attention. However, it is vitally important that EQA scheme participants have a record of their raw data. An example of the way in which this can be presented is shown in Figure 9, taken from a laboratory's monthly report in the UK NEQAS for alphafetoprotein. Information that can be gleaned from the table includes:

1   Cumulative bias and scatter of the bias (VAR) for the 6 months to date (-1.4 and 7.7, respectively).

2   Mean bias on each distribution. Distribution 96 shows high results ($+18.7\%$), indicating bias in the assay run and the need for the laboratory to examine the IQC data.

3   Stability of target (consensus mean) across distributions (e.g. pools T318, 307).

4   Repeatability of laboratory results on a single sample across distributions (e.g. pools T318, 307).

5   Bias related to concentration and sample type.

6   Laboratory error on each sample.

The importance of the latter cannot be understated, as statistics summarising performance should always be interpreted in relation to the raw data, and the clinical significance of the errors observed.

Limitations of EQA

- EQA scheme samples and patient samples not processed identically in laboratory.
- EQA scheme samples do not behave identically to patient samples in method.
- Difficult to assess both individual laboratory and method performance when a single target is used.
- May inhibit development of improved methods giving numerically different results.
- Laboratory performance may differ in different EQA schemes.

Table 9 Limitations and risks in EQA.

Although EQA is a powerful tool for improvement in quality of analysis it has limitations and can present some risks (Table 9).

The laboratory processing of EQA samples may not truly reflect the processing of patient samples, owing to their different packaging and presentation and the unique report document required for returning EQA results. Further errors might occur where the EQA scheme requires results in concentration units different from those normally used by the laboratory. The need for identity of behaviour between EQA and patient samples has been discussed above: differences may be due to alterations in the matrix during preparation of EQA samples, or due to preservatives added, and can be method-dependent.

Use of a single all-laboratory target provides an assessment of method performance, but where methods differ in specificity and give differing results, e.g. in the EQA of immunoassays for gonadotrophins, a consequence is that users of some methods have high bias, making it difficult to assess their performance. Use of method targets would make it easier to assess laboratory performance, but at the expense of assessing method performance. A combined approach to targeting EQA samples has been proposed (Thienpoint and Stockl, 1995), based on regular use of method targets, with occasional distribution of material with a RMV to assess method bias, and establish traceability of results.

The achievement of results near to EQA targets is important for IVD manufacturers, and for laboratories, especially where the data are used for licensing purposes. Immunodiagnostics is one of the most rapidly developing areas in laboratory medicine, and the dangers of new and possibly superior methods being discriminated against because of 'out-of-consensus' performance in EQA schemes must be recognised.

Finally, the validity of EQA data on method and laboratory performance may be challenged because performance data in different schemes do not agree. Such an observation is not suprising given the many factors outlined above that influence performance assessment in EQA, which include sample type and concentration, selection of target value, method mix, the duration of data collection, and the statistical calculation of the performance indices. Laboratories should evaluate EQA schemes against the principles set out in Table 7.

CONCLUSIONS

Quality assurance should be a core activity in the laboratory, whether in research, industry or health-care. A broad view of all the steps in the laboratory process having a bearing on the quality of the laboratory output is essential, and it should be recognised that the overall quality is only as good as the weakest part of the process. Immunoassay presents some particular challenges in QA, reflecting the wide range of analytes covered, the lack of reference methods, difficulties in calibration and the variety of immunoassay techniques used. The increasing use of automated immunoassay analysers with on-board facilities for IQC has brought about significant improvements in precision. However, method bias remains a significant cause of lack of agreement between immunoassay results in different laboratories. EQA schemes using validated targets are a powerful tool for identifying the causes of method bias, and for encouraging the development of methods that are correctly designed and calibrated.

ACKNOWLEDGEMENTS

I am grateful to many colleagues in the Department of Clinical Biochemistry, Royal Infirmary of Edinburgh, who have provided valuable advice and assistance, in particular E. Wilkinson, for advice on IQC of automated analysers. I am also grateful to colleagues in the UK NEQAS for providing data and for many helpful discussions on EQA, in particular A. Ellis, C. M. Sturgeon, J. G. Middle, F. MacKenzie and D. G. Bullock. I would also like to thank J. O. Westgard, University of Wisconsin, for advice on the QC Validator software.

REFERENCES

Bacon, R. R. A., Hunter, W. M. & McKenzie, I. (1983) The UK external quality assessment schemes for peptide hormones, objectives and strategy (and discussion). In: *Immunoassays for Clinical Chemistry* (eds Hunter, W. M. & Corrie, J. E. T.) pp. 669–683 (Churchill Livingstone, Edinburgh).

Commission of the European Communities (1995) *Proposal for a European Parliament and Council Directive on* in vitro *diagnostic medical devices* (draft) (Commission of the European Communities, Brussels).

Ellis, A. R., Seth, J., Sturgeon, C. M. *et al.* (1996) UK NEQAS for peptide hormones (review). *Proc. UK NEQAS Participants Mtg 1996* (in the press) (Association of Clinical Biochemists, London).

Eurachem Working Group (1995) *Quantifying Uncertainty in Analytical Measurement* (HMSO, London).

Franzini, C., Fraser, C. G. & Malvano, R. (eds) (1991) Analytical quality and diagnostic performance in immunoassay. *Annali Istitut. Superiore di Sanita* **27** (3).

Healy, M. J. R. (1979) Outliers in clinical chemistry quality control schemes. *Clin. Chem.* **25**, 675–677.

Jeffcoate, S. L. (1981) *Efficiency and Effectiveness in the Endocrine Laboratory* (Academic Press, London).

Lapworth, R. & Teal, T. K. (1994) Laboratory blunders revisited. *Ann. Clin. Biochem.* **31**, 78–84.

MacKenzie, F. (1995) UK NEQAS for thyroid hormones (review). *Proc. UK NEQAS Participants Mtg 1994* **1**, 219–224 (Association of Clinical Biochemists, London).

Middle, J. G. & Singh, G. K. (1995) UK NEQAS for steroid hormones (review). *Proc. UK NEQAS Participants Mtg 1994* **1**, 182–194 (Association of Clinical Biochemists, London).

Mugan, K., Carlson, I. H. & Westgard, J. O. (1994) Planning QC procedures for immunoassays. *J. Clin. Immunoassay* **17**, 216–222.

Seth, J. & Hanning, I. (1988) Factors associated with the quality of laboratory performance in the United Kingdom external quality assessment scheme for serum growth hormone. *Clin. Chim. Acta* **174**, 185–196.

Sturgeon, C. M. (1996) Interpretative exercises in EQA. *Proc. UK NEQAS Participants Mtg 1996* (in the press) (Association of Clinical Biochemists, London).

Thienpoint, L. M. & Stockl, D. (1995) EQA with accuracy-based kits: bringing together consensus/reference method targets and method dependent targets *Proc. UK NEQAS Participants Mtg 1994* **1**, 44–47 (Association of Clinical Biochemists, London).

Thompson, M. & Wood, R. (eds) (1993) *Harmonised Guidelines for Internal Quality Control in Analytical Laboratories* (International Union of Pure and Applied Chemistry (IUPAC)).

Westgard, J. O. (1994) Quality management. In: *Tietz Textbook of Clinical Chemistry* 2nd edn (eds Burtis, C. A. & Ashwood, E. R.) pp. 548–592 (W. B. Saunders & Co., Philadelphia).

Westgard, J. O. & Weibe, D. A. (1991) Cholesterol operational process specifications for assuring the quality required by CLIA proficiency testing. *Clin. Chem.* **37**, 1938–1944.

Westgard, J. O., Barry, P. L., Hunt, M. R. *et al.* (1981) A multi-rule Shewhart chart for quality control in clinical chemistry. *Clin. Chem.* **27**, 493–501.

Whitehead, T. P. (1977) *Quality Control in Clinical Chemistry* (John Wiley & Sons, Chichester).

World Health Organisation (1981) External quality assessment of health laboratories: Report on a WHO working group. *EURO Reports and Studies* (36 Regional Office for Europe, WHO, Copenhagen).

Chapter 11

Standardisation of Immunoassays

Ulf–Håkan Stenman

INTRODUCTION

Efforts to improve the standardisation of conventional clinical determinations have had a considerable impact, as can be seen from the results of external quality assessment schemes (EQAS). Standardisation of immunochemical assays is more complicated and, as shown by EQAS data, unsatisfactory for most analytes. During the pioneering stages of immunoassay development, in-house methods based mainly on reagents of limited availability were used. Now most immunoassays are performed with commercial reagent kits, and increasingly with automatic immunoanalysers. This places much of the responsibility for standardisation on reagent and instrument manufacturers. This may eventually help standardisation, but during the past decade there has been no clear improvement in between-laboratory agreement (Seth *et al.*, 1994).

Automation tends to limit flexibility of immunoassay design. Short assay times are used to reduce turnaround time and to increase capacity. This hampers optimisation, especially of inhibition assays. However, because of the need for cost containment, simplicity and expedience, laboratory staff may feel compelled to use their expensive analysers for as many available assays as possible, even if the quality of certain of the assays is unsatisfactory. The importance of accuracy in clinical chemistry needs to be emphasised, especially in the immunoassay field (Tietz, 1994).

Assay calibration constitutes part of the standardisation process. It consists of the transfer of the value of the primary standards to secondary standards and calibrators. The final calibration of an assay needs to be checked, and often adjusted, every time a new lot of reagents is introduced. For reagents' manufacturers this is a demanding process, the success of which can be evaluated by quality control schemes. Problems are revealed by the occurrence of large inter-assay and lot-to-lot variation.

The International Federation of Clinical Chemistry (IFCC) has initiated several programmes for immunoassay standardisation. This chapter is mainly based on experience gathered in connection with these. In addition to general aspects, I will deal with a limited number of analytes, the standardisation of which has been explored. The theoretical basis of immunoassay standardisation has been extensively dealt with in several Bergmeyer symposia organised by the IFCC (Kallner *et al.*, 1991, 1993). (*See* also Quality Assurance, Chapter 10.)

PRINCIPLES AND PRACTICE OF STANDARDISATION

The aim of standardisation of laboratory methods is to improve the comparability of results from various laboratories by improving accuracy, i.e. the results should be as close to the true value as possible. The expression 'harmonisation' is sometimes used as an alternative to standardisation. However, harmonised methods can give identical results, but they may all be biased. Whenever possible, the aim should be to achieve standardisation rather than harmonisation.

A prerequisite for standardisation is that standard and analyte are identical. If these conditions are not met, standardisation in its most strict sense is not possible (Ekins, 1991). For many immunoassays these conditions are not met, and although this complicates standardisation it does not prevent it. Another definition is that 'the standard should contain the analyte in a form identical to that found in the sample, or in a form that is similar enough to behave identically in the assay system'. These more realistic requirements can be met satisfactorily in most cases.

Organisations Involved in Standardisation

The Expert Committee on Biological Standardisation (ECBS) of the World Health Organisation (WHO) is responsible for the establishment of international standards and other reference materials for biological substances. The proceedings of the ECBS meetings are published in the WHO *Technical Report Series*. Member states of the World Health Assembly have agreed to adopt and use WHO standards (NIBSC, 1994). The WHO provides international standards for most polypeptide hormones and some tumour markers through the National Institute for Biological Standards and Control (NIBSC). Standards are also prepared by local and regional organisations, e.g. the Community Reference Bureau (BCR) of the European Community (EC) through its Measurement, Testing and Standards (MT & S) programme, the Centers for Disease Control (CDC), and the National Committee of the College of American Pathologists (CAP). The National Institute of Health (NIH) provides polypeptide hormone standards especially for research purposes. The IFCC has organised preparation of a standard for lipoproteins and serum proteins, which is available through CAP and M & TS. The International Society of Oncodevelopmental Biology and Medicine has initiated a programme for epitope mapping of tumour markers.

Standards alone do not guarantee comparability of immunoassay results, but they represent a key component. Standardisation further requires establishment of reference methods (Jeffcoate, 1991). The aspects of immunoassay standardisation are being pursued by various scientific societies, e.g. IFCC, the International Union of Pure and Applied Chemistry (IUPAC), the National Committee of Clinical Laboratory Standardisation (NCCLS), and the American and Canadian Societies for Clinical Chemistry (AACC and CSCC). These organisations also prepare some standards for analytes not available through WHO and Nordkem in the Nordic countries. In the United States, immunoassays need to be approved by the Food and Drug Administration (FDA). In Germany, the Institute for Standardisation and Documentation in Medical Laboratories (INSTAND) serves as a supervising organisation.

Standards and Reference Materials

The first biological standard was prepared for insulin by Sir Henry Dale 70 years ago. This standard was adopted by the League of Nations Health Organization, which was the precursor of the WHO. Since then, the content of insulin preparations have been expressed in international units (IU) of a series of international standards (IS), each of which has been calibrated against the preceding one (Jeffcoate, 1991). Subsequently, ISs have been prepared for most important polypeptide hormones and for other 'substances of complex molecular composition, whose identity, potency or safety cannot be completely characterised by physical and chemical methods alone' (NIBSC, 1994). The units to be used for an IS are assigned by the ECBS on the basis of an international collaborative study, in which the suitability of the proposed preparation to serve as an IS in different assays systems is also estimated. Bioassays are mainly used for estimation of the potency of polypeptide hormone standards and calibration of new standards against previous ones. Therefore the unit of IU usually indicates bioactivity, but is also used for analytes lacking known bioactivity. The standards are usually prepared in lots large enough to last for at least 10 to 20 years (NIBSC, 1994).

For analytical purposes, standards and reference preparations are used as calibrators to define common units for expression of results on an international level. In individual laboratories they are used to assess assay validity and as internal quality control specimens. They are also very valuable for quality assessment (Jeffcoate, 1991).

The term 'IS' supersedes the term international reference preparation (IRP) which has been used by the WHO for some standards. The present standard for human chorionic gonadotrophin (hCG) was initially called the (1st) IRP and was later adopted as the 3rd IS (Storring *et al.*, 1980). Although most IS preparations consist of pure antigens dissolved in a buffer containing a carrier protein, some standards, e.g. those for serum proteins, are serum-based materials (Whicher *et al.*, 1994).

Standards are classified as primary, secondary and tertiary. The primary standards are available in limited amounts and are intended to be used for 10 to 20 years. They are provided lyophilised with a carrier protein. The primary standards are used to calibrate secondary and tertiary standards, e.g. the calibrators used in routine assays. When available, ISs are used as primary standards. Secondary standards are used for maintenance of calibration once primary calibration has been established. Sufficiently pure preparations suitable for secondary standards are available from various manufacturers, which usually want to have alternative sources. Calibrated secondary standards may be available on a national basis, but the user is responsible for appropriate calibration of commercial preparations. For many analytes, standards approved by national or international organisations are not available.

The characteristics of the standards need to be carefully described and controlled. The ideal standard should be pure but still reflect possible heterogeneity of the analyte with respect to isoforms. This requirement is hard to fulfil, because removal of impurities by biochemical methods often requires that minor isoforms be lost during purification. Immunoaffinity chromatography can be used to extract all isoforms specifically, but the elution process often requires the use of denaturing conditions, which may cause irreversible modification. Proteins can also be produced by expression in cell systems, but the product still requires purification and glycosylation tends to be different from that in the native protein. The requirements for various types of standards are listed in Tables 1 and 2.

Units

The concentrations of analytes for which international standards are available are generally expressed in IU l^{-1}, whereas those of well defined substances, e.g. steroid and thyroid hormones, should be expressed in substance concentrations (mol l^{-1}) (Dybkaer, 1991; CSCC, 1992). However, the definition 'well defined substance' is not unambiguous, and the number of peptide hormones that can be sufficiently well defined is continuously increasing. Thus, although ISs for adrenocorticotrophic hormone (ACTH) and insulin are available, their concentrations are often expressed in mol l^{-1} or g l^{-1} rather than IU l^{-1}. The concentrations of well characterised tumour markers are mostly expressed in mass concentrations (g l^{-1}) whereas arbitrary units (U l^{-1}) are used for less well defined markers.

The expression of hormone concentrations in IU l^{-1} gives the impression that the concentration of biologically active hormone is measured, but it should be borne in mind that immunoassays do not measure bioactivity (Ekins, 1991). They actually reflect the molar concentration of an epitope or a combination of epitopes on the antigen, especially when assays based

---

a **Primary standard**

Limited availability from one source.
Time of use: 10–20 years.
Stored lyophilised.
Availability:
    One source.
    Various commercial manufacturers (low M_r substances).

b **Secondary standard**

Purified material, pooled serum (serum proteins), crude extract.
Prepared in:
    Buffer containing carrier protein.
Available from various sources.
Time of use: 1–5 years.
Value assignment:
    Immunoassay against primary standard.
Stored frozen below −70°C.

c **Tertiary standard or calibrators**

Prepared in:
    Serum or plasma.
    Artificial protein-based buffer.
Value assigned by:
    Immunoassay against secondary standard.
Time of use: between one and several years.
Stored frozen or in stabilised solution, possibly lyophilised.

Table 1 Requirements common to standards for various immunoassays. Preparation of calibrators for well defined substances of low relative molecular mass (low M_r) is often done without secondary standards, which, however, can still be used for maintenance of calibration.

on monoclonal antibodies are used. Thus substance concentrations (expressed in mol l^{-1}) reflect most closely what is measured. The molar content of pure proteins can be accurately determined by amino acid analysis even if the preparation is heterogeneous with respect to carbohydrate composition and isoelectric point. Gravimetric determination of the mass of glycoproteins is inaccurate, because they contain tightly bound water that is not removed by lyophilisation (Stenman *et al.*, 1993).

The next generation of hCG standards will be determined by amino acid analysis and expressed in mol l^{-1}. Conversion factors for the present 3rd international standard (3rd IS) can be established by cross-calibration with immunoassays (Stenman *et al.*, 1993). If an immunoassay detects molecular variants with different molecular mass but similar immunoreactivity, substance concentrations correctly reflect the concentrations of the various components. However, if the various molecular forms do not have equal immunoreactivity, substance concentrations will also be biased. This problem should be solved by using antibodies and standards with appropriate specificity (Stenman *et al.*, 1995).

Difficulties with standardisation may arise when standards are replaced. A new standard may change the potency estimates of diagnostic immunoassays, however carefully calibration is carried out. Calibration of hormone standards by bioassay is complicated. The assays are less reproducible than immunoassays. The carbohydrate composition of the hormone, which has little effect on immunoreactivity, strongly affects bioactivity and the effect is different for *in vitro* and *in vivo* assays (Jeffcoate, 1991; Stenman *et al.*, 1993). If calibration of new

---

a   **Polypeptides of known structure (hormones and tumour markers)**

Purest protein available.
Value assignment:
    Amino acid analysis (substance concentration).
    Gravimetry (mass concentration).
    Immunoassay against earlier standard (IU).
    (Bioassay, IU).

b   **Proteins of unknown structure (antibody-defined tumour markers)**

Partially purified or unpurified extract or body fluid.
Value assignment:
    Consensus agreement by international organisation (IU).
    By developer, arbitrary unit (U).

c   **Serum proteins**

Pooled serum (pure protein).
Value assignment:
    Consensus agreement by international organisation (IU).
    Immunoassay against pure proteins (mass concentrations).

d   **Low molecular mass compound (steroid, thyroid hormone)**

Chemically pure (>99%) substance.
Value assignment:
    Gravimetry (substance and mass concentration).
    Photometry.

Table 2 Requirements specific to primary standards for different types of immunoassays. Although the official primary standards (IS) for serum proteins consist of pooled serum, purified proteins (without official status so far) have been used to assign mass concentrations for various proteins in the international standards and reference preparations.

hormone standards is based on bioactivity, immunoassay calibration may change when a new standard is introduced. Code FSH 83/575, a recent standard for follicle-stimulating hormone (FSH), would have changed the calibration of FSH immunoassays by a factor of 4. However, replacement of the standards for prolactin, luteinising hormone (LH) and growth hormone have caused no or only minor changes (Jeffcoate, 1991).

Assay Calibration and Value Transfer

The process by which an assay is calibrated consists of several steps during which the value of the primary standard is transferred to the calibrators used in the final assay. This includes the selection of standards and assay methods, buffers and their matrices, control of dilution, statistical evaluation and quality control of the final result. When establishing a method, the values of the primary standards are transferred to secondary and tertiary standards and/or calibrators. Maintenance of calibration requires that part of the process is repeated every time a new batch of reagents is introduced. The calibration process is different for different types of analytes, e.g. serum proteins, polypeptide hormones or low molecular mass hormones bound to carrier proteins. Few reports are available on the procedures used by manufacturers (Dati, 1990). Therefore the following description is mainly based on reports of 'in-house' methods and on personal experience.

Serum Proteins

The preparation and application of standards for apolipoprotein AI and the major serum proteins has been carefully described (Marcovina *et al.*, 1993; Whicher *et al.*, 1994). This work was performed by international expert groups in collaboration with several reagent manufacturers. The standards are available from CAP and BCR and they can be directly used to assign values to the calibrators used in the assay kit. Values for most but not all clinically important serum proteins have been assigned to these standards. Value assignment for other proteins is planned (Whicher *et al.*, 1994).

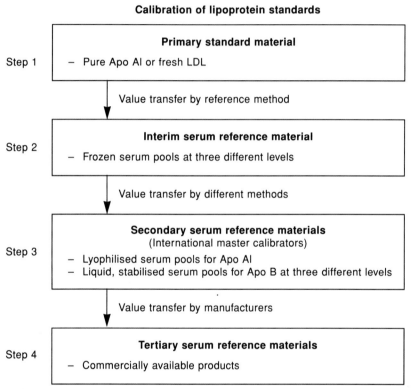

Calibration of lipoprotein standards

Step 1
Primary standard material
– Pure Apo AI or fresh LDL

Value transfer by reference method

Step 2
Interim serum reference material
– Frozen serum pools at three different levels

Value transfer by different methods

Step 3
Secondary serum reference materials
(International master calibrators)
– Lyophilised serum pools for Apo AI
– Liquid, stabilised serum pools for Apo B at three different levels

Value transfer by manufacturers

Step 4
Tertiary serum reference materials
– Commercially available products

Figure 1 Outline of procedures used to develop standards for apolipoprotein AI (modified from Marcovina *et al.*, 1993).

The steps involved in the preparation of apolipoprotein AI standards are described in Figure 1 (modified from Dati, 1990). Important aspects of this process included the use of weight correction for the dilutions, and determination of many dilutions of the secondary against the primary standards. Linearity over the range and regression through zero were required. Values assignment was based on the slopes of the regression lines (Whicher *et al.*, 1994).

The standards (or reference materials) for serum proteins and apolipoproteins differ from most other standards by being serum-based rather than purified proteins. Thus they can be used directly for the assignment of values to the final calibrators. Because the standards are serum-based, differences in matrix effects are largely eliminated. This probably explains why good between-method and between-laboratory accuracy has been obtained with these materials (Marcovina *et al.*, 1993; Whicher *et al.*, 1994).

Polypeptide Hormones and Tumour Markers

Although standards for polypeptide hormones have been available for more than 10 years, few assays can be considered to be properly standardised. This is mainly due to problems of transferring the value of the standard to the final calibrator, but differences in specificity also contribute to between-method bias (Seth *et al.*, 1994).

Primary and secondary standards are usually diluted in an artificial protein-based buffer. All reconstitutions and dilutions should be weight-corrected and the values assigned on the basis of the slope of the regression line for various dilutions (Whicher *et al.*, 1994). After reconstitution, the primary and calibrated secondary standards should be divided into aliquots and stored frozen below −70 °C in well stoppered glass vials. Evaporation through plastic tubes causes concentration during long-term storage. Once thawed, the aliquots should not be refrozen.

Although the secondary standards are usually prepared in a buffer with a low protein content (e.g. 0.5–1% albumin), the calibrators should be serum-based or prepared in a buffer with a protein content similar to that of serum. This places strict requirements on the assay method used for value transfer, i.e. it should be insensitive to matrix differences. Absence of matrix effects should be ascertained by assaying samples diluted in a sample of the zero calibrator. Ideally, a reference method should be used for value transfer but such methods have not been established for polypeptide hormones and tumour markers.

A calibrator matrix free of endogenous hormone can be obtained by using serum from patients with suppressed hormone levels. Alternatively, polypeptides can be removed from serum by immunoadsorption with specific antibodies. However, this procedure often leaves trace amounts of antibody in the serum, which disturb the assay. Animal sera or an artificial protein-based buffer are also used. These matrices have their own advantages and disadvantages (Rej and Drake, 1991). Human serum is most natural but, because of limited availability, the batch needs to be changed frequently, and each new batch will be slightly different. Animal sera can be prepared in large lots, but the properties may differ systematically from human serum and animal hormones may crossreact with human ones. Protein-based buffers are very reproducible but they lack most of the interfering substances of normal serum. If the volume of the sample is small (10–15%) in relation to the total assay volume, these effects are usually negligible. This approach requires that the assay is inherently sensitive, which is the case with certain nonisotopic assays.

The composition of the calibrators is often tuned to the characteristics of the assay. Thus calibrators for one assay may produce quite different results, if used in another assay (Rej and Drake, 1991). This lack of 'commutability' demonstrates the problems inherent in immunoassay calibration.

Steroid and Thyroid Hormones

Calibration of direct assays for protein-bound hormones is complicated because of interference by the binding proteins. Because the affinities of the binding proteins are similar to those of the antibodies used, dissociating substances have to be used to displace the hormones from their binding proteins during the assay. The effect of the binding proteins is hard to eliminate completely without interfering with antibody binding. Therefore serum-based calibrators need to be used. Steroid-free serum can be prepared by adsorption with charcoal, a procedure that nonspecifically removes low molecular mass substances. Calibrators are prepared by adding pure steroid dissolved in ethanol (about 1% of serum volume) to serum that has been charcoal-stripped to remove endogenous steroids. However, considerable bias may still be caused by abnormal binding protein concentrations. Thus, direct assays have been found to underestimate testosterone in samples with high sex hormone-binding globulin (SHBG) and overestimate it if the SHBG concentration is subnormal (Masters and Hahnel, 1989). However, this appears to be less of a problem in recent methods (Middle and Singh, 1994).

In addition to binding proteins, all the nonspecific factors affecting other immunoassays also plague steroid and thyroid hormone assays. Because the sample volume in relation to the total assay volume often has to be rather high to achieve adequate detection limits, nonspecific factors are important sources of error.

Calibration of extraction methods for steroid hormones is relatively simple. Standards are commercially available in pure form, and calibrators can be prepared by dissolving weighed amounts of standard in an organic solvent, usually ethanol, in which the content of steroid can be ascertained by photometry. Calibrators are prepared by diluting the stock solution. Steroid hormones are extracted from the sample after addition of a trace amount of tritiated steroid hormone, which is used for calculation of recovery. Both the extracted sample and the standards are evaporated to dryness, and reconstituted in buffer. Recovery is estimated by counting part of the reconstituted sample. Because interference by binding proteins is eliminated, extraction assays may be quite accurate, if they are not affected by crossreacting steroids (which may be eliminated by chromatographic purification). They may also be quite sensitive because the sample can be concentrated. However, precision is a problem because of the many steps involved.

Maintenance of Calibration

Maintenance of calibration is demanding because even minor changes in the assay may affect calibration. It is not only a change in calibrators but any change in the components that requires control, and sometimes adjustment, of calibration. A new batch of antibodies, label or matrix requires that the calibration is checked. A change of polyclonal antiserum usually requires complete recalibration of an assay but even a change in coating procedure or a new batch of labelled antibody or antigen requires checking of the calibration. Because the stability of biological reagents is limited, the calibration process needs to be repeated at regular intervals. The regular maintenance of calibration consists of comparison of the result against the secondary standard and a sufficiently large set of quality control samples. The procedures are different for commercial manufacturers and individual laboratories. As an example, on a laboratory scale, the same lot of calibrators can be stored frozen and used for years, whereas in commercial products, the calibrators are mostly provided in solution, and therefore their stability is limited.

Reference Methods

Reference methods (or reference measurement procedures) have proved to be suitable for the standardisation of many chemical determinations. A definitive method is a reference method with high precision and no systematic bias. Isotope dilution-mass spectrometry (ID-MS) is used as a definitive method for steroid hormones and some other low molecular mass antigens (Thienpont *et al.*, 1995). So far, this technique has been too expensive to be used on a large scale. Samples analysed by ID-MS are used for quality control, but the number of such samples available is insufficient for calibration. A network of reference laboratories is being established to improve standardisation of steroid hormone assays (Gosling *et al.*, 1993; Thienpont *et al.*, 1995).

Mass spectrometric methods for proteins are developing rapidly but are not yet suitable for quantitative determinations of low concentrations of polypeptides in complex biological samples. When a definitive method is not available, the best method available may be designated a reference method. For example, a reference method for apolipoprotein B has been suggested but has not achieved widespread use (Albers *et al.*, 1989; Marcovina *et al.*, 1993). The working group for standardisation of hCG assays has recommended development of reference methods for the different variants of hCG. Such a method should have a low detection limit and be insensitive to nonspecific interference and crossreaction with related compounds. It should be based on generally available, carefully characterised monoclonal reference antibodies. Although all key reagents would be the same, assay design could still cause bias. Therefore it may be necessary to establish a network of reference laboratories, such as those for steroid hormone assays, maintaining thoroughly validated reference methods (Stenman *et al.*, 1993).

Reference methods could be used to help the transfer of primary standard values and to establish serum panels made up of samples with properly assigned analyte concentrations. The working group for hCG standardisation plans to evaluate whether such a serum panel can reduce the problem of value transfer in hCG assays. Sera analysed by a 'reference method' are actually used for calibration by many manufacturers, but the reference method is usually the market leader for the assay in question. It is clear that a bias in this assay will have serious effects. Samples provided through EQAS programmes are also used to check calibration but, because the number of such samples is small, an abnormal matrix effect may cause considerable bias. Furthermore, the values assigned to such samples have not always been determined by an appropriate method. Therefore, availability of serum panels analysed by approved reference methods would be a better alternative.

Problems in Immunoassay Standardisation

Standardisation of immunoassays is complicated by several problems, e.g. protein heterogeneity, crossreactions, matrix effects and the need to measure concentrations close to the detection limit. The immunoreactivity measured is often a mixture of protein isoforms differing with respect to glycosylation, degradation (such as nicking and fragmentation) and complex formation.

Matrix Effects

Matrix effects are here defined as nonspecific factors that interfere with the reaction between antigen and antibody but are unrelated to the interference caused by the analyte. Although sometimes considered matrix effects, the interference caused by crossreacting substances, fragments and complexes of the antigen (Wood, 1991a) will here be considered separately. Matrix effects are highly dependent on assay format and antibody selection. They therefore affect various assays in different ways.

Matrix effects are caused by proteins, salt, phospholipids, complement, antibodies to immunoglobulins (rheumatoid factors and human anti-mouse antibodies (HAMA)) , drugs and substances that may contaminate the sample (reviewed in Weber *et al.*, 1990; Gosling, 1991; Wood, 1991b). The effect of these can be reduced by careful assay design, e.g. the use of high-affinity antibodies of certain subtypes or antibody fragments, a small ratio of sample to total assay volume, addition of immunoglobulin to the assay buffer, and optimal temperature and (long) incubation times.

The calibrators in immunoassays are usually prepared in a buffer with a matrix resembling that of the sample. This can be an antigen-free human serum, an animal serum lacking immunologically crossreacting antigen or an artificial buffer with a protein content similar to that of the sample. Because the composition of serum varies, a change in the batch of a serum-based matrix affects calibration. Therefore a matrix based on pure proteins is easier to maintain. However, for assay of hormones that are bound to serum protein it is hard to use any other matrix than human serum. It should be recognised that serum-based calibrators only equalise the matrix problem, they do not eliminate it.

The concentrations of total protein and salt in serum (and plasma) are fairly constant but in urine the salt concentration varies considerably. Increasing concentrations of salt exert an inhibitory effect on antigen-antibody reactions, the degree of which is antibody-dependent (Haskell *et al.*, 1983). This causes false low results in sandwich assays and falsely elevated results in inhibition assays. Osmolality is mainly due to salt concentration, and it is therefore fairly constant in serum. However, total protein concentration may vary by a factor of two, which can give rise to differences in matrix effects in assays relying on a large sample volume fraction. The effect of protein is mostly insignificant if the sample volume is less than 10–15% of the total incubation volume. However, a larger sample volume is often needed to maintain sensitivity. Reference methods should be based on assays with such a low detection limit that the sample volume in relation to total assay volume can be kept small enough to eliminate most matrix effects.

Heterophilic antibodies. Immunoglobulins in the sample can affect the results by reacting with the antibodies used in the assay. Patients with autoimmune disease often have rheumatoid factors (RF), i.e. immunoglobulins reacting with other immunoglobulins including those used in the assay. Heterophilic 'natural' antibodies against animal immunoglobulins are quite common, but in most cases their concentrations and affinity are low (Hunter and Budd, 1980; Boscato and Stuart, 1988). Specific human anti-mouse antibodies (HAMA) are often induced in patients injected with monoclonal mouse IgG for the purpose of radioimaging. In inhibition assays, these antibodies interfere with the function of the primary and/or second antibody, causing a false inhibition. In sandwich assays they usually link solid phase and detector antibody, causing a false positive response. Thus, heterophilic antibodies, RF and HAMA tend to cause a positive bias in immunoassays, but in rare cases the bias may be negative (Turpeinen *et al.*, 1995).

The effect of RF, heterophilic antibodies and HAMA can in most cases be reduced to an acceptable level by inclusion of sufficient amounts of animal immunoglobulin from the same species as the antibodies used in the assay. The interference can also be reduced by using Fab or F(ab′)2 fragments rather than intact reagent antibodies. However, if the sample contains antibodies against the idiotype of the reagent antibody, these methods are insufficient. Anti-idiotypic antibodies are often induced by immunisation with the antibody used in the original cancer antigen (CA) 125 assay, OC 125 (Turpeinen *et al.*, 1990). In this case correct results can only be obtained by removal of the immunoglobulins from the sample or by using an assay based on another solid-phase antibody (Turpeinen *et al.*, 1995).

Complement. The various complement factors react with antibodies. This interferes with the ability of the reagent antibodies to bind antigen and to react with the second antibodies used for separation. In sandwich assays this causes a false negative bias, and a positive one in inhibition assays. Mouse immunoglobulins of the $IgG2_a$ and $IgG2_b$ subtype are especially sensitive to complement effects (Børmer, 1989). Complement interference can be eliminated by heating the sample or by including chelating substances in the buffer, but many analytes are affected by heating, and chelators interfere with some nonisotopic labels such as europium chelates and enzymes. Therefore it is preferable to use antibodies or antibody fragments that are insensitive to complement effects.

Low molecular mass organic substances. Phospholipids have been reported to cause falsely elevated results in steroid assays by interfering with antigen binding. Many other factors, e.g. components derived from serum-separating gels, anticoagulants, detergents, drugs, uraemic toxins, free fatty acids and dyes used for reagent coding may also interfere in immunoassays (Weber *et al.*, 1990; Gosling, 1991; Wood, 1991b).

Antigen Heterogeneity and Crossreacting Substances

Prohormones, fragments and complexes. Protein hormones are typically heterogeneous and, in addition to the biologically active forms, prohormones, fragments and subunits often occur in the circulation. Analytical problems may be caused by, for example, fragments of parathyroid hormone (parathormone; PTH) and ACTH and prohormones of ACTH, big forms of prolactin and gastrin and splicing variants of growth hormone. Two-site sandwich assays with monoclonal antibodies greatly improve the possibilities of designing an assay to detect specifically a certain molecular form; as an example, sandwich assays to gonadotrophins based on one antibody to the β-subunit and one to the α-subunit will not detect free subunits. Assays using two antibodies to the amino-terminal and carboxy-terminal parts, respectively, of ACTH or PTH do not measure biologically inactive fragments. In most cases, assays measuring the biologically active forms are desirable but, for certain purposes, specific assays for a certain degradation product (e.g. the core fragment of hCG) may have important clinical applications. It is always highly desirable that the specificity of the assay is accurately specified. This requires standards not only for the biologically active hormones but also for clinically relevant degradation products (Stenman *et al.*, 1993). The problems associated with hCG, LH, carcinoembryonic antigen, prostate-specific antigen and steroid hormones are described below.

Genetic variants. Some serum proteins exist in various genetic variants that differ in their isoelectric points (e.g. α_1-antitrypsin) or in the degree of their polymerisation (e.g. haptoglobin). Although different proportions of the variants can affect the results obtained by immunoassays, this does not appear to be a problem with the immunoassays for serum proteins (Whicher *et al.*, 1994). The assays used for plasma protein determinations are usually based on polyclonal antisera, which are not likely to detect minor differences in protein structure. A genetic variant of luteinising hormone is not recognised by some monoclonal antibodies (see below) (Pettersson *et al.*, 1992). This case demonstrates a potential problem for immunoassays in general. However, changes in protein structure are likely to cause loss of function before they affect immunoreactivity. We do not yet know how much genetic variants cause discrepancies between results obtained by different assays.

Glycosylation variants. Differences in glycosylation and especially sialic acid content are a typical cause of glycoprotein heterogeneity. Variation in the numbers of sialic acid residues gives rise to variants differing with respect to isoelectric point and electrophoretic mobility.

However, antibodies are generally insensitive to these differences (Ekins, 1991), and therefore carbohydrate heterogeneity has little effect on immunoreactivity. However, a carbohydrate chain in a protein can modify or mask a peptide epitope thereby changing the immunoreactivity (Børmer, 1991; Pettersson et al., 1992). In contrast to the carbohydrate moiety of glycoproteins, those of mucins constitute major antigenic determinants (Hilgers et al., 1995).

Polymorphic antigens. Large differences in the results obtained for polymorphic antigens can be caused by apparently small differences in assay design. This is clearly demonstrated by assays for the mucin antigens CA 125, CA 19-9 and CA 15-3; for example, CA 15-3 produced by various tissues contains a variable number of tandem repeats of 20 amino acids (Hilgers et al., 1995). The antigens measured by these assays were identified by monoclonal antibodies prepared against tumour cells. They are large molecules of poorly defined structure, and the calibration materials for these are maintained by the company introducing the assays. Although most companies use the same standards and antibodies, the correlation between various assays is poor. This is probably due to differences in assay design (Yedema et al., 1992). Therefore, reference range values should be established for each method separately. Lipoproteins (Marcovina et al., 1994) and cytokeratin fragments (Bodenmüller, 1995) also display a high degree of polymorphism.

Effect of Assay Design

Assay design strongly affects detection limit, which within certain limits is inversely related to incubation time. By using high antibody concentrations in sandwich assays, maximal binding (and minimal detection limit) may be reached in minutes. In inhibition assays, the detection limit decreases with decreasing antibody concentrations provided that sufficiently long incubation times are used, i.e. usually hours and in some cases days. This is not compatible with rapid turnaround times and high capacity in automatic immunoanalysers, but in these the reaction rate can be increased by using higher assay temperatures (37 °C rather than room temperature) and efficient mixing. Therefore, it is often possible to achieve a certain detection limit with a shorter incubation time in an automatic analyser.

Because of their lower detection limits, immunometric sandwich assays have profoundly changed the clinical use of some analytes, e.g. LH (Apter et al., 1989) and thyroid-stimulating hormone (thyrotrophin; TSH) (Spencer et al., 1995). Sandwich assays also facilitate development of assays for specific forms of a hormone or fragment in a mixture of these, e.g. ACTH (Dobson et al., 1987) and PTH in serum (Wood, 1991b) and LH and hCG in urine (Stenman et al., 1990; Alfthan et al., 1992). Therefore, sandwich assays have now replaced conventional radioimmunoassay-type inhibition assays for most protein hormones and tumour markers. However, only antigens containing at least two independent epitopes can be measured by conventional sandwich assays. ACTH is the smallest peptide routinely measured, but insulin, although larger, is mainly determined by inhibition assays.

One-step versus two-step assays. The performance of a sandwich assay in two steps eliminates many potential problems. Crossreacting substances that react with the labelled antibody but not with the capture antibody can be removed with a washing step. This also eliminates hook effects and interference of sample constituents with the labelled antibody. However, because of longer assay times in two-step assays, one-step assays are mostly used. For analysis of problem samples, the option of performing an assay in two steps is very valuable, but with automated methods this is seldom possible. Two-step assays are also less prone to interference in assays for closely related substances, e.g. hCG and hCGβ, which share antigenic determinants The antigen present in excess (e.g. hCG) may interfere with measurement of the other antigen (hCGβ) by 'consuming' antibody to a common determinant (Alfthan *et al.*, 1988). The negative bias caused by this phenomenon may be hard to detect.

Kinetics. Large molecules react more slowly than smaller ones and this may cause a bias when molecular forms with different sizes are measured. For example, complexed prostate-specific antigen (PSA) (M_r 90K) may be underestimated in comparison with free PSA, when short incubation times are used (Strobel *et al.*, 1995).

STANDARDISATION OF SELECTED ASSAYS

Polypeptide Hormones

Chorionic Gonadotrophin (hCG)

The glycoprotein hormones present several problems for immunoassay standardisation. The four hormones, hCG, LH, FSH and TSH consist of a common α-subunit and a specific β-subunit. The β-subunits of LH and hCG are very similar, complicating development of specific assays. Antisera raised to intact glycoprotein hormones tend to crossreact with other members of the family because of the common α-subunit, and the first immunoassays measured LH and hCG together. Specific assays for hCG were first developed by immunisation with the free β-subunit (hCGβ) (Vaitukaitis *et al.*, 1972).

Monoclonal antibodies have greatly facilitated development of specific assays for hCG and its subunits but many problems still exist (Stenman *et al.*, 1993). A major question is whether an assay should measure both hCG and hCGβ or whether separate assays should be used. Although separate assays would be theoretically preferable, a combined assay has practical advantages (Mann *et al.*, 1993). Assays specific for intact hCG are available, but most hCG assays measure both hCG and hCGβ. Standardisation of these is complicated by a tendency to overestimate hCGβ (Stenman *et al.*, 1993). This is a problem if the assay is used to estimate the proportion of hCGβ to hCG. In pregnancy serum this proportion is usually below 3%, but storage of samples at room temperature may cause dissociation of hCG into subunits, which may be induced by nicking, i.e. proteolytic cleavage of the peptide chain (Birken *et al.*, 1991; Cole and Kardana, 1992). This is important when determination of hCGβ in maternal serum is used for detection of trisomy 21 in the foetus.

Nicked forms of hCG and hCGβ occur especially in cancer patients but also in pregnancy (Cole *et al.*, 1994). The gross conformation of nicked hCG is retained because of disulphide bonding but the reactivity with some antibodies is reduced. It is currently considered desirable that assays measure intact and nicked hCG (or hCGβ) equally (Cole and Kardana, 1992).

An important aim in the standardisation of hCG assays is to define the molecular forms and to develop specific assays. This requires pure standards for the various forms and development of reference methods. The presently used 3rd IS for hCG was calibrated by bioassay, and the units (IU) can be traced back to the 2nd and 1st IS. The concentrations of the hCGβ and hCGα standards are also expressed in IU although they lack hCG activity. One IU of these corresponds to 1 μg of the respective standards. For comparison, one IU of hCG is about 0.11 μg. The ratio of hCG to hCGβ is clinically important and calculation of the ratio should be based on molar concentrations (Alfthan *et al.*, 1992). Although the nicked forms of hCG (hCGn) and hCGβ (hCGβn) are not specifically assayed, availability of these is important for characterisation of assays for the intact forms (Stenman *et al.*, 1993).

A fragment of the hCGβ subunit of hCG called the core fragment (hCGβcf) occurs at high concentrations in urine of pregnant women. In men and nonpregnant women the urine concentrations are very low, but elevated levels are common in various types of cancer (reviewed in Stenman et al., 1993). This fragment is probably derived from degradation of hCG or hCGβ in the tubules of the kidney. On the basis of the correlation between the serum levels of hCGβ and the urine levels of hCGβcf, the elevation of hCGβcf in cancer patients is probably due to expression of hCGβ by the tumour (Alfthan et al., 1992). Because hCGβcf has potential use as a marker for several tumours, standardisation is important (Stenman et al., 1993).

Luteinising Hormone (LH)

Because of a high degree of homology between LH and hCG, crossreaction with hCG is a common feature of LH assays. LH and hCG have the same function; therefore a method measuring both hormones reflects total bioactivity. Because the hCG concentrations in men and nonpregnant women are very low (Stenman et al., 1987), the crossreaction of hCG in LH assays is a theoretical rather than a practical clinical problem. In spite of this, most assay manufacturers are aiming to develop LH-specific assays. Although the crossreaction of hCG in many assays is only 0.01–0.1%, the clinical advantage is limited. The slight crossreaction may even cause confusion, because a pregnant woman with an hCG level of 1,000–10,000 IU l^{-1} will have an apparent LH level of only about 10. Such levels are encountered in amenorrhea caused by a pregnancy that has not been recognised. If the LH assay also measures hCG, the condition can readily be recognised on the basis of the extremely high result. This example shows that high immunochemical specificity does not always provide better clinical utility.

LH assays with low hCG crossreaction are usually based on two monoclonal antibodies, reacting with LH subunits but which also recognise intact LH. Thus these assays also measure free β-subunits and in some cases its fragments. Because neither of these normally occur in serum, this is not a problem for serum assays. However, in urine, subunits and fragments may represent the majority of the LH immunoreactivity (Stenman et al., 1990).

Radioimmunoassay (RIA) methods do not measure LH levels below 1 IU l^{-1} but, with ultrasensitive sandwich assays based on monoclonal antibodies, the true serum levels in prepubertal children are in the range 0.0–0.15 IU l^{-1}. A 10–fold increase in serum LH coincides with the onset of puberty (Apter et al., 1989) and determination of LH by an ultrasensitive method appears to be the most accurate laboratory method of evaluating pubertal state (Haavisto et al., 1990). However, only a few methods can actually provide this sensitivity.

A potential problem of using monoclonal antibodies is that they may fail to recognise genetic variants of protein antigens. A genetic variant of LH shows strongly reduced immunoreactivity with certain monoclonal antibodies. This is due to a point mutation giving rise to a new glycosylation site. Apparently the additional carbohydrate chain blocks an antigenic determinant. With certain assays, homozygotes have unmeasurable LH concentrations and in heterozygotes the levels are reduced by 30–50%. The problem can be eliminated by careful selection of antibodies (Pettersson et al., 1992).

Thyroid-stimulating Hormone (Thyrotrophin; TSH)

The clinical utility of ultrasensitive TSH assays has stimulated the development of assays with continuously decreasing detection limits. So-called second- and third-generation assays have replaced the first generation RIAs. Second-generation assays have a detection limit around 0.1–0.2 IU l^{-1} and third-generation assays around 0.01–0.02 IU l^{-1} (Spencer *et al.*, 1995). Third-generation assays should be able reliably to measure subnormal TSH concentrations associated with hyperthyroidism, which facilitates the use of TSH as a first-line test for thyroid function. Standardisation of TSH assays is fairly good, but there is considerable variation in detection limit and reproducibility at low concentrations (McKenzie, 1994), and assay manufacturers tend to estimate the detection limit in an unrealistic fashion. For evaluation of an assay as a first-line test for thyroid function, the true detection limit should be estimated with clinical samples (Spencer *et al.*, 1995).

Steroid Hormone Assays

The assay of steroid hormones is complicated by the occurrence of closely related crossreacting compounds and by the presence in plasma of binding proteins. For urine assays, metabolites are the major problem. Initially, most steroid hormones were determined by RIA using tritiated tracers and extraction of the steroid with organic solvents. Often, crossreacting steroids were removed by chromatographic methods and, to correct for losses during pretreatment, recovery was estimated by adding a trace amount of tritiated steroid to the sample before extraction. Such methods were often quite accurate, but precision suffered from the many steps involved.

Currently, most steroid hormone determinations are direct assays. This has become possible through the development of more specific antisera and blocking substances that release the steroid from its binding protein(s). Although these methods reduce interference, they do not eliminate it, thus the binding proteins may still interact with tracer and analyte. To compensate for these problems, the standards are prepared by adding pure steroid to a serum-based matrix, from which the endogenous steroids have usually been removed by charcoal adsorption. This treatment also removes other low molecular mass compounds, which would crossreact or interfere nonspecifically with the assay. Therefore the standards do not correspond to the sample. In practice, this means that the standards have to be 'tweaked', i.e. the value assignment of the standards may not correspond to the actual content of steroid. Studies on direct assays for testosterone suggest that the SHBG concentration affects the results and that recovery of added steroid is much less than 100% (Masters and Hahnel, 1989). However, recent EQAS studies suggest that this problem has been reduced, although it still affects some assays (Middle and Singh, 1994).

In automatic immunoassays, the small isotopic label is replaced with a larger fluorophore or a very large enzyme. The reaction rate of such a label is different from that of the antigen in the sample and with short incubation times it is hard to reach binding equilibrium. Thus, although direct nonisotopic assays are simple to perform and may have good precision, accuracy is often a problem (Stenman *et al.*, 1991a; Middle and Singh, 1994).

Cortisol

Cortisol occurs in serum and urine at relatively high concentrations. Although this should simplify determinations, different assays show considerable variation (Middle and Singh, 1994). EQAS results with samples determined by mass spectrometry show that serum cortisol assays on average overestimate the true values by 10–15% with a range of −20% to +25%. The overestimation cannot be accounted for by crossreactions with other steroid hormones

(Gosling *et al.*, 1993), and because most assays are performed without extraction, interference by binding proteins in serum is the most likely cause. Various blocking agents are used to dissociate cortisol from cortisol-binding globulin (CBG), but assay manufacturers seldom reveal which substances are used and how completely the influence of protein binding has been eliminated.

Urine contains a large excess of steroid metabolites and conjugates that interfere with the assay of cortisol. Therefore, most assays require extraction of cortisol before immunoassay, but even this does not guarantee acceptable accuracy. Very few assays have been adequately validated for the assay of urinary cortisol, and the general standard of urinary cortisol determinations is poor (Holder, 1994). Comparative studies indicate that immunoassays overestimate the true concentration of cortisol by a factor of two in comparison with results obtained by mass spectrometry.

Oestradiol

Oestradiol is determined for different clinical purposes, which require assays with different characteristics. Monitoring of ovulation induction requires a large concentration range, about $0.1-15$ nmol l^{-1}. Because the results are used to direct therapy on a daily basis, turnaround time should be rapid, i.e. a few hours. Therefore direct assays are nearly exclusively used and automated analysers are gaining popularity. The performance of the first automatic methods was however disappointing, but some recent assays are acceptable. EQAS results also show that many RIAs also perform poorly (Middle and Singh, 1994).

Oestradiol determinations are also important for the estimation of pubertal development in girls and ovarian function in postmenopausal women. In prepubertal girls the oestradiol levels are below the detection limit of most assays, i.e. $20-30$ pmol l^{-1}, and in postmenopausal women the levels are below $100-110$ pmol l^{-1}. Some direct assays are claimed to have a detection limit in this range, but this has to be validated with clinical samples. At the moment there appear to be no commercial assays that fulfil these requirements. Therefore, extraction methods need to be used, but properly validated extraction methods are not commercially available either (Stenman *et al.*, 1991a). Such methods need to be established and validated in each laboratory performing oestradiol assays on paediatric samples.

Standardisation of Tumour Marker Assays

Carcinoembryonic Antigen (CEA)

Development of specific assays for carcinoembryonic antigen (CEA) is complicated by a family of CEA-related antigens. Normal crossreacting antigen (NCA) is produced by, for example, granulocytes and occurs at fairly high concentration in plasma. NCA-2 is apparently a foetal (glycosylation) variant of CEA, both of which are produced by adult and foetal colonic mucosa. In some cancer patients, part of the CEA produced is of the foetal (NCA-2) type. Currently available assays have negligible crossreaction with NCA but show variable reactivity with NCA-2 (Sturgeon *et al.*, 1994). This, along with the heterogeneity of CEA, explains the considerable differences in standardisation between CEA assays but it has no documented clinical significance (Børmer. 1991). Even various assays from the same manufacturer may be calibrated differently (Turpeinen *et al.*, 1992). An IS for CEA is available but the results are generally expressed in mass units.

Alphafoetoprotein (AFP)

Standardisation of alphafoetoprotein (AFP) assays is important because of its use for maternal screening for foetal trisomy 21 (Down's syndrome) during the second trimester. For screening purposes, the concentrations of AFP are usually converted to multiples of the median (MoM) of a reference population for each pregnancy week. Because of the very strong impact of even minor differences in calibration on the risk calculation, the reference values have to be established separately for each laboratory performing screening. In the IS for AFP one IU roughly corresponds to 1.2 μg.

Prostate-specific Antigen (PSA)

Prostate-specific antigen (PSA) is a serine protease of M_r 30K that forms complexes with protease inhibitors when it reaches the circulation. About 50–98% of the immunoreactive PSA in serum occurs in complex with α_1-antichymotrypsin (ACT). Most of the rest is free, but a small fraction is complexed with α_1-antitrypsin (Stenman *et al.*, 1991b). Serum also contains a PSA-α_2-macroglobulin (AMG) complex that is not measurable by conventional immunoassays (Zhou *et al.*, 1993). Currently available PSA assays differ in their capacity to recognise PSA-ACT. In the complex, some of the PSA epitopes are covered by ACT, which reduces the reactivity with polyclonal antibodies (Stenman *et al.*, 1991b).

Currently, PSA is almost exclusively determined by sandwich assays based on two monoclonal antibodies or one monoclonal and a polyclonal antibody. The latter ones tend to underestimate PSA-ACT but this is also the case with some monoclonal antibodies. In some assays this has been compensated for by calibrating the assay against a method measuring both components equally (Vessella *et al.*, 1992). However, some assays are quite differently calibrated (Zhou *et al.*, 1993). Another problem with PSA assays is the matrix of the calibrators. If purified PSA is added to serum, it forms complexes with ACT and AMG. Because the PSA-AMG complex is not detected by PSA assays, about 30–45% of the PSA becomes undetectable (Christensson *et al.*, 1990). Because of this, serum should be used as a matrix for PSA calibrators (Stenman *et al.*, 1995).

An international collaboration has resulted in the preparation of a reference standard for PSA, consisting of 10% free and 90% PSA-ACT. Assays calibrated with this standard will give similar results, even if they do not measure each form of PSA in an equimolar fashion. Use of this standard may rapidly improve comparability of the results obtained by various assays (Stamey, 1995). However, it should be recognised that this approach is harmonisation rather than standardisation. Only assays measuring PSA and PSA-ACT equally can be properly standardised (Stenman *et al.*, 1995). It is also of interest that human kallikrein-2 (hK2) is highly homologous to PSA and could therefore interfere in the assay (McCormack *et al.*, 1995); however, hK2 has not yet been determined in serum.

Because the proportion of PSA-ACT is higher in prostate cancer than benign prostatic disease, a further improvement in the diagnostic value of PSA can be achieved by measuring PSA and PSA-ACT separately and calculating the ratio of these (Stenman *et al.*, 1991b; Lilja *et al.*, 1994). Therefore, separate standards for these two forms are necessary.

PSA assays are increasingly used for prostate cancer screening. Even slight differences in calibration will have a large effect on the number of men who screen positive. Standardisation of PSA assays is therefore very important.

Serum Proteins

Reference preparations for determination of serum proteins have been prepared from lyophilised serum pools. In the first preparation (the WHO immunoglobulin standard, lot 67/86 issued in 1967), the content of IgG, IgA and IgM was defined to be 100 IU per ampoule. Mass values were later ascribed on the basis of mean values determined in 10 laboratories (Rowe *et al.*, 1972). Later standards were calibrated against the first one. The WHO reference preparation for six human serum proteins (WHO 6SP) was assigned values for albumin, α_1-antitrypsin, caeruloplasmin, α_2-macroglobulin, transferrin and complement C3c in IU. The mass units were determined later (Reimer *et al.*, 1981).

Although adequate for standardisation of assays based on immunodiffusion and rocket electrophoresis, early standards were less suitable for use in immunonephelometric and immunoturbidimetric methods because of turbidity. A working group appointed by IFCC developed the techniques required to prepare a new international reference preparation for proteins in human serum (RPPHS). Blood was collected under strictly controlled conditions and lipoproteins were removed by adsorption with silica before lyophilisation. Many laboratories participated in the determination of the concentrations of most clinically important serum proteins, i.e. albumin, α_1-acid glycoprotein (orosomucoid) α_1-antitrypsin, caeruloplasmin, haptoglobin, α_2-macroglobulin, transferrin and C3, C4, IgG, IgA, IgM and C-reactive protein, the concentrations of which were expressed in mass units (g l^{-1}) and, when possible, also in IU. The new standard changes the concentrations of certain proteins as compared to values obtained by earlier standards, e.g. those of α_1-acid glycoprotein (orosomucoid) α_1-antitrypsin, and IgM (Whicher *et al.*, 1994).

RPPHS is intended to be used for calibration of tertiary standards for routine determination of serum protein. It is available in Europe through BCR and in the United States through CAP.

Reference Values

If all assays were well standardised, the same reference values would be applicable to different assays. Because this is not the case, it is necessary to establish separate reference values for each assay, but this is seldom done in an appropriate way. Often reference values are taken from the literature, even if these have been established with a method giving results that differ substantially from those obtained with the method actually used. This practice is unacceptable. When establishing reference values, differences in sex, age and race must be taken into account. For some analytes, the season and social class also need to be considered (Solberg and Gräsbeck, 1989). For many analytes, e.g. sex steroids, it is self-evident that age and sex are considered, but in many cases in which this is important the problem is overlooked. For example, for PSA a cutoff value of 4 µg l^{-1} is commonly used although the concentrations in men over 70 years of age are roughly double those in men under 50.

Establishment of reference values could be the responsibility of the assay manufacturer. Method-specific reference values would provide crucial information about the characteristics of an assay; for example, the true detection limits of assays for LH and oestradiol would be shown by the values obtained in prepubertal girls.

Assay Characterisation

The following characteristics of an assay are usually described: specificity, detection limit, precision at various antigen concentrations, recovery of added antigen, linearity of the assay, reagent stability and influence of antigen excess (hook effect) (Vadlamudi *et al.*, 1991). The methods for estimation of these criteria vary, and mostly the figures provided are not representative for routine conditions (Spencer *et al.*, 1995). Useful crossreaction data are mainly provided for steroid and thyroid hormones, but the influence of binding proteins, which for these analytes is a major problem, are seldom provided. Crossreaction data for polypeptide hormones and serum tumour markers should be improved. This requires establishment of reference preparations for antigens, which as such may not be clinically useful (e.g. peptide hormone fragments and precursors; NCA and NCA-2 for CEA assays).

More accurate description of the specificity of monoclonal antibodies would facilitate evaluation of the suitability of an assay for a certain purpose. Techniques for epitope mapping and developing rapidly, and some analytes have already been carefully 'mapped' (Bidart *et al.*, 1993). When well characterised monoclonal reference antibodies become available, it will be possible to define the reactivity of antibodies used in an assay on the basis of their similarity with the reference antibodies. Reference laboratories could perform such characterisation.

Assay manufacturers usually provide information of 'expected values' but only occasionally adequately determined reference values. It is desirable that these should be included in any future information on assay characteristics.

FUTURE DEVELOPMENTS

The development of immunoassay technology is very rapid, and the trend is towards more automated methods and random access analysers. Although this reduces turnaround times it does not necessarily improve quality (Seth *et al.*, 1994; Wheeler, 1994). Standardisation of immunoassays has not reached the same maturity as that of conventional clinical chemistry, and it is unlikely that this will happen in the near future unless new procedures are introduced.

Standardisation is part of laboratory quality, and maintenance of quality is expensive. However, the effects of bad standardisation are much more expensive, but these costs accumulate in clinical departments and are therefore not easily calculated. Although standardisation is the responsibility of laboratory staff, poor standardisation mainly hampers the work of clinicians. It is conspicuous that a very ambitious effort to standardise PSA assays has been initiated and carried out by a urologist (Stamey, 1995).

Standardisation is dealt with by several bodies, none of whom takes responsibility for the whole process. The WHO is responsible for preparation of biological standards but cannot provide standards for all clinically important analytes. Other organisations complement the WHO, but there is no clear allocation of responsibilities. Because standardisation is an international rather than a national or regional problem, one international organisation should be responsible for the coordination of various standardisation projects.

The assays that have been or are being standardised are outnumbered by new ones appearing. The capacity to standardise is limited by lack of both economic and human resources. Standardisation is not 'sexy' science, for which large research grants are awarded. It is hard work, for which resources should be made available by society. It may even be necessary to seek actively for these resources in order to engage competent experts. The importance of standardisation is recognised by the MT & S programme of the European Community, but the results are not yet apparent in the case of immunoassays. Standardisation is also important for assay manufacturers, and some standardisation projects have become possible through support from industry.

The state of standardisation can be judged by the results of EQAS programmes. Although participation in such programmes is not mandatory, participation is widespread. However, poor performance and the use of poorly calibrated methods seldom lead to legal actions. Once the authorities realise the implications of poor quality and poor standardisation, accreditation of methods and laboratories is likely to become mandatory, unless laboratory staff eliminate the need for such measures by voluntary control.

The state of immunoassay standardisation demonstrates that standards and reference materials alone are not enough. Reference methods have proved their value in other fields of clinical chemistry, but at the Bergmeyer meetings industry representatives have not been enthusiastic about this approach. It is feared that differences in assay design cause too much bias even if the same standards and reference antibodies are used. Some assay manufacturers consider well characterised serum panels more useful (P. Seguin, CIS-Bio, personal communication). Although this approach may be considered to be a shortcut to standardisation, it deserves to be evaluated.

REFERENCES

Albers, J. J., Lodge, M. S. & Curtiss, L. K. (1989) Evaluation of a monoclonal antibody-based enzyme-linked immunosorbent assay as a candidate reference method for the measurement of apolipoprotein B-100. *J. Lipid. Res.* **30**, 1445–1458.

Alfthan, H., Haglund, C., Roberts, P. *et al.* (1992) Elevation of free β-subunit of human choriogonadotropin and core β fragment of human choriogonadotropin in the serum and urine of patients with malignant pancreatic and biliary disease. *Cancer Res.* **52**, 4628–4633.

Alfthan, H., Schröder, J., Fraser, R. *et al.* (1988) Choriogonadotropin and its beta subunit separated by hydrophobic-interaction chromatography and quantified in serum during pregnancy by time-resolved immunofluorometric assays. *Clin. Chem.* **34**, 1758–1762.

Apter, D., Cacciatore, B., Alfthan, H. *et al.* (1989) Serum luteinizing hormone concentrations increase 100-fold in females from 7 years to adulthood, as measured by time-resolved immunofluorometric assay. *J. Clin. Endocrinol. Metab.* **68**, 53–57.

Bidart, J.-M., Birken, S., Berger, P. *et al.* (1993) Immunochemical mapping of hCG and hCG-related molecules. *Scand. J. Clin. Lab. Invest.* **53** (**suppl. 216**), 118–136.

Birken, S., Gawinowicz, M. A., Kardana, A. *et al.* (1991) The heterogeneity of human chorionic gonadotropin (hCG): II, Characteristics and origins of nicks in hCG reference standards. *Endocrinology* **129**, 1551–1558.

Bodenmüller, H. (1995) The biochemistry of CYFRA-21 and other cytokeratin markers. *Scand. J. Clin. Lab. Invest.* **55** (**suppl. 221**), 60–66.

Børmer, O. P. (1989) Interference of complement with the binding of carcinoembryonic antigen to solid-phase monoclonal antibodies. *J. Immunol. Meth.* **121**, 85–93.

Børmer, O. P. (1991) Major disagreements between immunoassays of carcinoembryonic antigen may be caused by nonspecific cross-reacting antigen 2 (NCA-2). *Clin. Chem.* **37**, 1736–1739.

Boscato, L. M. & Stuart, M. C. (1988) Heterophilic antibodies: A problem for all immunoassays. *Clin. Chem.* **34**, 27–33.

Christensson, A., Laurell, C. B. & Lilja, H. (1990) Enzymatic activity of prostate-specific antigen and its reactions with extracellular serine proteinase inhibitors. *Eur. J. Biochem.* **194**, 755–763.

Cole, L. A. & Kardana, A. (1992) Discordant results in human chorionic gonadotropin assays. *Clin. Chem.* **38**, 263–270.

Cole, L. A., Kohorn, E. I. & Kim, G. S. (1994) Detecting and monitoring trophoblastic disease. New perspectives on measuring human chorionic gonadotropin levels. *J. Reprod. Med.* **39**, 193–200.

CSCC (1992) Canadian Society of Clinical Chemists position paper: Standardisation of selected hormone measurements. *Clin. Biochem.* **25**, 415–424.

Dati, F. (1990) Standardisation of commercial assays for serum Apo A-I and Apo B: A consensus procedure for the calibration of reference materials. *Scand. J. Clin. Lab. Invest.* **50 (suppl. 198)**, 73–79.

Dobson, S., White, A., Hoadley, M. *et al.* (1987) Measurement of corticotropin in unextracted plasma: comparison of a time-resolved immunofluorometric assay and an immunoradiometric assay, with use of the same monoclonal antibodies. *Clin. Chem.* **33**, 1747–1751.

Dybkaer, R. (1991) Scales for measurement based on an antigen-antibody reaction. *Scand. J. Clin. Lab. Invest.* **51 (suppl. 205)**, 55–62.

Ekins, R. (1991) Immunoassay standardisation. *Scand. J. Clin. Lab. Invest.* **51 (suppl. 205)**, 33–46.

Gosling, J. P. (1991) Standardisation of immunoassays for hapten analytes. *Scand. J. Clin. Lab. Invest.* **51 (suppl. 205)**, 95–104.

Gosling, J. P., Middle, J., Siekmann, L. *et al.* (1993) Standardisation of hapten immunoprocedures: Total cortisol. *Scand. J. Clin. Lab. Invest.* **216 (suppl.)**, 3–41.

Haavisto, A. M., Dunkel, L., Pettersson, K. *et al.* (1990) LH measurements by *in vitro* bioassay and a highly sensitive immunofluorometric assay improve the distinction between boys with constitutional delay of puberty and hypogonadotropic hypogonadism. *Pediatr. Res.* **27**, 211–214.

Haskell, C. M., Buchegger, F., Schreyer, M. *et al.* (1983) Monoclonal antibodies to carcinoembryonic antigen: Ionic strength as a factor in the selection of antibodies for immunoscintigraphy. *Cancer Res.* **43**, 3857–3864.

Hilgers, J., von Mensdorff-Pouilly, S., Verstraaten, A. *et al.* (1995) Quantitation of polymorphic epithelial mucin: A challenge for biochemists and immunologists. *Scand. J. Clin. Lab. Invest.* **55 (suppl. 221)**, 81–86.

Holder, G. (1994) The UK NEQAS for urinary free cortisol. *Proc. UK NEQAS Mtg* **1**, 200–204.

Hunter, W. M. & Budd, P. S. (1980) Circulating antibodies to ovine and bovine immunoglobulin in healthy subjects: A hazard for immunoassays (letter). *Lancet* **2**, 1136.

Jeffcoate, S. L. (1991) Role of reference materials in immunoassay standardisation. *Scand. J. Clin. Lab. Invest.* **51 (suppl. 205)**, 131–133.

Kallner, A., Magid, E. & Albert, W. (eds) (1991) Immunoassay standardisation. In: *Improvement of Comparability and Compatibility of Laboratory Assay Results in Life Sciences, 3rd Bergmeyer Conference. Scand. J. Clin. Lab. Invest.* **51** (**suppl. 205**).

Kallner, A., Magid, E. & Ritchie, R. (eds) (1993) Proposals for two immunomethod reference systems: cortisol and human chorionic gonadotropin. In: *Improvement of Comparability and Compatibility of Laboratory Assay Results in Life Sciences, 4th Bergmeyer Conference. Scand. J. Clin. Lab. Invest.* **53** (**suppl. 216**).

Lilja, H., Björk, T., Abrahamsson P.-A. *et al.* (1994) Improved separation between normals, benign prostatic hyperplasia (BPH) and carcinoma of the prostate (CAP) by measuring free (F), complexed (C) and total concentrations (T) of prostate specific antigen (PSA). *J. Urol.* **151**, 400A.

Mann, K., Saller, B. & Hoermann, R. (1993) Clinical use of hCG and hCGβ determinations. *Scand. J. Clin. Lab. Invest.* **53** (**suppl. 216**), 97–104.

Marcovina, S. M., Albers, J. J., Henderson, L. O. *et al.* (1993) International Federation of Clinical Chemistry standardisation project for measurements of apolipoproteins A-I and B. III. Comparability of apolipoprotein A-I values by use of international reference material. *Clin. Chem.* **39**, 773–781.

Marcovina, S. M., Albers, J. J., Kennedy, H. *et al.* (1994) International Federation of Clinical Chemistry standardisation project for measurements of apolipoproteins A-I and B: IV, Comparability of apolipoprotein B values by use of International Reference Material. *Clin. Chem.* **40**, 586–592.

Masters, A. M. & Hahnel, R. (1989) Investigation of sex-hormone binding globulin interference in direct radioimmunoassays for testosterone and estradiol. *Clin. Chem.* **35**, 979–984.

McCormack, R. T., Rittenhouse, H. G., Finlay, J. A. *et al.* (1995) Molecular forms of prostate-specific antigen and the human kallikrein gene family: A new era. *Urology* **45**, 729–744.

McKenzie, F. (1994) UK NEQAS for thyroid related hormones. *Proc. UK NEQAS Mtg* **1**, 219–224.

Middle, J. & Singh, G. (1994) UK NEQAS for steroid hormones. *Proc. UK NEQAS Mtg* **1**, 182–194.

NIBSC (1994) *Catalogue of Biological Standards and Reference Materials* (National Institute for Biological Standards and Control, Potters Bar, UK).

Pettersson, K., Ding, Y. Q. & Huhtaniemi, I. (1992) An immunologically anomalous luteinizing hormone variant in a healthy woman. *J. Clin. Endocrinol. Metab.* **74**, 164–171.

Reimer, C., Smith, S., Wells, T. *et al.* (1981) Collaborative calibration of three established reference preparations for specific proteins in human sera as secondary standards for IgA, IgM, and IgG. *J. Biol. Stand.* **9**, 393–400.

Rej, R. & Drake, P. (1991) The nature of calibrators used in immunoassays. *Scand. J. Clin. Lab. Invest.* **51** (**suppl. 205**), 47–54.

Rowe, D., Grab, B. & Anderson, S. (1972) An international reference preparation for human serum immunoglobulins, G, A and M: Content of immunoglobulins by weight. *Bull. World Health Org.* **46**, 67–79.

Seth, J., Ellis, A., Sturgeon, C. *et al.* (1994) The external quality assessment of peptide hormone assays in the 1990s: Scientific problems and priorities. *Proc. UK NEQAS Mtg* **1**, 205–209.

Solberg, H. & Gräsbeck, R. (1989) Reference values. *Adv. Clin. Chem.* **27**, 1–79.

Spencer, C. A., Takeuchi, M., Kazarosyan, M. *et al.* (1995) Interlaboratory/intermethod differences in functional sensitivity of immunometric assays of thyrotropin (TSH) and impact on reliability of measurement of subnormal concentrations of TSH. *Clin. Chem.* **41**, 367–374.

Stamey, T. A. (1995) 2nd Stanford Conf. on International Standardisation of Prostate-specific Antigen Immunoassays, September 1 and 2, 1994. *Urology* **45**, 173–184.

Stenman, U.-H., Alfthan, H., Ranta, T. *et al.* (1987) Serum levels of human chorionic gonadotropin in nonpregnant women and men are modulated by gonadotropin-releasing hormone and sex steroids. *J. Clin. Endocrinol. Metab.* **64**, 730–736.

Stenman, U.-H., Alfthan, H. & Turpeinen, U. (1991a) Method dependence of interpretation of immunoassay results. *Scand. J. Clin. Lab. Invest.* **51** (**suppl. 205**), 86–94.

Stenman, U. H., Bidart, J. M., Birken, S. *et al.* (1993) Standardisation of protein immunoprocedures. Choriogonadotropin (CG). *Scand. J. Clin. Lab. Invest.* **51** (**suppl. 205**), 42–78.

Stenman, U.-H., Leinonen, J., Alfthan, H. *et al.* (1991b) A complex between prostate-specific antigen and alpha 1-antichymotrypsin is the major form of prostate-specific antigen in serum of patients with prostatic cancer: Assay of the complex improves clinical sensitivity for cancer. *Cancer Res.* **51**, 222–226.

Stenman U.-H., Leinonen, J. & Zhang W.-M. (1995) Standardisation of determinations. *Scand. J. Clin. Lab. Invest.* **55** (**suppl. 221**), 45–51.

Stenman U.-H., Pettersson, K., Koskimies, A. *et al.* (1990) Changing ratio of free βLH to LH in urine during the menstrual cycle. *VII World Congress on Human Reproduction*, Helsinki 1990, Abstract 22.

Storring, P. L., Gaines-Das, R. E. & Bangham, D. R. (1980) International reference preparation of human chorionic gonadotrophin for immunoassay: Potency estimates in various bioassay and protein binding assay systems; and international reference preparations of α and β subunits of human chorionic gonadotrophin for immunoassay. *J. Endocrinol.* **84**, 295–310.

Strobel, S. A., Sokoloff, R. L., Wolfert, R. L. *et al.* (1995) Multiple forms of prostate-specific antigen in serum measured differently in equimolar- and skewed-response assays (letter). *Clin. Chem.* **41**, 125–127.

Sturgeon, R., Seth, J. & Al-Sadie, R. (1994) UK NEQAS for CEA and hCG: Improving performance? *Proc. UK NEQAS Mtg* **1**, 214–218.

Thienpont, L., Stöckl, D. & De Leenher, A. (1995) Isotope dilution-mass spectrometry and implementation of a common accuracy base for routine medical laboratory analysis: Practice and prospects (letter). *J. Mass Spectrom.* **30**, 772–774.

Tietz, N. W. (1994) Accuracy in clinical chemistry: Does anybody care? *Clin. Chem.* **40**, 859–861.

Turpeinen, U., Haglund, C., Roberts, P. *et al.* (1992) Comparability of three assays for carcinoembryonic antigen (letter). *Clin. Chem.* **38**, 1506–1507.

Turpeinen, U., Lehtovirta, P., Alfthan, H. *et al.* (1990) Interference by human anti-mouse antibodies in CA 125 assay after immunoscintigraphy: anti-idiotypic antibodies not neutralised by mouse IgG but removed by chromatography. *Clin. Chem.* **36**, 1333–1338.

Turpeinen, U., Lehtovirta, P. & Stenman U.-H. (1995) Determination of CA 125 by three methods in samples from patients with human anti-mouse antibodies (HAMA). *Clin. Chem.* **41**, 1667–1669.

Vadlamudi, S., Stewart, W., Fugate, K. *et al.* (1991) Performance characteristics for an immunoassay. *Scand. J. Clin. Lab. Invest.* **51** (**suppl. 205**), 134–138.

Vaitukaitis, J. L., Braunstein, G. D. & Ross, G. T. (1972) A radioimmunoassay which specifically measures human chorionic gonadotropin in the presence of human luteinizing hormone. *Amer. J. Obstet. Gynecol.* **113**, 751–758.

Vessella, R. L., Noteboom, J. & Lange, P. H. (1992) Evaluation of the Abbott IMx automated immunoassay of prostate-specific antigen. *Clin. Chem.* **38**, 2044–2054.

Weber, T. H., Käpyaho, K. I. & Tanner, P. (1990) Endogenous interference in immunoassays in clinical chemistry: A review. *Scand. J. Clin. Lab. Invest.* **50** (**suppl. 201**), 77–82.

Wheeler, M. (1994) Update on immunoassay automation. *Proc. UK NEQAS Mtg* **1**, 163–170.

Whicher, J. T., Ritchie, R. F., Johnson, A. M. *et al.* (1994) New international reference preparation for proteins in human serum (RPPHS). *Clin. Chem.* **40**, 934–938.

Wood, W. G. (1991a) Immunoassay external quality assessment in the Federal Republic of Germany. *Ann. Inst. Super. Sanita* **27**, 495–498.

Wood, W. G. (1991b) 'Matrix effects' in immunoassays. *Scand. J. Clin. Lab. Invest.* **51** (**suppl. 205**), 105–112.

Yedema, K. A., Thomas, C. M., Segers, M. F. *et al.* (1992) Comparison of five immunoassay procedures for the ovarian carcinoma-associated antigenic determinant CA 125 in serum. *Eur. J. Obstet. Gynecol. Reprod. Biol.* **47**, 245–252.

Zhou, A. M., Tewari, P. C., Bluestein, B. I. *et al.* (1993) Multiple forms of prostate-specific antigen in serum: Differences in immunorecognition by monoclonal and polyclonal assays. *Clin. Chem.* **39**, 2483–2491.

Chapter 12

Data Manipulation

Peter R. Raggatt

'Machine computation should never be thought to relieve the analyst of responsibility for reliability of his measurements' (Dudley *et al.*, 1985)

INTRODUCTION

It is self-evident that computerised processing of immunoassay data is advantageous. What is not self-evident is whether any particular computer method gives the correct result in all circumstances. My objective in this chapter is to provide the information needed to form a judgement about the correctness of immunoassay results calculated by computer.

Ideas on immunoassay data processing have been well developed for many years and it is fair to say that all the main questions were settled by about 1975 (for reviews, see Rodbard, 1974; Dudley *et al.*, 1985; Special Supplement: *Scandinavian Journal of Clinical Laboratory Investigations (1991)*), although there were some important contributions in the early 1980s. Although there has been little recent innovation in this field, it remains important because nearly every assay result is produced using a computer data-processing package. In 1993, an evaluation of five commercial software packages in the United States caused the authors to conclude that the packages showed 'numerous deficiencies' (Gerlach *et al.*, 1993). So why are there problems? The problems arise in part from fundamental properties of immunoassays, particularly their errors, and in part from the uses to which we wish to put them. Relatively sophisticated statistical thinking is required but this is uncongenial to our human characteristics, which demand a simple 'method' for all assays and a simple 'result' for each specimen. If the analysts are to take responsibility for their measurements they must have an understanding of the chemistry of their assays and also they must have an understanding of what the computer does to the data that they produce.

CHARACTERISATION OF A CALIBRATION CURVE

Immunoassay calibration curves have few characteristics that are constant but there are some and these are worth restating:

Nonlinear relationship between response and calibrator The parameter measured (the response) has a non-linear relationship to analyte concentration so that a more sophisticated method than drawing a straight line with a ruler must be used.

No single unique line fits the data There is more than one curved line that could pass through a set of calibrator points and so a choice of line must be made, which introduces the risk of bias in making this choice.

Relatively large assay errors with heteroscedasticity The assay errors that occur are large relative to the analyte levels that are being measured and this in turn means that there is significant uncertainty in just where the line should run even though its general shape is defined. These errors are not constant in every region of the assay's working range so that we are less certain about where to draw the line in some parts of the assay curve than in others. Furthermore the errors are not constant in every batch so that usually the curve must be drawn anew for every batch.

Many of these problems could be reduced by an increase in the number of calibrators ('standards') used; we could use calibrators that are more closely spaced and we could use many more replicates for each calibrator. However, costs forbid this. Overall we have to make some compromises and accept some degree of uncertainty. The science of immunoassay data processing depends on understanding the compromises.

CURVE-FITTING PROCEDURES

Having obtained some assay response data for a set of calibrators and realising that this data contains error both in the calibrator values and in the measured responses, we must compute the curve from which the unknowns will be calculated. This is often referred to as **curve-fitting**. There are two main choices of approach. The first is to reproduce mathematically what would be done with graph paper, a pencil and a ruler, i.e. an **empirical approach**. The second is to begin with some chemical theory that may reflect the molecular events that occur during the assay and derive an equation from this for the general shape of the curve. In either case, we may refer to the equation and any underlying assumptions as a **mathematical model** for the actual events. In theory there is a very large number of choices of curves and models; in practice there are perhaps eight distinct methods which fall into three groups.

Interpolation methods

Linear Interpolation

The simplest method is simply to join adjacent calibrator points with a straight line. For a continuous smooth curve, such as an immunoassay, this will clearly introduce significant errors unless the data points are very close together. However, it makes no prior assumptions and is unbiased in that it simply follows the experimental data. A further step would be to transform the data in some way, perhaps by taking logarithms of the response data, and then to carry out linear interpolation on the transformed data. If the transformation tends to line-arise the data, the fit will be better. Challand *et al.* (1976) showed that linear interpolation of the ratio of free radioactivity to bound radioactivity versus calibrator concentrations in a radioimmunoassay gave significantly less distortion (bias) than other methods. Nonetheless, the accuracy of each segment of the calibration line depends crucially on the accuracy and precision of the two calibration points that define it and is largely independent of the rest of the calibration curve; thus some segments could be accurate and others inaccurate. Ideally, each segment should have a quality control sample whose result falls within the segment so that the accuracy of each segment may be judged.

Curvilinear Interpolation and the Spline Function

Instead of using straight lines to join up the calibrators it is possible to use curved lines. By reference to the stencils or templates formerly used by architects to draw smoothly curved lines this is sometimes called the **French curves** method and the name clearly illustrates the arbitrary nature of this method. Mathematically this is carried out by calculating a curve for a series of short segments of the overall calibration curve. The equation used for each segment is usually a cubic polynomial: $y = a + bx + cx^2 + dx^3$, where y is the response and x is the concentration of the analyte. In order to calculate a cubic polynomial at least four independent data points are essential. Each of the short curves may then be modified in order to compel it to join smoothly to the next (**smoothing**). This involves recalculating all the curves repetitively until the joins between the segments and the fit of each segment to its data points are acceptable. The places where the curves join are called **knots**. In the original version of the method the knots are at the values of the calibrator concentrations; thus for a six-point calibration curve there will be four knots and five independent segments. This leads to a large number of degrees of freedom and a heavy data-processing load. A simpler version uses fewer knots, perhaps only two between the lowest and the highest calibrators, at arbitrary values. The mathematical test used for ensuring a smooth join at each knot is to ensure that the first derivative (slope) and the second derivative (rate of change of slope) of each of the two curves are the same at the place where they join. Because of the need for each segment to be recalculated until the join is smooth (**iteration**), a computer is essential.

The composite mathematical function obtained is called a **spline function**. Smoothed spline functions are reviewed by Wegscheider (1985). They were first described by Reinsch (1967, 1971) and then applied to immunoassay by Marschner *et al.* (1973) using a knot at every calibrator. Malan *et al.* (1978a,b) showed that use of fewer knots was advantageous for immunoassay and he suggests that the number of knots should be no more than one or two. In the early reports of use of this method the main limitation was the complexity of programming the large mainframe computer that was needed to achieve a realistically short computation time. The availability of fast personal computers (PCs) has made versions of the spline method readily available although methods vary in the sophistication of the smoothing used and in the rapidity of computation. All methods use smoothing but there are spline methods where additional smoothing factors are used, either preset or computed from the data, and which, for example, can test the curve to ensure that there is only one point of inflexion.

Curvilinear interpolation and the spline function are methods that will fit the experimental data closely no matter how unlikely the data points are on chemical grounds. Each segment is largely independent of the rest of the calibration curve and it is possible for some segments to be accurate and others not. Thus, ideally each segment should contain a quality control specimen so that it is independently controlled for accuracy. As each segment may depend on a very small number of data points and is largely independent of other parts of the calibration curve, even one moderate error in a data point will have a significant effect on the accuracy of the curve in that segment. An unsophisticated spline function, especially one with three or more knots, is quite capable of producing a curve with a wiggle in it, i.e. a curve that has more than one point of inflexion. Even though such a curve may be statistically the best-fit curve, it is impossible chemically and there must be error somewhere, for example in the assigned value of one of the calibrators or chance coincidence of two sizeable errors in measurement of the assay response for one calibrator. The spline function should thus be used with care and avoided unless the data is very precise and there are many calibrators. If it is desired that the line should follow the individual calibrator data points closely even if some of them are wrong, then the spline function will give the desired result.

Empirical models

Hyperbolic Model

The data is assumed to fit an equation of the form:

$$y = a + b(1/x)$$

where y is the assay response and x is the concentration of the analyte. Another version is an equation of the form:

$$(1/y) = p + q(x)$$

These equations give a smooth curve which may fit competitive immunoassay (e.g. radio-immunoassay, RIA) data well, at least for a limited range of values. However, it is hyperbolic, not sigmoid, and tends towards infinity at each end and thus is unlikely to give a good fit at the extremes of the calibration curve, especially the low calibrator end of a competitive immunoassay (Figure 1). It is very simple and by plotting the reciprocals of the calibrator values against the responses, or by plotting the ratio of binding at zero concentration/binding at each calibrator concentration (B_0/B) against calibrator values, a straight line is obtained (Hales and Randle, 1963) and a best fit can be obtained by least-squares linear regression. This seems

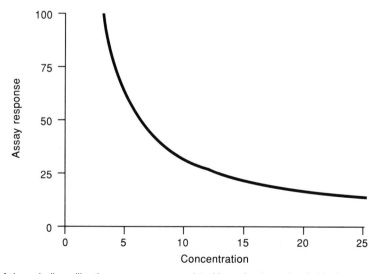

Figure 1 A hyperbolic calibration curve: $y = a + b/x$. Very simple and suitable for some competitive assays, e.g. RIA, but distorts errors.

simple and attractive. However, there is an important problem which also occurs in other curve-fitting methods: not only are reciprocals taken of the actual data but in effect reciprocals are also taken of the assay errors. Thus at the extremes of the calibration curve, where the errors are the greatest, taking reciprocals means that the errors are minimised and conversely in the middle of the calibration curve where the actual errors are smallest, taking reciprocals means that the effect of error is exaggerated. This is a general problem of the hyperbolic function as a curve-fitting model which, together with its lack of sigmoid shape, has limited its popularity.

Polynomial Model

The calibration curve is assumed to fit a curve of the form:

$$y = a + bx + cx^2 + dx^3 + \ldots\ldots px^n$$

where y is the assay response and x is the concentration of the analyte.

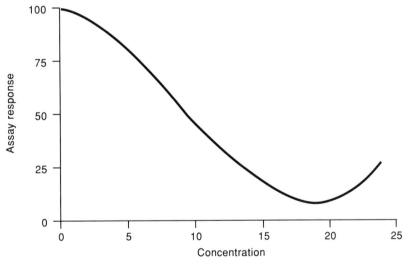

Figure 2 A cubic polynomial calibration curve: $y = a + bx + cx^2 + dx^3$. Simple and suitable for some competitive assays, e.g. RIA, but the curve may turn up at high levels producing ambiguous results unless truncated.

Most commonly a cubic is used (highest power three); higher powers may be used but require proportionately more data in order to get an unambiguous solution. This type of equation may be thought of as a straight line ($y = a + bx$) which is then modified by the addition or subtraction of the other terms, some of which are only significant at very high or very low values of x. A simple cubic has three mathematically possible values of x for each value of y; one will usually be negative (impossible) but it is quite possible mathematically to have two positive 'results' for a given assay response (Figure 2). For this reason it is essential to

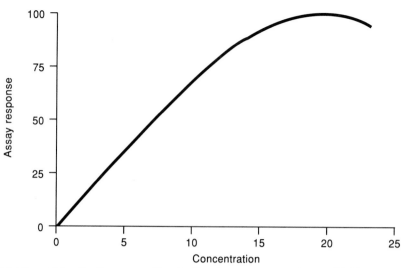

Figure 3 A polynomial calibration curve with a fractional power: $y = a + bx - cx^{3.5}$. Simple and suitable for some noncompetitive assays, e.g. IRMA, but is essentially linear at low levels.

truncate the calibration curve at suitable places such as those where the slope becomes zero (first derivative = 0). In the figure this is at a concentration of about 18. Provided that truncation is carried out sensibly, a cubic polynomial can be fitted to competitive immunoassay (e.g. radioimmunoassay) data rapidly and successfully. Immunometric (noncompetitive) assays, which have a portion of the calibration curve which is essentially a straight line, may not fit so well.

A further example of the polynomial is where the powers of x are not integers but are fractional powers. An example is: $y = a + bx + cx^p$ where p has a non integer value such as 2.75. If c is small and negative, this model may be seen as virtually a straight line at low levels of x but which then curves away from linearity at higher values of x. This model may fit immunometric (noncompetitive) assays well as it reproduces the virtually linear part of the calibration curve but then flattens off at higher analyte concentrations (Figure 3). As the curve approaches zero concentration it becomes linear and so cannot represent the flattening of the response which normally occurs at low concentrations in noncompetitive assays. Again truncation is necessary at high concentrations as the curve can turn downwards and give ambiguous results. Least-squares regression can be used for both integer and noninteger polynomials.

Log-logit model

Rodbard (Rodbard and Cooper, 1970; Rodbard and Lewald, 1970; Feldman and Rodbard, 1971) was principally responsible for introducing this model for immunoassay calibration curves in 1970. The logit is a general, mathematical transformation which was named by Berkson (1944, 1951) who claimed to have used it for various bioassays since the 1920s.

$$\text{logit}(z) = \ln\left(\frac{z}{1-z}\right)$$

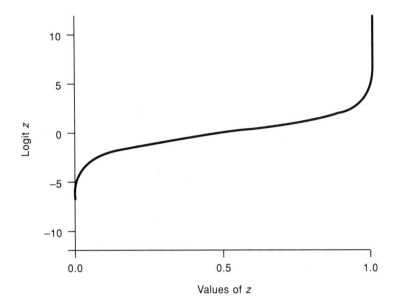

Figure 4 The logit function: $y = \ln(z/(1 - z))$. This symmetrical function can only be used for values of z between 0 and 1.0.

The logit function is a continuous sigmoidal function with a single point of inflexion (Figure 4). It will be seen that it resembles immunoassay standard curves in general shape and only has meaning for values of z between 0 and 1. To use this function for immunoassay it is necessary also to take logs of the calibration values and the calibration curve is assumed to fit a curve of the form:

$$\text{logit}(y) = a + b\ln(x)$$

where y is the assay response and x is the analyte concentration. The assay response must be expressed as fraction bound or as B/B_0 so that it has values between 0 and 1. The log-logit transformation is shown in Figure 5. Having transformed the response data by converting it into logits, it can be plotted against the log-transformed calibrator values and the best straight line can be computed by least-squares linear regression. It should be noted that the data for the zero calibrator (B_0) cannot be included as the log of zero has no real meaning; similarly, data for the 'infinite standard' or 'nonspecific binding' tubes in a radioimmunoassay cannot be included. With this limitation, the simple log-logit model fits many competitive immunoassays (e.g. radioimmunoassay) well in practice. Particular care should be taken not to extrapolate much beyond the lowest or highest calibrators as the assay zero and non-specific

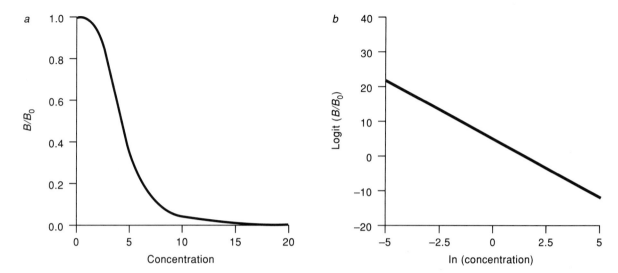

Figure 5 The log-logit transformation of an idealised competitive immunoassay calibration curve: *a*, the data simply plotted; *b*, the same data transformed using log of concentration and logit of assay response. Transformation into a straight line allows use of least-squares linear regression to get the best straight line from the data.

binding data can have no influence on the shape of the curve. Its other limitation arises from the fact that both the log function and the logit function are symmetrical and thus the log-logit curve is also symmetrical. Because of this, an immunoassay that produces an asymmetrical calibration curve may not fit the log-logit curve very well. Asymmetrical curves occur particularly in polyclonal radioimmunoassays that have been optimised for use at very low concentrations of antigen (e.g. very low antibody concentration), in assays in which the labelled antigen is chemically different from the unlabelled antigen and in immunometric assays.

Healy's Four-parameter Logistic Model

This model was developed by Healy (1972) to improve the log-logit model. The log-logit model produces two parameters: the slope and the intercept of the linear regression line. Healy added two more parameters to deal with the data for the assay zero (B_0) and the non-specific binding (blank) and expressed the model in the form:

$$y = a + b \left(\frac{\exp[c - d \ln x]}{1 + \exp[c - d \ln x]} \right)$$

where y is the assay response and x the analyte concentration. Note that this model can accept any measure of response, including radioactive counts etc., whereas the simple log-logit model requires the response to be expressed as a number between 0 and 1. In the four parameter model the parameters *a* and *b* are related to the nonspecific binding and to the B_0 (response at zero calibrator) while *c* and *d* are calculated by linear regression of logit response versus log concentration. Thus the blank and the B_0 are regarded as fixed but not error-free and are determined afresh for each assay. This model thus has significant advantages over the simple log-logit model and in particular the fit at the extremes of the calibration curve is usually better. However, the curve is still essentially symmetrical about the estimated dose corresponding to 50% maximum binding (ED_{50}) point as is the log-logit curve.

Five-parameter Logistic Model

The formula for the four-parameter model above can be modified by introduction of a fifth parameter:

$$y = a + b \left(\frac{\exp[c - d \ln x]}{1 + \exp[c - d \ln x]} \right)^m$$

The fifth parameter, *m*, allows some asymmetry to be introduced. If *m* = 1 the curve is identical to the four parameter model and is symmetrical about the ED_{50} point. Other values of *m* allow the curve to be asymmetrical and sometimes a significantly better fit to the experimental data is obtained. However, each additional parameter requires more data for the same degree of confidence and the five-parameter model may allow excessive flexibility if the number of data points making up the calibration curve is small. It may be preferable to choose a value for *m* for a particular method from a consensus of several independent 'good' batches and then to keep *m* constant for all future batches of that method rather than to determine m afresh for each batch.

The Law of Mass Action Models and Scatchard Plots

The reactions of antibody with antigen are chemical reactions and if they are allowed to continue until equilibrium is reached they can be described by the law of mass action. This approach is attractive as it is based on sound chemical theory and so is likely to be more reliable than any arbitrary model such as those described above. The law of mass action model is also valuable as it gives insight into the chemical events of immunoassay.

The linearisation of the first-order mass action law for chemical reactions in general was introduced by Scatchard (1949) and was first applied to radioimmunoassay by Berson and Yalow (1964). Ekins (*et al.*, 1968; Ekins and Newman, 1970; Malan *et al.*, 1978a) and Rodbard and Lewald (1970) are mainly responsible for the further development of the application of the law of mass action to immunoassay chemistry as a means of computing the calibration curve from chemical principles and for demonstrating that this does in practice account for many of the observed features of immunoassays. Further refinement and marketing of the model in readily accessible computerised form is associated with a team led by Wilkins (*et al.*, 1978a, b). Proponents of models based on the mass action law have pointed to the advantages of basing routine immunoassay data processing on mathematical representation of the actual chemical events rather than on whatever arbitrary model happens to fit the experimental data. A critical analysis of this approach when applied to real immunoassay systems, for example when using polyclonal antibodies, has been published more recently (Keilacker *et al.*, 1991).

For the chemical reaction:

$$Ab + Ag \Leftrightarrow AbAg$$

where Ab is an antibody, Ag is an antigen and AbAg is the antigen-antibody complex formed when antibody binds to antigen, the law of mass action shows that the concentrations of the reactants at equilibrium are related by:

$$K_a = \frac{[AbAg]}{[Ab][Ag]}$$

where K_a is a constant.

The molar concentrations of Ab Ag, and AbAg are shown by the convention [Ab], [Ag] and [AbAg]. K_a is the familiar equilibrium constant used to describe the binding affinity of an antibody for an antigen and has a high numerical value, perhaps 10^8–10^9, for antibodies that are of practical use in immunoassays. The units of the equilibrium constant are litres per mole, often printed as $l\ mol^{-1}$. The equilibrium constant for the reverse reaction, dissociation of antigen-antibody complex, is the reciprocal of the equilibrium constant for the forwards reaction.

The equation can be rewritten in the form:

$$\frac{[bound]}{[free]} = K_a(n - [bound])$$

where [bound] is the molar concentration of bound antigen; [free] is the molar concentration of unbound antigen; n is the maximum binding capacity of the antibody in moles per mass of antibody in the reaction tube; K_a is the equilibrium constant (litres/mole).

If the ratio of bound to free is plotted against the concentration of bound antigen, a straight line should be obtained; this is the **Scatchard plot** (Figure 6). Note that molar (mole per litre, $mol\ l^{-1}$) concentrations must be used throughout and the mass of the labelled antigen must not be neglected otherwise the value of the equilibrium constant obtained will be numerically incorrect. In practice, and especially with polyclonal antibodies, the Scatchard plot is often linear only over a limited concentration range.

It is valuable to restate the theoretical limitations that apply if the law of mass action, as stated in the simple form above, is to be true:

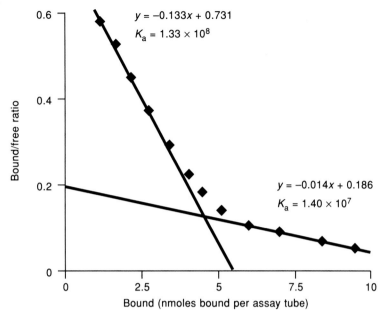

Figure 6 The Scatchard plot showing two binding species with $K_a = 1.33 \times 10^8$ and $K_a = 1.40 \times 10^7$, respectively.

1 The antigen must be present in homogeneous form consisting of only one chemical species.

2 The antibody must similarly be present in homogeneous form.

3 Both antigen and antibody must be univalent, i.e. only one molecule of antigen can react with one molecule of antibody.

4 The antigen and antibody must react according to the first-order mass action law and there may be no effects that modify the reactivity of either antibody or antigen, such as cooperativity or allosteric effects.

5 The antigen and antibody must react until equilibrium is reached and the equilibrium must be microreversible.

6 The measures of the bound and free concentrations must be true measures and must not be influenced by factors such as incomplete separation of bound and free fractions or nonspecific binding of the reacting species to the reaction tube.

These ideals may not be attainable. However, under the typical reaction conditions of a radioimmunoassay or other competitive immunoassay – ambient temperature, low antibody concentrations etc. – they may be approached fairly closely for at least some methods. It should be clearly understood that if the assay deviates from ideality then the ideal equation may not fit the experimental data and the law of mass action model may be unsatisfactory as a curve-fitting model. Even if the law of mass action model is satisfactory for computing results for a nonideal assay, any parameters obtained, such as equilibrium constant, will not be valid.

The requirement that the antigen should be homogeneous means that it must behave as if it were chemically homogeneous under the reaction conditions. An example of nonideality is use of a labelled antigen that is chemically different from the antigen being measured. Thus the binding of a tritiated steroid to antibody is identical to that of the nonradioactive steroid, but the binding of a steroid labelled with ^{125}I via a conjugated group may not be. However, careful matching of antibody and labelling method may permit near-ideal behaviour in practice. The requirements that the antibody should be homogeneous and univalent mean that it must behave as if it were chemically homogeneous under the reaction conditions. A solid-phase antibody must behave as if it were actually in the liquid phase. The antibody must behave as if it were a monoclonal Fab fragment, unable to bind a second molecule of antigen. For intact IgG antibodies, which have two antigen-binding sites, this will only be true over a limited concentration range; under conditions of antigen excess, binding to the second site will become significant. The use of polyclonal antibodies means the presence of species with a wide range of equilibrium constants and so the use of an equation that assumes a single binding species will result in departure from ideality.

The requirement of attaining equilibrium and microreversibility of the reaction may be quite difficult to satisfy practically, e.g. it is common practice to stop the reaction by separating bound and free fractions before true equilibrium has been reached. However, if longer incubation times are used, competing reactions may become significant, e.g. decomposition of one or more of the reactants. Some assay protocols require sequential addition of reagents; this manoeuvre may give a better assay on practical grounds but theoretically invalidates use of the mass action law to describe them. It is worth emphasising that Scatchard analysis will not give a valid measure of the equilibrium constant unless all the reactants are added simultaneously and unless equilibrium is reached. When a mass action law model is used to compute the calibration curve and read off unknowns, failure to satisfy the strict requirements will theoretically result in the fit being imperfect; it may nevertheless be of practical use. It may then be regarded as another arbitrary model but one that is based on an approximation to a theoretically valid model. Like all models, it is likely to fit some parts of the curve better than others.

In general, non-competitive immunoassays, such as immunometric or sandwich assays, cannot be described by simple mathematical methods based on the law of mass action , as the fundamental criteria do not apply. The capture antibody is in excess and is bound to a solid phase, the assay is noncompetitive and in effect the reaction proceeds in two stages.

The equation used in Wilkins' mass action law model for computing a noncompetitive or radioimmunoassay calibration curve (Wilkins *et al.*, 1978a, b) is:

$$y = \frac{2P(1-b)}{K_a + P + A + x \sqrt{(K - P + A + x)^2 + 4KP}} + b$$

where y is the fraction (or percentage) of label in the bound fraction, i.e. actual radioactivity in the bound fraction divided by the total radioactivity in the reaction tube; x is the concentration of antigen; K_a is the mass action law equilibrium constant; P is the concentration of antibody; A is the concentration of labelled antigen; b is the fraction of radioactivity in the bound fraction that is due to nonspecific binding.

In addition to the simple univalent reaction theory described above, Ekins (*et al.*, 1968; Malan *et al.*, 1978b) developed equations capable of describing multivalent binding; such equations are of course more complex. It must be realised that the more complex the equation and the greater the number of parameters, whether based on the law of mass action or not, the more data is required to achieve an unambiguous fit. Practically, some compromises and approximations are inevitable.

DETECTION OF OUTLIERS IN THE CALIBRATION CURVE AND WEIGHTING OF DATA

It is a common experience that sometimes one or more data points of an immunoassay calibration curve are 'out of consensus' with the other points. A pair of duplicates may not agree well or one point may lie well off the line which goes through all the other data points. It seems common sense that any calibrator points that are out of consensus should have less influence or weight than the points that appear to have less error, and it is a simple matter to reject points and simply remove them. The problems arise when we try to devise unbiased methods of assigning weight to individual points.

For all assays, there are many possible curves that would fit the data and we want to choose what is commonly called 'the best' by which is meant 'statistically unbiased'. The statistical criterion that is universally accepted is the least-squares criterion. This simply means that the best line is the one where the sum of the squares of the differences between the co-ordinates of the calculated line and those of the actual data points is at a minimum. When the sum of squares is calculated we may either give each data point the same weight, simply adding all the squares of the differences together, or each point may be weighted in some way, depending on its degree of reliability.

Consider first the familiar least-squares linear regression method used to compute the 'best' straight line through a set of data points. All the data points are used and it at first appears that all are given equal weight. However, outlying data points at the extremes of the data pool have a larger influence on the slope of the line than data points in the middle. The further away from the median a data point is, the greater its influence on the slope (Figure 7). If we plot a measure of the influence of outlying points on the slope of the least-squares linear regression line against the deviation from the mean of the pool of data points, the influence function is a straight line through the origin. A graph that plots a measure of the influence or weight of outlying points on the error of a resulting measurement, or the equation that represents it, is called an influence function (Hampel, 1974).

Data points that are out of consensus with the rest of the data pool are called outliers (Barnett and Lewis, 1984). Healy (1979) defined an outlier as 'an observation which departs from expectation to an improbable extent' and explained that we can detect an outlier only against a background of some theoretical or expected distribution of observations. In the case of random errors in immunoassay the simplest assumption is that errors are Gaussian and that if it were not for errors, all the data points would lie on a smooth line. If data are Gaussian we can define outliers as those data points outside mean $\pm m(SD)$ where m is some multiplier and SD is the appropriate standard deviation. Mean $\pm 3(SD)$ is commonly used although the value of m ought to be varied depending on the size of the sample and the degree of confidence required (Burnett, 1975).

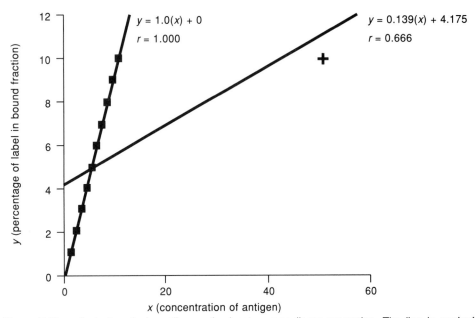

Figure 7 The effect of a single outlier on the least-squares linear regression. The line is markedly affected by adding a single data point (+) which is an outlier and is also at the extremity of the data. To avoid such bias, outliers must be given low weight.

Clearly some thought must be given as to what value for the standard deviation should be used. The expected errors in an assay are described by the precision profile and it is clear that the standard deviation varies from one part of the calibration curve to another, i.e. variance is nonuniform. The overall standard deviation at any calibrator value can be estimated from analysis of variance of the replicates of the calibrators and unknowns in the assay. However, this procedure requires the somewhat risky assumption that errors for calibrators and unknowns are similar. The alternative, determining the standard deviation from the data of the calibrators alone, means that the estimate of the standard deviation is usually a poor one because there are so few data points. Care must be taken that any data points that can be independently determined to be outliers do not influence the standard deviations so obtained; the method of Healy(1979) can be used. If a method has similar error characteristics from batch to batch then data from more than one batch can be combined.

Having defined outliers we can simply exclude them, i.e. give them zero weight. This procedure gives an influence function as shown in Figure 8 and the graph illustrates the arbitrary nature of this method. Data points that are 3.0(SD) from the mean are given the same weight as data points that are very close to the mean but data points which are 3.1(SD) from the mean are given zero weight.

There are some more subtle alternatives to the above procedure (Nicol *et al.*, 1985) and they can be described in terms of the influence function or weighting method they use. An example of an influence function which has been shown to be useful in immunoassay (Nicol *et al.*, 1985) is Ramsay's Eγ function shown in Figure 9. It can be seen that greatest weight is assigned to data points close to the mean and that for points away from the mean the assigned weight is less but never zero. However, the weights assigned by this function fall off quite rapidly, much more rapidly than with a Gaussian bell-shaped curve which might seem

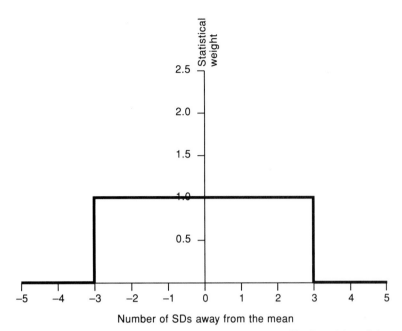

Figure 8 The influence for the procedure of rejecting data beyond 3 SDs but giving all data within this range equal weight.

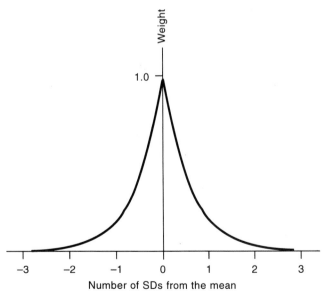

Figure 9 The influence curve using Ramsey's function. The weight given to data points that are away from the mean falls off rapidly but smoothly. Data far from the mean is given low but not zero weight.

more appropriate if the errors were expected to have a Gaussian distribution. Thus it is important to make a realistic decision on what influence function will be used to decide weighting.

Once the equation of the curve has been determined, the residuals should be calculated. The residuals are the differences between the computed values and the observed values; it is most helpful to express residuals both in the same units as the calibrators and as percentage differences. The overall 'goodness-of-fit' may be determined by comparing the mean of the squares of the residuals with the variance of the duplicates for the assay as a whole or some other measure of expected variance.

The procedure may be summarised as:

- Determining the expected dispersion of data for each calibrator.

- Testing the experimental data for each calibrator against this expectation to determine how likely each one is to be an outlier, and hence assigning a weight to each data point using the chosen influence function.

- Using the data points and their weights to determine the equation of the calibration curve using the chosen model and least-squares regression analysis.

- Analysing the residuals (the differences between the actual data points for the calibrators and those computed).

If the data used to construct the calibration curve are precise, then almost any of the above models will give a good fit and hence reliable results. However, when the data are imprecise and contain possible outliers, methods will perform differently and some will produce results with a degree of bias. The ability of a data analysis method to produce unbiased results even in the presence of outliers, which is a reflection of the weighting method used, has been termed **robustness** by Hawker and Challand (1981) and they have suggested that robustness ought to be the principal criterion by which a curve-fitting procedure is judged. Robustness can be tested by fitting the curve and then changing the response data for one or more points and recomputing the curve. Robust methods will show little change in the patient results for modest perturbations of the calibrator data. Methods of robust modelling of immunoassay data have been discussed recently in some detail by Normolle (1993).

COMPUTING THE RESULTS FROM THE EQUATION

The computation of the calibration curve is only the first step in processing the data of an immunoassay. Once the calibration curve is determined, the results for the unknown samples must be read off. This is relatively straightforward for some models and there is little to worry about except the size of errors made by the computer in calculating logs and exponents. However, solving a multiparameter equation may involve a significant amount of arithmetic. Consider the case of a simple cubic polynomial:

$$y = a + bx + cx^2 + dx^3$$

The parameters *a*, *b*, *c* and *d* have been determined by the curve-fitting process and all that remains is to solve the equation by setting *y* to the value of each of the measured responses for each assay tube in turn. Although there is an exact method to solve quadratic equations, there is no such equation for polynomials of higher powers or with fractional powers. The method which is used is arbitrary iteration in which an arbitrary trial value of *x*, e.g. the value of the middle calibrator, is inserted into the equation and the corresponding value of *y* is computed and compared with the value of *y* for which the equation must be solved. This initial value of *x* is then modified in the light of the difference to get a closer estimate, and the calculation is repeated; the process is one of successive approximation (iteration) and is repeated many times to obtain the best estimate. There are a small number of techniques for solving equations by iterative methods. Although totally arbitrary methods of estimating the change in *x* required to get a better solution in each cycle of the iteration may be used, they may not be very efficient. Instead, the next best estimate may be calculated using the Newton theorem. This states that if x_0 is an approximate solution to the function $f(x)$ and if $f'(x)$ is the first derivative of $f(x)$, then $x_0 + f(x_0)/f'(x_0)$ is a better approximation.

The process by which the computed value of *x* approaches the true value, which actually fits the equation for the value of *y* concerned, is called **convergence** and methods may differ greatly in the efficiency with which they converge on the true value and hence the speed with which they produce results. For example, beginning with a value of *x* that is in the middle of the standard curve may appear to be more efficient than starting always from one end; using the Newton theorem is more efficient than changing *x* by a constant percentage each cycle. The problems of nonconvergence have been examined in the context of the four-parameter logistic model by Normolle (1993).

A method of solving complex equations that shares the iterative approach but which may converge much more rapidly is the **simplex method** (Nicol *et al.*, 1986). A simplex is a geo-

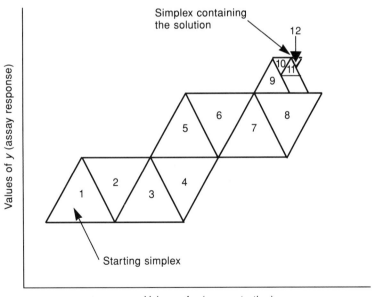

Figure 10 The simplex method of finding a solution to a complex equation, The vertices of the triangle represent possible solutions to the equation. The simplex advances towards the correct solution and when it overshoots, the simplex is reduced in size and the search continues until a solution of acceptable precision is achieved.

metric figure that has one more vertex than the number of dimensions in which it exists; for example, in two dimensions a simplex is an equilateral triangle and in three dimensions a simplex is a regular tetrahedron. The dimensions represent the variables of the equation to be solved, which in the case of immunoassay data are the value of the response y and the corresponding analyte concentration x. Thus the appropriate simplex is a triangle. The method involves evaluation of the equation to be solved for different values corresponding to each vertex of the simplex. The value that produces the 'worst' solution is rejected and the simplex is geometrically reflected over the centroid of the remaining vertices to form a new simplex; the value of the equation is evaluated at the new vertex produced and compared with the other unchanged vertices. The cycle is then repeated (Figure 10). If there is 'overshoot' so that the new vertex gives a worse solution than the previous one, then the size of the simplex is reduced, e.g. halved, and the process continued. This ensures that the iteration converges efficiently towards the final solution, making large steps at first and then smaller and smaller steps as the solution is reached.

Whichever iterative method is used, there must be a rule that decides when the iteration is stopped and the result accepted. Now that fast computers are readily available, many methods simply iterate 100 times and accept the result obtained after 100 cycles. However, it is possible, and more efficient, to test for convergence, for example by terminating the iteration when the value of x differs from that in the previous cycle by less than 1% or when a result of a desired degree of numerical precision has been reached. Some curves, especially spline curves with many knots, may allow two possible solutions which are close to the true solution and if the test for convergence is unsophisticated it is possible for the iteration simply to oscillate between them.

In the case of a simple cubic polynomial there are three mathematically possible values of x (concentration) for each value of y (assay response) but only one will be an allowable result and a choice must be made (Figure 2). The same will be true for many complex equations. In the case of a composite curve such as a spline function, a decision has to be made as to which segment of the curve should be used for each individual data point.

DETECTION AND MEASUREMENT OF ERRORS

Immunoassay, like all analytical procedures, has inherent errors and these errors can be classified into three kinds.

Systematic errors These may be due to use of calibrators whose assigned values are incorrect or whose purity is unsuitable, or to use of antibodies or other reagents of unsuitable specificity.

Gaussian errors These familiar errors are readily described by standard deviation, coefficient of variation and precision profile and, for any measurement, confidence limits can be calculated. Such errors are small but relatively frequent and are due to the cumulative effect of small random errors at each stage of the assay and in the measurement of the response. In theory, Gaussian errors can be deconstructed into their components, such as pipetting error, counting error etc., and independent estimates of these errors should allow prediction of confidence limits (Rodbard and Lewald, 1970; Delaage *et al.*, 1992). This may be helpful in identifying which errors ought to be reduced but this approach does not allow prediction of the random way in which errors coincide or cancel out for individual samples. The experimental approach of observing total error is of more practical use. The confidence limits for any result will be determined by the average standard deviation at that level obtained from the precision profile. If the sample was assayed in duplicate, each singleton is an independent estimate and the mean of the singletons is the best estimate.

Catastrophic errors These are also random errors and are only different from Gaussian errors in that they are much greater in size and much less frequent. If expressed in terms of the standard deviation, they are so many multiples of the standard deviation away from the mean that the probability of such errors occurring is extremely remote according to the Gaussian distribution. Nevertheless they do occur and the rate of occurrence of such errors is an important property of the method. Sometimes the partial cause of a catastrophic error is known, such as the situation when a substantial antigen-antibody complex falls out of a particular tube during separation in a solid-phase immunoassay. It is self-evident that the Gaussian distribution cannot describe such rare events except over a very long period of time.

These catastrophic errors have been defined (World Association of Societies of Pathology, 1979) as 'a reported value which is so far from the true value that it may lead to undesirable and possibly harmful medical decisions or actions'. This is in some ways a very strict definition but it relies on medical (human) criteria rather than wholly scientific criteria and it leaves a class of errors that are too large and infrequent to be described by the Gaussian distribution but that are yet not large enough to fit the above medical definition. It seems a practical response to describe all non-Gaussian errors as catastrophic errors. They are also of course outliers within the definition given earlier in this chapter.

It is a common experience that such catastrophic errors do occur and so it has been customary to carry out immunoassays using duplicates because duplicate assay is a reasonably powerful test for catastrophic errors. Assay using replicates also reduces Gaussian error because the mean of the replicates is a better estimate of the true value than a singleton estimate would be, i.e. the within-batch and between-batch imprecision, as measured by the standard deviation, will be smaller than if singleton assay had been used:

$$SD_{replicates} = \frac{SD_{singletons}}{\sqrt{number\ of\ replicates}}$$

Thus, changing from assay in singleton to assay in duplicate decreases the standard deviation by a factor of 1.414 (or by approximately 30%) as well as providing a method of detecting catastrophic errors.

Assay in duplicate gives a means of calculating the within-batch imprecision, which can be expressed as a precision profile. The use of duplicates to estimate standard deviation in immunoassays was described by Rodbard *et al.* (1968) and by Healy (1972) but has been popularised by Ekins (1983). With modern computers there is every reason why precision profile should be calculated routinely for every assay batch that is carried out in duplicate and the precision data accumulated from batch to batch (Raggatt, 1989).

Sadler and Smith (1990) have shown how reliable confidence limits for results can be obtained from precision profile data and have emphasised the value of analysis of the large amount of valuable data that accumulates from routine assays. They point out that imprecision data based on small numbers of batches, such as is commonly given in research papers or commercial reagent documentation, is of low reliability as a means of judging the long-term performance of a method. Robison-Cox (1995) has recently pointed out that it is possible to be over-optimistic about confidence limits if they are determined from the characteristics of a single batch, especially when there are multiple batches as is usual in diagnostic tests. There is a confidence interval for the result of each unknown but, in addition, the calibration of each batch has error and therefore there is a confidence interval for the determination of the calibration curve. Another way of expressing this is to say that we usually accept the calibration curve as truly and accurately calibrating that batch, despite knowing that the calibration varies slightly from batch to batch. Nevertheless we refer the patient results to a fixed normal reference range. Robison-Cox (1995) offers some solutions to this problem.

Knowledge of the within-batch standard deviation gives an objective means of detecting outliers using mean $\pm m(SD)$ with a value for the standard deviation which is appropriate to the mean of the duplicates. This method is closely similar to the method of using the percentage difference between duplicates because D_{max}, the maximum allowable percentage difference between the duplicates, is given by:

$$D_{max} = \frac{2m(SD)}{mean} \, 100 = 2m(CV)$$

D is the percentage difference between the duplicates;

m is a multiplier (Burnett, 1975);

SD is the standard deviation appropriate to the value of the mean;

and CV is the corresponding coefficient of variation.

It should be noted that the standard deviation used should be one that is unbiased by the presence of outliers; the method of Healy (1979) can be used.

In addition to the above method of detecting outliers, it is valuable to detect pairs of duplicates where the individual singleton values would have different clinical meanings. When a pair of duplicates straddle the upper limit of normal, the one would be interpreted as 'normal' and the other would be interpreted as 'elevated'. Thus this is a misclassification error (Raggatt, 1989) and fits the medical definition of a catastrophic error (World Association of Societies of Pathology, 1979). In practice, a result just outside the normal range would usually be considered as 'borderline'. Poor agreement between duplicates when both would be interpreted in the same way, e.g. both interpreted as 'abnormal', may be relatively unimportant by the medical definition but may still represent a catastrophic error.

Thus there are methods of detecting catastrophic errors and, if a large series of data is considered, it is possible to measure the rate of occurrence of catastrophic errors. The ability

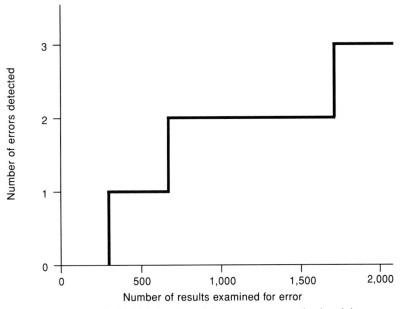

Figure 11 Sequential analysis. Multiple batches of the assay are examined and the occurrence of any catastrophic errors that are detected is plotted against the sequence number when they occurred. In this example, 3 errors occurred in 2000 results examined and they occurred after 350, 650 and 1,650 results, respectively. The 'average rate of error' of about 2 errors per 1000 is beginning to become apparent but will require much more data before it is certain.

to classify results as 'good' (Gaussian error only) or 'bad' (catastrophic error) indicates that the binomial distribution is appropriate to describe the occurrence of these errors and their frequency. It is then possible to apply the method of sequential analysis to determine the confidence limits for error rates and to determine the number of pairs of duplicates that must be examined in order to be reasonably sure that a given error rate is not exceeded (Raggatt, 1989).

Comparative error rate data may be extremely useful in judging the merits of various methods and it will be appreciated that it is possible to have a method with apparently good within-batch and between-batch imprecision determined on small numbers of samples or with a defined material such as commercial quality control serum but which also has an unacceptable rate of catastrophic errors for patient samples. In order to accumulate the large amounts of data that are needed to measure rates of such errors, the data in every assay batch should be examined for errors. Many curve-fitting programs already do this and any duplicates with poor agreement are flagged. In order to carry out error analysis it is only necessary to record the numbers and characteristics of any errors flagged and to cumulate this data from batch to batch. Once the errors are recorded, and by definition they are relatively infrequent, it is possible to carry out the sequential analysis with a pocket calculator and graph paper (Raggatt, 1989) and so obtain a statistically reliable estimate of catastrophic error rate (Figure 11).

Another type of catastrophic error can occur where the concentration of the substance being measured, or of another substance present in the sample, is so high that a result is produced that is totally erroneous. In turbidimetric assays for serum proteins, which measure the change in light scattering due to formation of large particles of antigen-antibody complex, if the concentration of antigen is very high indeed so that the molar ratio of antigen to antibody is high, a different stoichiometry becomes dominant and so produces a misleadingly low result. This problem cannot be detected by assay in duplicate but it can be detected by monitoring the initial rate of reaction, which is much higher than normal because of the high antigen concentration, or by assay of all samples both neat and in a suitable dilution. Similarly the extremely high concentrations of human chorionic gonadotrophin (HCG) in a pregnancy serum may interfere in some immunometric assays for luteinising hormone (LH); here the problem arises because one of the antibodies, but not the other, can react with HCG and the antibody is in effect swamped and so unavailable to form the sandwich with LH. A falsely low result is obtained. This is different from simple crossreactivity where the HCG can react with both antibodies so giving a falsely high result. Clearly there can be no general method of detecting all such problems.

USE OF STORED CALIBRATION CURVES

At first sight it appears that each batch of an assay is a new creation, different from and totally unrelated to all previous batches. If the curve-fit is done with graph paper and pencil, or the computerised equivalent, this may be literally true as there is no objective way in which experience of previous batches can be incorporated. However, more careful thought reveals that most of the components, especially the antibodies, will be the same in each batch and their equilibrium coefficients are unchanging. The labelled component may vary a little from batch to batch, especially if it is radioactive, but nevertheless it has been carefully chosen and purified and must be fundamentally the same chemical compound in every batch. The dilutions, reaction times and temperatures are all constant. Thus it would appear that there must be some underlying commonality between all batches using the same reagents and therefore we should be able to use data from previous batches to help the calibration of future batches. This is now common practice for some nonradioactive methods. The calibration curve's fundamental shape and characteristics are determined once and for all and for each subsequent assay batch the predetermined calibration curve is used. The same curve may be used in every batch in the same way as an extinction coefficient is used in a spectrophotometric assay. A refinement is to adjust the predetermined curve up or down a little by use of one calibrator and a blank.

The common practice of determining the calibration curve totally independently for each batch, using the very limited data from perhaps six calibrators each assayed in duplicate, has grown up because our reagents are in fact more variable and our assays less well optimised than they should be and because our curve-fitting methods are unduly arbitrary. It can be argued that we are imposing limitations on assay performance by an excessively empirical approach to curve-fitting and that this approach conceals evidence for changing assay characteristics which would be revealed if we could express the accumulated experience for each method in a useful way.

A way of using the accumulated experience of a method is to use the mathematical characteristics of the curve-fitting method as quality control parameters. For example, one could record the values of the four parameters of a Healy four-parameter curve-fit for each batch. However, the complex shape of most immunoassay calibration curves means that for any one batch and any one mathematical model there are a large number of possible curves that fit the data within a given range of error and change in one parameter may be compensated by change in another. Hence some of the parameters may appear to be unstable as quality con-

Nature of imprecision

Stored curve better

Less imprecision with a stored calibration curve than with a separate calibration curve each batch

1) Accuracy error in the values assigned to the calibrants.
2) Random errors in pipetting the calibrants.
3) Errors in manipulating calibrant tubes and in separation of bound and free fractions etc.
4) Errors in measuring the signals for the calibrant tubes.
5) Errors in computing the calibration curve.

Stored curve worse

More imprecision with a stored calibration curve than with a separate calibration curve each batch

6) Accuracy error (bias) in pipetting the unknown samples (if the same bias error is made for calibrants and unknowns it is neutralised).

Stored curve the same

Same imprecision with a stored calibration curve as with a separate calibration curve each batch

7) Random errors in pipetting the unknown samples.
8) Errors in manipulating unknown tubes and in separation of bound and free fractions etc.
9) Errors in measuring the signals for the unknown tubes.
10) Errors in computing the results for the unknowns from the calibration curve.

Table 1 The effect of using a stored calibration curve: Classification of assay imprecision according to whether it is associated with use of a stored calibration curve or with use of a independent calibration curve in every assay batch. Note that the table refers to imprecision not bias (inaccuracy). Whether one type of error is numerically greater than another can only be determined experimentally.

trol parameters. If a model based on the law of mass action is used, the parameters may be more stable, and hence more useful, as they represent physicochemical realities. The concentrations at the ED_{50} of the curve, and similar parameters, are useful in nearly all competitive assays but comparable points are harder to define in noncompetitive assays.

It is rarely realised that use of a stored standard curve to calibrate successive batches must inherently improve between-batch imprecision compared to calibrating each batch afresh. If the same stored standard curve is used in each batch, the calibration process will make no contribution to overall between-batch imprecision. However, if each batch has its own calibration curve there will inevitably be some experimental error in determining that curve and thus the overall between-batch imprecision will be worse. Examples of this can be found with the improved between-batch imprecision found for several particle-enhanced light-scattering immunoassays that have calibration stabilities in excess of six months. (Medcalf *et al.*, 1990; Holownia *et al.*, 1997; Thakkar *et al.*, 1997). This is illustrated in Table 1.

The one source of error where the stored curve is not superior is the variability of accuracy of pipetting from one batch to the next. If the pipetting procedure results in dispensing 100 µl in one batch and 105 µl in the next, but with similar imprecision, this may have little effect with an integral calibration curve because the same volume of both calibrants and unknowns would be dispensed. However, if the stored curve was based on 100 µl, then dispensing 105 µl for unknowns will introduce a 5% bias error in results.

Some thought must be given to the reliability of the process by which the stored curve is determined. Mathematical aspects of this are discussed by Robison-Cox (1995). If we take the statistical view that the mean of all independent batches is the best estimate of the 'true value' then the use of a separate calibration curve for each batch will result in the best estimate but only when all the data are combined, for example obtaining the mean value for a quality control serum. In this sense, the 'best estimate' is the most accurate (least biased) estimate. This estimate will of course have imprecision and confidence limits. Unless a stored calibration curve is similarly based on a large sample of standard curves, it risks having some bias. If a single 'calibration run' is used to define the stored calibration curve and this calibration run is biased from the true value, all batches using that stored curve will have equal bias. The bias will be greater or smaller and positive or negative, depending on chance when the stored curve was determined. It should not be a surprise that some apparent shift in accuracy is observed when the stored standard curve is redetermined, especially if no more effort is expended than would be used for a single normal batch. The key issues are the robustness to bias of the process whereby the stored standard curve is determined and acceptance that use of stored standard curves requires additional vigilance and regular checking of the accuracy of pipetting.

In some cases the manufacturer will have made a once-and-for-all calibration for the particular batch of reagents. The manufacturer will have in effect fixed the bias of that assay for all users and, if the reagents are good, all users should agree on the results. These results may still have significant bias from the 'true' value. This phenomenon can be seen clearly in method bias reported by external quality control schemes and applies equally to conventional calibration and to use of stored standard curves. The danger is that one method will dominate the market and thus impose its bias on all users. We need to be very critical about the process of calibration.

Stored standard curves will usually use a constant mathematical function to determine the shape of the curve and this function may have some of its parameters fixed. Other parameters such as the zero or blank and the slope, or an equivalent measure of response per dose, may be checked in each batch. This is often described as 'two-point calibration'. If two-point calibration is used we have a position that is intermediate between running a full standard curve in each batch and using a stored curve totally. Clearly two-point calibration is a safer compromise and reduces the worry that the curve is steadily shifting as the reagents age and it is able to compensate for shifting accuracy of pipetting.

CONCLUSIONS

The processing of the data of an immunoassay should consist of:

1   Computing the calibration curve from the calibrator data using an unbiased method that takes into account the relative reliability of each individual data point by means of weighting and a suitable mathematical model followed by calculating and analysing the residuals for each data point.

2   Analysis of the characteristics of the curve such as the B_0, the ED_{50}, the nonspecific binding, the mean square of the residuals, the correlation coefficient of the regression analysis and any useful parameters from the equation of the curve.

3   Calculating the values of the unknown samples and applying appropriate truncation so that a reliable result is obtained for each.

4   If any samples were assayed in duplicate, calculating the precision profile by analysis of the duplicates. This data can be accumulated from batch to batch.

5   Determining the confidence limits for each result by use of the precision profile or other data.

6   Analysis of the quality control data given by the assay to determine its overall reliability.

7   Analysis of the data for any catastrophic errors and accumulating such data from batch to batch so that a composite analysis of catastrophic error rate is obtained. Any results showing catastrophic errors will be rejected.

8   Long-term analysis of trends in the method for changes in accuracy, in calibration curve parameters, of average imprecision and of rates of catastrophic errors.

REFERENCES

Barnett, V. & Lewis, T. (1984). *Outliers in Statistical Data* (Wiley, Chichester, USA).

Berkson, J. (1944) Application of the logistic function in bioassay. *J. Amer. Statist. Assoc.* **39**, 357–365.

Berkson, J. (1951) Why I prefer logits to probits. *Biometrics* **7**, 327–339.

Berson, S. A. & Yalow, R. S. (1964) *The Hormones: Physiology, Chemistry and Applications*, Vol 4. (eds Pincus, G. Thiman, K. V. & Astwood, E. B.) pp. 557–630 (Academic Press, New York).

Burnett, R. W. (1975) Accurate estimation of standard deviations for quantitative methods used in clinical chemistry. *Clin. Chem.* **21**, 1935–1938.

Challand, G. S., Spencer, C. A. & Ratcliffe, J. G. (1976) Observations on the automated calculation of radioimmunoassay results. *Ann. Clin. Biochem.* **13**, 354–360.

Delaage, M., Compiano, J. M., Artus, A. *et al.* (1992) Statistical properties of immunoanalytic system. *J. Immunol. Meth.* **150**, 103–110.

Dudley, R. A., Edwards, P., Ekins, R. P. *et al.* (1985) Guidelines for immunoassay data processing. *Clin. Chem.* **31**, 1264–1271.

Ekins, R. P. & Newman, G. B. (1970) Theoretical aspects of saturation analysis. *Acta Endocrinol. (Kbh)* **147** (**suppl.**) 11–36.

Ekins, R. P. (1983) The precision profile: Its use in assay design, assessment and quality control. In: *Immunoassays in Clinical Medicine* (eds Hunter, W. M. & Corrie, J. E. T.) pp. 76–105 (Churchill-Livingstone, Edinburgh)

Ekins, R. P., Newman, G. B. & O'Riordan, J. L. H. (1968) In: *Radioisotopes in Medicine* (eds Hayes, R. L., Goswitz, F. A. & Murphy, B. E. P.) pp. 59–100, (US Atomic Energy Commission, Oak Ridge, Tennessee).

Feldman, H. & Rodbard, D. (1971) Mathematical theory of radioimmunoassay. In: *Competitive Protein Binding Assays* (eds Daughaday, W. H. & Odell, W. D.) pp. 158–203 (Lippincott, Philadelphia).

Gerlach, R. W., White, R. J., Deming, S. N. *et al.* (1993) An evaluation of five commercial immunoassay data analysis software systems. *Anal. Biochem.* **212**, 185–193.

Hales, C. N. & Randle, P. J. (1963) Immunoassay of insulin with insulin-antibody precipitate. *Biochem. J.* **88**, 137–146.

Hampel, F. R. (1974) The influence curve and its role in robust estimation. *J. Amer. Statist. Assoc.* **69**, 383–393.

Hawker, F. & Challand, G. S. (1981) Effects of outlying standard points on curve-fitting in radioimmunoassay. *Clin. Chem.* **27**, 14–17.

Healy, M. J. R. (1972) Statistical analysis of radioimmunoassay data. *Biochem. J.* **130**, 207–210.

Healy, M. J. R. (1979) Outliers in clinical chemistry and quality control schemes. *Clin. Chem.* **25**, 675–677.

Holownia, P., Bishop, E., Newman, D. J. et al. (1997) Adaptation and validation of a particle enhanced assay for percent glycated hemoglobin to a DuPont Dimension® analyser. *Clin. Chem.* **43**, 76–84.

Keilacker, H., Besch, W., Woltanski, K. P. et al. (1991) Mathematical modelling of competitive labelled-ligand assay systems. Theoretical re-evaluation of optimum assay conditions and precision data for some experimentally established systems. *Eur. J. Clin. Chem. Clin. Biochem.* **29**, 555–563.

Malan, P. G., Cox, M. G., Long, E. M. R. et al. (1978a). Curve-fitting to radioimmunoassay standard curves: spline and multiple binding site models. *Ann. Clin. Biochem.* **15**, 132–134.

Malan, P. G., Cox, M. G., Long, E. M. R. et al. (1978b). Development in curve-fitting procedures for radioimmunoassay using a multiple binding site model. In: *Computing in Clinical Laboratories* (ed. Siemaszko, F.) pp. 282–290 (Pitman Medical, Tunbridge Wells, UK).

Marschner, I., Erhardt, F. & Scriba, P. C. (1973) Calculation of the radioimmunoassay standard curve by spline function. In: *Radioimmunoassay and Related Procedures in Clinical Medicine and Research* pp. 111–112 (International Atomic Energy Agency, Vienna).

Medcalf, E. A., Newman, D. J., Gilboa, A., et al. (1990) A rapid and robust particle-enhanced turbidimetric immunoassay for serum β_2-microglobulin. *J. Immunol. Meth.* **129**, 97–103.

Nicol, R., Smith, P., & Raggatt, P. R. (1985) A robust microcomputer routine for the identification of outlying and influential points in radioimmunoassay standard curves. *Comput. Biomed. Res.* **18**, 334–346.

Nicol, R., Smith, P., & Raggatt, P. R. (1986) The use of the simplex method for the optimisation of non-linear functions on a laboratory microcomputer. *Comput. Biol. Med.* **16**, 145–152.

Normolle, D. P. (1993) An algorithm for robust non-linear analysis of radioimmunoassays and other bioassays. *Statist. in Med.* **12**, 2025–2042.

Raggatt, P. R. (1989) Duplicates or singletons? An analysis of the need for replication in immunoassay and a computer program to calculate the distribution of outliers and the precision profile from assay duplicates. *Ann. Clin. Biochem.* **26**, 26–37.

Reinsch, C. H. (1967) Smoothing by spline functions. *Numer. Math.* **10**, 177–183.

Reinsch, C. H. (1971) Smoothing by spline functions II. *Numer. Math.* **16**, 451–454.

Robison-Cox, J. F. (1995) Multiple estimation of concentrations in immunoassay using logistic models. *J. Immunol. Meth.* **186**, 79–88.

Rodbard, D. (1974) Statistical quality control and routine data processing for radioimmunoassay and immunometric assays. *Clin. Chem.* **20**, 1255–1270.

Rodbard, D. & Cooper, J. A. (1970) A model for the prediction of confidence limits in radioimmunoassay and competitive protein binding assays. In: In vitro *Procedures with Radioisotopes in Medicine* pp. 659–673 (International Atomic Energy Agency, Vienna).

Rodbard, D. & Lewald, J. E. (1970) Computer analysis of radioligand assay and radioimmunoassay data. *Acta Endocrinol. (Kbh)* **147** (**suppl.**), 79–103.

Rodbard, D., Rayford, P. L., Cooper, J. A. *et al.* (1968) Statistical quality control of radioimmunoassay. *J. Clin. Endocrinol.* **28,** 1412–1418.

Sadler, W. A. & Smith, M. H. (1990) Use and abuse of precision profiles: Some pitfalls illustrated by computing and plotting confidence intervals. *Clin. Chem.* **36,** 1346–1350.

Scand. J. Clin. Lab. Invest (1991) **205,** (**suppl.**), special issue.

Scatchard, G. (1949) The attractions of proteins for small proteins and molecules. *Ann. N.Y. Acad. Sci.* **51,** 660–672.

Thakkar, H., Newman, D.J., Holownia, P. *et al.* (1997) Development and validation of a Particle turbidimetric assay for urine albumin on the DuPont aca® analyser. *Clin. Chem.* **43,** 109–113.

Wegscheider. W. (1985). Use of cubic spline functions in solving calibration problems. In: *Trace Residue Analysis* American Chemical Society Symposium Series Vol. 284 (ed. Kurtz, D. A.) pp. 167–181 (American Chemical Society, Washington DC, USA).

Wilkins, T. A., Chadney, D. C., Bryant, J. *et al.* (1978a). Non-linear least-squares curve fitting of a simple theoretical model using a mini-computer. *Ann. Clin. Biochem.* **15,** 123–135.

Wilkins, T. A., Chadney, D. C., Bryant, J. *et al.* (1978b). Non-linear least-squares curve fitting of a simple statistical model to radioimmunoassay dose-response data using a mini-computer. *Radioimmunoassay and Related Procedures in Medicine* pp. 399–423 (International Atomic Energy Agency, Vienna)

World Association of Societies of Pathology (1979) Analytical goals in clinical chemistry: Their relationship to medical care. *Amer. J. Clin. Pathol.* **71,** 624–630.

Chapter 13

An Overview of Immunoassay Automation

Eileen G. Gorman, Rene Arentzen, William Bedzyk and Lee Anne Cassidy

INTRODUCTION

The Changing Context for Immunoassay Automation

Antibodies, whether they be polyclonal, monoclonal, digested fragments or one of several recombinant species, are by definition the cornerstones of immunoassays. Measurement of analytes which occur at very low concentrations in order to guide patient management, places stringent demands on our ability to monitor the antibody-analyte reaction. Other chapters describe in detail antibody production and assessment (Chapters 3 and 8), the current status and potential role of antibody engineering as applied to immunodiagnostic assays (Chapter 4), antibody-analyte reaction kinetics (Chapter 5), and the various detection methods (Chapters 14–20). In this chapter, therefore, we will briefly describe the technologies but will focus on the strategies involved in the engineering and integration of immunochemistry with automated instrument systems.

Since we last addressed the topic of immunoassay automation in 1993 (Gorman *et al.*, 1993), many automated immunoassay systems have come into wide use in the clinical laboratory. Several comprehensive reviews of the various systems have been published in the past 5 years (e.g. Truchaud *et al.*, 1991; Ng, 1991; Wild, 1994; Chan, 1992, 1996). In fact, *The Journal of Clinical Immunoassay* (1991) dedicated an entire issue to the subject. Recently, Wild (1994) published an impressive catalogue of immunoassay systems, describing many in detail and following on from a similar book by Chan (1992). Chan (1996) has updated his views in a useful new book on general laboratory automation. New systems that focus on work-station consolidation and laboratory productivity continue to be introduced. Because most of the published work focuses on the features related to components unique to heterogeneous immunoassays, notably the need for washing and separation, we have taken a different approach. We will address the aspects of system integration from the perspective of the location of the technology: in the reagent or in the instrumentation.

Because clinical chemists focus on the final result, many of the features and technologies required to produce a high-quality, reportable result are transparent to the laboratory worker and physician. Researchers in industry and academia still search for improved methods to perform homogeneous assays for analytes needing high assay sensitivity. This is because of the benefits of a solution-phase reaction, technology transportable to many instruments, reagent costs and production costs of unique reagent delivery systems. Assay performance in a fully integrated system, however, is influenced by the same factors for both heterogeneous and homogeneous systems: reactant metering, timing, temperature, reagent concentration and detection method. These issues will also be important to the new generation of technologies, which may eventually replace the immunoassay as the means for measuring low-concentration analytes. Furthermore, automation of sample processing prior to analysis is surfacing as a major factor for productivity (Godolphin *et al.*, 1990). Although this and compatible interfaces for automated systems are major future trends, they are beyond the scope of this chapter.

We will focus both on reagent and instrument characteristics, which interact and contribute to the overall accuracy of the result. System integration has become an overriding design issue. In addition, cost containment issues impinge on testing as well as instrument and reagent design, and will affect all future products being developed. The current trend is to adapt chemistry analysers to perform immunoassays to allow more routine analytes measured by immunoassay to become integrated into the routine laboratory. The consolidation of three instruments into the Abbott AxSym® (Smith *et al.*, 1995) system illustrates this trend.

The Quest for High Sensitivity at Low Cost

The laboratory environment in major geographical markets has changed considerably. Budgetary and medical outcome concerns in the United States, United Kingdom and Germany are all driving factors of cost containment. Although the laboratory is only a small contributor to the total cost of patient care, it is an easily identifiable unit which is often targeted for initial cost containment. In addition, the growing markets of Asia and India present different cost design, delivery and operating challenges for suppliers.

Because complex instrumentation is developed and introduced for laboratory use by companies keen to make profits, the economic climate influences system availability. Lower reimbursement rates demand lower costs for reportable results. This in turn drives the demand for lower reagent costs. As a result, the debate concerning cost containment for medical care over the past several years has influenced the technologies that have been introduced for clinical use. This in turn affects both laboratory and patient care. Accuracy, precision goals, medical relevance and improved distillation of the information available in treating the patient have been addressed (Hamilton *et al.*, 1991; Witte, 1993). The use of data, not its acquisition, has become an important issue (Altschulter, 1994). Increasingly, the debate is becoming centred on the balance between cost containment and improvement in medical outcome (Witte, 1995). One recurring theme throughout the debate is the need for systems to include links to the entire medical decision process and the required synthesis of information. This focus on cost containment is not unique to the US; massive changes in official health policies have also occurred in Germany (Müller, 1994).

There is still a strong desire for homogeneous assay technologies capable of detecting very low analyte levels. Although it is possible to design a system that can produce a digoxin result in less than 10 minutes using a heterogeneous assay mode, such assays are inherently more expensive than the homogeneous assay format. Heterogeneous assays require more reagents, thus increasing raw material and manufacturing costs and, most importantly, more complex instrumentation is required. These factors combine to increase the cost of a reportable result and ultimately may increase the cost of patient management. This is well illustrated by Danese and colleagues (1996) in a study of the cost effectiveness of detecting and treating subclinical hypothyroidism. They studied the cost of total patient management as related to the cost of thyroid stimulated hormone (thyrotrophin; TSH) testing. Screening adults is very sensitive to the cost of TSH testing because TSH assays are substantially more expensive than other comparable thyroid tests. However, there are important questions about the overall costs of the patient episode and the benefits of such screening. Despite the need for a more holistic approach, the goal of a less expensive means of producing results continues to drive research into homogeneous assay formats (Singh *et al.*, 1994) as illustrated by the recent development of luminescent oxygen channelling assay (LOCI™) by Ullman *et al.* (1996).

The elegant EMIT® technology pioneered by SYVA in the 1970s (Rubenstein *et al.*, 1972) continues to be applied to analytes present in nanomolar levels, such as cyclosporin (Schumann *et al.*, 1993) and digoxin (Knight *et al.*, 1995). Light-scattering assays, enhanced for improved sensitivity by the use of latex particles, gold sols and particle counting, are also widely applied (Bangs, 1990). These technologies represent a class of immunoassay designs adaptable to many automated spectrophotometers in use in the laboratory. Transportability of reagent technology to many instrument systems has led to the addition of analytes traditionally detected by immunoassays to many general chemistry analysers. Thyroxine and C-reactive protein (CRP) are two examples (Jaggon and Price, 1987; Price *et al.*, 1987). This has enabled work-station consolidation and faster turnaround for analytes processed in this way.

The design of an automated immunoassay system is a compilation of many different factors (such as instrument design, reagent design and antibody selection) integrated into a reliable, easy-to-use system. The major difference between an immunoassay and a routine chemistry assay is the use of an antibody-analyte reaction to detect and quantify an analyte of interest in a sample. The technologies surrounding that antibody-analyte reaction are important when designing an immunoassay system. The key differentiating factor for immunoassay systems lies with incorporation and investment in technology in two main areas: consumable supply and instrumentation.

In principle, it would be possible to develop a technology with one detection system using competitive and sandwich immunoassays to cover the analytical detection range. In fact, the use of anti-idiotypic antibodies for hapten analytes would eliminate the need for the competitive assay format (Barnard and Kohen, 1990). Over the past three decades, many different technologies have been developed. The enormous cost of developing totally new technologies and the movement to work-station consolidation have resulted in instrument systems capable of handling several technologies.

Researchers and users often lose sight of the fact that direct assay systems, those used for enzyme detection, provide very sensitive analytical measurements. Figure 1 illustrates this in an immunoassay sensitivity continuum showing the molar concentration of analyte detected by technology. For comparison, note the molar concentration of enzymes routinely measured, such as lipase and amylase. These analytes require approximately the same analytical detection capability usually associated with analytes currently requiring high-sensitivity immunoassays.

System automation requires the engineering of reagents and hardware. This integration provides convenience of use but introduces design constraints. In general, the design of an analytical system distributes the technology between the reagent design and the instrument design because the system includes both chemistry and instrument components required to produce a reportable result. If the advanced technology is mainly in the supplied reagent, the reproducibility must be built into the assay components during manufacturing. If the technology is concentrated in reagent processing on the instrument system, instrument performance will be the key to test result imprecision and overall quality. In addition, instrument system maintenance, whether performed automatically or by the operator, becomes a more crucial part of the reliability of the produced result.

The best approach to the *de novo* design of an automated immunoassay analyser involves selection of the assay technology first, followed by instrument design, the interrelationship between the two reflecting a high level of integration between reagent and instrument. An early example was the development of flourescence polarisation immunoassay (FPIA) technology followed by the development of the TD_x. More recently there has been the introduction of the Boehringer Mannheim Diagnostics Elecsys immunoassay system where the original electro-chemiluminescent detection work was pioneered by Bard and co-workers (Faulkner, 1977) in the 1970s. The application of this work to a commercial system by Blackburn *et al.* (1991) and subsequently by Boehringer Mannheim is a relatively recent event (Hoyle *et al.*, 1996). It illustrates the time and expense needed for translation from invention to routine use in the clinical laboratory. Thus, the system is based on requirements imposed by the assay format(s), whether homogeneous and/or heterogeneous, while also providing the optimal signal detection system(s). Although design from the ground up would theoretically be preferred, implementing immunoassays on an existing clinical analyser, with existing compo-

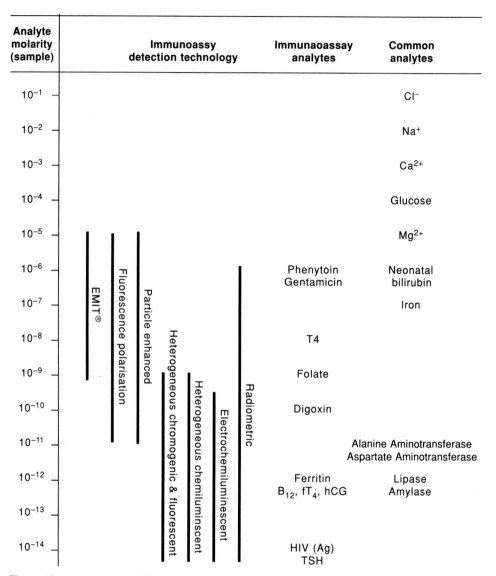

Figure 1 Immunoassay sensitivity continuum.

nents, poses a completely different set of problems. With an increasing move to work-station consolidation, manufacturers have taken the route of adapting technologies to existing instruments or to early instrument introduction followed by more sophisticated integration in a later version of the instrument family.

The addition of homogeneous immunoassays based on particle enhanced turbidimetric inhibition immunoassay (PETINIA), CEDIA® EMIT® or similar technologies to analysers running only colorimetric and enzyme-mediated chemistries is, in general, only limited by the reagent delivery capability and detection method existing on the system. Contrarily, addition of heterogeneous immunoassays to such analysers requires addition of a separation system. A digoxin immunoassay using magnetic particles, involving no sample pretreatment, was re-

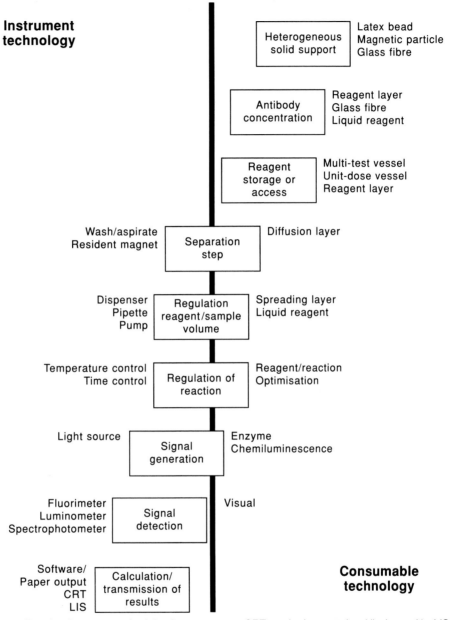

Figure 2 Functional steps required for immunoassay. CRT, cathode ray tube (display unit), LIS, laboratory information system.

cently introduced for the Dimension® clinical chemistry system (Dade International) (Stille *et al.*, 1995), the first heterogeneous assay to be implemented on a system previously capable of running only general chemistries and homogeneous immunoassays. The reagents are configured to be handled by the instrument fluidics (magnetic particle slurry), in conjunction with a relatively simple modification to the instrument (i.e. the addition of a magnet for separation).

305

Figure 2 illustrates the functional steps required for immunoassays. A particular design will place technology at different phases of an assay and not all steps are required by all assay designs. For example, homogeneous assays do not require a solid support. Representative examples of technologies used for each step in assay processing are also given. Nevertheless, production of accurate, reliable, comprehensive reagent systems (e.g. incorporating antibody, means of separation and several different reagents into a single unit consumable) requires considerable manufacturing expertise. In contrast, a highly integrated reagent design relies on the instrument to deliver the required components accurately and precisely to reach an equal level of performance.

THE CONSUMABLE

Definition

The term consumable, used in the context of clinical chemistry systems, refers to that part of the system that is disposed of after use. This includes a unit-dose consumable and a unit, such as a cup or tab, which holds enough reagents to run a single test for a specific analyte. Consumable also refers to bulk reagents, packaged in a multi-test format, which reside on the analyser for testing a specific analyte, several analytes, or all analytes. This section is particularly concerned with the technology associated with consumables needed for immunoassays.

High Complexity in the Consumable

The most basic form of an immunoassay consumable is demonstrated by common over-the-counter pregnancy tests. These products are ready for use by an untrained, but highly motivated operator, and are a totally comprehensive immunoassay system incorporating sample regulation, all reagents, visible detection and quality assurance into a single consumable which needs no ancillary instrumentation (*see* Chapters 22 and 23). Many analytes measured by immunoassays, however, require more than a qualitative answer and occur at much lower concentrations in blood than human chorionic gonadotrophin (hCG), the hormone detected in over-the-counter pregnancy tests.

Immunoassay systems incorporate varying components of the required elements (e.g. antibody, support, reagents and detection) into the consumable. A highly comprehensive consumable design may incorporate all of these elements and therefore require a simple, yet specific, instrument design. In contrast, systems that use a very basic consumable design are typically dependent on a precise, intricate instrument to deliver the required elements for the immunoassay system.

In general, unit-dose, high-complexity consumables are easy to use, require simple (or no) on-board inventory management, no preparation and are easy to dispose of. The Hybritech ICON® format and Johnson and Johnson Surecell®, for example, require no automation and are at one end of the spectrum. However, the Hybritech ICON QSR® uses a battery-powered reflectance meter to provide a quantitative result (Payne *et al.*, 1994). Bulk reagents, on the other hand, often require reagent metering, off-line and/or on-board refrigeration and possibly reconstitution prior to use. This processing may occur automatically or may be done by the operator prior to use on the instrument.

With a single-use consumable, such as the Dade International aca® discrete clinical analyser test pack or the Behring Opus® (Crowley and Bauduin, 1994) test system, little can be done to improve the reagent performance, mixing, dispersion, etc., as this is all controlled during the manufacturing process. Problems associated with the performance of a single method are often associated with the consumable lot as opposed to the system and are, therefore, the responsibility of the manufacturer.

A unit-dose consumable also allows for greater flexibility in method design. A method design with predetermined instrument parameters is subject to many more system restrictions compared to one that can attempt to incorporate any type of reagent needed for the method into the consumable. The size of the analyser, the number of on-line reagents and the stability of the assay reagents all come into play when designing the reagent/consumable system.

However, the physical design of the consumable can pose some obstacles in method design. Some reagents may be more stable in multi-test or bulk liquid form and may require a higher degree of accuracy from the complementary instrument to perform optimally. Furthermore, the use of dry reagents (tablets, powders, cakes) requires complex and expensive manufacturing processes.

Manufacturers and operators must also consider the costs and liabilities associated with designing, manufacturing and using highly complex consumables. Obviously, the greater the number of system functions incorporated into the consumable, the more difficult the manufacturing process of that unit and the higher the cost. However, there are also potential savings in skilled operator costs albeit with a reduction in the level of expertise in the work force. In effect this reflects a transfer of responsibility from operator to manufacturer.

HOMOGENEOUS IMMUNOASSAYS

Assays that do not require a separation step are known as homogeneous immunoassays. These assays use turbidimetric, colorimetric, fluorometric and luminescent detection schemes and, in some cases, can be adapted to many analysers. For example, turbidimetric and colorimetric assays may be adapted to any instrument possessing a spectrophotometer; however, adapting a fluorescent or luminescent assay to the same instrument would require addition of a new detector technology.

Light scattering, in the form of turbidimetric or nephelometric detection, has been used to detect immunoglobulins and other serum proteins. In addition, the use of latex particles and gold sol to amplify the signal has extended this technology to hapten analytes. Bangs (1990) and others have discussed the adaptation of latex particle assays to many systems including the Dade International, Beckman and Bayer/Technicon systems (*see* also Chapter 18).

Reagents used in homogeneous immunoassays, such as the Microgenics CEDIA® (cloned enzyme donor immunoassay) (Coty *et al.*, 1992) reagents, may be packaged in a multi-test format as opposed to unit-dose. This methodology can be considered as an example of low-level integration between consumable and instrument technology, because the technology can easily be adapted to many different instrument systems. Because the technology is designed into the reagents, CEDIA® assays can, in principle, be run on any analyser which can accurately dispense 2–4 reagents and possesses a spectrophotometer. In fact, the Microgenics CE-DIA® reagent kits have been adapted to over 20 different clinical chemistry systems and have allowed laboratories to run immunoassays on routine chemistry analysers.

The SYVA/Behring EMIT® (enzyme multiplied immunoassay technique) technology (Rubenstein *et al.*, 1972) follows a similar principle for measuring low molecular mass compounds such as drugs. Again, the inclusion of all assay components required allows the EMIT® technology to be used in multi-test reagent kits. EMIT® reagents in multi-test units are used both on high-volume and unit-dose analyser systems.

Similarly, fluorescence detection can be used in homogeneous assay formats, e.g. fluorescence polarisation immunoassay (FPIA) (*see* Chapter 16). Fluorometric immunoassays are identical in principle and design to colorimetric assays except that a fluorometer, as opposed to a spectrophotometer, is required for signal detection. Adapting fluorometric assays to existing colorimetric-only systems, therefore, will be subject to severe hardware constraints.

HETEROGENEOUS IMMUNOASSAYS

The Solid Support

Automation of the separation step in a heterogeneous immunoassay has been one of the predominant difficulties that have been overcome in the past few years. Heterogeneous immunoassays require antibody, analyte or analyte analogue to be attached to a solid support. The solid support acts as an anchor for the capture reagent in the steps required for a heterogeneous immunoassay: specific binding, washing to remove unwanted components, analyte concentration and, sometimes, development of the signal to be measured. In most systems, the analyte-specific solid phase is part of the consumable (*see* also Chapter 8).

Solid support selection is influenced by the available technology and overall system design. Incorporation of antibody into the consumable results in less dependence on the instrument itself for method performance. Characteristics of the solid support include low adhesion to nonspecific proteins, strong binding of specific capture reagents, maintenance of support structure and properties during wash steps, large surface area and good washing properties.

Various solid supports are used in immunoassay systems today. These include, glass or plastic tubes (ES300, Boehringer Mannheim Corporation), plastic microtitre wells (Amerlite® and Vitros™ Immunodiagnostic system, Johnson and Johnson Clinical Diagnostics), solid glass-fibre matrix (Stratus® Systems, Dade International), polystyrene or latex beads of various diameters (IMMULITE® immunoassay system, Diagnostic Products Inc.) and magnetic particles (ACS 180® Chiron/Ciba Corning; ACCESS® Immunoassay System, Sanofi; AIA® 600 and AIA® 1200, Tosoh Medics Inc.). Just as the choice of detection chemistry dictates certain instrument requirements, so does the choice of solid support material. For example, solid support magnetic particles impose the need for a magnet for separation and wash steps.

Sensitivity Of Automated Heterogeneous Assays

Overall sensitivity of an immunoassay system is dependent on several factors including the method used to detect the antibody-analyte binding event, the signal-to-noise ratio, the concentration of antibody and the antibody binding constant. Ekins and Chu (1991) discuss this topic in detail, providing a good summary and historical perspective (*see* also Chapter 9). It is now generally accepted that the greater the solid support surface area available for the antibody-analyte reaction to occur and the greater the rate of this reaction, the more sensitive the assay. Solid surface supports such as glass tubes, $\frac{1}{4}$-inch polystyrene beads or microtitre plates generally have low surface area, which limits the amount of antibody immobilised, and thus leads to relatively low analyte capture.

In addition, antibody immobilisation onto solid supports often leads to inactivation of a relatively large percentage of the analyte-binding sites. Two major technologies, both resulting in random attachment, are currently used to couple antibody molecules onto solid supports; passive adsorption and chemical fixation. In order to increase the number of antibody active sites available to react with analyte, the design must decrease the amount of binding site inactivation due to the coupling reaction and/or increase the solid support surface area. To address the first point, some systems use 'universal' particles (e.g. avidin-coupled particles) to help orient the antibody binding sites. Another method to orient antibody binding sites uses covalent coupling to the solid support through carbohydrate moieties found in the antibody Fc region (Evans *et al.*, 1991; Zara *et al.*, 1995). Theoretically, this is one application where genetically engineered antibody molecules could be used in immunoassay systems; however, nothing has yet been commercialised.

Increasing the solid support surface area has been, to date, the approach used to increase the number of antibody active sites available to react with analyte. Thus, reducing the size of the solid support, usually in the form of microparticles, increases the analyte capture rate and theoretically increases the immunoassay sensitivity. Once again, however, the larger the total surface area, the greater the chance of nonspecific binding and a decrease in the signal-to-noise ratio. Use of solid support systems, such as free-floating, microsized particles (colloidal suspensions), not only expands the surface area but allows for faster kinetics (approaching diffusion-controlled reactions). For example, antibody-bound magnetic or paramagnetic particles act as the solid phase and provide both high surface area and easy dispersion for subsequent reaction and wash steps. These particles can also be treated as a liquid for purposes of transport by the instrument fluidics. In the recently introduced Elecsys system (Boehringer Mannheim Corporation), magnetic particles are used both to concentrate the captured analyte at the electrode surface and to perform a separation step in the reaction vessel. Once the analyte is concentrated at the electrode surface, the luminescent signal is generated by application of a current across the reaction cell. This approach eliminates the need for transport of the captured analyte to another instrument location prior to development of a signal which is then translated to analyte concentration.

Most immunoassay systems use standard competitive binding or sandwich assay formats to detect the analyte in a sample. After incubating the antibody-bound particles with analyte, the particles can easily be separated in the reaction vessel such that the unbound analyte in solution can be aspirated to waste. The particle/analyte complex is then resuspended for a wash or second incubation. Because of their relatively small size, magnetic particles can be incorporated into cost-effective, multi-test reagent containers for high-volume analytes. Examples of systems that use magnetic particles include ACS 180® (Chiron/Ciba-Corning), ACCESS® immunoassay system (Sanofi), AIA®-600 and AIA®-1200 (Tosoh), VISTA® Immunoassay System (Behring/SYVA), AuraFlex™ immunoassay system (Anagen) and Elecsys (Boehringer Mannheim Corporation).

Magnetic supports can range in size from microscopic particles (100 nm–20 μm) to 1.5-mm beads. Again, the smaller the particles, the higher the surface area and the greater the ease of wash and resuspension phases. The particles are made of chromium dioxide or iron oxides such as magnetite or ferrite, and, in the case of the Tosoh AIA beads, polymer beads coated with ferrite (Loebel, 1994).

Suspensions of relatively large (10–20 μm) magnetic particles settle under gravity and typically require agitation for binding reactions. Likewise, automation of particle-based immunoassays may be complicated by the compatibility of the solid support with microanalytical devices that could clog when large beads are used. A recent development in biomagnetic separations are the ferrofluids (Immunicon Corporation) which are dense colloidal dispersions of magnetic particles in the nanometre size range (DePalma, 1995). Binding kinetics are diffusion-controlled because these small (80–120 nm) ferrofluidic particles behave essentially like fluids. Thus, ferrofluids can be handled as liquids, offering surface areas significantly greater than those of relatively large magnetic particles. More surface area per volume also enables smaller reaction volumes. The potential benefits of low reaction volumes include higher assay sensitivity and better precision due to a higher signal-to-noise ratio. Lower reagent cost should also be possible.

The magnetic field strength needed to separate magnetic particles from the reagents will dictate the specific requirements of the analyser's resident magnet. In the competitive binding format of the ACCESS® immunoassay system (Sanofi), for example, sample (analyte) is incubated with antibody-tagged magnetic particles and analyte and alkaline phosphatase conjugate. Following an appropriate incubation period, the antibody-tagged magnetic particles and the labelled and unlabelled analyte are moved to a wash carousel. Each vessel then goes through a series of wash steps in which a resident magnet pulls the magnetic particles with bound analyte to one side while the unbound fraction is aspirated to waste. Particles are then resuspended in buffer solution and substrate is added to the antibody-bound fraction of the analyte. The resulting luminescence, measured by a sensitive photomultiplier, is inversely proportional to the analyte concentration in the sample (Alpert, 1994).

Reagent Consumable

As previously discussed, heterogeneous immunoassay systems incorporate the antibody into the consumable, usually attached to a solid support. Other reagents required to perform the assay are in the form of a liquid, tablet, freeze-dried powder or thin-film layer either in a multitest or unit-dose format. Systems that incorporate the required reagents into a unit-dose consumable typically require a less sophisticated instrument design and more sophisticated reagent manufacturing capabilities. DuPont pioneered this approach with the aca® discrete clinical analyser (Caffo, 1993). Ready-to-use analytical test packs, with accurately metered reagents, are processed by the automated spectrophotometer.

The unique design of the OPUS® immunoassay analyser (Behring Diagnostics) incorporates the required buffers and reagents into a unit-dose, multilayer film reaction vessel (Loebel, 1991). The OPUS® consumable is one of the best commercial examples of a highly integrated consumable. Behring Diagnostics employs a multilayered design that does many of the basic steps required of an immunoassay system. The consumable tab is the reagent delivery device, incorporating a spreading layer to distribute the sample evenly, all necessary reagents, the solid antibody support, the separation technology (similar to washing) and reagents required to generate the signal.

The OPUS® multilayer film module is used to detect small molecular mass compounds. During the assay, a 10 μl sample containing the analyte of interest is dispensed onto the module and a spreader layer evenly distributes the sample onto the film's surface. The sample comes into contact with a blocking layer that releases the analyte from any binding proteins and retains all large molecules on the surface. The analyte then passes through an optical screen to the signal layer where it competes with fluorescent-labelled antigen for antibody-binding sites. Any unbound analyte diffuses out of the signal layer through the optical screen, whereas bound antigen remains in the signal layer. The bound analyte is excited by a halogen lamp. The emitted light or amount of fluorescence generated is inversely proportional to the sample analyte concentration (Loebel, 1991; Crowley and Bauduin, 1994).

The AIA® 600 and AIA®-1200 (Tosoh) systems incorporate an alkaline phosphatase conjugate in a unit-dose reagent cup in freeze-dried form; on-board bulk diluent is added to hydrate the reagent and bound enzyme is detected using a fluorescent substrate (Lehrer *et al.*, 1992). The IMMULITE® immunoassay system (Diagnostic Products Corp.) also uses a single test reagent format for the capture antibody while providing a novel means of separating free from bound label (Babson, 1991).

In several other systems, the reagents are packaged in multi-test formats designed to work on batch or random-access instruments. Although still assay-specific, the performance of the assay is now somewhat dependent on the instrument design and its ability to deliver accurate amounts of reagent. Examples of heterogeneous immunoassay systems using reagents in multi-test format include the ACCESS® immunoassay system (Sanofi), the ACS:180® (Chiron/Ciba-Corning), ImX® and AxSym® systems (Abbott) and Stratus® (Dade International).

DETECTION CHEMISTRY

A key aspect of any immunoassay system performance is the detection chemistry (how the reagents translate the antibody-analyte reaction into an easily measured signal). During the past few years, extensive research efforts have been directed to better detection techniques. A recent Oak Ridge Conference (1995) highlighted some efforts dedicated to this critical role in immunoassay systems. This part of the immunoassay system is dependent on the capabilities of both the reagents and the instrument. Current technologies used to detect immunoassay reactions include colorimetric, turbidimetric, fluorescent, luminescent(chemi- and bio-), as well as electrochemical (mostly amperometric) and optical immunosensor methods (Glazier and McCurley, 1995).

Colorimetric detection is based on the measurement of colour formation resulting from an enzyme-substrate reaction and is used in both heterogeneous and homogeneous assays . An example of a heterogeneous format is the Boehringer Mannheim ES 300 analyser which uses both competitive and sandwich assay formats. In the competitive format, antibody- or streptavidin-coated tubes are used as the solid phase. Sample (analyte) and enzyme-labelled analyte are incubated in the coated tube until apparent equilibrium is reached. After a wash step, unbound analyte (labelled and unlabelled) is aspirated to waste and a substrate solution is added to initiate colour development. Following incubation, the final solution is aspirated into a quartz flow-through cuvette for absorbance measurement (Duncan *et al.*, 1991).

Colorimetric applications of homogeneous assay formats have been described above in the overviews of the CEDIA® (Boehringer Mannheim Corporation) and EMIT® (Behring/SYVA) technologies.

Another detection method, fluorescence, can be used in either heterogeneous or homogeneous assay formats (e.g. FPIA). A basic heterogeneous fluorometric assay follows the same principles as a colorimetric assay except for the substrate used. A common substrate in fluorometric enzyme immunoassays is 4-methylumbelliferyl phosphate (4-MUP) in conjunction with alkaline phosphatase as the enzyme label. A fluorometer, as opposed to a spectrophotometer, is required for signal detection. The need for a fluorometer in place of a spectrophotometer is obvious, though other instrument functions may also be affected. Use of time-resolved fluorescence, for example, would require additional incubation time (and possibly space) prior to signal measurement plus a pulsed light source..

Bioluminescent, chemiluminescent and electrochemiluminescent signal generation methods are characterised by luminescent compounds emitting light during the course of a biochemical, chemical or electrochemical reaction. Properties inherent to the luminescent reactions make them well suited for immunoassay detection because of the extremely low light intensity that can be detected. Kricka (1991) reviewed these detection systems. Weeks addresses luminescence immunoassays in this volume (Chapter 17). For even more information on luminescence, including use in immunoassay detection systems, the reader is referred to Campbell *et al.*, 1994.

The kinetics of the light-emitting system chosen has implications for automation. In the flash-type chemistries, the light is emitted within seconds of initiating the reaction. The reaction vessel must therefore be in place for detection when the flash occurs. In the glow-type chemistries, with light-intensity measurements made from minutes to hours after initiation of the reaction, the reaction must be held for detection at a later time. Reaction detection, therefore, can be separated in time from the immediate binding reaction. As a result, instrumentation can be designed to process the detection at a time after the capture or binding event. This may provide for sample processing and then transfer to a different station for detection. The flash-emitting systems require that the reaction takes place in the detection module. Neither has been demonstrated to be clearly superior; however, hardware design will be affected by the choice of the light-generating system.

Signal detection in each case incorporates a high-sensitivity photomultiplier, free of interfering light, on the particular analyser. In enhanced reactions, the signal is improved by adding other chemicals to increase the signal intensity or duration. Greater assay sensitivity and low background noise have made heterogeneous assays using chemiluminescent detection (such as the Chiron/Ciba-Corning ACS180®) popular. In contrast, bioluminescent and electrochemiluminescent assays are more recent developments.

Claims are being made for femtomolar sensitivity for electrochemiluminescent labels that can be coupled to low and high molecular mass analytes (Blackburn *et al.*, 1991; Hoyle *et al.*, 1996). If this can be accomplished in routine use, this technology will challenge conventional sandwich immunoassays.

CONSUMABLE REVIEW

Table 1 reviews several important system characteristics for immunoassay analysers. Most of the systems profiled were introduced within the past five years and represent the most contemporary system designs currently on the market.

High Complexity in the Instrument

In contrast to immunoassays using single-use highly complex consumables on relatively simple instruments, assays using multiple-test or bulk consumables require more complex instrumentation. Such instruments need to be capable of storing reagents under appropriate conditions, usually refrigerated, without any effect on reagent integrity (degradation, contamination, or change in concentration). In addition, reagents typically need to be dispensed with high accuracy and precision.

	Assay format	Detection chemistry	Consumable support	Consumable reagents	random access	Reagent stability	Sample (in μl)	TTFR (min)	Throughput (tests per h)	Min. cal. Stability (points)
Abbot AxSYM®	Heterogeneous	Fluorescent MEIA	Glass fibre	Unit-dose	Yes	112 h on-board	100–150	8–30	75–120	30 days (2†)
Anagen Auraflex™	Heterogeneous	Fluorescent EIA	Magnetic particle	Unit-dose*	Yes	90 days on-board	5–75	17–65	Up to 72	30 days (2†)
Bayer Immuno-1®	Homo-heterogeneous	Latex agglutination EIA	Magnetic particle	Multitest	Yes	60 days on-board	2–65	7–35	Up to 120	30 days (6)
Behring OPUS®	Heterogeneous	Fluorescent EIA	Multilayer film	Unit-dose	Yes	7 days on-board	10	6–27	80	2–6 weeks (6)
BMD Elecsys®	Heterogeneous	Electrochemical	Paramagnetic particle	Multitest	Yes	6 weeks on-board	15–50	9–18	100–120	6 weeks (2)
Chiron/CCD ACS®: 180	Heterogeneous	Chemiluminescence	Magnetic particle	Multitest	Yes	40 h on-board	10–200	15	180	1–2 weeks (2†)
Dade International aca® PLUS	Heterogeneous	EIA	Magnetic particle	Unit-dose	Yes	6–12 months off-line only	100–300	25	30	60–90 days (3–5)
Dade Dimension® RxL Heterogeneous Module‡	Heterogeneous	Cascade EIA	Magnetic particle	Multitest	Yes	30 days On-line	30–150	15	168	30–60 days (3–6)
Dade Stratus® II	Heterogeneous	Fluorescent EIA	Glass fibre	Unit-dose*	No	1–2 months off-line only	200	8–10	70	2 weeks (6)
DPC Immulite®	Heterogeneous	Chemiluminescent EIA	Latex bead	Unit-dose*	Yes	30 days on-board	5–75	45–75	120	2 weeks (2†)
J&J VITROS System‡	Heterogeneous	Chemiluminescent	Coated well	Multitest	Yes	2 months on-board	10–80	40?	80–100	28 days (1–3)
Sanofi Access®	Heterogeneous	Chemiluminescent EIA	Magnetic particle	Multitest	Yes	30 days on-board	10–100	20–55	50–100	28 days (6)
Syva 30-R™	Homogeneous	EMIT®	None	Multitest	Yes	Up to 2 months	2–20	10	314	Up to 4 weeks (1–6)
Tosoh AIA-600® (1200)	Heterogeneous	Fluorescence EIA	Magnetic particle	Unit-dose*	Yes	24 h on-board	10–100	50–62	60 (120)	30 days (2–6)

* Generic system reagents (wash, buffers, etc.) are also used.
† Two-point calibration adjustment based on a full factory-generated curve stored in the system.
‡ J&J VITROS Immunodiagnostic System and Dade Dimension® RxL subject to FDA approval at time of publication.
TTFR = Time to First Result.
Min. Cal = Minimum calibrations stability, the minimum length of time that a method will maintain a calibration curve. This is usually a manufacturer's claim.

Table 1 Summary of the system characteristics for immunoassay analysers.

On the majority of automated analysers, reagents are dispensed as liquid solutions or suspensions. Not all reagents used in immunoassays, however, can be stored as a solution or suspension for an extended length of time because of reagent instability, even when refrigerated. Thus, some type of preparation may be required depending on the form of the reagent(s). Usually the addition of water to a freeze-dried solid, powder or tablet(s) is all that is needed. In some cases, mixing is required to guarantee complete dissolution of the solid material and produce a homogeneous solution. On fully automated random-access instruments, this may be accomplished by mechanical stirring, ultrasonic mixing, or mixing by pumping or pipetting and dispensing. Although this latter approach appears attractive from an instrument manufacturing viewpoint because of its relatively low cost and complexity, it puts high demands not only on instrument design and performance, but also on method development.

From a system perspective, immunoassay automation involves the total package of hardware, software and assay chemistry. The underlying assay technology determines the need for the hardware components and the software control of those components. It dictates the number of reagents necessary for each test and may also impose constraints on how these reagents can be combined and stored in a multiple-test consumable. Depending on the flexibility of the instrument design, the assay chemistry used in a nonautomated environment may have to be reoptimised to match instrument resource availability in order to maximise throughput. Total design goals may require suboptimal conditions for some parameters. It is important to know and understand the sensitivities of the assays to, among other factors, reagent storage, assay temperature, analyte configuration, reagent evaporation or dilution, reagent delivery, sample delivery and mixing characteristics. Multiphasic cooptimisation of components and performance, with final system performance the goal, has been applied to this process (Krouwer *et al.*, 1988). Because total system integration and performance become paramount, it may not be possible to operate at the optimum for each parameter. For example, compromises may be made in timing of specific events to improve system throughput (Aarts *et al.*, 1995).

Reagent Storage

Reagents must be stored during manufacturing, shipping, in the laboratory prior to use and in some cases, once opened, on-board the instrument. Factors affecting the quality of the stored reagent include container design, temperature and stability when sealed, after opening and, if required, during preparation. Storage on and off the instrument is also important.

Variation in reagent concentration and integrity depends largely on the multiple-test consumable design and on how reagents are stored and dispensed. Evaporation from open storage containers, dilution by condensation, or carryover of liquids, including water, by pipetting are some of the most frequently encountered problems. Any change in reagent concentration is critical when, for example, a small change in the concentration of an antibody-enzyme conjugate reagent leads to a large shift in assay result. In this case, method robustness might be improved by dilution of the antibody-conjugate reagent. If this significantly reduces reagent stability in a multiple-test consumable, expiration time for this reagent should be reduced; alternatively, multiple smaller reagent quantities can be prepared.

The use of enzyme cascades for signal amplification (Obzansky *et al.*, 1991) requires extremely accurate delivery of the enzyme reagents. Some enzymes cannot be combined in one reagent for reasons of storage and/or incompatibility. This is especially true when the signal gain for each enzyme reagent in the cascade is large and strongly affected by small variations in the delivery volume. Thus, accuracy of reagent delivery can have a greater than expected impact on the ultimate assay signal.

ASSAY TEMPERATURE

Variation in assay temperature can be one cause of poor method precision. Although the effect of temperature on enzyme kinetics and antibody-analyte binding is generally understood, the potential impact on certain physical parameters of molecules, such as the molar extinction coefficient, is less well recognised. Variation of assay temperature by 0.5 °C may produce an effect on the kinetics of most enzyme or antibody-analyte binding reactions. The absorbance of reporter molecules, however, can also be affected, resulting in poor imprecision (Southwell *et al.*, 1994).

Although assay temperature under dynamic conditions can typically be maintained at ± 0.2 °C or better on modern automated analysers, researchers should be aware of the time it takes to reach the steady-state temperature. Not only does this depend on the temperature desired, but also on the reagent temperature at reaction initiation. Refrigerated components will require time to reach thermal equilibrium. In addition, the time required to reach the steady-state temperature may not be the same for different assays on the same instrument because of varying temperature coefficients of antibodies, different reagent volumes, and varying reaction times.

CONCENTRATION OF REACTION COMPONENTS

Most consumable containers are designed to prevent reagent evaporation during shipment and storage. However, once the reaction vessel on board the system is open to that environment, many new sources of variability can significantly affect precision (e.g. total reaction volume, method used to control temperature, and variation in the assay components concentration due to evaporation or condensation). For instance, the evaporation from an open container is strongly enhanced when temperature control is accomplished by forced air circulation rather than a water bath with near-stagnant air over the container. The evaporation rate increases with the displacement rate of air over the container (Holman, 1981). In addition, the smaller the reaction volume and the longer the reaction time, the greater the potential for evaporation and the effect on precision, which can reduce some of the potential advantages of small reaction volumes on assay kinetics. Some instrument systems use lids to minimise evaporation from reagent containers. For example, the Chiron/Ciba-Corning ACS:180® system includes disposable, slotted reagent covers.

Although the impact of evaporation can be limited by instrument and assay design, environmental factors affecting evaporation, such as room temperature and relative humidity, are typically less well controlled.

SINGLE OR MULTIPLE-USE REACTION VESSELS

The choice between disposable and reusable reaction vessels must be carefully balanced, not only in terms of direct consumable cost but, more importantly, from the perspective of instrument design and potential impact on assay performance. Nonspecific binding to the vessel surface and ease of cleaning will affect the design and choice of materials for reusable vessels. Fully automated analysers using reusable reaction containers need to have on-board wash, rinse and dry stations. This requires the instrument to be connected to a local water supply line to meet the high volume of water required. Furthermore, the waste generated has to be treated as a biohazard requiring special disposal provisions. In addition, heterogeneous immunoassays may complicate the cleaning process because of their use of a solid phase.

In contrast, single-use reaction containers, although treated as biohazard waste, may eliminate the need for plumbing and generate much less liquid waste. On-board production of disposable reaction vessels requires additional instrument functionality. Creation of the reaction vessel on-board eliminates the need to reload premanufactured consumables, allowing longer instrument run-time between operator interventions.

Finally, if an assay result is measured optically and directly in the reaction vessel, strict quality control of the disposable container, whether single- or multiple-use and produced on- or off-line, is essential for system performance. This can be accomplished on-line by establishing an optical baseline.

REAGENT DELIVERY

Accuracy and precision of reagent delivery is critical to the accuracy and precision of the assay. Few immunoassays can be designed such that accuracy and precision are robust with regard to under- and over delivery of all assay components. The greater the number of reagent deliveries to the reaction vessel, the higher the potential impact on precision. Hardware used for fluid delivery is dictated by the volumes required by the assays and is independent of the assay methodology. For example, sample volumes ranging from 10 to 50 µl should not be handled by a delivery system designed for accuracy and precision in the 100–1,000 µl range. Generally, better precision is attained when the syringe or pipetting system covers a narrow volume range. Delivery systems should be capable of delivering homogeneous solutions with varying viscosities as well as heterogeneous suspensions. Tubing lengths and the number of valves and couplings must be kept small to minimise the time and volume required for flushing between deliveries. This will improve overall throughput and reduce the chance of cross-contamination.

Pipetting systems may allow the use of disposable pipette tips (e.g. Behring Opus®) (Loebel, 1991). This can prevent cross-contamination and may provide greater accuracy and precision of reagent delivery. However, drawbacks include increased cost per test, increased solid waste and increased system complexity. The possibility of using the pipette tip as a probe for ultrasonic mixing is also eliminated. Conversely, a semi-permanent reagent probe tip requires an effective wash and/or rinse procedure between reagent deliveries. This can usually be combined with flushing of the delivery system.

Carryover

Most users are aware of the potential for sample carryover on an automated system. This, however, is only one source of carryover-related inaccuracy. In the following discussion, carryover is defined as the effect of one assay on another whether the same method or not.

Reagent aspiration from a multiple-test consumable can result in undesired reagent carryover on the outside of the probe. This volume varies with the nature, temperature and viscosity of the reagent, the design and material of the probe and the distance below the surface at which reagent aspiration occurs. If an assay is highly sensitive to small volume variations of a particular reagent, provision has to be made to eliminate carryover. Wiping or washing the external probe surface has been applied. In fact, lids on reagent vessels are often designed to prevent changes in concentration by evaporation, but also to wipe the probe as it is inserted into and withdrawn from the vessel. For example, the Sanofi ACCESS® uses a unique lid-stock material which serves as an evaporation barrier and a probe wipe.

Carryover of one reagent into another can be caused by multiple reagent aspiration from the consumable without intermediate wiping or washing of the external probe surface. Stacked reagent aspiration, i.e. aspiration of more than one reagent prior to delivery to the reaction vessel, should be avoided if possible. If stacked reagent delivery is required by the integration of the assay design on a particular instrument, the potential for reagent cross-contamination increases. Such cross-contamination may cause or accelerate deterioration of the affected reagent and/or jeopardise assay performance. Multiple-test consumables are especially susceptible to this source of reagent instability.

Reagent carryover from one assay into another, whether an assay mixture or reagent component, can also result from inadequate delivery system flushing. This may occur particularly with high viscosity reagents and the resulting cross-contamination can lead to serious assay performance problems.

Water carryover into a reagent in a multiple-test consumable can occur because of water adhering to the external probe surface after flushing the delivery system. Water may also collect on the lid or sealing surface of the multiple-test consumable. This usually results from condensation formed on the sealing surface of the refrigerated reagent consumables stored in high relative humidity. As the probe travels through the lid, water may be carried into the reagents remaining in the consumable vessel, resulting in reagent dilution.

SAMPLE DELIVERY

With increasing work-station consolidation and market demands to minimise or eliminate sample processing before the sample is placed into the processing chamber, level sensing has become more important. A detailed discussion of the available technologies is beyond the scope of this chapter; however, absorbance, capacitance, resistance and frequency measurements have been described. Irrespective of the technology, designers must be aware of the potential for sample interference if components of the tube used to draw the specimen are added to the reaction chamber (e.g. serum separation gel).

Accuracy and precision are much more critical for sample than for reagent delivery because the assay results correlate directly with the sample volume, although reagent addition will be more critical for competitive versus noncompetitive assays. Because sample volumes are typically much smaller than reagent volumes, sample carryover of even very small volumes on the external probe surface can produce inaccurate results and significant imprecision. It is critical, therefore, that the design of the sample delivery system allows for the best possible imprecision as dictated by the imprecision of the hardware components. An efficient cleaning step, providing the greatest possible precision in sample volume delivery, has to be an integral part of sample aspiration from either primary tubes, sample cups or other containers.

MIXING OF ASSAY COMPONENTS

To guarantee homogeneous assay mixtures, whether solutions or suspensions, automated analysers use a mechanism to mix the assay components after reagent(s) and sample delivery. In simple one-reagent assays, mixing usually occurs after sample addition. Assays with multiple reagent deliveries or pre-incubations may require several mixing steps as time progresses. Because sample volume is typically a small fraction of the total assay volume, mixing after sample addition is a virtual necessity.

In an effort to adapt existing systems to process tests that have previously been performed in a heterogeneous mode, pretreatment or preprocessing may be required. The Abbott TD_x® FPIA system uses an operator-performed pretreatment to improve the digoxin assay sensitivity. The Dade International aca® PLUS system provides automation of the reaction incubation and washing to allow analytes requiring the sensitivity delivered by heterogeneous assays to be performed with the aca® system. In this case, the captured sandwich is added to the test pack for development of the colorimetric signal. Instrument geometry allows the detection of the signal in the presence of the chromium dioxide solid phase (Allard *et al.*, 1995).

Mixing of the assay reaction can be accomplished by mechanical stirring using a paddle, by pumping using a 'sip-and-spit' or with ultrasonic energy through cavitation. The latter two mixing actions can be carried out with either a standard fluid-handling system or a modified system in which the pipette tip or probe is attached to an ultrasonic horn. The inclusion of a device for mixing with a mechanical paddle stirrer also requires a method to clean the paddle.

Mixing can cause aerosol formation, some forms of mixing being more prone to this than others. Likewise, foaming or bubble formation in the reaction mixture can contribute to inaccurate detection measurements.

FUTURE DIRECTIONS IN AUTOMATION

The demand for rapid turnaround time, short time to first result, and the integration of chemistry, immunoassay, infectious-disease, endocrinology and haematology tests onto the same work-station will introduce analyte-specific issues to instruments. The basics that we have discussed will all apply. We expect many of the specific components needed to prevent erroneous results to be incorporated into the consumable. This will be the case for instruments that already exist and for which the repertoire is being expanded to incorporate testing that was once considered to be special but is now becoming routine.

There is a clear trend in the field of automated clinical analysers towards designing smarter instruments, capable of self-diagnosis or remote diagnosis by modem. Some instruments already include the ability to dilute a sample automatically when the analytical result exceeds the assay range. Future systems will incorporate the ability to define follow-up testing, referred to as reflex testing, according to a user-defined testing protocol (e.g. TSH used as the primary thyroid test, followed by further testing (such as free thyroxine) only when abnormal predetermined TSH values are observed). The downloading of data from automated clinical analysers to central or remote computers is already commonly used in laboratory information systems (LIS). These systems could be augmented by expert systems to improve productivity and quality in a clinical laboratory (Gendler, 1995). However, these developments in automated data handling are less frequently applied for routine diagnosis of system performance, including instrument performance, operating software and consumables.

We can expect to see incorporation of such self-diagnostic features and remote communications in new generations of smart instruments. In fact, the OPUS® Magnum Immunoassay System (Behring Diagnostics Inc.) and the IMMULITE® Immunoassay System (Diagnostic Products Inc.) incorporate bidirectional interfaces with host query allowing remote system diagnostics. Other features may include:

1   *Advanced built-in instrument diagnostics*

    Runs periodic and automatic diagnostic routines.

    Uses built-in expert systems for self-diagnosis and operator-assisted troubleshooting.

    Uses built-in modem for remote system performance assessment and troubleshooting.

2   *Advances in calibration routines* The trend is towards less operator intervention. The Hitachi 911 routine chemistry instrument provides a calibrator and quality control sample wheel on the instrument. The operator fills the appropriate cups at the beginning of the shift. The instrument automatically samples according to preprogrammed parameters. The AxSym® and the Elecsys claim factory calibration. Although operator calibration is still required, fewer points are tested than typically required to linearise immunoassay curves.

    Calibration consumes test equivalents. The trend for the future is less testing to verify calibration; less frequent calibration has already been used to minimise operator involvement. For example, the Ektachem® systems use very infrequent calibration (6 months) to overcome a cumbersome calibration scheme.

3   *Advanced built-in reagent quality control (QC)* In addition to the more commonly used QC of reagent solutions or suspensions prepared on-board from tablets or lyophilised solids, an advanced reagent QC protocol might be used for every test and may have the following features:

    Specific for each method and consumable lot.

    Self-learning, automatically establishing QC limits.

IMPLICATIONS FOR THE FUTURE

As manufacturers continue to focus on immunoassays, new and more complex consumable designs will continue to arise. In addition, there is a move to less complex instrumentation because of the lack of qualified laboratory personnel and cutbacks in personnel costs. An ideal system in this environment would incorporate an elegant consumable into an easy-to-use, cost-effective system. The marriage of immunoassay techniques with such state-of-the-art diagnostic techniques as biosensors and DNA probes also holds promise for the continued development of consumables in the *in vitro* diagnostics market.

Sophisticated, multi-test, homogeneous reagent systems such as PETINIA, CEDIA® and EMIT® will continue to play an important role as laboratories look for ways to add more cost-competitive reagents onto high-throughput systems. The expansion of these homogeneous immunoassay formats into the detection of high-molecular weight compounds, and their adaptation to various high-throughput analysers could have a dramatic effect on the current market for unit-dose, high-complexity reagents used on low-throughput analysers.

Miniaturisation of analytical components, functional parts and systems is also a clear trend (Harrison *et al.*, 1993; Lammerink *et al.*, 1993; van der Schoot *et al.*, 1993; Jacobson *et al.*, 1994); (*see* also Chapter 23). This approach will revolutionise test methodology and delivery systems. It will make hand-held devices more convenient and versatile.

In addition, the first signs of commercial automated assays for DNA probes, polymerase chain reaction (PCR) and ligase chain reaction (LCR) are beginning to appear (Birkenmeyer and Armstrong, 1992; Thomas *et al.*, 1995). These systems also promise to change the type and level of automation in the clinical laboratory.

CONCLUSION

When instrumentation was initially introduced for immunoassays, the technologies needed for sensitivity and specificity were the most important factors. These factors are no longer the technical limits and challenges. Total system integration of the consumable and instrument processor is now crucial to the future needs of the laboratory staff. New technologies will be adapted to existing systems; however, the basic physicochemical principles will determine success. Cost and size constraints will determine development and implementation of new technologies. The ability to integrate consumables and instruments into systems that overcome the constraints imposed by the sample and/or reagents will be a differentiating factor. Furthermore demonstration of consistent, reliable manufacture of instruments and reagents, to assure analytical performance as claimed, will be essential.

ACKNOWLEDGEMENTS

We thank D. M. Obzansky, T. C. O'Brien, D. Dietzen and M. T. Largen for editorial review. We also thank M. Rule and L. Duffy for administrative assistance.

REFERENCES

Aarts, R. J., Lindsey, J. S., Corkan, L. A. *et al.* (1995) Flexible protocols improve parallel experimentation throughput. *Clin. Chem.* **41**, 1004–1010.

Allard, W. J., Obzansky, D. M. & Vaidya, H. C. (1995) Assay with signal detection in the presence of a suspended solid support. *U S Patent* No. 5,434,051.

Alpert, N. L. (1994) ACCESS® immunoassay system. *Clin. Instrum. Syst.* **13**, 1–7.

Altshulter, C. H. (1994) Data utilization, not data acquisition, is the main problem. *Clin. Chem.* **40**, 1616–1620.

Babson, A. L. (1991) The Cirrus IMMULITE® automated immunoassay system. *J. Clin. Immunoassay* **14**, 83–88.

Bangs, L. B. (1990) Latex immunoassays. *J. Clin. Immunoassay* **13**, 127–131.

Barnard, G. & Kohen, F. (1990) Idiometric assay: Noncompetitive immunoassay for small molecules typified by the measurement of estradiol in serum. *Clin. Chem.* **36**, 1945–1950.

Birkenmeyer, L. & Armstrong, A. S. (1992) Preliminary evaluation of the ligase chain reaction for specific detection of *Neisseria gonorrhoeae. J. Clin. Microbiol.* **30**, 3089–3094.

Blackburn, G. F., Shah, H. P., Kenten, J. H *et al.* (1991) Electrochemiluminescence detection for the development of immunoassays and DNA probe assays for clincal diagnostics. *Clin. Chem.* **37**, 1534–1539.

Caffo, A. L. (1993) The complete chemistry system: Du Pont aca® analyzer. *Clin. Chem.* **39**, 1313.

Campbell, A. K., Kricka, L. J. & Stanley, P. E. (1994) *Bioluminescence and Chemiluminescence: Fundamentals and Applied Aspects* (Wiley, New York).

Chan, D. W. (ed.) (1992) *Immunoassay Automation: A Practical Guide* (Academic Press, New York).

Chan, D. W. (1996) Immunoassay automation: From concept to system performance. In: *Handbook of Clinical Automation, Robotics, and Optimization* (ed. Kost, G. J.) (Wiley, New York.)

Coty, W. A., Loor, R., Bellet, N. *et al.* (1992) *Wien Klin Wochenschr Suppl.*, **191**, 5–11, CEDIA®-Homogeneous immunoassays for the 1990s and beyond.

Crowley, H. J. & Bauduin, M. A. (1994) PB Diagnostics Opus®, Opus® Plus and Opus® Magnum. In: *The Immunoassay Handbook* (ed. Wild, D.) pp. 197–203 (Stockton Press, London).

Danese, M. D., Powe, N. R., Sawin, C. T. *et al.*(1996) Screening for mild thyroid failure at the periodic health examination, a decision and cost effectiveness analysis. *J.A.M.A.* **276**, 285–292.

DePalma, A. (1995) Biomagnetic separations touted for their scalability and efficiency. *Gen. Engng. News* **15**, 6.

Duncan, T., Engelberth, L. & LaBrash, B. (1991) The Boehringer Mannheim ES 300 immunoassay system. *J. Clin. Immunoassay* **14**, 105–110.

Ekins, R. P. & Chu, F. W. (1991) Multianalyte microspot immunoassay: Microanalytical 'compact disk' of the future. *Clin. Chem.* **37**, 1955–1967.

Evans, S., Kirchick, H. & Goodnow, T. (1991) Radial Partition Immunoassay. In: *Principles and Practice of Immunoassay.* (eds. Price, C. P., Newman, D. J.) pp. 610–643, Stockton Press, London.

Faulkner, L. R. (1977) Techniques of electrogenerated chemiluminescence. In: *Electroanalytical Chemistry* Vol. 10 (ed. Bard, A. J.) pp. 1–95, (Marcel Dekker, New York).

Gendler, S. M. (1995) LIS expert systems: Feature evaluation. *Amer. Clin. Lab.* **14**, 12.

Glazier, S. A. & McCurley, M. F. (1995) Biosensor applications for bioprocess monitoring and drug analysis. *BioPharm* **8**, 38–50.

Godolphin, W., Bodtker, K., Uyeno, D. *et al.* (1990) Automated blood-sample handling in the clinical laboratory. *Clin. Chem.* **36**, 1551–1555.

Gorman, E. G., Hochberg, A. H. & Tseng, S. Y. (1993) Automation of high-sensitivity immunoassays. *Lab. Robotics Automation* **5**, 129–141.

Hamilton, D. R., Thomas, A. T. & Pijar, M. L. (1991) User reporting under the safe medical devices act of 1990. *J. Clin. Immunoassay* **14**, 222–226.

Harrison, D. J., Fluri, K., Seiler, K., *et al.* (1993) Micromaching a miniaturized capillary microsystem for flow injection analysis on a chip. *Science* **261**, 895–897.

Holman, J. P. (1981) *Heat Transfer* 5th edn. (McGraw-Hill, New York).

Hoyle, N. R., Eckert, B. & Kraiss, S. (1996) Electrochemiluminescence: leading edge technology for automated immunoassay analyte detection. *Clin Chem.* **42**, 157.

Jacobson, S. C., Hergenroeder, R., Koutny, L. B. *et al.* (1994) High-speed separations on a microchip. *Anal. Chem.* **66**, 1114–1118.

Jaggon, R. & Price, C. P. (1987) Performance characteristics of a light scattering immunoassay for thyroxine on a discretionary analyser. *J. Auto. Chem.* **9**, 97–99

Knight, R. N., DeLaurentis, M. & Santomauro, L. (1995) Evaluation of a digoxin assay. *Amer. Clin. Lab.* **4**, 8–10.

Kricka, L. J. (1991) Chemiluminescent and bioluminescent techniques. *Clin. Chem.* **37**, 1472–1481.

Krouwer, J. S., Stewart, W. N. & Schlain, B. (1988) A multi-factor experimental design for evaluating random-access analyzers. *Clin. Chem.* **34**, 1894–1896.

Lammerink, T. S. J., Elwenspoek, M. & Fluitman, J. H. J. (1993) Integrated micro-liquid dosing system. *Proc. 1993 Inst. Elect. Electron. Engrs Micro Electro Mechanical Systems (MEMS)*, 254–259 (Institute of Electrical and Electronic Engineers Piscataway, N.J.).

Lehrer, M., Miller, L. & Natale, J. (1992) The OPUS system. In: *Immunoassay Automation: A Practical Guide* (ed. Chan, D. W.) (Academic Press, New York).

Loebel, J. E. (1991) TOSOH AIA–1200/AIA–600 automated immunoassay analyzers. *J. Clin. Immunoassay* **14**, 94–102.

Loebel, J. E. (1994) Tosoh AIA®-600 and AIA®-1200. In: *The Immunoassay Handbook* (ed. Wild, D.) pp. 228–232 (Stockton Press, London).

Müller, B. (1994) Laboratory diagnostics in light of massive changes in official health policies. *Clin. Chem.* **40**, 1658–1662.

Ng, R. H. (1991) Theme: CLAS review of automated immunoassay instruments. *J. Clin. Immunoassay* **14**, 53–136.

Oak Ridge Conference (1995) *Clin. Chem.* **41**, 1327–1406.

Obzansky, D. M., Rabin, B. R., Simons, D. M. *et al.* (1991) Sensitive, colorimetric enzyme amplification cascade for determination of alkaline phosphatase and application of the method to an immunoassay of thyrotropin. *Clin. Chem.* **37**, 1513–1518.

Payne, G. P., Saewert, M. & Harvey, S. (1994) Hybritech Icon® and Tandem® Icon QSR®. In: *The Immunoassay Handbook* (ed. Wild, D.) pp. 175–178, (Stockton Press, London).

Price, C. P., Trull, A. K., Berry, D. *et al.* (1987) Development and validation of a particle-enhanced immunoassay for C-reactive protein. *J. Immunol. Meth.* **99**, 205–211.

Rubenstein, K. E., Schneider, R. S. & Ullman, E. F. (1972) Homogeneous enzyme immunoassay: A new immunochemical technique. *Biochem. Biophys. Res. Commun.* **47**, 846–851.

Schumann, G., Peterson, D., Hoyer, P. F. *et al.* (1993) Monitoring cyclosporin A (Ciclosporin, INN) concentrations in whole blood: Evaluation of the EMIT™ assay in comparison with HPLC and RIA. *Eur. J. Clin. Chem. Clin. Biochem.* **31**, 381–388.

Singh, P., Moll F, III. Lin, S. H. *et al.* (1994) Starburst™ dendrimers: Enhanced performance and flexibility for immunoassays. *Clin. Chem.* **40**, 1845–1849.

Smith, J., Osikowicz, G., Tayi, R. *et al.* (1995) Abbott AxSYM™ Random and continuous access immunoassay system for improved workflow in the clinical laboratory. *Clin. Chem.* **39**, 2063–2069.

Southwell, F. R., Arentzen, R., Barger, J. D. *et al.* (1994) Development and analytical performance of a revised GGT method for the DuPont Dimension® clinical chemistry system. *Clin. Chem.* **40**, 1122.

Stille, D. K., Zuk, P J., Wiedenmann, R. K., *et al.* (1995) Development of an automated digoxin assay for the DuPont Dimension® Clinical Chemistry System. *Clin. Chem.* **41,** S131.

Thomas, B. J., MacLeod, E. J. & Taylor-Robinson, D. (1995) Evaluation of a commercial polymerase chain reaction assay for *Chlamydia trachomatis* and suggestions for improving sensitivity. *Eur. J. Clin. Microbiol. Infect. Dis.* **14,** 719–723.

Truchaud, A., Capolaghi, B., Yvert, J. P. *et al.* (1991) New trends for automation in immunoassays. *Pure Appl. Chem.* **63,** 1123–1126.

Ullman, E. F., Kirakossian, H., Switchenko, A. C. *et al.* (1996) Luminescent Oxygen Channeling Assay (LOCI™): Sensitive, broadly applicable homogenous immunoassay method. *Clin. Chem.* **42,** 1518–1526.

van der Schoot, B. H., Jeanneret, S., van der Berg, A. *et al.* (1993) Microsystems for flow injection analysis. *Anal. Meth. Instrum.* **1,** 38–42.

Wild, D. (ed.) (1994) *The Immunoassay Handbook.* (Stockton Press, London).

Witte, D. (1993) Medically relevant laboratory-performance goals: A listing of the complexities and a call for action. *Clin. Chem.* **39,** 1530–1543.

Witte, D. (1995) Measuring outcomes: why now? *Clin. Chem.* **41,** 775–780.

Zara, J., Pomato, N., McCabe, R. P. *et al.* (1995). Cobra venom factor immunoconjugates: Effects of carbohydrates-directed versus amino group-directed conjugation. *Bioconjugate Chem.* **6,** 367–372.

Chapter 14

Radiolabelled Immunoassays

Ray Edwards

INTRODUCTION

Radiolabelled immunoassays use reagents incorporating radioisotopes as tracers to monitor the distribution of free and bound antigen in radioimmunoassays (RIA) or free and bound antibody in immunoradiometric assays (IRMA). Radioisotopes have been used as tracers to monitor both chemical and biological systems since 1913, when George Charles de Hevery used a natural radioisotope of lead to investigate the solubility of lead salts in water and later the uptake of lead into growing plants.

The available natural radioisotopes were somewhat limiting in terms of experimental use and the invention and application of the cyclotron, i.e. charged particle accelerator, in the early 1930s, did much to enhance the availability and range. However, manufactured radioisotopes became plentiful only with the development of nuclear reactors in the 1950s, which produced fission products using neutron bombardment.

Radioisotopes have been widely used in medicine. The list is extensive, with more than 100 different ones having been used since 1945. The most significant medical radioisotopes are chromium-51 (^{51}Cr), iodine-131 (^{131}I), phosphorous-32 (^{32}P), iron-59 (^{59}Fe) and technetium-99m (^{99}Tc). Radioisotopes are used in therapy, diagnosis *in vivo* and *in vitro*, and sterilisation of medical supplies. The latter accounts for the most extensive use of gamma radiation.

Radioisotopes were introduced into immunoassays in 1960 (Yalow and Berson, 1960). Although earlier immunoassays, e.g. using red blood cells and subsequent haemagglutination (Arquila and Statvitsky, 1956), were similar in principle to the radiolabelled assays, the use of a radioisotope proved a major advance and improved detection significantly. Development of radioimmunoassays can be traced back to the mid-1950s. At this time, work was proceeding in two centres, one in London and the other in New York. Solomon Berson and Rosalyn Yalow were investigating the metabolic fate of intravenously administered ^{131}I-labelled insulin at the Veterans Administration Hospital in New York. Their studies showed that, although the insulin disappeared rapidly from the blood of normal subjects and diabetic patients not treated with insulin, it persisted for a longer period in the bloodstream of patients who had received insulin therapy for more than a few weeks. This proved to be due to the presence of antibodies to insulin in those patients receiving therapy. Their initial studies demonstrated that the binding of the ^{131}I-insulin to antibody was inhibited in a quantitative manner by the presence of unlabelled insulin. These simple findings were to be the basis of their method now familiar as a RIA.

In the other centre, the radioisotope unit of the Middlesex Hospital Medical School in London, Roger Ekins was working on a new theory for the measurement of endogenous hormones at levels consistent with those found in blood. Unable to buy expensive radiolabelled thyroxine, Ekins had to wait for several years to apply his method to the measurement of thyroxine in serum. Monitoring the radioactivity in serum from a patient with thyroid carcinoma metastases he found that some of the 138 mCi of ^{131}I administered to the patient had been incorporated into thyroxine *in vivo*. Using this radiolabelled thyroxine and thyroxine-binding globulin as a high-affinity binding reagent, the measurement of thyroxine was demonstrated. The technique, called saturation analysis (Ekins, 1960), was a general procedure using a specific binding protein and thus included all immunoassays.

Attempting to optimise sensitivity and precision in radiolabelled immunoassays led Miles and Hales (1968) to formulate the principles of assays using labelled antibodies, referred to as 'immunoradiometric' assays (IRMA) where the label was a radioisotope. The use of highly purified antibodies coupled to a radioactive tracer increased sensitivity and improved precision. Subsequent developments, in 1970, incorporating an additional antibody coupled to a particle or other solid phase and referred to as the 'two-site' IRMA or 'sandwich' assay (Haberman, 1970; Addison and Hales, 1971; Wide, 1971) further improved precision and hence sensitivity. The exponential growth in the application of radiolabelled-immunoassays was accompanied by numerous symposia, workshops and colloquia seeking to clarify and consolidate both theoretical and practical aspects. The proceedings of many of these meetings have been published (e.g. Wolstenholme and Cameron, 1962; Hayes *et al.*, 1968; International Atomic Energy Agency, 1970, 1974, 1978, 1982 and 1986; Kirkham and Hunter, 1971; Hunter and Corrie, 1983) and are a useful source of information. In addition, there have been a number of reviews (e.g. Chard, 1978; Edwards, 1985, 1990; Bolton and Hunter, 1986).

THEORY OF RADIOACTIVITY

Radioactivity is the emission of subatomic particles and radiation from unstable atomic nuclei when they decompose or 'decay' spontaneously, and may proceed through more than one state before reaching the ground state, or state of lowest energy. The term radioisotope refers to those isotopes of a chemical element that share the same chemistry but are radioactive, e.g. ^{123}I, ^{125}I, ^{131}I, and are radioisotopes of the element iodine (atomic mass 127). They all behave chemically as iodine. The term radionuclide refers to radioactive nuclear species with their electron clouds but without invoking their elemental relationship.

Radioactive decay is complex and difficult to summarise. However, most commonly, radioactive decay involves the emission of one or more of the following:

1   alpha particles;

2   beta particles;

3   gamma rays.

Radioisotope	Half-life	Major radioactive emission
^{3}H	12.3 years	β
^{14}C	5,730 years	β
^{57}Co	270 days	γ
^{75}Se	120.4 days	γ
^{123}I	14.3 days	β
^{125}I	60.2 days	γ
^{131}I	8.05 days	β/γ

Table 1 Radioisotopes used in radiolabelled immunoassays.

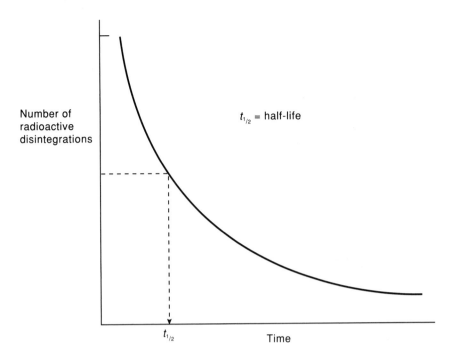

Figure 1 Diagram of the half-life of a radioisotope. Radioactive decay is exponential and the time taken for the amount of a radioactive substance to decrease to one-half of its original value is always constant and is specific for each radioisotope.

Alpha particles are helium ions with two positive charges and low penetrating power. Beta particles are essentially electrons, usually negatively charged (negatron) or a positively charged positron. Gamma rays are a form of electromagnetic radiation like radio waves, light or X-rays. Specifically gamma rays are photons. The emission of X-rays may also accompany radioactive decay, usually when decomposition proceeds through an intermediate 'excited' state or a state with a higher energy level. Radioactive decay is a random event and it is not possible to predict when any given atom will disintegrate. The number of atoms likely to decay in a given infinitesimal time interval $(dN)/dT$ is proportional to the number of atoms (N) present. This is expressed as:

$$\frac{-dN}{dT} = \lambda N$$

Unit	Symbol	Definition
Becquerel	Bq	1 disintegration per second = 2.7×10^{-11} Ci
Curie (old unit)	Ci	= 3.7×10^{10} Bq

Table 2 Units of radioactivity.

where λ is the decay constant. The decay constant is different for each radioisotope and is a feature of that radioisotope. Disintegration falls exponentially with time as does the number of parent nuclei. The term 'parent nuclei' refers to the radioactive unstable nuclei; daughter refers to nuclei produced from the disintegration process, some of which may be radioactive intermediate states. As the rate at which radioisotopes decay is exponential, the half-life ($t_{\frac{1}{2}}$) is equal to $0.693/\lambda$. The half-life (Figure 1), or the time taken for the number of parent nuclei to fall to half the number present at zero time, i.e. the time taken for half the number of radioactive nuclei to disintegrate, is characteristic for each radioisotope. Radioisotopes that have been used in radiolabelled immunoassays, together with their respective half-lives are given in Table 1. The units of radioactivity are given in Table 2. The original unit of activity, the curie (Ci), defined as the amount of radioactive substance equivalent to one gram of ^{226}Ra giving rise to 3.7×10^{10} disintegrations per second, has now been superseded by the becquerel (Bq).

DETECTION OF RADIOACTIVITY

Radiation is detected and measured by a number of different methods that depend on the property of radiation to cause the following:

1 ionisation in gases;

2 emission of light from sensitive material;

3 blackening of a photographic emulsion or glass.

Different types of detectors are suitable for different radioisotopes. The fundamental mechanism underlying the operation of radiation detectors is the dissipation of energy by a charged particle in a suitable medium and the distribution of this energy among atoms and molecules of the detecting material.

Ionisation Detectors

These detectors rely on the dissipation of energy to knock electrons out of atoms to produce ions and electrons. Commonly, gases are used as the ionising medium. Where a gas is ionised in a high electric field, the effect is to ionise more atoms and a multiplication of the signal is achieved. Proportional counters may lead to a multiplication factor of 10^6. At this level the output signal is still proportional to the initial energy and thus the detector retains discrimination. At much higher values of gas multiplication, the output becomes independent of the initial signal as is found in the Geiger-Müller counter tube.

Fluorescent or Light Detectors

Fluorescent detectors depend on the conversion of distributed energy of the primary ionising particle into light. This light is then used to generate photoelectrons from the cathode of a photomultiplier tube. The photoelectron current is multiplied in the tube to give an adequately large output signal. The various detection media that convert energy of moving electrons into light are called phosphors. Detectors using phosphors are referred to as scintillation counters.

There are two types of scintillation counter used for radioimmunoassays: (1) the scintillation crystal or 'gamma' counter; (2) the liquid scintillation or 'beta' counter, indicating the type of radiation each is appropriate for.

The principal features of a scintillation counter are as follows: charged particles arising from the radioactive disintegrations are absorbed by the phosphor and converted into light. When the light strikes the photocathode of a photomultiplier tube, the energy is converted into photoelectrons. Photocathodes in scintillation counters are usually constructed from semiconducting compounds of antimony and alkali metals such as caesium, sodium and potassium.

Electrons from the cathode are accelerated in an electric field and strike an electrode coated with a secondary emitting material. Each electron striking this surface with an energy between 1 and 500 eV knocks out further electrons that can be accelerated in turn onto subsequent electrodes or dynodes. This process can be repeated through a series of dynodes. The photomultiplier is a linear amplifier giving an output proportional to the primary photoelectron signal. The primary signal can be multiplied by a factor of up to 10^6.

In liquid scintillation, the phosphors are fluorescent organic materials derived from benzene and typified by anthracene and naphthalene. Samples are solubilised or mixed in a liquid medium containing toluene in which is dissolved an efficient organic phosphor such as p-terphenyl derivatives. Optimally, mixed phosphors are used. In this situation, energy is transferred from molecule to molecule without radiation until emission of light occurs from the molecules having the highest emission probability. In the case of a mixture of anthracene and naphthalene, the emission of light has the characteristic of anthracene but with the longer decay time of naphthalene. A common form of interference in this type of detection is quenching. Quenching is the reduction of fluorescent efficiency caused by competition between routes for energy dissipation. It is often caused by oxygen or chlorine. Plastic phosphors are similar in principle to the liquid phosphors. For example, organic fluorophors are dissolved in polymerised polyvinyltoluene to form a solid plastic phosphor.

Inorganic phosphors form the basis of scintillation crystal detectors. They are transparent insulating crystals containing a small proportion of a suitable impurity. When radiation is absorbed by such crystals, excess energy from the excited impurity centre is emitted as photons of energy. Gamma counters use thallium-activated sodium iodide crystals. Crystals of different sizes are optimal for different radioisotopes. Larger crystals are most efficient for radioisotopes with higher energy. Because they are hygroscopic, these crystals are hermetically sealed in a can with a window for coupling to a photomultiplier tube. To maximise the collection of fluorescent light, all surfaces of the crystal, except the one facing the window, are covered with white diffusing titanium oxide.

Photographic Emulsion or Glass Detectors

The systems described above involve transient effects, leaving the instruments capable of continuous or repeated detection. The absorption of radiation by a photographic film leads to a more permanent change. The distribution of energy causes the disruption of bonds between silver and bromine atoms. The subsequent development process leads to darkening of the atomic silver. Glass will also blacken under intense radiation. The degree of darkening of the photographic film or glass can be used to determine exposure to radiation and its degree. The radiation 'film' badge is an example of this type of detector.

APPLICATION OF RADIOISOTOPES TO RADIOIMMUNOASSAY

A number of different radioisotopes have been used as tracers in radioimmunoassays (Table 1) although the current practice is to use either ^{125}I or ^{3}H. The first published radioimmunoassay (Yalow and Berson, 1960) used ^{131}I, which has a relatively short half-life and consequently a higher activity, i.e. a higher number of disintegrations per unit time. This was useful as it enabled the measurement of small aliquots of reaction medium, dictated by the use of paper electrophoresis strips which have a limited loading capacity for separating free and antibody-bound analyte. ^{131}I was also readily available at a relatively high level of radioisotope purity.

Because antibody binding sites are extremely specific, it would seem logical that the best choice of radioisotope would be one that replaces its nonradioactive isotope in the tracer molecule; for example, replacing ^{3}H for hydrogen or using ^{125}I for molecules containing iodine as in thyroxine or triiodothyronine. In practice, if the substitution is made in a part of the molecule away from the antibody binding site, the choice of radioisotope can be governed by other considerations, such as half-life, availability, high activity and radiochemical purity. The larger the tracer molecule, the more easily this can be achieved.

Iodine-125

When ^{125}I with good radiochemical purity became commercially available, it rapidly became the radioisotope of choice representing a practical combination of high activity and reasonable reagent shelf-life.

Because the iodine atom is relatively large, about the size of a benzene ring, it proved unsuitable for many small molecules, such as steroids, as it interfered with antibody binding. The exceptions were those few molecules such as thyroxine that have endogenous iodine. ^{3}H, another readily available radioisotope, became widely used for small molecules. The use of ^{3}H introduces certain constraints, particularly the need for relatively expensive liquid scintillation detection. In 1968, an elegant technique was published (Oliver *et al.*, 1968), which permitted the use of ^{125}I to label small molecules without compromising immunoreactivity. It involved the synthesis of a suitably modified analogue, incorporating the radioactive iodine into an appropriate group like a histidyl or a tyrosyl group, attached to the molecule through a side chain at a point not directly bound by the antibody (Figure 2). In practice, this technique proved successful for virtually all small molecules, requiring only the judicious identification of appropriate positions to introduce side chains for the analogues. This approach has even

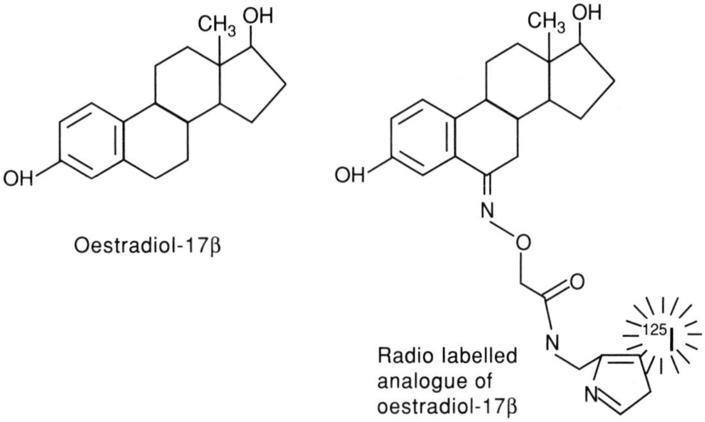

Figure 2 Schematic representation of a radiolabelled analogue, a conjugate of oestradiol-17β-6(carboxymethyl)oxime and ^{125}I-histamine, for use as a tracer. The radioisotope is incorporated in an appropriate way to permit the binding of the antibody to the most significant epitopes, i.e. the A- and D-rings.

allowed the use of extremely large molecular tracers, such as enzymes with relative molecular weights greater than 50,000 to be attached to analytes with molecular masses of only a few hundred.

In recent years, ^{125}I has become the most commonly used radioisotope in RIAs and IRMAs. Tritium ^{3}H is now used for relatively few assays, but is particularly useful where the incorporation of iodine is not practical because of a lack of suitable analogues or because it leads to an unstable tracer.

Multihead Gamma counter

The widespread use of ^{125}I was a potent factor in the introduction and success of the multi-head detector. Because of the relatively low energy of ^{125}I , much smaller crystals could be used, in turn requiring less lead shielding to reduce the background radiation, allowing for several heads to be assembled in a single instrument. Up to this time, gamma counters were traditionally expensive instruments with large crystals to accommodate a variety of radioisotopes, a lot of lead shielding, the ability to detect energy wavelengths over a continuously variable range, and complex automated sample handling facilities. The use of a manually operated, simple instrument dedicated to the measurement of low-energy radioisotopes such as ^{125}I was extremely economic in terms of cost and time and proved to be very popular with many laboratory users. In 1977, at St Bartholomew's Hospital, London, a single 16-headed gamma counter, with consequent high throughput, replaced eight automated gamma spectrophotometers, with a capital cost saving of approximately 20-fold. Being a manual instrument, it was also not subject to the frequent breakdown problems associated with the complex automated sample-handling facilities. In essence, gamma counting is extremely efficient and economical when compared to other forms of detection.

Dual Radioisotopic Assays

Gamma radiations from different radioisotopes display different energy spectra. It is possible to take advantage of this difference and discriminate the radioactivity associated with specific radioisotopes. The concept of assaying two components in a biological medium simultaneously using tracers labelled with two different radioisotopes was introduced in 1966 (Morgan). This 'dual' radioimmunoassay measured both growth hormone and insulin using ^{125}I and ^{131}I. Dual assays are perhaps best exemplified by the Becton Dickinson SimulTRAC® range using ^{125}I and ^{57}Co. ^{57}Co was introduced originally as an appropriate tracer for vitamin B_{12} (cobalamin) which has an endogenous cobalt atom. These types of assay are most appropriate for the measurement of those analytes that are measured in the same sample, such as thyroid-stimulatinghormone/free thyroxine, luteinising hormone/follicle-stimulating hormone and vitamin B_{12}/folate.

Homogeneous Assays

Because the radioactive process is unaffected by external conditions, radiolabelled assays have often been considered as unsuitable for nonseparation protocols, i.e. homogeneous assays. However, the detection of low-energy radioisotopes such as tritium (Hart and Greenwald, 1979) can be interfered with or altered. Amersham's scintillation proximity assay (SPA) is an example of homogeneous immunoassays, involving the use of beads impregnated with scintillant which are coupled to binding proteins, such as antibodies. In principle, the bound radioactive tracer allows emitted radiation energy to interact with the scintillant and thereby produce light which is detected in conventional liquid scintillation counters. The energy from unbound or free radioactive tracers, being at a distance from the bead, does not react with the fluoromicrospheres.

Homogeneous radiolabelled immunoassays are also possible if scintillant is localised in or at the surface of a microtitre plate e.g. Wallac ScintiStrip or DuPont NEM Flashplate. In the ScintiStrip a scintillant is an integral part of the polystyrene used to manufacture microtitre plates, whereas for the Flashplate it is precoated onto the surface of the 96-well plate. These products are available coated with second antibody or other specific binding protein for use with a primary antibody of choice.

Using these principles, homogeneous radiolabelled immunoassays have been developed for a variety of uses including steroid hormones (Siitari and Oikari, 1992) and prostaglandins (Udenfriend, 1985). These assays have demonstrated sensitivities from 10^{-19} mol l^{-1} to 10^{-20} mol l^{-1}.

PREPARATION OF RADIOLABELLED REAGENTS

Radioiodination

Iodine is readily incorporated into many molecules; a fact that has undoubtedly contributed significantly to the ubiquitous use of radioactive iodine as a tracer in radiolabelled immunoassays. The reactive species is cationic iodine, produced by the oxidation of an iodide ion (*see* Figure 3). Early methods of radioiodination, e.g. relying on the diffusion of gaseous oxi-

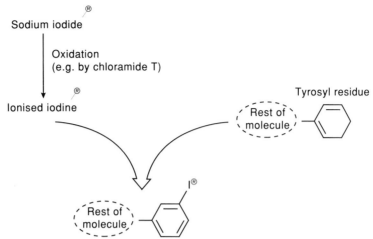

Figure 3 Simple radioiodination by oxidation of radioactive iodide.

dant (e.g. chlorine) or of gaseous radioiodine following oxidation, must have been difficult to control and were more hazardous and undoubtedly less efficient than current methods. The introduction of the mild soluble oxidant chloramine T (Hunter and Greenwood, 1962) was an important step. This led to a general method for the efficient production of radioiodinated tracer with high specific activities (Greenwood *et al.*, 1963). The major difficulty with this type of approach is the damaging effect of the oxidant on the molecule being labelled. To reduce or eliminate this, a variety of alternative methods have been tried, such as electrolytic oxidation of the radioactive sodium iodide (Pennisi and Rosa, 1969). The most practical and efficient alternative methods use either lactoperoxidase (Marchalonis, 1969) or Iodogen (Fraker and Speck, 1978). Enzymic radioiodination using lactoperoxidase can be as efficient and yet avoid some of the damaging effects of other methods. Because the enzyme itself incorporates radioiodine and may prove difficult to separate from the intended radiolabelled product, it can be used attached to a solid-phase material (David, 1972). The solid-phase enzyme can be easily separated from the reaction mixture.

Iodogen is the trade name for 1,3,4,6-tetrachloro-3α,6α-glycoluracil and is insoluble (or, rather, sparingly soluble) in aqueous medium. A convenient method uses Iodogen coated onto tubes or vials. Iodogen is deposited on the walls following evaporation of an organic solution. Studies comparing the various methods for radioiodination can be misleading as each method is not always optimised before use. When methods are optimised to give products of equal specific activity, solid-phase lactoperoxidase is less damaging than chloramine T which, in turn, is less damaging than Iodogen (Edwards *et al.*, 1983).

Conjugation Labelling

Some molecules, without appropriate groups such as tyrosine, cannot be radioiodinated directly. In such cases, so-called conjugation labelling may prove suitable. In this method, a molecule containing an appropriate group is radioiodinated and conjugated to the tracer molecule (Oliver *et al.*, 1968; Nars and Hunter, 1973). Conjugation labelling is typified by the Bolton and Hunter reagent (1973). Radioiodinated *N*-succinimidyl-3-(4-hydroxyphenyl) propionate,

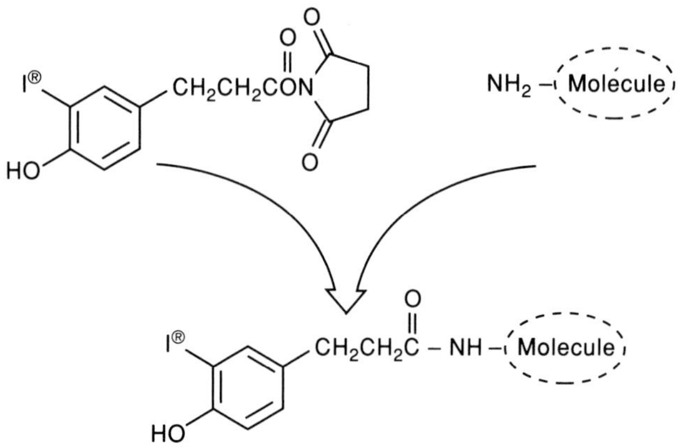

Figure 4 Conjugation labelling using 'Bolton and Hunter' reagent (*N*–succunimidyl–3– (4–hydroxy–5–{^{125}I} iodophenyl) proprionate) which reacts with the free amino group of the molecule to be radiolabelled.

an active ester, reacts with the primary amino groups on the tracer molecule, forming a radiolabelled conjugate (Figure 4). Conjugation labelling can be useful in those situations where direct radioiodination leads to a loss of immunoreactivity, for example, where the incorporation of radioiodine occurs at a site that interferes with antibody binding, or where the antigen is susceptible to damaging effects of radioiodination. Conjugation labelling has proved particularly successful with small molecules, allowing a radioiodine atom to be incorporated without interfering with antibody binding.

Production of Tritiated Tracers

Tritium-labelled compounds are produced either by direct chemical synthesis or by radioisotope exchange reactions. Typical chemical syntheses involve catalytic reduction of unsaturated compounds or dehalogenation using tritium gas, or reduction of intermediate compounds with tritiated borohydride. Radioisotope exchange reactions entail exposing the compound to tritium gas or tritiated water under conditions that promote the exchange of tritium for hydrogen. In general, very few laboratories are suitably equipped to produce their own tritiated tracers with sufficiently high specific activities for RIA, i.e. >50 Ci nmol^{-1} (1.85 × 10^{12} Bq nmol^{-1}). Many are available routinely from commercial sources and some companies, e.g. Amersham International plc., provide a custom labelling service for unusual or research requirements.

Although many tritiated tracers are available commercially and the shelf-life of the radioisotope is very long, their use may involve some additional work. At the specific activities appropriate for RIA, tritiated tracers often require regular repurification, which may involve complex steps as technically demanding as those required for the regular production of radioiodinated tracers.

Detection Limits

The terms 'detection limit' and 'assay sensitivity' are synonymous in this context and are intended to indicate the minimum quantity of analyte measurable with statistical significance in the specified assay. More specifically, assay sensitivity is defined as a significant variation in response, here 2–3 SD, from the signal at zero analyte concentration.

Clearly, detection limit depends on a number of different constraints coming together to give a final figure for a given method under specified conditions. Basically, in any RIA or IRMA, the detection limit relates to the error in signal measurement, the equilibrium constant (K_a) of the reaction and technical errors, such as in pipetting and in separation.

Signal Measurement

The error in signal measurement is made up of a number of factors. There are the errors associated with measuring radioactivity or the 'counting error'; the efficiency and specificity of the instrument; and the type of radioisotope and the specific activity (i.e. the signal per unit mass) of the tracer. There is a simple relationship between counting error and the number of counts measured, as illustrated in Figure 5. The counting error, a function of the probability of an unstable nucleus disintegrating or decaying, is calculated as follows:

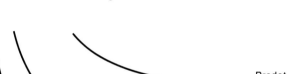

$$\text{Counting error} = \sqrt{\text{number of counts}}$$

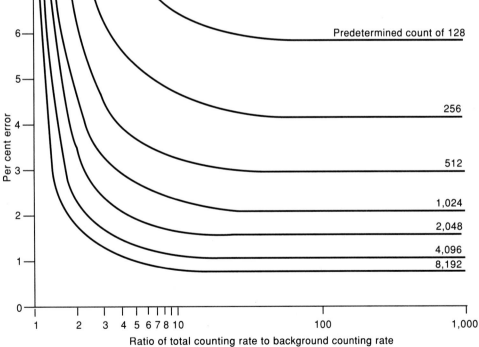

Figure 5 Diagram of the relationship between the error in the count rate and the total counts for different background counts (expressed as a ratio). The background will contribute significantly to the error when it is greater than one-tenth of the sample count rate.

This error, although seemingly a constant factor, is in practice variable because it is constrained by time. Where time is a limiting factor, the counting error will rise. Some counting strategies call for the accumulation of a specific number of counts – clearly inappropriate, as it does not relate the counting error to the overall precision (Ekins, 1974). Data processing programs can be used to terminate the measurement of each sample when the counting error has reached a specified proportion of the error at the appropriate point on the precision profile.

The efficiency and specificity of most instruments, particularly gamma counters, are usually very good. The background measurement is almost negligible. This is particularly so, as special precautions are taken to construct instrument components, specifically photomultiplier tubes, from materials with a minimal amount of radioactive contamination. Glass with the minimum amount of potassium-40 is used or occasionally fused silica is substituted for tube envelopes. By the use of appropriate shielding and instrument design, it is a relatively simple matter to eliminate, or reduce to a negligible level, signals arising from background radiation.

Obviously, differences in performance between units of a multiheaded instrument may compromise the overall precision of an assay, but in practice this sort of error is minimal, either because of careful matching of scintillation units (or heads) during manufacture or because the instruments have microprocessor-controlled facilities to monitor and adjust settings of individual units to a common performance.

In general, specificity of signal measurement with radiolabelled immunoassays depends on addition of a specific purified radioisotope to the reaction medium and the complete absence of any other radioisotope in the biological medium. Because gamma radiation from a specific radioisotope has a spectrum with sharp distinct peaks, the selection of signals at specified wavelengths improves the specificity and considerably reduces background measurement.

Although the two radioisotopes in a 'dual' assay are discriminated by appropriate adjustment of the spectrophotometer windows, some spillover of counts from each radioisotope into the signal of the other is inevitable (Figure 6). The spillover may well be as high as 3% and would increase the overall error. Although this would effectively limit potential sensitivity, it would not necessarily compromise the practical application and any worsening in precision could be compensated by more efficient generation of results.

Specific Activity

Specific activity of a tracer is a function of both the type of radioisotope and the degree of substitution. As stated before, the specific activity of each radioisotope is inversely proportional to its half-life. The specific activities of the two common radioisotopes used in radioimmunoassays and that of ^{14}C ^{131}I are given in Table 3.

Specific activity of the tracer is a direct consequence of the ratio of radioisotope to carrier molecule in the tracer and the activity of the radioisotope. An increase in specific activity of the tracer increases potential assay sensitivity; however, a considerable increase in specific activity only results in a minimal improvement in sensitivity (Ekins *et al.*, 1968). In addition, the stability and immunoreactivity of the tracer may be effectively reduced by damage incurred during the radiolabelling procedure, especially when attempting to achieve very high specific activities (Bolton and Hunter, 1986). Radiolysis, i.e. the damage to a carrier molecule

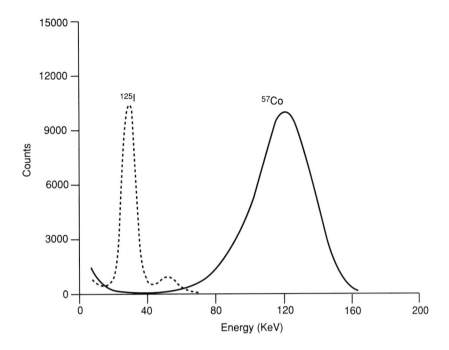

Figure 6 The pulse-height spectrum of ^{125}I and ^{57}Co illustrating the energy resolution into specific detection for each radioisotope. The diagram also indicates the 'spillover' of the higher-energy radioisotope into the lower-energy channel compromising the precision. It is possible to correct for spillover.

Radioisotope	Half-life	Specific activity	
		*GBq per milliatom	Ci per milliatom
^{3}H	12.3 years	1.07×10^{3}	28.9
^{125}I	60.2 days	8.05×10^{4}	2,176
^{131}I	8.05 days	5.90×10^{5}	16,000
^{14}C	5,730 years	2.3	6.2×10^{-2}

*Gigabecquerel = 1×10^{9} Bq.

Table 3 Approximate specific activities of radioisotopes used in radio-labelled immunoassays (assuming 100% isotopic abundance).

arising from radioactive decay of the radioisotope, may become a significant factor when specific activity is high or when tracer is stored at high concentration. The practical manifestations of this type of damage is often increased nonspecific binding and concomitant loss of sensitivity. In practice, the ratio for tracers labelled with ^{125}I need seldom exceed 1:1.

Sensitivity and Optimal Assay Conditions

Maximum sensitivity can be predicted from a theoretical consideration of optimal assay conditions. Several different theoretical approaches have been published, but these are sometimes contradictory (Ekins, 1976). Without resolving all aspects of controversy, the publications of Ekins and co-workers (Ekins *et al.*, 1968; Ekins, 1974, 1976; Jackson *et al.*, 1983; Jackson and Ekins, 1986) have proved accurate and useful in practice and have been validated by the empirical approach. It is clear from the work of Ekins (*see* Chapter 9) that potential detection limits for RIAs and IRMAs are different.

Detection Limits for Radioimmunoassay

Assay sensitivity for all radioimmunoassays is constrained mainly by the equilibrium constant of the reaction (K_a-value) and technical errors of reagent manipulation, e.g. pipetting and separation (Jackson and Ekins, 1986). It is very rare, if ever, that the K_a-value for antibody reactions exceeds 10^{12} l mol^{-1} and consequently this figure can be taken as a limit. Practically, it is difficult to reduce technical imprecision to less than 1% and again this represents a limit. It follows that predicted assay sensitivity will be limited to approximately 10^{-14} mol l^{-1} regardless of the tracer used (Jackson and Ekins, 1986). In practice, the lower limit for ^{125}I radioimmunoassays is usually of the order of 10^{-12} mol l^{-1}, and 10^{-10} mol l^{-1} for tritium. Because tritiated tracers depend on liquid scintillation detection, these radioimmunoassays are subject to the further constraint of quenching, which can be increased by factors such as haemolysis in the sample.

Detection Limits for Immunoradiometric Assays

Essentially, the sensitivity of these assays is limited by nonspecific binding of the labelled antibody, precision of separation and the affinity of the labelled antibody (Ekins, 1976). With similar constraints quoted for radioimmunoassays in the preceding section, a potential sensitivity of 10^{-16} mol l^{-1} is predicted by theoretical considerations. However, as already stated, the use of ^{125}I has a detection limit of about 10^{-14} mol l^{-1}. Clearly the potential increase in sensitivity offered by the immunoradiometric assay is only fully available using tracers with infinite specific activity (*see* Chapter 9 this volume). One important consideration from the above indicates that the practical limitation on sensitivity, given the constraints already mentioned, is the error in the nonspecific binding. With suitable solid-phase separation and efficient washing steps, the nonspecific binding can be reduced to a negligible quantity, removing or minimising a major constraint (see Chapter 8). Using this approach, a simple immunoradiometric assay for urine growth hormone has a sensitivity in practice of 3×10^{-14} mol l^{-1} (Hourd and Edwards, 1989).

LABORATORY PRACTICE AND REGULATION

The handling and use of radioisotopes in the UK is regulated and supervised to a very high standard. As a consequence, laboratory practice related to their use also conforms to a high standard. Each employer has the responsibility to prepare 'local regulations' and to elect a 'radiation protection adviser' to assist and advise in their implementation.

(i) The Ionising Radiations Regulations, 1985. (HMSO, UK).

(ii) Approved Code of Practice, 1985. The protection of persons against ionising radiations arising from any work activity. (HMSO, UK).

(iii) Guidance notes for the protection of persons against ionising radiations arising from medical and dental use, 1988. (HMSO, UK).

(iv) Ionising Radiation (Protection of Persons undergoing Medical Examination or Treatment) Regulations, 1988. (HMSO, UK). These publications are based on the following:

(v) Recommendations of the International Commission on Radiological Protection (ICRP).

(vi) Euratom Directive; Basic Safety Standards for Radiation Protection in the European Community.

(vii) The Health and Safety at Work Act, 1974. (UK).

(viii) The Radioactive Substances Act, 1960 and 1993. (UK).

(ix) The Federal Code of Regulations; together with reports from the National Council of Radiation Protection (NCRP) (USA).

Table 4 Radiation protection regulations.

Local regulations (e.g. St Bartholomew's Hospital, 1987) are based on the publications listed in Table 4.

The intention of these regulations is to make users aware of certain recommended dose limits, to ensure that the doses of ionising radiation received by classified persons are assessed in order to comply with the limits and to ensure that users demonstrate such compliance. In addition, *The Radioactive Substances Act*, 1960, legally controls the disposal of radioactive waste.

A dose received is a function of the specific radioisotope and the type and energy of its radiation, the distance over which the radiation travels and the medium through which it travels. The units of 'dose' are given in Table 5.

Two basic areas of work are designated by the above regulations, and are referred to as 'supervised areas' and 'controlled areas'. These areas are categorised by the amount of radio-

SI unit of dose	Symbol	Definition	Equivalent old units
Gray (adsorbed dose)	Gy	1 Gy = 10^{-2} joules of energy absorbed per kg of material irradiated.	100 rad
Sievert	Sv	Measure of absorbed dose and its radiobiological effectiveness (RBE). $Sv = Gy \times Q$ (for X and γ radiation $Q =1$)	100 rem
Röentgen	R	Measure of X or γ radiation expressed in terms of amount of ionisation produced in air. $1R = 2.58 \times 10^{-4}$ coulombs per kg air.	

Table 5 Dosage units for exposure to radioactivity.

	Supervised	Controlled
Dose equivalent rate	>2.5 µSv h^{-1}	>7.5 µSv h^{-1}
Total amount of radioactivity present		
(1) ^{125}I*	>1 × 10^8 Bq (2.7 mCi)	>3 × 10^8 Bq (8.1 mCi)
(2) ^{3}H**	>1 × 10^{10} Bq (270 mCi)	>3 × 10^{10} Bq (810 mCi)

*   Group III: medium radiotoxicity also includes ^{75}Se, ^{57}Co, ^{35}S.

**   Group IV: low radioactivity.

NB Average radiolabelled immunoassays use <5 µCi of tracer.
10 µCi of ^{125}I-tracer would give a dose-equivalent rate of 0.15 µSv h^{-1}.

Table 6 Regulated laboratory area dose limits.

^{3}H	3 GBq	(81 mCi)
^{125}I	1 MBq	(27 µCi)
^{14}C	90 MBq	(2.4 mCi)

Table 7 Annual limits on intake.

Tissue	Occupationally exposed	General public
Whole body	50 mSv per yr	5 mSv per yr
Individual organs and tissues (excluding eyes)	500 mSv per yr	50 mSv per yr
Lens of eye	150 mSv per yr	15 mSv per yr

Table 8 Dose limits as recommended by the ICRP.

activity present or the maximum dose, e.g. as listed in Table 6. Both categories of regulated activity are relatively similar and normally would only apply to radioiodination procedures or the production of tracers and would not apply to analytical procedures. However, with unsealed radioactive sources, as used in radiolabelled immunoassays, body organs or tissues may be irradiated following ingestion, inhalation or surface contamination of the skin. The annual limit on intake, or the amount of radioisotope taken internally which produces the annual dose limit, varies for different isotopes (*see* Tables 7 and 8). The derived limits for surface or skin contamination are very low, being 30 Bq cm^{-2} for iodine-125 and 300 Bq cm^{-2} for tritium. Most laboratories using radiolabelled immunoassays would be designated as supervised areas on the basis of the derived limits of intake or surface contamination. It is also a useful practice as it leads to better control, particularly of contamination and its subsequent detrimental effects on detection and precision.

Laboratory Design

Important aspects of controlled or supervised areas are those of design and layout. Some salient features of good laboratory design are listed below:

1   A continuous and impervious surface, e.g. melamine laminate, should cover benches from a raised (5 mm) front edge to an upstand 150 mm high at the walls.

2   Floors should be covered with welded vinyl sheets, which overlay the walls to a height of 100 mm. Welds should have a high proportion of PVC (e.g. 50%).

3   Stainless steel sinks must be used for disposal of liquid waste. Drainage should use high-density polyethylene or polypropylene with S- or P-type traps, and should connect directly to main drains, without branching, and with appropriate labelling.

4   Surfaces of walls and ceilings should be smooth and nonporous, e.g. high-quality gloss paint.

5   The laboratory must have good ventilation. The IAEA (International Atomic Energy Agency, Vienna) recommend at least 12 air changes per hour.

6   Separate writing areas, handwashing facilities and a separate room for refreshments must be provided.

7   Lockable cupboards must be provided.

The general layout of the laboratory should allow for easy supervision and monitoring of access. Proper laboratory design should always involve a consultative process, particularly with the 'radiation protection adviser'. The local rules may well require additional constraints on high-activity areas such as radioiodination suites.

Dose Limits

Examples of the dose limits recommended by the ICRP are given in Table 8. These dose limits were set at levels where there are negligible harmful effects. The background dose of 10 μCi

Source	Dose
Annual background dose in:	
Kerala, India (Monazite)	3.7–28 mSv
Brazil (Monazite)	5 mSv
France (Granite)	1.6–2.2 mSv
Cornwall, UK (Granite)	7.8 mSv
Average annual dose in UK	2.5 mSv
Dose from single transatlantic flight	0.04 mSv
Dose from an X-ray examination	up to 10 mSv
Average dose for radioimmunoassays	approximately 0.03 mSv

Table 9 A comparison of doses.

^{125}I (unshielded), equivalent to a large assay batch, at a distance of 1 metre is 0.15 μSv per hour. As the distance increases, the dose diminishes considerably (inverse square law) and, making certain assumptions, it is possible to estimate the average dose for a 'radioimmunoassayist'. This dose, compared with background doses from different localities throughout the world and other sources (Table 9), clearly indicates that radiolabelled immunoassays do not present any hazard from direct radiation. Of the two main radioisotopes used in radiolabelled immunoassays, ingestion would only be a problem with ^{125}I (Table 6). This should only be a potential hazard in radioiodination procedures with large amounts of radioiodine.

CONCLUDING PERSPECTIVES

Performance

Potentially, radiolabelled immunoassays are applicable to the measurement of almost any substance that is found in a biological medium, within the range 10^{-6} mol l^{-1} to 10^{-14} mol l^{-1}. This range includes many substances of biological and physiological interest and radiolabelled immunoassays have been successfully applied to many areas and have, for many years, represented a high standard of performance. The high precision found in radiolabelled immunoassays is undoubtedly related to the negligible radioactive background in biological samples. In addition, the disintegration process of radioisotopes is not affected by factors common to biological media, such as pH, ionic strength, turbidity, colour, substrates, inhibitors, etc. Many of these factors may affect or interfere with the detection of alternative labels, particularly those dependent on optical measurement.

As Ekins has elegantly demonstrated, the detection limit of radioiodinated tracers is not limiting in the practical application of an RIA compared to other limiting reagent immunoassays. However, it does become a constraint for the IRMA technique. A few of the alternative labels are capable of extending the working sensitivity of the labelled antibody technique, especially when used in conjunction with solid-phase systems designed to reduce the non-specific binding of tracers.

A restraint on counting time may represent a practical constraint on precision and sensitivity for radiolabelled immunoassays operating at the limit of sensitivity. However, in general this is not a problem, particularly when using multihead detectors.

Convenience

The ease with which radioiodine is introduced into such a variety of molecules and the availability of so many tritiated tracers has made radiolabelled tracers an excellent choice for many immunoassays. In particular, the convenience and simplicity of 'in-house' preparation of radioiodinated tracers has ensured that they have become the foundation for a considerable amount of research and development work. In some areas, such as clinical endocrinology, many radiolabelled immunoassays have served as definitive reference methods. Equipment for radiolabelled immunoassays is widely available and is not usually a constraint.

The difference in wavelength of gamma radiation emission from different radioisotopes is often sufficient virtually to resolve the specific detection of each using quite simple scintillation equipment. This property confers to radiolabelled immunoassays the convenience of specifically measuring more than one analyte in a single assay. Only a relatively few other systems share this potential.

The specific resolution of energy from two different radioisotopes would also allow for an application of Ekins's dual-label, 'radiometric', microspot immunoassay. This revolutionary principle involves the use of labelled 'sensor' antibodies and differently labelled 'developing' reagent, either antigen or antibody. Measuring a ratio of the two or the fractional binding site occupancy gives an analytical system essentially independent both of antibody concentration and of sample volume (Ekins, 1992).

Reagent-coated microtitre plates are considered by many to be an extremely convenient format for high-throughput assays. Radiolabelled immunoassays are readily adapted to this format.

Economics

In general, radioiodinated tracers and gamma counters are cheaper to buy and use than many alternatives (Edwards, 1990). The additional cost of liquid scintillation counting and subsequent disposal of waste scintillant associated with tritiated tracers may mean that they do not offer any particular cost advantage. Often, the use of 'alternative' tracers will incur additional expense and, in some cases, will double the cost of basic components.

Safety and Legislation

Legislation relating to the use of radioisotopes is a significant consideration in respect of radiolabelled immunoassays. However, publications referring to the use of radiolabelled immunoassays as a 'health hazard' clearly need further discussion. The data presented earlier in this chapter indicate that the health hazard incurred in using radiolabelled immunoassays is relatively minor, if not negligible, and has often been misrepresented and exaggerated. It is difficult to equate or compare radiotoxicity to other forms of toxicity, and many laboratories use highly toxic chemicals that could cause much more harm than radioiodine or tritium.

Although the production of radioiodinated tracers using high levels of radioactivity must always be practised and monitored with caution, considerable experience in this area indicates that there are no harmful effects. The very low levels of radioactivity used in the analytical methods clearly present no danger to the operator, unless the combined tracers from several assays are totally ingested. It is possible that the ubiquitous buffer component sodium azide represents a greater health hazard following ingestion than the radioisotope.

The presence of legislation may represent a constraint in some circumstances; however, in the clinical environment, where many medical radioisotopes are indispensable, the additional use of radiolabelled immunoassays should not present a significant problem. In conclusion, in the author's view, radiolabelled immunoassays have excellent characteristics with specific advantages that will ensure their continued use for many years.

REFERENCES

Addison, G. M. & Hales, C. N. (1971) *Horm. Metab. Res.* **3**, 59.

Arquila, E. R. & Statvitsky, A. B. (1956) *J. Clin. Invest.* **35**, 458.

Bolton, A. E. & Hunter, W. M. (1973) The labelling of proteins to high specific radioactivities by conjugation to a ^{125}I-containing acylating agent. *Biochem. J.* **133**, 529–538.

Bolton, A. E. & Hunter, W. M. (1986) Radioimmunoassay and related methods. In: *Handbook of Experimental Immunology* Vol.1 (ed. Weir, D. M.) pp. 26.1–26.56 (Blackwell Scientific Publications, Oxford).

Chard, T. (1978) *An Introduction to Radioimmunoassay and Related Techniques.* (North-Holland Publishing, Amsterdam).

David, G. S. (1972) Solid-state lactoperoxidase: A highly stable enzyme for simple, gentle iodination of proteins. *Biochem. Biophys. Res. Commun.* **48**, 464.

Edwards, R. (1985) *Immunoassay: An Introduction* (William Heinemann Medical Books, London).

Edwards, R. (1990) Radioimmunoassay. In: *Peptide Hormone Secretion* pp. 71–95 (IRL Press, Oxford).

Edwards, R., Lalloz, M. & Pull, P. I. (1983) Radioiodination of proteins by three procedures: Solid-phase lactoperoxidase, chloramine-T and Iodogen. In: *Immunoassays for Clinical Chemistry* (eds Hunter, W. M. and Corrie, J. T.) pp. 277–285 (Churchill Livingstone, Edinburgh).

Ekins, R. P. (1960) The estimation of thyroxine in human plasma by an electrophoretic technique. *Clin. Chim. Acta.* **5**, 453.

Ekins, R. P. (1974) Automation of radioimmunoassay and other saturation assay procedures. In: *Radioimmunoassay and Related Procedures in Medicine.* pp. 91–109 (International Atomic Energy Agency, Vienna).

Ekins, R. P. (1976) General principles of hormone assay. In: *Hormone Assays and their Clinical Application* (eds Loraine, J. H. & Bell, E. T.) pp. 1–72 (Churchill Livingstone, Edinburgh).

Ekins, R. P. (1992) *Development of Radioimmunoassay and Related Procedures* Proceedings Symposium, Vienna, 1991, 3 (International Energy Agency, Vienna).

Ekins, R. P., Newman, G. B., & O'Riordan, J. L. H. (1968) Theoretical aspects of 'saturation' and radioimmunoassay. In: *Radioisotopes in Medicine: In vitro Studies* Proceedings Symposium, Oak Ridge, 1967. (eds Hayes, R. L., Goswitz, F. A. & Pearson-Murphy, B. E.) pp. 59–100 (US Atomic Energy Commission).

Fraker, P. J. & Speck, J. C. (1978) Protein and cell membrane iodination with a sparingly soluble chloramide, 1,3,4,6-tetrachloro-3α,6α-diphenylglycoluril. *Biochem. Biophys. Res. Commun.* **80**, 849.

Greenwood, F. C., Hunter, W. M., & Glover, J. S. (1963) The preparation of ^{131}I–labelled human growth hormone of high specific radioactivity. *Biochem. J.* **89**, 114–123.

Haberman, E. (1970) *Z. Klin. Chem. Klin. Biochem.* **8**, 51.

Hart, H. E. & Greenwald, E. D. (1979) Scintillation proximity assay (SPA): a new method of immunoassay. *Molec. Immunol.* **16**, 265–267.

Hayes, R. L., Goswitz F. A. & Pearson-Murphy, B. E. (eds) (1968) *Radioisotopes in*

Medicine: In vitro *studies* Proceedings Symposium, Oak Ridge, USA (US Atomic Energy Commission).

Hourd, P. & Edwards, R. (1989) Measurement of human growth hormone in urine: Development and validation of a sensitive and specific assay. *J. Endocrinol.* **121**, 167–175.

Hunter, W. M. & Corrie, J. E. T. (eds) (1983) *Immunoassays for Clinical Chemistry* Proceedings Workshop, Edinburgh, 1982 (Churchill Livingstone, Edinburgh).

Hunter, W. M. & Greenwood, F. C. (1962) Preparation of Iodine-131 labelled human growth hormone of high specific activity. *Nature* **194**, 495–496.

International Atomic Energy Agency (1970) In vitro *Procedures with Radioisotopes in Medicine* Proceedings Symposium, Vienna (International Atomic Energy Agency, Vienna).

International Atomic Energy Agency (1974) *Radioimmunoassay and Related Procedures in Medicine* Proceedings Symposium, Istanbul, 1973 (International Atomic Energy Agency, Vienna).

International Atomic Energy Agency (1978) *Radioimmunoassay and Related Procedures in Medicine* Vol. 1 & 2 Proceedings Symposium, Berlin 1977 (International Atomic Energy Agency, Vienna).

International Atomic Energy Agency (1982) *Radioimmunoassay and Related Procedures in Medicine* Proceedings Symposium, Vienna, 1982 (International Atomic Energy Agency, Vienna).

International Atomic Energy Agency (1986) *Nuclear Medicine and Related Radionuclide Applications in Developing Countries* Proceedings Symposium, Vienna, 1985 (International Atomic Energy Agency, Vienna).

Jackson, T. M. & Ekins, R. P. (1986) Theoretical limitations on immunoassay sensitivity. *J. Immunol. Meth.* **87**, 13–20.

Jackson, T. M., Marshall, N. J., & Ekins, R. P. (1983) Optimisation of immunoradiometric (labelled antibody) assays. In: *Immunoassays for Clinical Chemistry* (eds Hunter, W. M. & Corrie, J. T.) pp. 557–575 (Churchill Livingstone, Edinburgh).

Kirkham, K. E. & Hunter, W. M. (eds) (1971) *Radioimmunoassay Methods Proceedings Workshop*, Edinburgh 1970 (Churchill Livingstone, Edinburgh).

Marchalonis, J. J. (1969) An enzymatic method for the trace iodination of immunoglobulins and other proteins. *Biochem. J.* **113**, 299–305.

Miles, L. E. M. & Hales, C. N. (1968) Labelled antibodies and immunological assay systems. *Nature* **219**, 186.

Morgan, C. R. (1966) Immunoassay of human insulin and growth hormone simultaneously using ^{131}I and ^{125}I tracers. *Proc. Soc. Exp. Biol. Med.* **123**, 230–233.

Nars, P. W. & Hunter, W. M. (1973) A method for labelling oestradiol-17 with radioiodine for radioimmunoassays. *Endocrinology* **57**, xlvii–xlviii.

Oliver, G. C., Parker, B. M., Brasfield, D. L. *et al.* (1968) The measurement of digitoxin in human serum by radioimmunoassay. *J. Clin. Invest.* **47**, 1035.

Pennisi, F. & Rosa, U. (1969) Preparation of radioiodinated insulin by constant current electrolysis. *J. Nuc. Biol. Med.* **13**, 64–70.

Siitari, H. & Oikari, T. (1992) In: *Liquid Scintillation Spectrometry* (eds Noakes, J. E., Schönhofer, F. & Polach, H.) pp. 301–305 (Radiocarbon, 1993).

St Bartholomew's Hospital (1987) Local radiation protection rules – radionuclide laboratories. Local Rules compiled for St Bartholomew's Hospital, London.

Udenfriend, S., Gerber, L. D., Brink, L. & Spector, S. *et al.* (1985) *Scintillation Proximity Radioimmunoassay Utilizing I-125-Labeled Ligands* Proc. Natl Acad. Sci. USA, **82**, pp. 8672–8676.

Wide, L. (1971) Solid phase antigen–antibody systems. In: *Radioimmunoassay Methods.* (eds Kirkham, K. E. and Hunter, W. M.) pp. 405–416, (Churchill Livingstone, Edinburgh).

Wolstenholme, G. E. W. & Cameron, M. P. (eds) (1962) *Immunoassay of Hormones* Ciba Foundation Colloquia on Endocrinology (Churchill Livingstone, London).

Yalow, R. S. & Berson, S. A. (1960) Immunoassay of endogenous plasma insulin in man. *J. Clin. Invest.* **39**, 1157–1175.

Chapter 15

Enzyme Immunoassay: with and without Separation

James P. Gosling

INTRODUCTION

In 1971 enzymes were first introduced as alternatives to radioisotopes in immunoassays (Van Weeman and Schuurs, 1971), and they have since become the most versatile and popular class of labelling substance for nonisotopic immunoassays. Enzyme-immunoassays have been the primary subject of quite a large number of books, symposium volumes (Maggio, 1980; Malvano, 1980; Ishikawa et al., 1981; Avrameas et al., 1983, 1992; Ngo and Lenhoff, 1985; Tijssen, 1985; Kemeny and Challcombe, 1988; Ternynck and Avrameas, 1988; Wreghitt and Morgan-Capner, 1990; Crowther, 1995) and reviews (Wisdom, 1976, 1981; Voller et al., 1978; Oellerich, 1984; Ishikawa, 1987; Ishikawa et al., 1989; Ngo, 1991), and an important concern in other books and reviews (Voller et al., 1981; Langone and Van Vunakis, 1982; Collins, 1985, 1988; Ngo, 1987; Albertson and Haseltine, 1988; Howanitz, 1988; Morris et al., 1988; Gosling, 1990, 1993).

ENZYMES

Enzymes are biological catalysts; by lowering activation energy they accelerate chemical reactions without themselves being changed in the process. Almost all enzymes are high molecular mass proteins or glycoproteins and the part of the enzyme that interacts with the reactants is called the active site. Like all true catalysts, enzymes do not affect the state of equilibrium of a reaction; they just permit equilibrium to be attained much more rapidly.

The activities of some enzymes are very impressive. Each molecule of the exceptionally fast enzyme catalase can break down $>10^7$ molecules of H_2O_2 a second. Enzymes are also specific; any one enzyme catalyses only one type of reaction with structural and stereospecific selectivity for every reactant.

Classification and Terminology

There are many thousands of different kinds of enzyme. Some have simple common names, such as catalase or peroxidase, that tell us little about their functions. Most, such as β-D-galactosidase or acetlycholinesterase have names that indicate the reaction catalysed and something of the substrate specificity.

In addition, a rational naming and numbering system has been devised by the Enzyme Commission of the International Union of Biochemistry. The six main classes are oxidoreductases, transferases, hydrolases, lyases, isomerases and ligases. Each enzyme is given a number, for example peroxidase is EC 1.11.1.7. The first three numbers define major class, subclass and sub-subclass, respectively, while the last number indicates the order in which an enzyme was added to the sub-subclass list. Recently, a total of 3,196 enzyme activities had been classified (Webb, 1992), being an increase of 29% over the previous 8 years. It is important to be aware that this classification system is not primarily concerned with the structure, origin or exact biological properties of enzymes, and that enzymes from different species with greatly different susceptibilites to inhibitors and heat stabilities may be designated by the same number, for example both lactoperoxidase and horseradish peroxidase are EC 1.11.1.7. Nevertheless, this system helps greatly in the avoidance of ambiguity and, along with its biological origin and source of supply, the EC number should be quoted for every enzyme of importance in research articles and reports.

The reactants entering enzyme-catalysed reactions are termed substrates, and those leaving are termed products. Many enzymes in metabolism use one or more of a limited range of co-substrates that act as carriers of electrons, reducing equivalents (e.g. nicotinamide adenine dinucleotide, NAD^+), phosphate (adenosine triphosphate, ATP) or acetyl groups (coenzyme A) etc. These are termed coenzymes and in metabolism are converted back to their original forms in other reactions. Many enzymes require tightly bound organic cofactors that are termed prosthetic groups (e.g. haem or flavin adenine dinucleotide, FAD). Metal ions such as Mg^{2+} or Fe^{2+} are also important cofactors and may associate tightly or loosely with the enzyme, or form an essential complex with a coenzyme or substrate. An enzyme missing a prosthetic group or tightly bound metal ion is called an apoenzyme, while a complete enzyme is called a holoenzyme.

Enzyme Kinetics

The activity of an enzyme is measured by preparing a pH-buffered solution of the enzyme, substrate(s) and any cofactor(s). The reaction is timed from when the last component (enzyme or substrate) is added. Then while the activity is constant, the change in concentration of a substrate, a product or a coenzyme is measured either continuously for a short time or after a fixed number of minutes and the activity expressed as moles of substrate converted per second. Specific enzyme activity is commonly expressed as μmol per min per mg protein present in the enzyme solution being assayed, and is useful for monitoring the progress of enzyme purification.

In normal enzyme assays and in classical enzyme kinetic studies the total molar concentration of enzyme $[E_T]$ is very low compared to the concentrations of substrates and soluble cofactors. In a case where there is a single substrate (S) and a single product (P) the catalysed reaction may be expressed as follows:

$$E + S \Leftrightarrow ES \Rightarrow E + P$$

E and S bind together reversibly with a certain affinity to form a complex ES, and [ES] determines the velocity (v) of the overall reaction giving P (and free E).

After enzyme and substrate are combined in the reaction mixture the concentration of the enzyme substrate complex [ES] increases and the concentration of free enzyme $[E_F]$ decreases, but the system soon reaches a steady state in which [ES] is constant (Figure 1a). The rate constants governing the individual forward and reverse reactions combine to give the steady-state Michaelis constant (K_m) with units of mol l^{-1}.

With $[E_T]$ constant, the steady-state [ES] is dependent on [S] up to a concentration of [S] that effectively saturates all molecules of the enzyme and gives the maximum initial velocity (V_{max}) of the reaction (Figure 1b). For many simpler enzymes experimentally determined

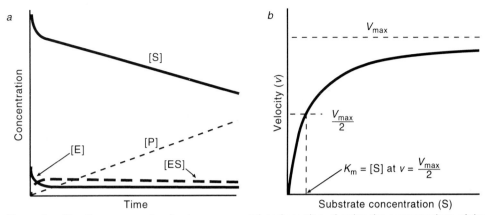

Figure 1 *a*, The time course of a simple enzyme-catalysed reaction, showing the concentrations of the single substrate [S], the single product [P], free enzyme [E] and enzyme-substrate complex [ES]. The first part of the time course is exaggerated to depict the progressive attainment of the steady-state [ES]. The steady reaction velocity, *v* (e.g. moles converted per second), is represented by the slope of the substrate or product concentration plot. Increasing the initial [S] at constant [E] will increase [ES] and consequently *v* (see below). Correspondingly, as the reaction progresses and [S] is used up both [ES] and *v* will gradually decrease. *b*, The dependence of the reaction velocity *v* on [S] for a similar enzyme-catalysed reaction. At extremely high [S] *v* approaches a maximum indicated by V_{max}. When the plot of *v* against [S] is truly hyperbolic, the Michaelis-Menten constant, K_m, is defined as [S] when *v* = $V_{max}/2$. Put simply, the lower the K_m the greater the affinity of substrate for the active site.

hyperbolic substrate dependence curves like that in Figure 1b correspond exactly to plots of *v* against [S] where *v* is calculated from [S] with the Michaelis-Menten equation:

$$v = \frac{V_{max}[S]}{[S] + K_m}$$

Note that the K_m corresponds to the substrate concentration necessary to give half the V_{max} (Figure 1b), and that the lower the K_m the greater the apparent affinity of the enzyme for its substrate. K_m and V_{max} are estimated graphically from the results of experiments like this. For enzymes with more than one substrate or with cofactors, the K_m for each substrate, coenzyme or other cofactor may be obtained by varying its concentration and measuring the reaction velocity, while maintaining the concentrations of all other substrates and cofactors in excess. Many enzymes, particularly those acting as control points, have much more complex kinetics and most of those used for immunoassays have individual kinetic peculiarities.

The turnover number of an enzyme, also referred to as its k_{cat}, is the maximum number of moles of substrate that one mole of enzyme can convert to product per second, given that each enzyme has one active site. It is calculated as follows:

$$k_{cat} = \frac{V_{max}}{[E_T]}$$

A compound that inhibits the catalytic activity of an enzyme may act reversibly or irreversibly. Reversible inhibitors may compete with substrate for occupancy of the active site or (as in the case of metabolic allosteric inhibitors) bind to other sites. Often they bind specifically with high affinity, as indicated by a low inhibition constant (K_i, units of mol l^{-1}). Irreversible inhibitors are chemically reactive agents that form more or less permanent complexes with a susceptible group at the active site. Although specific for this group, unless they are structurally complementary to the active site they may bind with very low affinity. Irreversible enzyme inhibitors such as acetazolamide (inhibits carbonic anhydrase, EC 4.2.1.1), methotrexate (inhibits dihydrofolate reductase, EC 1.5.1.3) and a *p*-amidinophenylester of cinnamate (inhibits thrombin, EC 3.4.21.5) have been used as labelling substances in the development of enzyme-mediated separation-free immunoassays (see below).

Enzyme Assays

Enzyme assays are usually performed with excess concentrations of substrates and cofactors (at least 5–10 times the K_m in each case if there is no substrate inhibition and if the substrate is sufficiently soluble and inexpensive) at suitable temperatures and pH and in the absence of inhibitory substances. Soon after the reactants are mixed together the 'initial' velocity of the reaction is established, and this is usually linear until sufficient product accumulates to cause product inhibition in susceptible enzymes, or until the substrate becomes limiting. When enzymes are assayed with a fixed reaction time (say 10–30 min), no such activity-limiting condition should have had time to become established before the end of the incubation, and the velocity should be constant over the whole period. A 'kinetic assay' is when the rate of formation of a reaction-dependent chromogen (or fluorogen etc.) is continuously monitored; this may be technically much more complex but can allow a wider range of activities to be measured.

Increasing temperature increases the k_{cat} until the heat lability of the enzyme protein causes the rate of increase to falter, halt and become negative. Assay temperatures should be chosen so as to maximise activity while ensuring stability during the time of incubation.

As proteins, enzymes maintain their structures and are stable only within a limited range of pH. Within this range both k_{cat} and K_m often depend on pH, because of effects on ionising groups at the active site or on reactants, or even because of changes in the tertiary structure of the enzyme. The optimum pH range for an enzyme may be relatively broad or quite narrow, and the best pH for the routine measurement of the activity of an enzyme may represent a compromise between its optimum pH and pH optima for the activities, solubilities, extinction coefficients etc. of other reactants.

Advantages and Limitations as Labelling Substances

The general suitability of a labelling substance depends on it having a combination of advantageous physicochemical properties. Of the nonisotopic labelling substances, enzymes are measurable by the greatest variety of methods and, with secondary amplification, are measurable in the smallest molecular quantities (see below). This means that enzymes are perhaps the most versatile class of labelling substance and they are indeed used in a wide range of assay formats, from the most simple and easily performed to the most sensitive and automated.

Therefore, enzymes score very well under the criteria for a good labelling substance, except that they are invariably of high molecular mass. Large enzyme-containing conjugates diffuse slowly and may have a greater tendency to bind nonspecifically to, for example, reaction vessels than some other labels. In addition, although properly stored enzyme conjugates usually have shelf-lives measured in years, enzymes are more susceptible to inactivation by environmental factors than are fluorescent or chemiluminescent compounds.

The Variety of Enzymes

Enzymes are perhaps the most varied class of labelling substances and perusal of relevant journals and volumes of the Immunoassay Kit Directory (Seth, 1996) indicates that the most common enzyme label in immunoassays is horseradish peroxidase, with alkaline phosphatase

Enzyme	Source	EC number	References
Acetylcholinesterase	*Electrophorus electricus*	3.1.1.7	*a*
Alkaline phosphatase	Calf Intestine	3.1.3.1	*b*
Catalase	Liver	1.11.1.6	*c*
β-D-Galactosidase	*E. coli*	3.2.1.23	*d*
Glucoamylase	*Rhizopus niveus*	3.2.1.3	*e*
Glucose oxidase	*Aspergillus niger*	1.1.3.4	*f*
Glucose-6-phosphate dehydrogenase	*Leuconostoc Mesenteroides*	1.1.1.49	*g*
β-Lactamase	Bacillus species	3.5.2.6	*h*
Lysozyme	Egg white	3.2.17	*i*
Peroxidase	Horseradish	1.11.1.7	*j*
Pyrophosphatase	*E. coli*	3.6.1.1	*k*
Urease	Jack bean	3.5.1.5	*l*

Table 1 Some enzymes used as immunoassay labels. References: *a*, Oellerich, 1984; Frobert and Grassi, 1992. *b*, Brown *et al.*, 1984; Hosada *et al.*, 1985; Shimizu *et al.*, 1985; Valkirs and Barton, 1985; Bronstein *et al.*, 1989; Ishikawa *et al.*, 1989; Schaap *et al.*, 1989; Christopolous and Diamandis, 1992; Hadas *et al.*, 1992; Cook and Self, 1993; Koshkinen *et al.*, 1995; Mares *et al.*, 1995; Roberts and Jackson, 1995; Satoh *et al.*, 1995; Van Kamp *et al.*, 1996. *c*, Oellerich, 1984. *d*, Ishikawa, 1987; Freytag *et al.*, 1984; Takayasu *et al.*, 1985; Pauillac *et al.*, 1993; Ruan *et al.*, 1993. *e*, Ishikawa, 1973. *f*, Oellerich, 1984. *g*, Jaklitsch, 1985; Beresini *et al.*, 1993; Yamamoto *et al.*, 1995. *h*, Saha and Das, 1991; Prabhasankar *et al.*, 1993. *i*, Rubenstein *et al.*, 1972. *j*, Boitieux *et al.*, 1984; Munro and Stabenfeldt, 1984; Thorpe *et al.*, 1985; Abdul-Ahad and Gosling, 1987; Ishikawa, 1987; Ikemoto *et al.*, 1993; Larue *et al.*, 1993; Aoyagi *et al.*, 1995; Chegini *et al.*, 1995; Henderson *et al.*, 1995; Ohkaru *et al.*, 1995; Rabitzsch *et al.*, 1995; Spiehler *et al.*, 1996. *k*, Peuravuori and Korpela, 1993. *l*, Lo *et al.*, 1988.

in second place, confirming a survey carried out in 1990 (Gosling, 1990). These enzymes are even more dominant in commercial enzyme-immunoassay (EIA) kits (Seth, 1996), and no other enzyme seems likely to challenge their positions in the near future. Table 1 lists a selection from the large number of enzymes that have been tested in immunoassay labels.

Horseradish Peroxidase

The popularity of 'hydrogen-peroxide oxidoreductase' from *Amoracia rusticana* (horseradish peroxidase (HRP)) is largely due to the sensitivity of its colorimetric and luminometric assay systems, its suitability for diverse conjugation procedures and its relatively small molecular size. Its disadvantages are its susceptibility to a wide range of inhibitors, relative fragility and complex reaction kinetics.

The high specific activity isoenzyme C of HRP from *A. rusticana* is a 308-residue, 44,000 M_r glycoprotein, with four disulphide bridges, six lysines, eight O-linked carbohydrate chains (making 20% by weight) and a protoporphyrin IX haemin prosthetic group. The Reinzeitszahl (RZ) number quoted for preparations of purified HRP is the ratio of the optical absorbances at 403 nm and 275 nm, and is a measure of haemin content rather than of specific enzyme activity. However, the absorbance of a pure enzyme solution with a 10 mm pathlength at 403 nm (22.5 for 1% *w/v*, 227 μmol l^{-1}) can be used to estimate enzyme concentration. Pure HRP is stable when stored dry at $-20\,°C$ and solutions of enzyme conjugates can be stable for years when stored frozen (a suitable storage medium used in my own laboratory is 1.36 mol glycerol, 10 mmol sodium phosphate, 30 μmol bovine serum albumin, 20 μmol cytochrome *c* per litre, pH 7.4).

The substrate is hydrogen peroxide and only a limited range of other peroxides are acted upon. The reaction is as follows:

$$H_2O_2 + 2DH \Rightarrow 2H_2O + 2D$$

where DH and D represent the reduced and oxidised hydrogen donor, respectively. The kinetics of HRP are complex as it is subject to substrate inhibition; high concentrations of peroxide cause oxidative inactivation of an intermediate form of the enzyme participating in the reaction. This means that a carefully chosen concentration, rather than excess substrate, should be used in assays for HRP activity. Hydrogen peroxide has a molar extinction coefficient (10 mm path) of 43.6 at 240 nm and the working stock concentration can therefore be checked. The final concentration used is usually in the range 2–6 mmol l^{-1}. Preparation of stock solutions of hydrogen peroxide should be done carefully, as the inadvertent addition of an extra drop may be sufficient to cause inhibition.

In contrast to the the relatively tight substrate specificity, a very wide range of compounds can act as efficient hydrogen donors. To measure HRP activity, donors are used that have oxidised forms with very high optical extinction coefficients, or that are fluorescent or undergo luminescent decay. However, o-phenylenediamine (OPD), one of the most efficient donors, is a mutagen. The most popular colorimetric donors, 2,2'-azino-di-[3-ethylbenzthiazoline-6-sulphonate] (ABTS), OPD and 3,3',5,5'-tetramethylbenzidine (TMB) (apparently the least toxic) are all available in tablet form, which reduces the possible risk from airborne particles generated when making solutions. Complete assay solutions with TMB and hydrogen peroxide are also available commercially (Kirkegaard and Perry Labs, Gaithersburg, MD, USA). (See also below under Measuring Enzyme Activity.)

Alkaline Phosphatase

Alkaline phosphatase (AP) is more formally named 'orthophosphoric monoester phosphohydrolase, alkaline optimum'. The enzyme used for immunoassays is a dimeric, zinc-containing, 140,000 M_r glycoprotein purified from calf intestine. It is easily conjugated as it has many free amino groups that are not necessary for catalytic activity, and an isoelectric point of 5.7. Inhibitors of AP include inorganic orthophosphate, which may be present in buffers, wash-solutions or as a contaminant of substrate, zinc chelators, borate, carbonate and urea. It has an activity pH optimum of 9.5–10.5, depending on substrate, substrate concentration and ionic strength, and is rapidly inactivated at pH <6 because of loss of Zn^{2+}. When secondary binding sites for divalent metal ions on the enzyme are occupied, by Mg^{2+} for example, both substrate-binding sites are catalytically active. The conditions needed for long-term storage at $-20\,^{\circ}C$ are 50% glycerol, 5 mmol l^{-1} $MgCl_2$, 0.2 mmol l^{-1} $ZnCl_2$ and a pH of 8.0–8.3 maintained by 10 mmol l^{-1} Tris-HCl.

Alkaline phosphatase catalyses the dephosphorylation of a wide variety of phosphate esters of primary alcohols, phenols and amines. The most common substrate is *p*-nitrophenol phosphate, giving a highly coloured nitrophenol product. Other substrates when dephosphorylated yield products that are insoluble and coloured, fluorescent (or act as cofactors for fluorescence), luminescent or electrically conductive. (See below under Measuring Enzyme Activity.)

Although AP gives labels with molar specific activities one-tenth or less than HRP when assayed colorimetrically, AP is popular because of its comparative ruggedness and the many and varied methods for its measurement, including multistage assays which greatly increase specific activity (see below also).

Others

β-D-galactosidase is sometimes favoured when a low detection limit is required and when equipment for fluorometric determination of the end point is available (Paulliac *et al.*, 1993; Ruan *et al.*, 1993). Acetylcholinesterase and β-lactamase are characterised by very high turnover numbers (14,000 and 2,000 respectively) and good long-term stability, and they have had many applications (e.g. Saha and Das, 1991; Frobert and Grassi, 1992; Prabhasankar *et al.*, 1993). Glucose-6-phosphate dehydrogenase is used in labels for EMIT assays (Jaklitsch, 1985; Beresini *et al.*, 1993).

Enzymes in Secondary Labels

Quite often the label determined at the end of an immunoassay procedure is not the primary label and some primary-secondary label combinations used in enzyme-immunoassays are listed in Table 2. This approach to labelling started with the use of a labelled 'second' anti-

Secondary label	Primary label	References
Anti-FITC–enzyme	Anti-analyte–FITC	*a*
Anti-'species' IgG–enzyme	Same 'species' anti-analyte (IgG)	*b*
Avidin–enzyme	Anti-analyte–biotin	*c*
Biotin–enzyme + avidin	Anti-analyte–biotin	*d*
Protein A (or G)–enzyme	Anti-analyte (IgG)	*e*

Table 2 Some enzyme immunoassays with secondary labels. References: *a*, Harmer and Samuel, 1989. *b*, Casl and Grubb, 1993; Monaghan *et al.*, 1993; Guérin-Marchand *et al.*, 1994; Rothwell *et al.*, 1995. *c*, Avrameas, 1992; Baly *et al.*, 1993; Yang and HayGlass, 1993; Rønne *et al.*, 1994; Mares *et al.*, 1995; Jørgensen *et al.*, 1996. *d*, Avrameas, 1992. *e*, Reis *et al.*, 1988; Vincent and Samuel, 1993.

body in solid-phase immunoassays for antigen. For example, if the analyte binds to immobilised (solid phase, sp) sheep antibody (SAb) and unlabelled rabbit antibody (RAb) is used to complete the sandwich (sp-SAb—**Ag**—RAb), the concentration of the bound rabbit antibody may be determined with a labelled goat antibody (GAb) raised against rabbit whole IgG or its Fc fragment (sp-SAb—**Ag**—RAb—GAb-HRP). Here the constant region of the rabbit IgG can logically be said to be the primary 'labelling substance'. Alternatively, protein A/enzyme conjugate, or protein A/enzyme chimeric protein (Sun and Lew, 1992), can be used as a general-purpose reagent for the quantification of immobilised Fc.

The use of biotin conjugated to antibody (or antigen/hapten) as primary label, with labelled avidin or streptavidin as a secondary label, is a logical, universally applicable extension of the above approach. The concentration of biotinylated antibody can be determined by means of avidin conjugated to an enzyme. The use of the avidin-biotin combination is usually justified by citing the high affinity of streptavidin or avidin for biotin ($K_a = 10^{15}$ l mol^{-1}), but the affinities of avidin and an anti-biotin monoclonal antibody for biotinylated proteins have been reported to be similar and much lower than for free biotin (Vincent and Samuel, 1993). Fluorescein isothiocyanate (FITC) is also used to prepare primary labels (rather than to prepare fluorimetric labels), and the concentration of FITC-antigen or FITC-antibody is then determined by means of enzyme-labelled monoclonal antibody to FITC (Harmer and Samuel, 1989).

Multienzyme Complexes

A recurring approach to maximising the final signal obtained in immunoassays is to attempt to attach multiple molecules of the final labelling substance to each immune complex to be detected (Durbin and Bodmer, 1987; Avrameas, 1992). This may be achieved by manipulation of the biotin-avidin system (Avrameas, 1992), or, in enzyme-immunoassays, by the use of antibodies to the labelling enzyme. For example, in an assay for lymphocytic antigens (**Ag**) (Durbin and Bodmer, 1987) three reagents were used: mouse antibody to antigen (Mab1); complexes of enzyme and mouse anti-enzyme antibodies ([MAb2-β-D-galactosidase]$_n$); and rabbit anti-mouse IgG as bridging molecule (RAb). These were used with the intention of bringing about the association of multiple copies of the enzyme with each analyte molecule to be detected (sp-lymphocyte-**Ag**—MAb1—RAb—[MAb2-β-D-galactosidase]$_n$.

Sample (with complement components)
+ Reagent 1 (labelled liposomes with enzyme)

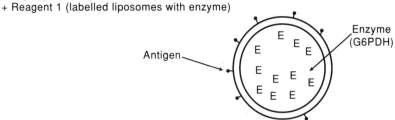

Antigen

Enzyme
(G6PDH)

+ Reagent 2 (antibodies, substrate, coenzyme)

G6P

NAD+

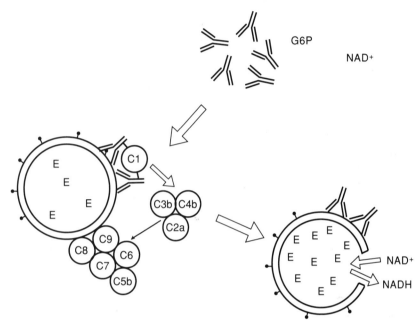

NAD+

NADH

Figure 2 Principle of a liposome-based separation-free assay system for total complement activity. Reagent 1 contains *N*-dinitrophenylaminocaproyldipalmitoylphosphatidylethanolamine-labelled (DNP-labelled) liposomes loaded with glucose-6-phosphate dehydrogenase (G6PDH, shown above as E). Reagent 2 contains anti-DNP antibody, glucose-6-phosphate (G6P) and NAD+. Sample, reagent 1 and then reagent 2 are mixed. Antibody binds to the DNP groups on the surface of the liposomes. Complement (C1–9) when present is activated by these bound antibodies resulting in damage to the liposomes and the escape of enzyme (E) into the general medium. The rate of appearance of NADH is continuously monitored at 340 nm indicating the total enzyme activity released, which is proportional to total complement activity in the sample. Reproduced from Yamamoto *et al.*(1995) with some adaptations.

In general, attempts to amplify the signal by assembling large label-containing complexes are inherently limited by steric effects and by high nonspecific binding of label. Therefore, although such tactics may be advantageous under certain circumstances, they are not usually considered relevant to the development of immunoassays with very low detection limits.

Alternatively, the use of liposomes, loaded with many enzyme molecules, as primary labelling substances (Canova-Davis *et al.*, 1986; Yamamoto *et al.*, 1995) may lead to amplification when the lysis of each vesicle releases many copies of the trapped enzyme (Figure 2). Such assays are usually 'separation-free'.

Enzyme	Assay method	Substrate etc.	References
Alkaline phosphatase	Amplified colorimetric	NADP etc.	a
		FADP etc.	b
	Amplified electrometric	NADP etc.	c
	Amplified fluorimetric	NADP etc.	d
	Colorimetric	4-Nitrophenyl-phosphate	e
	Electrochemical	1-Naphthyl phosphate	f
		p-Amino-phenyl phosphate	g
	Fluorometric	4-Methyl-umbelliferyl phosphate	h
	Luminometric	Adamantyl-1,2-dioxyethane	i
		Phenylphosphate-substituted dioxetane	j
	Radiometric	[³H]Adenosine monophosphate	k
	Time resolved (TR) fluorimetric	5-Fluorosalicyl phosphate	l
	Visual assessment	Bromochloroindoxyl phosphate (BCI)	m
		Indoxylphosphate	n
β-D-galactosidase	Colorimetric	2-Nitrophenyl-β-D-galactoside	o
	Fluorometric	4-Methylumbelliferyl-β-D-galactoside (MUG)	p
	Luminometric	Lactose with enzyme-coupled system	q
	Photodensitometry	MUG	r
Horseradish peroxidase	Colorimetric	H_2O_2 and o-phenylene-diamine (OPD)	s
		H_2O_2 and tetramethyl-benzidine	t
		H_2O_2, 3-methyl-2-benzothiazolinone hydrazone (MBTH) and 3-(dimethylamino) benzoic acid (DMAB)	u
	Electrochemical	H_2O_2 and iodide	v
	Fluorometric	3-p-Hydroxyphenyl- propionic acid	w
	Luminometric	Luminol	x
	Photodensitometry	H_2O_2 and OPD	y
	Visual assessment	H_2O_2 and 4-chloro-1-naphthol	z

Table 3 Assay methods for the principal enzymes used in immunoassays. References: *a*, Self, 1985. *b*, Obzansky *et al.*, 1991. *c*, Stanley *et al.*, 1988. *d*, Cook and Self, 1993. *e*, Ishikawa, 1987; Koshkinen *et al.*, 1995; Mares *et al.*, 1995; Roberts and Jackson, 1995; Satoh *et al.*, 1995. *f*, Athey *et al.*, 1993. *g*, Hadas *et al.*, 1992. *h*, Van Kamp *et al.*, 1996. *i*, Bronstein *et al.*, 1989. *j*, Schaap *et al.*, 1989. *k*, Harris *et al.*, 1979. *l*, Christopoulos and Diamandis, 1992. *m*, May, 1988. *n*, Valkirs and Barton, 1985. *o*, Ishikawa, 1987. *p*, Ruan *et al.*, 1993. *q*, Takayasu *et al.*, 1985. *r*, Labrousse and Avrameas, 1987. *s*, Howard *et al.*, 1989; Larue *et al.*, 1993; Monaghan *et al.*, 1993; Guérin-Marchand *et al.*, 1994; O'Rorke *et al.*, 1994; Rønne *et al.*, 1994; Aoyagi *et al.*, 1995; Henderson *et al.*, 1995; Ohkaru *et al.*, 1995; Rothwell *et al.*, 1995. *t*, Madersbacher and Berger, 1991; Ikemoto *et al.*, 1993; Madersbacher *et al.*, 1993; Mares *et al.*, 1995; Jørgensen *et al.*, 1996; Spiehler *et al.*, 1996. *u*, Geoghegan, 1985. *v*, Boitieux *et al.*, 1984. *w*, Tuuminen *et al.*, 1991. *x*, Thorpe *et al.*, 1985; Kricka *et al.*, 1996. *y*, Labrousse and Avrameas, 1987. *z*, Achord *et al.*, 1991; Houts, 1991.

MEASURING ENZYME ACTIVITY

The versatility of enzymes as labelling substances has much to do with the range of ways, each with certain advantages, by which enzyme activity may be measured. A wide variety of assay methods has been developed for each of the longer established and most widely used labelling enzymes (Table 3). The simplest and least expensive of these will be considered first.

Visual Assessment

Enzyme assays that generate a change in colour density, shade, area or location (or any other visible physical or optical characteristic) have been used for many qualitative and semiquantitative EIA procedures that are not dependent on instrumentation. Such visible end-point methods are sold over the counter for home use as, for example pregnancy tests, or are used in doctors' surgeries, or beside the hospitalised patient, and if inexpensive are of great value in all situations where laboratory facilities are poor or unavailable. If the colour change is permanent the assay device may be retained as a record of the result.

Used in conjuction with a simple instrument, such as a reflectance-colorimeter (Achord *et al.*, 1991), quantitative results may be calculated with reference to a standard, and an easily interpreted, printed result prepared. Although the principle of latex agglutination and the use of labelling substances such as highly coloured latex beads or colloidal-gold particles are also used to give immunoassays with visible end points, the most widespread and sensitive of such immunoassays use enzyme-containing labels (May, 1988; Achord *et al.*, 1991; Houts, 1991).

Most visible end-point enzyme-immunoassays, such as AccuLevel®, competitive, immunochromatography assays for drugs (Houts, 1991) or two-site ICON® immunoconcentration assays for antigens (Achord *et al.*, 1991), are carried out on a paper strip or a membrane (*see* Chapter 22). To ensure stable colour development the enzyme-substrates used must be converted to highly coloured insoluble product, which precipitates onto, and remains associated with, the paper or membrane.

Colorimetry

Colorimetric determination is the most common of all the methods used to measure the end point of enzyme-immunoassays because it is simple, well understood and more than adequate for most applications. Efficient, and sometimes highly sophisticated, microtitre plate readers are often already available in the users laboratory. In my own laboratory we have developed colorimetric horseradish peroxidase immunoassays with low detection limits for many steroids (Howard *et al.*, 1989; O'Rorke *et al.*, 1994) and proteins (Abdul-Ahad and Gosling, 1987; Monaghan *et al.*, 1993).

The limitations of a colorimetric end point are directly related to the fundamental limitations of colorimetry itself. By use of a colorimeter the intensity of the monochromatic light not absorbed by the sample is measured, so that to estimate low concentrations of chromogen small differences in intensity must be measured at high light intensity, thus limiting the lower detection limit. Also, the relationship between optical absorbance and the intensity of transmitted light is logarithmic, so that at high chromogen concentrations relatively large differences in optical absorbance correspond to very small differences in the intensity of unabsorbed light, thus limiting the precision of measurements. Therefore, it is usually advisable to design enzyme-immunoassays so that only optical absorbance readings in the range ~0.1 to ~1.5 are used. This would give a dynamic range of about 15, which is particularly constraining for reagent excess immunoassays.

However, extension of this dynamic range is made possible by simultaneous monitoring of absorbance at two or more wavelengths (Shimuzu *et al.*, 1985; Madersbacher and Berger, 1991; Madersbacher *et al.*, 1993). If wavelengths are chosen that correspond to the peak of the chromogen absorption peak and to a point low-down on its side, simple computation allows the effective range of the assay to be greatly increased. For example (Shimuzu *et al.*, 1985), *p*-nitrophenol (formed by alkaline phosphatase from *p*-nitrophenol phosphate) absorbs maximally at 405 nm but at 450 nm the molar extinction coefficient is about 20 % of that at 405 nm, so that dual measurements at these wavelengths can extend the range of enzyme activity readings by about a factor of five. With horseradish peroxidase and 3,3′,5,5′-tetramethylbenzidine (TMB) as cosubstrate, reading at the same two wavelengths allowed extension of the measuring range of an immunoenzymometric assay (IEMA) by a factor of about three (Madersbacher and Berger, 1991). Alternatively, the dynamic range of the colorimetric determination of enzyme activity may be extended by means of kinetic recording techniques as opposed to fixed time measurements. However, the ranges achieved in these ways may still be limited compared to the dynamic range possible with other enzyme assay methods such as time-resolved fluorometry (Christopoulos and Diamandis, 1992).

Fluorometry

Fluorometric measurements of very small concentrations of a pure fluorescent compound are precise because they are measured relative to an absence of light and very sensitive light detection systems can be used. Time-resolved fluorometric measurements reduce interference from contaminating fluorescent compounds thus enabling much of the theoretical potential of fluorometry to be exploited (Christopoulos and Diamandis, 1992). The potential of fluorometric measurements of enzyme activities in enzyme immunoassays has long been realised. Ishikawa (1987) tabulated the smallest detectable amounts of some enzymes used for immunoassays as determined with different assay systems. With 10-min incubations and a volume of 150 µl, amounts of, 25, 1,000 and 10,000 amol horseradish peroxidase, β-D-galactosidase and alkaline phosphatase, respectively, could be determind colorimetrically. Fluorometrically these limits decreased to 5, 0.2 and 10 amol, respectively. The Abbott IMx® automatic immunoassay analyser depends on fluorometric measurment of 4-methyl-umbelliferone formed from 4-methyl-umbelliferyl phosphate by the action of alkaline phosphatase (Van Kamp *et al.*, 1996).

Luminometry

Although luminometric assay methods have been developed for alkaline phosphatase (Bronstein *et al.*, 1989; Schaap *et al.*, 1989) and β-D-galactosidase (by means of an enzyme-coupled system, (Takayasu *et al.*, 1985), luminometric determination of horseradish peroxidase (Thorpe *et al.*, 1985) is more common.

By 'enhanced' luminescence determination is meant the addition of certain compounds to the assay buffer that enhance and prolong light emission from a luminescent reaction catalysed by the enzyme. For example, some phenol derivatives, including *p*-indophenol and *p*-phenylphenol, increase light emission from the peroxidase-catalysed oxidation of luminol by >1,000–fold and prolong light emission over several minutes. This obviates the need for initiation of the light-emitting reaction in the counting chamber of the luminometer and enables photographic determination of the end-point (De Boever *et al.*, 1983; Thorpe *et al.*, 1985).

Electrometry

The electrometric determination of enzyme activity has a number of inherent properties that could be highly advantageous for some immunoassay applications. Variably cloudy or coloured and even opaque solutions and containers can be monitored electrometrically, and the detection element can, potentially, be a tiny, remotely located probe. Electrometric immunoassays are reviewed in Chapter 19. Substrates yielding an electrochemically detectable product are used and the continuous operation of the enzyme leads to a large amplification of the measured signal as compared to the use of electrochemically detectable substances themselves in the label. Some electrometric enzyme immunoassays incorporate an extra amplification step (Stanley *et al.*, 1988) (*see* below).

Multistage Assay Systems

The impressive amplification method for the measurement of alkaline phasphatase developed by Colin Self (Self, 1985; Cook and Self, 1993) depends on the dephosphorylation of NADP$^+$ to NAD$^+$ (Figure 3). The NAD$^+$ then enters a specific redox cycle that cannot use NADP$^+$, where it is reduced by alcohol dehydrogenase to NADH, which is reconverted to NAD$^+$ by diaphorase with the concomitant reduction of *p*-iodonitrotetrazolium violet reagent to an intensely purple formazan dye. The NAD$^+$ is thus continuously cycled with the formation of more formazan with every turn of the cycle, giving approximately 100 times more 'colour'

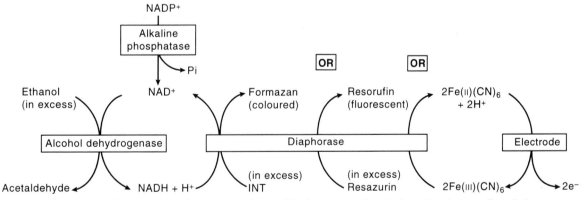

Figure 3 Colorimetric, fluorometric and amperometric amplification assays for alkaline phosphatase. For all three types of assay, the coenzyme nicotinamide adenine dinucleotide phosphate (NADP$^+$) acts as substrate for the phosphatase and is dephosphorylated to NAD$^+$. Present in excess are two enzymes, an NAD-specific alcohol dehydrogenase and diaphorase (a lipoyl dehydrogenase which also catalyses the NAD$^+$-dependent reduction of a range of substrates), ethanol as substrate for the alcohol dehydrogenase and diaphorase substrate. As NAD$^+$ is formed, a cycle begins that leads to the accumulation of acetaldehyde and diaphorase product. Therefore, the greater the activity of the phosphatase, the faster the cycle turns and the more diaphorase product is formed, with many molecules of product formed for each molecule of NAD$^+$ participating in the cycle. For the colorimetric assay the diaphorase substrate is iodonitrotetrazolium violet (INT) and this is reduced to the intensely red-coloured formazan. For the fluorometric assay the substrate is resazurin which is reduced to resorufin, a highly fluorescent compound. For the amperometric assay the substrate for diaphorase is ferricyanide which on reduction can then act to reduce a platinum electrode.

than a direct assay with *p*-nitrophenyl phosphate. Since it was first patented in 1982 this system has been quite widely applied in research and commercial enzyme-immunoassays for antigens and antibodies. It is now licensed to Dako Diagnostics Ltd. Two variations that have since been introduced concern the determination of the end point. Stanley *et al.* (1988) used amperometric determination of ferricyanide reduced by the diaphorase and reoxidised at the electrode, and Cook and Self (1993) used fluorimetric determination of resorufin, formed from nonfluorescent resazurin in the NADH-dependent diaphorase-catalysed reaction. The fluorescent system greatly extended the range of measurements and enabled the measurement of less than one-thousandth of an attomole (1 zeptomole) of alkaline phosphatase per micro-titre well and, consequently, the measurement of down to 17 amol l^{-1} of proinsulin by IEMA.

Another highly sensitive, multistage colorimetric assay for alkaline phosphatase, called the Rabin Cascade, was developed by Obzansky *et al.* (1991) and is in commercial use. The phosphatase converts the substrate, flavin adenine dinucleotide phosphate (FADP), to FAD which combines with excess holo-D-amino acid oxidase (EC 1.4.3.3) to give active oxidase. The oxidase then acts continuously to convert amino acid substrate, oxygen and H_2O to keto acid, ammonia and H_2O_2, which then acts as substrate for excess peroxidase to generate coloured product. This system can detect 5–10 fmol alkaline phosphate per tube.

CONJUGATION PROCEDURES

To prepare conjugates of antibodies, antigens or haptens with enzymes, the method of conjugation used should be particularly mild so as to maintain both immunological and enzymatic activities. It should also give conjugates that are stable.

Enzyme-Protein Conjugates

Glutaraldehyde Methods

Glutaraldehyde, a five-carbon dialdehyde, makes a versatile homobifunctional reagent that is very simple to use for linking together proteins via lysine ε-amino and N-terminal groups. Coupling procedures with glutaraldehyde may be carried out in one or two steps. One-step methods are not generally favoured for making labels because too many large aggregates and homoconjugates are produced. In two-step procedures one of the proteins (the enzyme for example) is first allowed to react with glutaraldehyde, the excess reagent is removed, and only then is the second protein (IgG for example) added and the conjugate allowed to form (Avrameas *et al.*, 1978). The coupling efficiency is greater and higher activtiy is retained than with one-step methods, although the recovey of enzyme activity may be still very low (<10%).

Periodate Oxidation of Glycoproteins

The oxidation of glycoproteins (e.g. horseradish peroxidase) with sodium periodate cleaves vicinal glycols of the carbohydrate residues to generate dialdehydes capable of reacting with free amino groups on other protein molecules to form Schiff-base linkages. After coupling, the Schiff-base linkages may be reduced with sodium borohydride. The method has been opti-

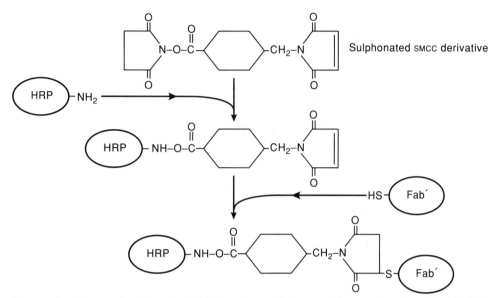

Figure 4 The conjugation of Fab' to horseradish peroxidase with *N*-succinimidyl-4-(*N*-maleimidomethyl)cyclohexane-1-carboxylate (SMCC). The cyclohexane bridge is claimed to give stability to the maleimide group. A sulphonated derivative of SMCC with improved water solubility is also available (Pierce, Rockford, Illinois, USA). *m*-Maleimidobenzoyl-*N*-hydroxysuccinimide ester (MBS) has the same reactive groups but a benzoyl bridge. In the first step SMCC is reacted with a protein containing available free amino groups, and no free sulphydryl group, in this case horseradish peroxidase (HRP). The consequent maleimide-substituted HRP is then reacted with the sulphydryl-containing protein, in this case Fab'. Both reactions proceed efficiently under mild conditions which facilitate full retention of enzyme and antigen-binding activities.

mised by Tijssen and Kurstak (1984) who reported 90% coupling efficiency and 90% retention of peroxidase activity.

Heterobifunctional Reagent Methods

Heterobifunctional reagent methods use reagents that can react with two different functional groups, one on each of the two proteins to be conjugated. The functional groups used are α- or ε-amino (lysine), sulphydryl (cysteine), imidazole (histidine) and phenolic (tyrosine) groups (Table 4). Although most proteins and most peptides have free amino groups, free sulphydryl groups are relatively rare in intact proteins and peptides, with the important exceptions of Fab' and β-D-galactosidase from *Escherichia coli*. The reaction sequence for the conjugation of an Fab' to an enzyme with free amino groups by means of a heterobifunctional coupling reagent is shown in Figure 4. Fab'-enzyme conjugates can retain full immunological activity because of the favourable geometry of the linkage and can retain full enzymatic activity because of the mildness of the reaction conditions (Ishikawa *et al.*, 1983; Abdul-Ahad and Gosling, 1987). The absence of the Fc from such conjugates greatly reduces binding to sample components. High specific activity, low nonspecific binding conjugates prepared in this way have enabled the development of assays for antigens and specific antibodies with detection limits down to 0.02 amol per tube (Ishikawa, 1987; Ishikawa *et al.*, 1989). The use of Fv fragments in immunoassays may further reduce nonspecific binding and interference from rheumatoid factors, complement and heterophilic antibodies (*see* Chapter 4).

Acronym	Name	Group 1 reacts with	Group 2 reacts with
ABDP	*N*-(4-aminobenzoyl)-*N*'-(pyridyldithiopropionyl)-hydrazine	–SH	–OH (tyrosine)
DPEM	*N*-[β-(4-diazophenyl)ethyl]maleimide (Geoghegan, 1985)	Phenol and imidazole	–SH
	Glutaraldehyde	–NH$_2$	–NH$_2$
HSAB	*N*-hydroxysuccinimidyl-4-azidobenzoate	–NH$_2$	–Unspecific
MBS	*m*-Maleimidobenzoyl-*N*-hydroxysuccinimide ester	–NH$_2$	–SH
SMCC	Succinimidyl-4-(*N*-maleimidomethyl) cyclohexane-1-carboxylate	–NH$_2$	–SH
SATA	*N*-hydroxysuccunimide S-acetylthioacetic acid (inserts protected –SH)	–NH$_2$	
SPDP	*N*-succinimidyl-3-(2-pyridyldithio)propionate (inserts protected –SH)	–NH$_2$	
–	2-Iminothiolane (Traut's reagent) (inserts –SH)	–NH$_2$	

Table 4 Reagents for protein-protein coupling, and for inserting sulphydryl groups into proteins. These are available from various suppliers including Pierce, Rockford, New Hampshire, USA; Boehringer Mannheim, Mannheim, Germany; and Pharmacia, Uppsala, Sweden.

Free sulphydryl groups may be generated by reductive cleavage of native cystine residues with reagents such as dithiothreitol or mercaptoethylamine, or may be introduced chemically. One of a number of available reagents (Table 4) may be used, often with a second step to remove the protective group and expose the sulphydryl.

Chimeric Proteins as Conjugates

Recombinant DNA technology may also be used to prepare protein-protein conjugates. Fusion of the genes for an enzyme and a binding protein can be done in such a way that one long polypeptide is synthesised; when this is correctly folded it contains catalytic and binding domains linked by a peptide bridge. Single-chain Fv fragments of antibodies (*see* Chapter 4) are very suitable for such applications.

Composite proteins such as these are called chimeric proteins after the mythical composite monster. However, their development is quite expensive and, because of inefficient folding, the initial yield of product with full catalytic and binding activites can be quite limited. Such methods may have greatest promise for the preparation of bulk reagents that have many applications, e.g. chimeric protein A/alkaline phosphatase for use as a second label (Sun and Lew, 1992).

Enzyme-labelled Haptens

The most popular procedures for the preparation of enzyme-hapten conjugates link haptens to free amino or sulphydryl groups, but other groups including phenolic, imidazole or carboxyl (glutamic or aspartic acid) can be the linkage site on the enzyme. On the hapten a carboxyl or an amino group is most commonly used and, if necessary, one may be added by derivitisation. In addition, a spacer group four to six atoms long between the hapten and the enzyme is usually necessary to allow adequate immunological recognition. A wide variety of common steroids (Steraloids, Wilton, NH, USA; Sigma Chemical Company, St Louis, MA, USA) and other haptens derivatised by the addition of potential bridging groups are available commercially. A range of haptens, including oestriol, oestradiol-17β, digoxin, theophylline, triiodothyronine and thyroxine, with both bridging groups and active functions already attached, are available from Boehringer Mannheim, Germany (Immunologicals for the Diagnostic Industry Catalogue).

In an EIA for hapten, the type of spacer group and its site of attachment to the hapten molecule may be the same in the enzyme-hapten conjugate as in the hapten-protein immunogen used to raise the antibody (homology) or they may be different (heterology). Heterology may concern the bridging group and/or the site of attachment. Site- or bridge-heterology decreases the affinity of the antibody for the enzyme-hapten conjugate and it used to be widely claimed that heterology is a necessary precondition for an EIA with a low detection limit. But most hapten EIAs are homologous and some of these have very low detection limits (Gosling, 1990).

The optimum hapten:enzyme ratio in conjugate for an EIA should be investigated each time by preparing a range of test conjugates starting with different ratios of reactant molarities. Often an incorpration ratio of 1:1 is suitable and a higher ratio results in a decrease in sensitivity (Hosada *et al.*, 1985). Determination of the ratio for hapten/horseradish peroxidase conjugates can be by spectral differences if such exist (as they do for steroids such as progesterone), but radioactive hapten may be used as a quantifiable tracer, or an immunoassay may be used to estimate the accessible haptens. The recovery of enzyme activity should be, or be near, 100%, and there should be negligible nonspecific binding; conjugates not meeting these criteria should normally be rejected for use in high-performance assays. The most usual coupling procedures for haptens and enzymes are the mixed anhydride and active-ester procedures.

Mixed Anhydride Procedure

Here a carboxyl group in the hapten is first converted to an acid anhydride that is then allowed to react with a protein amino group. In our own laboratory we have often successfully used the procedure described by Munro and Stabenfeldt (1984), by which the hapten reacts with isobutyl chloroformate in the presence of N-ethylmorpholine for two minutes at −20 °C, and is then transferred to react with the protein at the desired molar ratio of hapten:enzyme. It is important to maintain the pH of the protein near its isoelectric point, for example with horseradish peroxidase a pH of 8.0 should be maintained for efficient incorporation of hapten.

Active-ester Procedure

Here carbodiimide is used to enable the formation of an active N-succinimidyl ester from the carboxyl-containing hapten and N-hydroxysuccinimide (Hosada *et al.*, 1985) (Figure 5). This

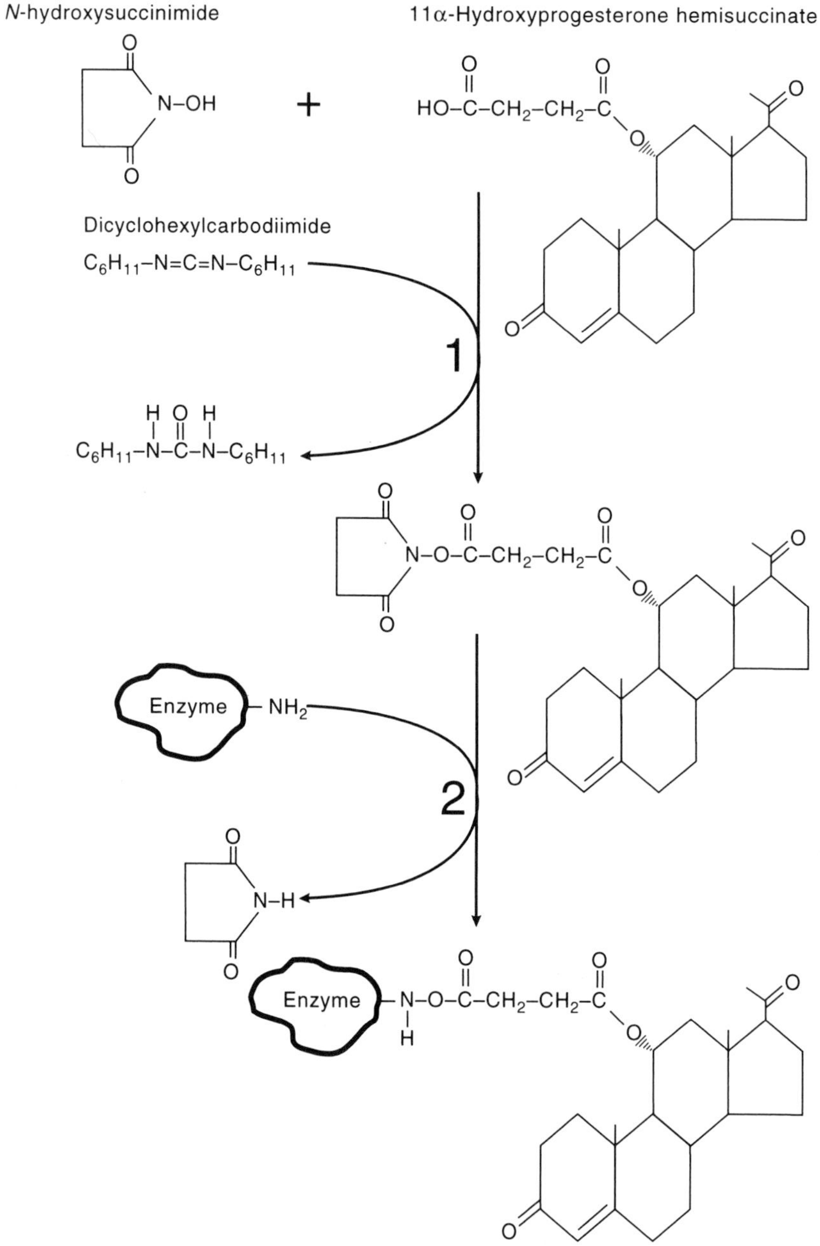

Figure 5 Active-ester procedure for the conjugation of steroid hapten to an enzyme or protein. This procedure is carried out in two steps (1 and 2 above), the first to generate the active-ester derivative of the carboxyl-containing hapten, which can then be used directly or stored until needed, and the second for the reaction of the activated hapten with the protein. Step 1: 11α-Hydroxyprogesterone hemisuccinate, the steroid to be conjugated, is reacted with N-hydroxy succinimide in the presence of dicyclohexylcarbodiimide in dioxane at room temperature (14–20 °C) for at least 2 h, with stirring. As the carbodiimide is transformed to *N,N*-dicyclohexyl urea, the NHS active-ester of the 11α-hydroxyprogesterone hemisuccinate is formed. The NHS ester is then isolated after dilution with water and extraction with ethyl acetate, and can be stored until needed. This procedure also removes residual carbodiimide, which could deactivate the protein during step 2, and facilitates the adjustment of the molar ratio of hapten to enzyme for step 2. Step 2: The active ester and enzyme (or carrier protein if an immunogen is being synthesised) are mixed together in 10 mmol/l^{-1} phosphate buffer, pH 7.0 and allowed to react at 4 °C overnight, before the conjugate is separated from the reactants by means of dialysis (with removal of precipitate by centrifugation) and gel filtration chromatography on Sephadex G 25.

procedure is similar to that described by Tijssen (1985), who reviewed many of the alternative approaches. The intermediate active-ester derivative of the hapten to be conjugated can be used directly or, more effectively, isolated in solid form. A range of such activated derivatives of steroid and thyroid hormones is available commercially from Boehringer Mannheim (Mannheim, Germany).

CLASSIFICATION OF ENZYME IMMUNOASSAYS

According to the 'antibody occupancy principle' of Ekins (Ekins and Chu, 1991; Chapter 9), when an immunoassay relies on the observation of binding sites unoccupied by analyte, the total number of sites available must be small to minimise error in the (indirect) estimation of occupied sites (reagent-limited assays); but when an immunoassay depends on the observation of sites occupied by analyte, errors may be minimised by the use of relatively large numbers of sites (reagent-excess assays). Essentially all current commercial and research enzyme-immunoassays can be classified as reagent-excess or reagent-limited (Table 5). Note that

Class	Analyte type	Subclass	References
Reagent excess	Antibodies	Labelled* antibody, two-site	a
	Antigens	Labelled* antibody, two-site	b
	Haptens	Labelled* antibody	c
		Selective antibody	d
Reagent limited	Antibodies	Labelled antibody	e
	Antigen or haptens	Labelled* antibody	f
		Labelled antigen or hapten	g
	Haptens	Labelled hapten, separation-free	h
	Haptens, free	Labelled 'analogue'	i
		Labelled antibody	j

*Directly or indirectly labelled.

Table 5 Classification of enzyme immunoassays. References: *a*, Thomas and Morgan-Capner, 1991; Frobert and Grassi, 1992; Kemeny, 1992; Goldblatt *et al.*, 1993; Lappalainen *et al.*, 1993; Ngai *et al.*, 1993; Olivieri *et al.*, 1993; Ward *et al.*, 1993; Underwood, 1993; Koshkinen *et al.*, 1995; Satoh *et al.*, 1995. *b*, Harris *et al.*, 1979; Valkirs and Barton, 1985; Abdul-Ahad and Gosling, 1987; Baly *et al.*, 1993; Casl and Grubb, 1993; Cook and Self, 1993; Ikemoto *et al.*, 1993; Larue *et al.*, 1993; Monaghan *et al.*, 1993; Peuravouri and Korpela, 1993; Ruan *et al.*, 1993; Yang and HayGlass, 1993; Rønne *et al.*, 1994; Aoyagi *et al.*, 1995; Ohkaru *et al.*, 1995; Rabitzsch *et al.*, 1995. *c*, Freytag *et al.*, 1984. *d*, Self *et al.*, 1994; Mares *et al.*, 1995. *e*, Ekins and Chu, 1991. *f*, Pauillac *et al.*, 1993; Ylätupa *et al.*, 1993; Yonezawa *et al.*, 1993; Henderson *et al.*, 1995; Roberts and Jackson, 1995; Rothwell and Kamanna, 1995. *g*, Munro and Stabenfeldt, 1984; Howard *et al.*, 1989; Saha and Das, 1991; Prabhasankar *et al.*, 1993; Wallemacq *et al.*, 1993; Yie *et al.*, 1993; O'Rorke *et al.*, 1994; Chegini *et al.*, 1995; Henderson *et al.*, 1995; Mares *et al.*, 1995; Spiehler *et al.*, 1996. *h*, Rubenstein *et al.*, 1972; Jaklitsch, 1985; Zuk *et al.*, 1985; Canova-Davis *et al.*, 1986; Henderson *et al.*, 1986; Chen *et al.*, 1987; Beresini *et al.*, 1993; Dasgupta *et al.*, 1993; Marenbloom and Oberhardt, 1995; Ngo, 1995. *i*, Kunst *et al.*, 1988. *j*, Christofides, 1992.

separation-free assays are indicated under reagent-limited assays for haptens; these will be discussed separately in the next section.

Reagent-excess Assays

Assays for Antibodies

Most routine immunoassays for the quantification of specific antibodies are reagent-excess and the majority of these use enzyme-containing labels (Kemeny, 1992). Most often, diluted test serum is added to excess antigen immobilised on a solid phase (sp-Ag), and the amount of specific antibody that binds (or is 'captured', sp-Ag—**Ab**) may then be quantified by the use of labelled antibodies that specifically bind to the constant region of the immunoglobulin class or classes of interest (e.g. sp-Ag—IgG_1—Ab-enzyme).

Alternatively, and much less frequently, an 'antigen capture' approach may be used. In such assays, immobilised anti-immunoglobulin-class antibodies (sp-Ab) first adsorb relevant immunoglobulins from the sample (sp-Ab– IgA_1, added antigen is then specifically 'captured' only by the antibodies of interest (sp-Ab—IgA_1—Ag), and the amount of antigen bound is finally determined by, for example, the use of a labelled antibody to the antigen (sp-Ab–IgA_1—Ag—Ab-enzyme). In one such assay (Olivieri *et al.*, 1993) F(ab')$_2$ fragments of an antibody against human IgG_1 were immobilised and excess antigen with enzyme-labelled antibody were used (sp-F(ab')$_2$—IgG_1—Ag—Ab-peroxidase). 'Antigen capture' assays may be preferable for specific antibodies of the minor immunoglobulin classes, as antibodies of other classes do not interfere because they are discarded after the first step. In addition, because the antigen capture may act as an immunoaffinity purification step, they may operate well with impure antigen, and the structural and antigenic integrity of the antigen may be better preserved than if it is coated directly onto the solid phase (Satoh *et al.*, 1995).

The affinity of the immunoglobulin synthesised in response to an infection increases as the infection develops. Therefore, both IgM and early IgG antibodies have, in general, lower affinity for pathogen antigens than the IgG antibodies that represent chronic infection or immunity. This situation is exploited in the use of 'protein-denaturing immunoassay' or 'avidity enzyme-linked immunosorbent assay (avidity ELISA)', which are designed to detect only high-affinity antibodies (Thomas and Morgan-Capner, 1991; Lappalainen *et al.*, 1993; Ward *et al.*, 1993). For example (and briefly), diluted patient sera are placed in contact with solid phase coated with pathogen antigen and, instead of the usual washing step, a protein denaturant solution such as 6 mol l^{-1} urea is used to elute both nonspecifically adsorbed proteins and lower-affinity specific antibodies, before thorough washing and the determination of the remaining bound antibody with labelled anti-Ig or anti-IgG antibody (sp-Ag—**Ab**—Ab-enzyme, where **Ab** represents only 'high-affinity' antibody (Lappalainen *et al.*, 1993)). However, the validity of such methods has been questioned (Underwood, 1993) and more careful development and validation procedures may be needed (Goldblatt *et al.*, 1993).

Assays for Antigens

Such assays are almost always two-site sandwich assays equivalent to immunoradiometric assay (IRMA), immunofluorometric assay (IFMA) and immunochemiluminometric assay (ICLMA) and are best referred to as IEMA. The acronym ELISA is very loosely used and, outside certain limited contexts (e.g. reagent-excess assays for specific antibodies, often conveys little about the mechanism of the assay so described.

Normally, labelled antibody against the analyte (e.g. Ab-enzyme) is the principal reagent. To separate bound label (e.g. **Ag**—Ab-enzyme) from free, any of a range of adsorption or precipitation reagents can be used, but usually the antigen-label complex is removed by means of excess immobilised antibody which binds to a separate antigenic site on the analyte. This results in the now 'classical' two-site assay complex in which antigen is sandwiched between two antibodies (e.g. sp-Ab—**Ag**—Ab-enzyme), and plotting the concentration of labelled antibody bound against the concentration of analyte (**Ag**) gives a direct, nonlinear standard curve. Therefore, specificity is determined by the combined selectivity of two antibodies and such assays are observed to be inherently more specific than single-site assays. However, precautions must be taken to ensure that the use of excess reagents does not lead to high nonspecific binding of label, or degradation of assay specificity (Boscato *et al.*, 1989). It follows that all candidate analytes for such assays must have two antigenic determinants that can be recognised simultaneously, which excludes simple steroids, small peptides with less than 15–20 amino acid residues and most drugs. The most sensitive of such assays in routine use are capable of detecting <1 amol of analyte (Ishikawa, 1987; Gosling, 1990; Cook and Self, 1993).

A very large number of variations on the basic two-site sandwich assay for antigen have been described. These include indirect labelling (see above) and the use of enzyme conjugates with antibody fragments to decrease nonspecific binding (Ishikawa *et al.*, 1983, 1989; Abdul-Ahad and Gosling, 1987; Ishikawa, 1987; Aoyagi *et al.*, 1995; Koshkinen *et al.*, 1995). In addition, assay schemes and formulations have been developed that are suitable for a wide variety of applications, from highly sensitive thyroid-stimulating hormone (TSH) assays (e.g. Bronstein *et al.*, 1989) to home pregnancy detection kits (e.g. Achord *et al.*, 1991).

Immunoblotting, for which enzymes are often used as labelling substances, is a one-site excess-reagent immunoassay, and many of the same strategies and tactics are used (Stott, 1989).

Assays for Haptens

Because the two-site assays described above are unsuitable for analytes with a molecular mass <200 and because of the inherent limited sensitivity of competitive assays (Avrameas *et al.*, 1978), much effort has been put into the invention of reagent-excess assays for haptens. In one such system (Freytag *et al.*, 1984), analyte was incubated with a calculated excess of labelled antibody (usually Fab' or F(ab')$_2$) and unoccupied labelled antibody was removed by means of excess immobilised analyte before the label associated with analyte was determined. Note that, although the reagents used here and for labelled-antibody competitive assays may be exactly equivalent, the use of excess label and the determination of the analyte-label complex (**Ha**—Ab-peroxidase, and not immobilised label, sp-Ha—Ab-peroxidase) alters completely the character of the assay. A recent variant of this approach involved a label with acridinium ester (Piran *et al.*, 1995).

Self *et al.* (1994) and Barnard and Kohen (1990) have taken another approach to designing reagent-excess immunoassays for small molecules, and an EIA for oestradiol designed in this way has been described (Mares *et al.*, 1995). Figure 6 shows the three stages of an assay of this kind for oestradiol (Barnard and Kohen, 1990). Development of such assays is inherently expensive because two types of anti-idiotypic antibody are needed and these are only suitable for one primary anti-analyte antibody. When an assay for another analyte is to be developed, two new anti-idiotypic antibodies must be prepared and characterised. In addition,

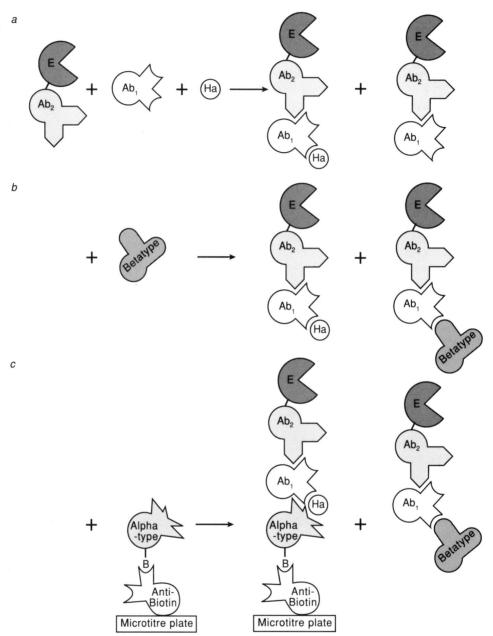

Figure 6 A flow diagram of an idiometric immunoenzymometric assay for oestradiol. Five separate antibodies were used: (1) affinity-purified, anti-oestradiol 2F$_9$, an IgG2a hybrid monoclonal antibody produced by a rat mouse hetero-hybridoma (Ab$_1$); (2) mouse anti-rat F(ab′)2 conjugated to AP (E-Ab$_2$); (3) 'betatype' anti-idiotypic antibody 1D$_5$ that can bind to 2F$_9$ idiotype only when it is not complexed to oestradiol; (4) biotinylated 'alphatype' anti-idiotypic antibody that can bind to 2F$_9$ idiotype even if it is complexed to oestradiol; (5) anti-biotin antibodies coated on the microtitre wells. *a*, In glass tubes 125 μl standard (50-2,500 pg ml^{-1}) or unknown was added to anti-oestradiol (1) and label (2) giving a total volume of 500 μl, mixed and incubated at room temperature for 45 min. *b*, Betatype (3) in 20 μl was added, mixed and incubated for 15 min. *c*, Aliquots (220 μl) were transferred to microtitre wells that had biotinylated alphatype (4) bound to the walls via anti-biotin (5), and incubated for 30 min at room temperature. After washing the activity of bound AP was measured colorimetrically with *p*-nitrophenyl phosphate. Absorbance was directly proportional to oestradiol concentration as is the case for standard curves in two-site IEMA. Reproduced with permission from Mares *et al.* with adaptations.

the lower detection limit of this new type of assay (~10 fmol per well, 10 pmol l^{-1}, 28 pg ml^{-1}) (Mares *et al.*, 1995) is still not better than that of the best competitive assays (~400 amol per well) (Gosling, 1990).

However, a quite different alternative approach, but still involving the measurment of enzyme activity as the end-point, may prove more promising in the long term. That is recombinant-cell bioassay (RCB) by which transgenic yeast cells expressing a suitable receptor and with suitable responsive control genes quantitatively respond to analyte by synthesising a marker enzyme. Such an assay has been developed for oestradiol (Klein *et al.*, 1994) and used to measure oestrogen in childhood (Klein *et al.*, 1994) and in breast cancer patients receiving the aromatase inhibitor letrozole (Klein *et al.*, 1995). Its detection limit was 59 amol per tube, or 73 fmol l^{-1} with 800-µl samples. The addition of the versatility of antibodies (as opposed to receptors with their many inherent limitations) to such systems could be truly revolutionary.

Reagent-limited Assays

Assays for Antibodies

Although most assays for specific antibodies are 'reagent-excess' (see above), limited-reagent assays can offer certain advantages for some applications (Kemeny, 1992). For example, if antibodies that bind only to a specific region of an antigen (a specific epitope) must be determined, a monoclonal antibody that binds to the same region is selected and labelled. In the assay, the specific antibodies in the sample (**Ab**) are allowed to compete with a limited concentration of the labelled antibody (Ab-enzyme) for the antigen immobilised on a solid phase (sp-Ag). The two possible final complexes are sp-Ag—Ab-enzyme and sp-Ag—**Ab**. Plotting the concentration of labelled antibody bound to the immobilised antigen against the concentration of analyte (**Ab**) gives an inverse standard curve.

Assays for Antigens or Haptens

Enzyme-labelled-antibody reagent-limited assays for antigen or hapten have the advantage that labelled antigens or haptens with undesirable properties (e.g low solubility in aqueous media) may be avoided. However, immobilised analyte must also be present in a constant, limited amount in each assay vessel. The primary (mouse) antibody does not have to be directly labelled but can be measured with peroxidase conjugated to goat anti-mouse IgG (Rothwell *et al.*, 1995). This approach works well with highly purified monoclonal or affinity-purified polyclonal antibodies, as only then is the nonspecific binding of label not enhanced by contamination with irrelevant antibodies. In a recent study (Henderson *et al.*, 1995) both antibody-coated (hapten-bovine serum albumin and peroxidase-hapten) and antigen-coated (peroxidase-antibody) formats of a competitive EIA were developed to measure oestrone-3-glucuronide; and the coated antigen format had the lower detection limit (1.1 pg per well, 2.3 fmol per well).

Enzyme-labelled antigen or labelled-hapten assays for antigens or haptens, respectively, are equivalent, to 'classical' radioimmunoassay (RIA). The labelled analyte is formed by tagging the analyte, or a derivative of the analyte, with an enzyme. After incubation of a limited concentration of label with a limited concentration of analyte-specific antibody and analyte, antibody-bound label and free label are separated to allow the bound enzyme to be determined. Plotting the the concentration of label bound to antibody (sp-Ab—**Ag**-enzyme) against the concentration of analyte (**Ag**) gives an inverse, nonlinear standard curve.

Competitive, labelled-hapten EIAs are very important for the measurement of low molecular mass analytes such as steroids or melatonin (Chegini *et al.*, 1995) or drugs such as cocaine (Spiehler *et al.*, 1996). The detection limits of all reagent-limited immunoassays may be maximised by the use of high specific activity label, but the smallest amount of analyte detectable is ultimately limited by the affinity of the antibody used (Ekins and Chu, 1991). The most sensitive of these assays used enzyme-containing labels and can detect <1 fmol analyte (Gosling, 1990).

Immunoassays to measure free hormones are also reagent-limited and they may involve the use of 'analogue of analyte'–enzyme (Kunst *et al.*, 1988) or antibody-enzyme conjugates (Christofides *et al.*, 1992).

SEPARATION-FREE ENZYME-MEDIATED ASSAYS

Basic Considerations

Separation-free enzyme-mediated assays all have features that result in modulation of the signal from the label by the binding reaction, thereby allowing binding to be monitored without the necessity for a separation step. Not all actually have an enzyme in the label, rather the labelling substance may be a prosthetic group or an enzyme fragment (see below). Most other separation-free immunoassays have fluorescent labels or depend on end points related to agglutination and precipitation.

An ideal separation-free or 'homogeneous' assay requires 100% modulation by the binding reaction of the activity of the label. In practice this is very difficult to achieve and separation-free assays generally have poorer detection limits than immunoassays with separation steps. Homogeneous assays suitable for very high molecular mass protein analytes have not become very popular because they are not usually clearly superior to precipitation immunoassays. The presence of sample in the assay mixture throughout the procedure also maximises the potency of interfering substances and background signal. Nevertheless, enzyme-mediated separation-free immunoassays are characterised by simplicity and speed and are widely used in monitoring blood and urine levels of therapeutic drugs and of drugs-of-abuse when very low detection limits ($<10^{-10}$ mol l^{-1}) are not required.

EMIT®

EMIT is a registered name of the Syva Corporation and is an acronym for 'enzyme-multiplied immunoassay technique'. EMIT® is almost as old as competitive EIA and dates from the classic paper of Rubenstein *et al.* (1972). For the original assay the enzyme label was a lysozyme-morphine conjugate (Morph-Lyz) with an incorporation ratio of 2:1 to 4:1. This conjugate was fully active and could hydrolyse a suspension of bacterial cells, but this activity could be sterically inhibited by the binding of a specially selected anti-analyte antibody (Ab—Morph-Lyz). With the antibody and conjugate present in limited amounts and the concentration of morphine varied, the more morphine present the greater the [Ab–**Morph**] and [Morph-Lyz] and the smaller the [Ab—Morph-Lyz]. Consequently, the enzymatic activity of the assay mixture was proportional to the concentration of analyte. The operation of the assay was astonishingly simple; after a brief incubation, substrate was added, incubated for a few minutes, the turbidity measured at 436 nm and the results calculated.

The invention of EMIT is one of the most important milestones in the history of immunoassays. In one stroke radioisotopes were avoided, procedures simplified, 'turn-around times' greatly reduced and automation on clinical chemistry analysers made feasible.

However, lysozyme has a low k_{cat} (only 0.5 molecules of substrate converted per second), the turbidimetric assay is insensitive and this enzyme is found in the urine samples often used for drug analysis. However, alternative enzymes were adopted and the system refined. Dehydrogenases, particularly glucose-6-phosphate dehydrogenase from *Leuconostoc mesenteroides*, were found to be suitable because when conjugated to hapten, their activities could also be inhibited by antibody-induced steric and conformational changes. With malate dehydrogenase (EC 1.4.1.37) conjugates, binding of antibody can give either an inhibition or an activation depending on the length of the bridging group linking the hapten to the enzyme. Activation is also dependent on the hapten being sufficiently hydrophobic to have good affinity for the active site and it is inherently limited by the high background activity of the conjugate (Jaklitsch, 1985). Therefore, most current EMIT assays use glucose-6-phosphate dehydrogenase conjugates with the binding of antibody causing inhibition and increasing amounts of analyte giving increasing enzyme activity (Beresini *et al.*, 1993).

These assays are mainly for the measurement of low molecular mass analytes such as drugs of abuse (down to about 1 mg l^{-1}, 5 µmol l^{-1} for amphetamine/methamphetamine) (Dasgupta, 1993) and therapeutic drugs (down to about 30 µg l^{-1}, 30 nmol l^{-1} for cyclosporine) (Beresini *et al.*, 1993). Because a very comprehensive range of EMIT assays for different drugs are available, they are widely used in drug-abuse treatment programmes, clinical laboratories, emergency rooms and forensic laboratories.

CEDIA®

To devise cloned enzyme donor immunoassay (CEDIA®), recombinant DNA technology was exploited to produce new strains of *E. coli* synthesising inactive variants of the 540,000 M_r tetrameric enzyme β-D-galactosidase (Henderson *et al.*, 1986; Khanna, 1991; Engel and Khanna, 1992). These were of two complementary kinds, large ~113,000 M_r inactive fragments of the enzyme monomer (enzyme acceptors, EA) and smaller 70–90-residue peptides homologous to the amino-terminal sequence of the same protein (enzyme donors, ED). Those fragments and peptides of interest could associate to give functional monomer, leading to the formation of active enzyme.

Pairs of complementary fragments, EA and ED, were produced that were stable, reassociated readily to give fully active enzyme, and in which the ED contained a cysteine sulphydryl group or other group that could be readily conjugated to hapten/analyte without affecting effective reassociation. The formation of active enzyme is multistepped and maximum activity is not attained immediately, although a great excess of EA leads to substantial activation within minutes.

The binding of specific anti-hapten/analyte antibody to ED-analyte conjugate severely reduces the ability of ED-analyte to contribute to enzyme reactivation and this is the basis for CEDIA. In the assay tube, free analyte and a limited amount of ED-analyte interact with a limited number of antibody binding sites and the greater the total amount of analyte present

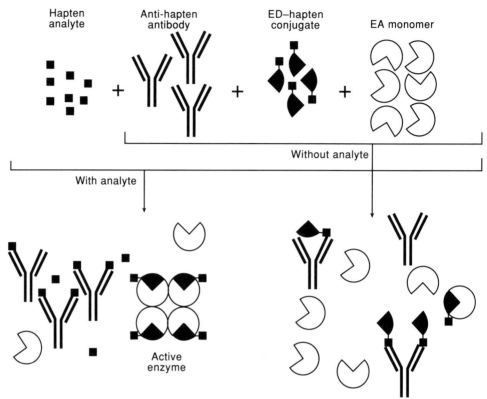

Figure 7 The principle of CEDIA. The large (inactive) enzyme acceptor protein (EA, 113,000 M_r) and the small enzyme donor polypeptide (ED, about 90 amino acid residues) can spontaneously associate to form monomers that then aggregate to give active β-D-galactosidase. The ability to reactivate EA is retained by ED–hapten conjugate but binding of ED–hapten by anti-hapten antibody prevents reassociation. In the diagram (adapted from Khanna (1985)) the effect of anti-hapten antibody in preventing reassociation is inhibited by the presence of free hapten.

the more free ED-hapten is available to activate EA (Figure 7). The linking of two molecules of hapten/analyte to each donor peptide can improve the signal:background ratio by making enzyme activation more susceptible to inhibition, but more antibody must also be used to give a substantial improvement, making this innovation unsuitable when a lower detection limit is necessary. Like EMIT, CEDIA is suited to automation by means of many general-purpose clinical analysers.

The ability of ED-analyte to interact successfully with EA is dependent both on the ED and the analyte, and for each new analyte a range of EDs with different sequences, positions for attachment of analyte and linking groups must be tested. The antibody must also be carefully selected, both on normal criteria of affinity and specificity for analyte, and on suitability for CEDIA. The most suitable antibodies give linear response curves and this is regarded as an important advantage when the assays are to be performed on analysers with only linear line-fitting software. CEDIAs are available for the important relevant therapeutic drugs and most have lower detection limits above or about 10^{-9} mol l^{-1}.

CEDIA has some weak points that must be taken into account. Both EA and ED are less resistant to normal physicochemical stresses and degrade more readily than intact natural proteins. Precautions must be taken to ensure their stability during transport and storage, such as the addition of antioxidants and heavy-metal chelators to reagent mixtures. ED in the label, being a small polypeptide without stable compact structure, is very susceptible to proteolytic degradation by sample components, although protease inhibitors are routinely added to mini-mise this. The central reaction of CEDIA is the self-assembly of multimeric, active β-galactosidase and this complex process must be protected against significant outside physical and chemical influences, particularly variable or erratic influences.

Cofactor-labelled Assays

The cofactor in question may be a coenzyme such as NAD^+ or a prosthetic group, in which case the assay may be called prosthetic group labelled immunoassay (PGLIA) (Ngo, 1985). A version of PGLIA that is commercially available is called apoenzyme reactivation immu-noassay systems (ARIS®). For ARIS the label is analyte-conjugated through a bridging mol-ecule to FAD. Inactive glucose oxidase apoenzyme can quite easily be prepared by removing the bound FAD from holoenzyme, and the analyte-FAD used in ARIS is capable of binding to, and reactivating, the apoenzyme. In addition, when a suitable antibody binds to the ana-lyte part of the label, this prohibits its binding to apoenzyme. Consequently, when the assay is properly configured, enzyme activity depends on the concentration of free label and the greater the concentration of analyte the greater the activity. ARIS dry-reagent assays for ther-apeutic drugs have been developed (Sommer *et al.*, 1985) and have been used in automated equipment.

With PGLIA, as with other assays with cofactor labels, care must be taken to avoid inter-ference from cofactor or related nucleotides and vitamins endogenous to patient samples.

Immunochromatography Assays

Enzyme immunocapillary migration (Glad and Grubb, 1981) or immunochromatography assays (Zuk *et al.*, 1985; Chen *et al.*, 1987) are homogeneous immunoassay systems based on the principle of 'enzyme channelling', in which the concentration of analyte is related to the distance along a chromatographic strip that colour develops rather than to the intensity of colour development. The original immunocapillary migration system of Glad and Grubb (1981) for the determination of C-reactive protein was a multistep adaptation of a sandwich ELISA in which analyte was extracted from sample as it migrated along a strip of cellulose acetate. Later an analogous system allowing one-step operation and based on the use of cellu-lose strips with immobilised antibody to analyte was developed (Chen *et al.*, 1987).

This led to the AccuLevel system for therapeutic drug measurement procedure for patient-side testing developed by the Syva Corporation. Central to the method is a 4 mm by 90 mm strip of paper onto which antibody to theophylline (or another drug) has been evenly immo-bilised. The test is started by mixing 12 µl whole blood obtained from a pinprick with 1 ml buffer containing theophylline-horseradish peroxidase conjugate and glucose oxidase. The bottom centimetre of the strip is immersed in this solution to allow capillary flow. Theophyl-line (free and conjugated) from the mixture flows past the immobilised antibodies and binds, and this continues until all the theophylline is bound or the top of the strip is reached. There-fore, the greater the concentration of theophylline the higher up the paper strip immobilised theophylline-peroxidase conjugate will be found. After about 10 minutes the paper is removed and developed by exposure to glucose and 4-chloro-1-naphthol. Because the paper is evenly

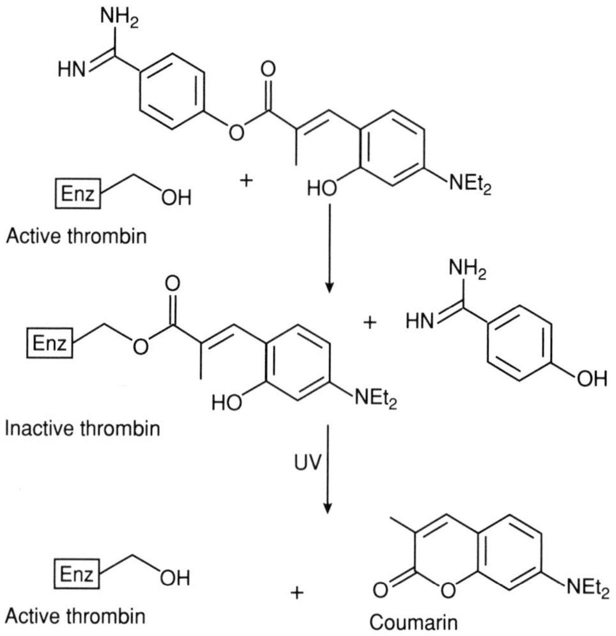

Figure 8 The 'irreversible' inhibition of thrombin and its UV-dependent reactivation. The inhibitor, the *p*-amidinophenyl ester of cinnamate, reacts with serine hydroxyls at the active sites of serine proteases, including thrombin, to give a stable, inactive complex. However, the ester linkage of the complex is sensitive to higher-energy photons and illumination with UV light induces the release of coumarin with the restoration of the serine residue and full enzyme activity. In the separation-free, immunoassay system of Marenbloom and Oberhardt (1995) this is exploited to ensure the inactivation of the enzyme until the end point is to be determined. Reproduced with permission from Marenbloom and Oberhardt (1995) with alterations.

impregnated with glucose oxidase, colour is only fully developed where the peroxidase is immobilised and the height of the coloured column measured in millimetres can be converted to mg l^{-1} of theophylline with the help of a calibration table.

Other Systems

Recently a novel homogeneous immunoassay system for whole blood samples was outlined that may be useful for quantitative point-of-care measurements (Marenbloom and Oberhardt, 1995). This method is loosely analagous to EMIT in that binding sterically inhibits analyte-enzyme activity and it incorporates a potentially powerful amplification assay of enzyme activity. The enzyme used is thrombin, but after synthesis of conjugate, and before its use in the assay, its activity is completely inhibited by a *p*-amidinophenyl ester of cinnamate, an efficient 'irreversible' inhibitor of serine proteases such as thrombin. However, exposure of the inhibited enzyme to ultraviolet light causes photoisomerisation and release of the inhibitor and restoration of protease activity (Figure 8). The thrombin activity of conjugate can also be doubly inhibited by the binding of anti-analyte antibody. The end-point is the clotting of an aliquot of control plasma containing paramagnetic iron oxide particles (PIOP) in an instrument used to measure coagulation time by monitoring PIOP movement in an oscillating magnetic field.

In Marenbloom and Oberhardts' paper a model assay for biotin is described in which the label is a thrombin-biotin conjugate (biot-Throm). The conjugate is fully active before being inhibited with the cinnamate ester, but the UV-induced restoration of this activity is sterically inhibited by the binding of anti-biotin antibody (Ab—biot-Throm). With the antibody and conjugate present in limited amount, and the concentration of biotin varied, the more biotin present the greater the [Ab—biot] and [biot-Throm] and the smaller [Ab—biot-Throm]. After incubation for two minutes and UV irradiation for 30 seconds to activate biot-Throm, the clotting time is measured and is inversely proportional to the concentration of biotin.

Many other separation-free enzyme-mediated immunoassay schemes involving the use of inhibitors, substrates and so on have been published, some of which are reviewed in Khanna (1985), Ngo and Lenhoff (1985), and by myself (1990).

MULTIANALYTE ASSAYS

There are obvious practical advantages to the simultaneous determination of a number of analytes in single samples, especially if all results are required at the same time in order to make a diagnosis. The screening of blood donations is an important example. However, the greatly increased complexity associated with multianalyte assays may be exponentially related to the number of analytes. Testing for susceptibility to crossreactions and interference, optimisation of assay concentration ranges, control of manufacture and routine quality control by the user are only some of the areas that require more formalised and rigorous procedures.

Most multianalyte EIA rely on the use of multiple enzymes to distinguish between intermixed binding sites, and it is difficult to measure even two enzymatic labels colorimerically because near-UV/visible absorption bands are broad. In addition, the usual labelling enzymes require quite different conditions for full activity, e.g. the pHs of assays for HRP, β-galactosidase and AP are 5–6, 6–8 and 9–10, respectively. AP is also rapidly inactivated at low pH. This inevitably results in the use of less favoured enzymes, substrates and/or severely compromised assay conditions for EIAs that are, in addition, limited to dual analytes.

Early attempts included an assay for two thyroid hormones with kinetic measurement of AP and β-galactosidase (Blake *et al.*, 1982), and a separation-free substrate-labelled fluorescent immunoassay (SLFIA) for two therapeutic drugs (Dean *et al.*, 1983). In a dual 'IE/RMA', two quite different labels were used: AP and ^{125}I for the determination of total and IgA-conjugated α_1-microglobulin (DeMars *et al.*, 1989). More recently, dual-analyte double-enzyme EIAs have been developed for the measurement of specific antibodies against human immunodeficiency virus and hepatitis B virus (with HRP and AP) (Porstmann *et al.*, 1993), and for the measurement of α-fetoprotein and free hCGβ for prenatal screening of Down's syndrome (Macri *et al.*, 1992; Spencer *et al.*, 1993).

An alternative approach is to use only one enzymatic label (or even different labels containing the same enzyme) but to have spatially distinct groups of specific binding sites; this has the advantage that the number of analytes determined is limited only by the number of groups of sites. Immunoconcentration assays are readily adapted in this way to include calibration and control readings and to allow the detection of dual analytes. Donohue *et al.* (1989) described a 'panel testing' IEMA system with a nitrocellulose membrane embossed to form an array of 5×6 small regions on which different capture proteins are immobilised. Another multianalyte IEMA with many spatially distinct groups of binding sites has been in widespread use for a number of years. The MAST® system uses 38 individual allergen-coated cellulose threads mounted in a special pipette-like test chamber to measure picomole amounts of allergen-specific IgE against up to 35 different allergen classes. The binding of anti-human IgE/peroxidase conjugate to the threads is detected by means of a peroxidase-dependent enhanced-luminescent reaction and a special cassette that holds a Polaroid instant film packet and up to five sets of threads (Brown *et al.*, 1984).

CONCLUSION

The popularity of enzymes as labelling substances in 'in-house' immunoassays has as much to do with their suitability for use in microtitre plates, and on the ready availability of conjugation reagents, plate-reading colorimeters etc., as with their versatility and their intrinsic virtues. The choice of enzymes has also been supported by the lack of (or relatively recent) availability of reagents for the simple preparation of high-quality chemiluminescent or time-resolved flourescent labels. In the commercial domain the choice of a labelling substance and end-point method is largely determined by research and development resources, the availability and cost of licences, the availability and cost of bulk conjugates and other reagents, and marketing considerations. These often favour the choice of enzymatic labels.

Comparisons of immunoassay technologies (e.g. Madersbacher *et al.*, 1993; Ryall *et al.*, 1993) can be very useful although they usually have serious limitations. Certain relevant methods or methodological variants may be absent. For example, enzyme immunoassays may be found wanting with respect to lower detection limit or range (Madersbacher *et al.*, 1993) but these limitations may be abolished by an alternative method of end-point determination (Christopoulos and Diamandis, 1992; Cook and Self, 1993). If enzymes have important practical limitations these are more likely to be related to their relative fragility, large size (with consequent lower diffusion rates) and a variable tendency to bind nonspecifically, and to the costs of measures needed to overcome or minimise these.

Therefore, the wise professional user of immunoassays also keeps abreast with the state of standardisation of immunoassays (Chapter 11) and with reports of well established and competent external quality assessment schemes (EQAS) (Chapter 10). Although EQAS have limitations, it is clear from their collective findings that good comparability and precision are not the prerequisite of any one methodology.

Enzymatic analysis started in the 1950s with routine measurement of metabolites; EIA and microtitre plate ELISA appeared in the 1970s and the recent and revolutionary polymerase chain reaction (PCR) seems already to be omnipresent. Enzymes are also extensively used as auxiliary reagents for immunoassays whether to prepare antibody fragments, promote iodination or activate luminescent labels, or in the recombinant DNA procedures that are essential to continued innovation in immunoassay methodology. For recombinant cell bioassay (RCB) (discussed above) enzymes serve as reporter molecules. Therefore, purified enzymes and enzymatic reagents will long continue to contribute to antibody-based and other binding protein-based measurement of clinical analytes, probably in an ever increasing variety of ways.

REFERENCES

Abdul-Ahad, W. G. & Gosling, J. P. (1987) An enzyme-linked immunosorbent assay (ELISA) for bovine LH capable of monitoring fluctuations in baseline concentrations. *J. Reprod. Fert.* **80**, 653–661.

Achord, D., Oayne, G. & Saewert, M. (1991). Immunoconcentration. In: *Principles and Practice of Immunoassay 1st edn.* (eds Price, C. P. and Newman, D. J.) pp. 584–609, Stockton Press, New York.

Albertson, B. D. & Haseltine, F. P. (1988) *Non-radiometric Assays: Technology and Application in Polypeptide and Steroid Hormone Detection* (Alan R. Liss, New York).

Aoyagi, K., Miyake, Y., Urakami, K. *et al.* (1995) Enzyme immunoassay of immunoreactive progastrin-releasing peptide(31–98) as tumor marker for small-cell lung carcinoma: Development and validation. *Clin. Chem.* **41**, 537–543.

Athey, D., Ball, M. & McNeill, C. J. (1993) Avidin-biotin based electrochemical immunoassay for thyrotropin. *Ann. Clin. Biochem.* **30**, 570–577.

Avrameas, S. (1992). Amplification systems in immunoenzymatic techniques. *J. Immunol. Meth.* **150**, 23–32.

Avrameas S., Dreut P., Masseyeff, R. *et al.* (eds) (1983) *Immunoenzymatic Techniques* (Elsevier, Amsterdam).

Avrameas, S., Nakane, P. K., Paramichail, M. *et al.* (1992) Enzyme immunoassay techniques. *J. Immunol. Meth.* **150** parts 3–4.

Avrameas, S., Ternynck, T. & Guesdon, J. L. (1978) Coupling of enzymes to antibodies and antigens. *Scand. J. Immunol.* **8** (**suppl. 7**), 7–20.

Baly, D. L., Allison, D. E., Krummen, L. A. *et al.* (1993) Development of a specific and sensitive two-site enzyme-linked immunosorbent assay for measurement of inhibin-A in serum. *Endocrinology* **132**, 2099–2108.

Barnard, G. & Kohen, F. (1990) Idiometric assay: A non-competitive immunoassay for haptens typified by the measurement of serum estradiol. *Clin. Chem.* **36**, 1945–1950.

Beresini, M. H., Davalian, D., Alexander, S. *et al.* (1993) Evaluation of EMIT® cyclosporine assay for use with whole blood. *Clin. Chem.*, **39**, 2235–2241.

Blake, C., Al Bassam, M. N., Gould, B. J. *et al.* (1982) Simultaneous enzyme immunoassay of two thyroid hormones. *Clin. Chem.* **28**, 1469–1473.

Boitieux, J.-L., Thomas, D. & Desmet, G. (1984) Un système potentiometric en phase heterogene pour le dosage enzymo-immunologique du 17β-oestradiol. *Clin. Biochem.* **17**, 151–156.

Boscato, L. M., Egan, G. M. & Stuart, M. C. (1989) Specificity of two-site immunoassays. *J. Immunol. Meth.* **117**, 221–229.

Bronstein, I., Voyta, J. C., Thorpe, G. H. G. *et al.* (1989) Chemiluminescent assay of alkaline phosphatase applied in an ultrasensitive enzyme immunoassay of thyrotropin. *Clin. Chem.* **35**, 1441–1446.

Brown, C. R., Higgins, K. W., Frazer, K. *et al.* (1984) Simultaneous determination of total Ig and allergen-specific IgE in serum by the MAST chemiluminescent assay system. *Clin. Chem.*, **31**, 1500–1505.

Canova-Davis, E., Redemann, C. T., Vollmer, Y. P. *et al.* (1986) Use of a reversed-phase evaporation vesicle formulation for a homogeneous liposome immunoassay. *Clin. Chem.* **32**, 1687–1691.

Casl, M.-T., & Grubb, A. O. (1993) A rapid enzyme-linked immunosorbent assay for serum amyloid A using sequence-specific antibodies. *Ann. Clin. Biochem.* **30**, 278–286.

Chegini, S., Ehrhardt-Hofman, B., Kaider, A. *et al.* (1995) Direct enzyme-linked immunosorbent assay and a radioimmunoassay for melatonin compared. *Clin. Chem.* **41**, 381–386.

Chen, R., Li, T. M., Merrick, H. *et al.* (1987) An internal clock reaction used in a one-step enzyme immunochromatographic assay of theophylline in whole blood. *Clin. Chem.* **33**, 1521–1525.

Christofides, N. D., Sheehan, C. P. & Midgley, J. E. M. (1992) One-step, labelled-antibody assay for measuring free thyroxin. 1. Assay development and validation. *Clin. Chem.* **38**, 11–18.

Christopoulos, T. K. & Diamandis, E. P. (1992) Enzymatically amplified time-resolved fluorescence immunoassay with Terbium chelates. *Anal. Chem.* **64**, 342–346.

Collins, W. P. (ed.) (1985) *Alternative Immunoassays* (John Wiley & Sons, Chichester).

Collins, W. P. (ed.) (1988) *Complementary Immunoassays* (John Wiley & Sons, Chichester).

Cook, D. B. & Self, C. H. (1993) Determination of one thousandth of a attomole (1 zeptomole) of alkaline phosphatase: Application in an immunoassay of proinsulin. *Clin. Chem.* **39**, 965–971.

Crowther, J. R. (1995) *ELISA: Theory and Practice* (Humana Press, New York).

Dasgupta, A., Saldana, S., Kinnaman, G. *et al.* (1993) Analytical performance evaluation of EMIT® II monoclonal amphetamine/methamphetamine assay: More specificity than EMIT® d.a.u. monoclonal monoclonal amphetamine/methamphetamine assay. *Clin. Chem.* **39**, 104–108.

De Boever, J, Kohen F & Vandekerckhove D. (1983) Solid-phase chemiluminescence immunoassay for plasma estradiol-17β during gonadotropin therapy compared with two radioimmunoassays. *Clin. Chem.*, **29**, 2068–2072.

Dean, K. J., Thompson, S. G., Burd, J. F. *et al.* (1983) Simultaneous determination of phenytoin and phenobarbitol in serum or plasma by substrate-labeled fluorescent immunoassay. *Clin. Chem.* **29**, 1051–1056.

DeMars, D. D., Katzmann, J. A., Kimlinger, T. K. *et al.* (1989) Simultaneous measurement of total and IgA-conjugated α1-microglobulin by a combined immunoenzyme/immunoradiometric assay technique. *Clin. Chem.* **35**, 766–772.

Donoghue, J., Bailey, M., Gray, R. *et al.* (1989) Enzyme immunoassay system for panel testing. *Clin. Chem.* **35**, 1874–1877.

Durbin, H. & Bodmer, W. F. (1987) A sensitive micro-immunoassay using β-galactosidase/anti-β-galactosidase complexes. *J. Immunol. Meth.* **97**, 19–27.

Ekins, R. P. & Chu, F. W. (1991) Multianalyte microspot immunoassay: Microanalytical 'compact disk' of the future. *Clin. Chem.* **37**, 1955–1967.

Engel, W. D. & Khanna, P. L. (1992) CEDIA *in vitro* diagnostics with a novel homogeneous immunoassay technique: Current status and future prospects. *J. Immunol. Meth.* **150**, 99–102.

Freytag, J. W., Lau, H. P. & Wadsley, J. J. (1984) Affinity-column-mediated immunoenzymometric assay: Influence of affinity-column ligand and valency of antibody-enzyme conjugates. *Clin. Chem.* **30**, 1494–1498.

Frobert, Y. & Grassi, J. (1992) Screening of monoclonal antibodies using antigens labelled with acetylcholinesterase. In: *Methods in Molecular Biology* pp. 65–78 (Humana Press Totowa, N.J.).

Geoghegan, W. D. (1985) The Ngo-Lenhoff (MBTH-DMAB) peroxidase assay. In: *Enzyme-mediated Immunoassay* (eds Ngo, T. T., Lenhoff, H. M.) pp. 451–465 (Plenum Press, New York).

Glad, C. & Grubb, A. O. (1981) Immunocapillary migration with enzyme-labelled antibodies: Rapid quantification of C-reactive protein in human plasma. *Anal. Biochem.* **116**, 335–340.

Goldblatt, D., van Etten, L., van Milligen, F. J. *et al.* (1993) The role of pH in modified ELISA procedures used for the estimation of functional antibody affinity. *J. Immunol. Meth.* **166**, 281–285.

Gosling, J. P. (1990) A decade of development in immunoassay methodology *Clin. Chem.* **36**, 1408–1427.

Gosling, J. P. (1993) Advanced Immunoassays In: *Immunotechnology* (eds Gosling, J. P. & Reen, D. J.) pp. 91–106 (Portland Press, London).

Guérin-Marchand, C., Batard, T., Brodard, V. *et al.* (1994) DMISA (dissociated membrane immunosorbent assay), a new ELISA technique performed with blotted samples. *J. Immunol. Meth.* **167**, 219–225.

Hadas, E., Soussan, L., Rosen-Margalit, I. *et al.* (1992) A rapid and sensitive heterogeneous immunoelectrochemical assay using disposable electrodes. *J. Immunoassay* **13**, 231–252.

Harmer, I. J. & Samuel, D. (1989) The FITC-anti-FITC system is a sensitive alternative to biotin-streptavidin in ELISA. *J. Immunol. Meth.* **122**, 115–121.

Harris, C. C., Yolken, R. H., Kroken, H. *et al.* (1979) Ultrasensitive enzymatic radioimmunoassay: Application to detection of cholera toxin and rotavirus. *Proc. Natl Acad. Sci. USA* **76**, 5336–5339.

Henderson, D. R., Friedman, S. B., Harris, J. B. *et al.* (1986) 'CEDIA', a new homogeneous immunoassay system. *Clin. Chem.,* **32**, 1637–1641.

Henderson, K. M., Camberis, M. & Hardie, A. H. (1995) Evaluation of antibody- and antigen-coated enzymeimmunoassays for measuring oestrone-3-glucuronide concentrations in urine. *Clin. Chem. Acta* **243**, 191–203.

Hosada, H., Takasaki, W., Arihara, S. *et al.* (1985) Enzyme labelling of steroids by *N*-succinimidyl ester method: Preparation of alkaline phosphate-labelled antigen for use in enzyme immunoassay. *Chem. Pharm. Bull.* **33**, 5393–5398.

Houts, T. (1991) Immunochromatography. In: *Principles and Practice of Immunoassay 1st edn.* (eds Price C. P. & Newman D. J.) pp. 563-583, Stockton Press, New York.

Howanitz, J. H. (1988) Immunoassay: Innovations in label technology. *Arch. Pathol. Lab. Med.* **112**, 775–779.

Howard, K., Kane, M., Madden, A. *et al.* (1989) Direct solid-phase enzymoimmunoassay of testosterone in saliva. *Clin. Chem.* **35**, 2044–2047.

Ikemoto, M., Ishida, A., Tsunekawa, S. *et al.* (1993) Enzyme immunoassay of liver-type arginase and its potential clinical application. *Clin. Chem.* **39**, 794–799.

Ishikawa, E., Imagawa, M., Hashida, S. *et al.* (1983) Enzyme-labelling of antibodies and their fragments for enzyme immunoassay and immunohistochemical staining. *J. Immunoassay* **4**, 209–327.

Ishikawa, E. (1973) Enzyme immunoassay on insulin by fluorimetry of insulin-glucoamylase complex. *J. Biochem.* **73**, 1319–1321.

Ishikawa, E. (1987) Development and clinical application of sensitive enzyme immunoassay for macromolecular antigens: A Review. *Clin. Biochem.* **20**, 375–385.

Ishikawa, E., Kawai, T., & Miyai, K. (eds) (1981) *Enzyme Immunoassay* (Igaku-Shoin, Tokyo).

Ishikawa, E., Hashida, S., Tanaka, K. *et al.* (1989) Methodological advances in enzymology: Development and applications of ultrasensitive enzyme immunoassays for antigens and antibodies. *Clin. Chim. Acta* **185**, 223–230.

Jaklitsch, A. (1985) Separation-free enzyme immunoassay for haptens. In: *Enzyme mediated Immunoassay* (eds Ngo., T. T. & Lenhoff, H. M.) (Plenum Press, New York) pp. 33–55.

Jørgensen, P. E., Vinter-Jense,. L. & Nexø, E. (1996) An immunoassay designed to quantitate different molecular forms of rat urinary epidermal growth factor with equimolar potency: Application on fresh rat urine. *Scand. J. Clin. Lab. Invest.* **56**, 25–36.

Kemeny, D. M. (1992) Titration of antibodies. *J. Immunol. Meth.* **150**, 57–76.

Kemeny, D. M. & Challcombe, S. J. (eds) (1988) *ELISA and Other Solid Phase Immunoassays: Theoretical and Practical Aspects* (John Wiley & Sons, Chichester).

Khanna, P. (1991) Homogeneous enzyme immunoassay. In: *Enzyme mediated Immunoassay* (eds Ngo, T. T. & Lenhoff, H. M.) pp. 326–364 (Plenum Press, New York).

Klein, K. O., Baron, J., Colli, M. J. *et al.* (1994) Estrogen levels in childhood determined by an ultrasensitive recombinant cell bioassay. *J. Clin. Invest.* **94**, 2475–2480.

Klein, K. O., Demers, L. M., Santner, S. J. *et al.* (1995) Use of ultrasensitive recombinant cell bioassay to measure estrogen levels in women with breast cancer receiving the aromatase inhibitor, letrozole. *J. Clin. Endocrinol. Metab.* **80**, 2658–2660.

Koshkinen, S., Hirvonenm M, & Tölö, H. (1995) An enzyme immunoassay for the determination of anti-IgA antibodies using polyclonal human IgA. *J. Immunol. Meth.* **179**, 51–58.

Kricka, L. J., Ji, X., Thorpe, G. H. G. *et al.* (1996) Comparison of 5-hydroxy-2,3-dihydrophthalazine-1,4-dione and luminol as cosubstrates for detection of horseradish peroxidase in enhanced chemiluminescence reactions. *J. Immunoassay* **17**, 67–84.

Kunst, A., Seidenschwarz, E., Bürk, H. *et al.* (1988) New one-step enzyme immunoassay for free thyroxin. *Clin. Chem.* **34**, 1830–1833.

Labrousse, H. & Avrameas, S. (1987) A method for the quantification of a colored or fluorescent signal in enzyme immunoassays by photodensitometry. *J. Immunol. Meth.* **103**, 9–14.

Langone, J. J. & Van Vunakis, H. (eds) (1982) *Immunochemical Techniques: Part D Selected Immunoassays. Meth. Enzymol.* **84**.

Lappalainen, M., Koskela, P., Koskiniemi, M. *et al.* (1993) Toxoplasmosis acquired during pregnancy: Improved serodiagnosis based on avidity of IgG. *J. Infect. Dis.* **167**, 691–697.

Larue, C., Calzolari, C., Bertinchant, J.-P. *et al.* (1993) Cardiac-specific immunoenzymometric assay of troponin I in the early phase of acute myocardial infarction. *Clin. Chem.*, **39**, 972–979.

Lo, C. Y., Notenboom, R. H. & Kajioka, R. (1988) An assessment of urease-based enzyme-linked immunosorbent assay. *J. Immunol. Meth.* **114**, 127–137.

Macri, J. N., Spencer, K. & Anderson, R. (1992) Dual analyte immunoassay in neural tube defect and Down's syndrome screening. *Ann. Clin. Biochem.* **29**, 390–396.

Madersbacher, S. & Berger, P. (1991) Double wavelength measurement of 3,3′,5,5′-tetramethylbenzidine (TMB) provides a three-fold enhancement of the ELISA measuring range. *J. Immunol. Meth.* **138**, 121–124.

Madersbacher, S., Shu-Chen, T., Schwarz, S. *et al.* (1993) Time-resolved immunofluorimetry and other frequently used immunoassay types for follicle-stimulating hormone compared by using identical monoclonal antibodies. *Clin. Chem.*, 39, 1435–1439.

Maggio, E. T. (ed.) (1980) *Enzyme-immunoassay* (CRC Press, Boca Raton).

May, K. (1988) In-home testing. In: *Complementary Immunoassays* (ed. Collins, W. P.) pp. 451–465 (John Wiley & Sons, Chichester).

Malvano, R., (ed.) (1980) *Immunoenzymatic Assay Techniques* (Martinus Nijhoff, The Hague).

Marenbloom, B. K, & Oberhardt, B. J. (1995) Homogeneous immunoassay of whole blood samples. *Clin. Chem.* 41, 1385–1390.

Mares, A., DeBoever, J., Osher, J. *et al.* (1995) A direct non-competitive idiometric enzyme immunoassay for serum oestradiol. *J. Immunol. Meth.* 181, 83–90.

Mares, A., DeBoever, J., Stans, G. *et al.* (1995) Synthesis of a novel biotin-estradiol conjugate and its use for the development of a direct, broad range enzyme immunoassay for plasma estradiol. *J. Immunol. Meth.* 183, 211–19.

Monaghan, D. A., Power, M. J, & Fottrell, P. F. (1993) Sandwich enzyme immunoassay of osteocalcin in serum with use of an antibody against human osteocalcin. *Clin. Chem.* 39, 942–947.

Morris, B. A., Clifford, M. N., & Jackman, R. (eds) (1988) *Immunoassays for Veterinary and Food Analysis* (Elsevier, London).

Munro, C., & Stabenfeldt, G. (1984) Development of a microtitre plate enzyme immunoassay for the determination of progesterone. *J. Endocrinol.* 101, 41–49.

Ngai, P. K. M., Ackermann, F., Wendt, H. *et al.* (1993) Protein A antibody-capture ELISA (PACE): An ELISA format to avoid denaturation of surface-adsorbed antigens. *J. Immunol Meth.* 158, 267–276.

Ngo, T. T. (1985) Prosthetic group labelled enzyme immunoassay. In: *Enzyme-Mediated Immunoassay* (eds Ngo, T., & Lenhoff, H. M.) pp. 73–84 (Plenum Press, New York).

Ngo, T. T. (ed.) (1987) *Electrochemical Sensors in Immunological Analysis* (Plenum Press, New York).

Ngo, T. T. (1991) Enzyme systems and enzyme conjugates for solid-phase ELISA. In: *Immunochemistry of Solid-Phase Immunoassay* (ed. Butler, J. E,) pp. 85–104 (CRC Press, Boca Raton).

Ngo, T. T. & Lenhoff H. M. (eds) (1985) *Enzyme-mediated Immunoassay* (Plenum Press, New York).

O'Rorke, A., Kane, M. M., Gosling, J. P. *et al.* (1994) Development and validation of a monoclonal antibody enzymeimmunoassay for the measurement of progesterone in saliva. *Clin. Chem.* 40, 400–410.

Obzansky, D. M., Rabin, B. R., Simons, D. M. *et al.* (1991) Sensitive, colorimetric enzyme amplification cascade for determination of alkaline phosphatase and application of the method to an immunoassay of thyrotropin. *Clin. Chem.* 37, 1513–1518.

Oellerich, M. (1984) Enzyme-immunoassay: A Review. *Eur. J. Clin. Chem. Clin. Biochem.* 22, 895–904.

Ohkaru, Y., Asayama, K., Ishii, H. *et al.* (1995) Development of a sandwich enzyme-linked immunosorbent assay for the determination of human heart type fatty acid-binding protein in plasma and urine by using two different monoclonal antibodies specific for human heart fatty acid-binding protein. *J. Immunol. Meth.* 178, 99–111.

Olivieri, V., Beccarini, I., Gallucci, G. *et al.* (1993) Capture assay for specific IgE: An improved quantitiative method. *J. Immunol Meth.* 157, 65–72.

Pauillac, S., Halmos, T., Labrousse, H. *et al.* (1993) Production of highly specific monoclonal antibodies to monensin and development of a microELISA to detect this antibiotic. *J. Immunol. Meth.* **164**, 165–173.

Peuravuori, H. & Korpela, T. (1993) Pyrophosphatase-based enzyme-linked immunosorbent assay of total IgE in serum. *Clin. Chem.* **39**, 846–851.

Piran, U., Riordan, W. J. & Livshin, L. A. (1995) New noncompetitive immunoassays of small analytes. *Clin. Chem.* **41**, 986–990.

Porstmann, T., Nugel, E., Henklein, P. *et al.* (1993) Two-colour combination enzyme-linked immunosorbent assay for the simultaneous detection of HBV and HIV infection. *J. Immunol. Meth.* **158**, 95–106.

Prabhasankar, P., Ragupathi, G., Sundaravadivel, B. *et al.* (1993) Enzyme-linked immunosorbent assay for the phytotoxin thevetin. *J. Immunoassay* **14**, 279–296.

Price, C. P. & Newman, D. J. (eds) (1991) *Principles and Practice of Immunoassay 1st edn* (Stockton Press, New York).

Rabitzsch, G., Mair, J., Lechleitner, P. *et al.* (1995) Immunoenzymometric assay of human glycogen phosphorylase isoenzyme BB in diagnosis of ischemic myocardial injury. *Clin. Chem.* **41**, 966–978.

Reis, K. J., Von Mering, G. O., Karis, M. A. *et al.* (1988) Enzyme-labelled type III bacterial Fc receptors: A versatile tracer for immunoassay. *J Immunol. Meth.* **107**, 273–280.

Roberts, C. J. & Jackson, L. S. (1995) Development of an ELISA using a universal method of enzyme-labelling drug-specific antibodies. Part 1: Detection of dexamethasone in equine urine. *J. Immunol. Meth.* **181**, 157–166.

Rønne, E., Behrendt, N., Plough, M. *et al.* (1994) Quantitation of the receptor for urokinase plasminogen activator by enzyme-linked immunosorbent assay. *J. Immunol. Meth.* **167**, 91–101.

Rothwell, T. C., Kamanna, V. S., Jin, F.-Y. *et al.* (1995) Characterisation of a monoclonal antibody (HB–22) and development of an ELISA for human apolipoprotein A-1. *Clin. Chem.* **41**, 1150–1158.

Ruan, K.-H., Kulmacz R. J., Wilson, A. *et al.* (1993) Highly sensitive fluorimetric enzyme immunoassay for prostaglandin H synthase solubilized from cultured cells. *J. Immunol. Meth.* **162**, 23–30.

Rubenstein, K. E., Schneider, R. S. & Ullman, E. F. (1972) Homogeneous enzyme immunoassay: A new immunochemical technique. *Biochem. Biophys. Res. Commun.* **47**, 846–851.

Ryall, R. G., Gjerde, E. M., Gerace, R. L. *et al.* (1993) Modifying an enzyme immunoassay of immunoreactive trypsinogen to use time-resolved fluorescence. *Clin. Chem.* **39**, 224–228.

Saha, B. & Das, C. (1991) Development of a highly sensitive enzyme linked immunosorbent assay for human serum progesterone using penicillinase. *J. Immunoassay* **12**, 391–412.

Satoh, M., Treadwell, E. & Reves, W. H. (1995) Pristane induces high titers of anti-Su and anti-nRNP/Sm autoantibodies in BALB/c mice: Quantitation by antigen capture ELISAs based on monospecific human autoimmune sera. *J. Immunol. Meth.* **182**, 51–62.

Schaap, A. P., Akhavan, H. & Romano, L. J. (1989) Chemiluminescent substrates for alkaline phosphatase: Application to ultrasensitive enzyme-linked immunoassays and DNA probes. *Clin. Chem.* **35**, 1863–1864.

Self, C. H. (1985) Enzyme amplification: A general method applied to provide an immunoassisted assay for placental alkaline phosphatase. *J. Immunol. Meth.* **76**, 389–393.

Self, C. H., Dessai, J. L. & Winger, L. A. (1994) High-performance assays of small molecules: Enhanced sensitivity, rapidity, and convenience demonstrated with a noncompetitive immunometric anti-immune complex assay system for digoxin. *Clin. Chem.* 40, 2035–2041.

Seth, J. (ed) (1996, continuously updated) *The Immunoassay Kit Directory* (Kluwer Academic Publishers, Dordrecht, The Netherlands).

Shimizu, S. Y., Kabakoff, D. S., Sevier & E. D. (1985) Monoclonal antibodies in immunoenzymetric assays. In: *Enzyme-mediated Immunoassay* (eds Ngo, T. T., Lenhoff, H. M.) pp. 433–451 (Plenum Press, New York).

Sommer, R., Nelson, C. & Greenquist, A. C. (1985) Dry-reagent strips for measuring phenytoin in serum. *Clin. Chem.* 32, 1770–1774.

Spencer, K., Macri, J. N., Anderson, R. W. *et al.* (1993) Dual analyte immunoassay in neural tube defect and Down's syndrome screening: Results of a multicentre clinical trial. *Ann. Clin. Biochem.* 30, 394–401.

Spiehler, V., Fay, J., Fogerson, R. *et al.* (1996) Enzyme immunoassay validation for qualitative detection of cocaine in sweat. *Clin. Chem.* 42, 34–38.

Stanley, C. J., Cox, R. B., Cardosi, M. F. *et al.* (1988) Amperometric enzyme-amplified immunoassays. *J. Immunol. Meth.* 112, 153–161.

Stott, D. I. (1989) Immunoblotting and dot blotting. *J. Immunol. Meth.* 119, 153–187.

Sun, S. & Lew, A. M. (1992) Chimaeric protein A/protein G and protein G/alkaline phosphatase as reporter molecules. *J. Immunol. Meth.* 152, 43–48.

Takayasu, S., Maeda, M. & Tsuji, A. (1985) Chemiluminescent enzyme immunoassay using β-D-galactosidase as the label and the bis(2,4,6-trichlorophenyl)oxalate-fluorescent dye system. *J. Immunol. Meth.* 83, 317–325.

Ternynck. T. & Avrameas, S. (1988) *Techniques Immunoenzymatiques* (Editions INSERM, Paris).

Thomas, H. I. J. & Morgan-Capner, P. (1991) The use of antibody avidity measurements for the diagnosis of rubella. *Rev. Med. Virol.* 1, 41–50.

Thorpe, G. H. G., Kricka, L. J., Mosely, S. B. *et al.* (1985) Phenols as enhancers of the chemiluminescent horseradish peroxidase-luminol-hydrogen peroxide reaction: Application in luminescence monitored enzyme immunoassays. *Clin. Chem.* 31, 1335–1341.

Tijssen, P. (1985) *Practice and Theory of Enzyme Immunoassays* (Elsevier, Amsterdam).

Tijssen, P. & Kurstak, E. (1984) Highly efficient and simple methods for the preparation of peroxidase and active peroxidase-antibody conjugates for enzyme immunoassays. *Anal. Biochem* 136, 451–457.

Tuuminen, T., Palomäki, P., Rakkolainen, A. *et al.* (1991) 3-p-Hydroxyphenylpropionic acid: A sensitive fluorogenic substrate for automated fluorimetric enzyme immunoassays. *J. Immunoassay* 12, 29–46.

Underwood, P. A. (1993) Problems and pitfalls with measurement of antibody affinity solid phase binding in the ELISA. *J. Immunol. Meth.* 164, 119–130.

Valkirs, G. E. & Barton, R. (1985) ImmunoConcentration™: A new format for solid phase immunoassays. *Clin. Chem.* 31, 1427–1431.

Van Kamp, G. J., Bon, G. G., Verstraeten, R. A. *et al.* (1996) Multicenter evaluation of the Abbott IMx® CA 15-3™ assay. *Clin. Chem.* 42, 28–33.

VanWeeman, B. K., & Schuurs, A. H. W. M. (1971) Immunoassay using antigen-enzyme conjugates. *FEBS Lett.* 15, 232–236.

Vincent, P. & Samuel, D. (1993) A comparison of the binding of biotin and biotinylated macromolecular ligands to an anti-biotin monoclonal antibody and to streptavidin. *J. Immunol. Meth.* **165**, 177–182.

Voller, A., Bartlett, A. & Bidwell D. E., (eds) (1981) *Immunoassays for the 80s* (MTP Press, Lancaster).

Voller, A., Bartlett, A. & Bidwell, D. E. (1978) Enzyme immunoassays with special reference to ELISA techniques. *J. Clin. Path.* **31**, 507–520.

Wallemacq, P. E., Firdaous, I. & Hassoun, A. (1993) Improvement and assessment of enzyme-linked immunosorbent assay to detect low FK506 concentrations in plasma or whole blood within 6 hours. *Clin. Chem.* **39**, 1045–1049.

Ward, K. N., Gray, J. J., Joslin, M. E. *et al.* (1993) Avidity of IgG antibodies to human herpesvirus-6 distinguishes primary from recurrent infection in organ transplant recipients and excludes cross-reactivity with other herpesviruses. *J. Med. Virol.* **39**, 44–49.

Webb, E. C. (1992) *Enzyme Nomenclature 1992: Recommendations of the International Union of Biochemistry and Molecular Biology on Nomenclature and Classification of Enzymes* (Academic Press, San Diego).

Wisdom, G. B. (1976) Enzyme-immunoassay. *Clin. Chem.* **22**, 1243–1255.

Wisdom, G. B. (1981) Recent progress in the development of enzyme immunoassays. *Ligand Rev.* **3**, 44–49.

Wreghitt, T. G. & Morgan-Capner, P. (eds) (1990) *ELISA in the Clinical Microbiology Laboratory* (Public Health Laboratory Service, London).

Yamamoto, S., Kubotsu, K., Kida, M. *et al.* (1995) Automated homogeneous liposome-based assay system for total complement activity. *Clin. Chem.* **41**, 586–590.

Yang, X. & Hay Glass, K. T. (1993) A simple, sensitive, dual mAb based ELISA for murine gamma interferon determination: Comparison with two common bioassays. *J. Immunoassay* **14**, 129–148.

Yie, S.-M., Johansson, E. & Brown, G. M. (1993) Competitive solid-phase enzyme immunoassay for melatonin in human and rat serum and rat pineal gland. *Clin. Chem.* **39**, 2322–2325.

Ylätupa, S., Partanan, P., Haglund, C. & Virtanen, I. (1993) Competitive enzyme immunoassay for quantification of the cellular form of fibronectin (EDAcFN) in blood samples. *J. Immunol. Meth.* **163**, 41–47.

Yonezawa, S., Kambegawa, A. & Tokudome, S. (1993) Covalent coupling of a steroid to microwell plates for use in a competitive enzyme-linked immunosorbent assay. *J. Immunol. Meth.* **166**, 55–61.

Zuk, R. F., Ginsberg, V. K., Houts, T. *et al.* (1985) Enzyme immunochromatography: A quantitative immunoassay requiring no instrumentation. *Clin. Chem.* **31**, 1144–1150.

Chapter 16

Fluoroimmunoassay

Peter Wood and Geoff Barnard

INTRODUCTION

In this chapter we deal with the use of fluorophores both in hetero- and homogeneous fluoro-immunoassays (FIAs). Heterogeneous FIAs are defined as techniques using antigen or antibody labelled with a fluorophore and requiring separation of bound from free tracer before fluorescence measurement. Homogeneous or nonseparation FIAs are defined as procedures in which the extent of the antigen-antibody reaction can be quantified without separation of the free tracer from the antibody-bound fraction. These methods can be classified into limited-reagent immunoassay systems (fluoroimmunassay, FIA) and excess-reagent immunometric methods (immunofluorometric assay, IFMA) by analogy with the terms radioimmunoassay (RIA) and immunoradiometric assay (IRMA).

Historically, to be accepted as a substitute for radioisotope-labelled immunoassay systems, any alternative tracer had to provide methods with specificity, accuracy and precision equal to or better than existing methods and also have the potential for increased assay sensitivity and convenience. It was also envisaged that the availability of a convenient system for 'in-house' labelling of antigens and antibodies with a new tracer would lead to the gradual replacement of iodination procedures used in assay development.

Antibodies labelled with fluorophores have been used since 1941 in histological immunofixation techniques (Coons et al., 1941) but immunoassay applications have taken longer to develop. Over the past 15 years, the introduction of fluorescent probes into heterogeneous immunoassay systems has provided some alternative methods for analytes such as drugs or proteins that are present at relatively high concentrations in blood. Detection limits for these methods tend to be high because of background fluorescence and quenching problems, and they have not gained widespread popularity.

The use of time-resolved fluorescence techniques using europium chelates and specialised counting equipment has provided methods that are viable alternatives to existing RIA and IRMA methods. The commercial dissociation-enhanced lanthanide fluorescence immunoassay (DELFIA®) system (Wallac Ltd) can be used for in-house immunoassay development.

Homogeneous FIA methods using fluorescence polarisation have gained widespread popularity for the assay of therapeutic drugs using the Abbott TD$_x$ and Cobas Fara analysers.

Basic Theory of Fluorescence

Fluorescent molecules can absorb energy in the form of radiation and emit this as photons. Absorbed light excites the electron field of the molecule from its ground state singlet (S_0) to a higher state (S_1, S_2 etc.; Figure 1). Energy may be lost from nonradiative conversion (for example, as heat), by radiative transition to the ground state (fluorescence) or through a semi-stable triplet state (phosphorescence) (Sidki and Landon, 1985).

Some rare earth ions, particularly of europium (Eu^{3+}) and terbium (Tb^{3+}) form highly luminescent chelates with suitable organic ligands. In this case, light absorption by the ligand is followed by energy transfer from the excited singlet state through its triplet state to the resonance energy levels of the lanthanide ion (Soini and Hemmilä, 1979).

The wavelength of emitted light is always longer than that of the excited energy because of energy losses before emission. This wavelength difference (the 'Stokes's shift') is generally small – in the region of 30–50 nm for fluorescent organic molecules – but is greater for phosphorescent molecules (e.g. 150 nm for erythrosin) and much greater for luminescent lantha-

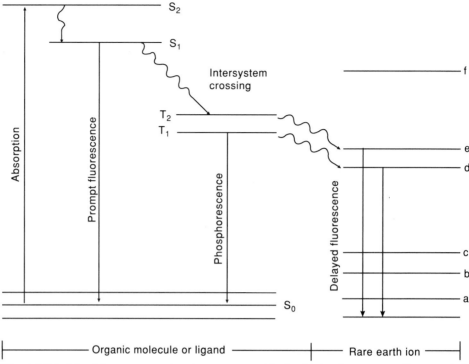

Figure 1 Principle of fluorescence, phosphorescence and lanthanide ion fluorescence. S_0, ground state singlet level; S_1, S_2, excited singlet levels; T_1, T_2, triplet levels; a–f, resonance levels of the rare earth ion; →, radiative transition; ↝, nonradiative energy transfer. Nonradiative energy loss to the ground state is also possible (not shown).

nide chelates (over 200 nm for europium and samarium) (Hemmilä, 1988). The decay times for phosphorescence (10^{-4} to 1 s) and lanthanide chelate luminescence (10^{-5} to 10^{-2} s) are much longer than for fluorescent organic molecules (10^{-9} to 10^{-8} s) and this factor has permitted the development of time-resolved fluorescence techniques. Fluorescent probes can also be classified in terms of quantum yield (the ratio of absorbed to emitted light energy). Both quantum yield and decay time are dependent on temperature, polarity and pH of the solvent, concentration of fluorophore ('inner filter' effects) and on other quenching effects (Wieder, 1978). Tables 1 and 2 list the characteristics of the main fluorescent probes that have been used in FIA and IFMA methods.

Theory of Time-resolved Fluorescence

Problems of high background fluorescence and quenching have limited the sensitivity of FIAs or IFMAs using conventional fluorescent probes. Time-resolved fluorescence measurement has permitted the development of assay methods with much lower detection limits, making them a realistic alternative to ^{125}I-labelled methods and competitive with enzyme and luminescence assays (Hemmilä, 1985a).

The sequence of events during one measurement cycle is illustrated in Figure 2. Excitation occurs with a flash of light lasting less than 1 μs. Background fluorescence in the sample due

Probe	Excitation max. (nm)	Emission max. (nm)	Decay time (ns)	Quantum yield
Fluorescein	492	520	4.5	0.85
Rhodamine B-Isothiocyanate	550	585	3.0	0.7
Lissamine-rhodamlne B-sulphonyl chloride	530,565	595	1.0	–
Umbelliferones	380	450	–	–
Dansylchloride	340	480–520	14.0	0.3
Anilino-naphthaline sulphonic acid (ANS)	385	471	16.0	0.8
Fluorescamine	394	475	7.0	0.1
2-methoxy 2,4 diphenyl -3(2H) furanone (MDPF)	390	480	–	0.1
N-(3-Pyrene)- maleimide (NPM)	340	375,392	100.0	–
Lucifer yellow	430	540	–	–
Porphyrins	400–410	619–633	–	–
Chlorophylls	430–453	648–669	–	–
Phycobiliprotein	550–620	580–660	–	0.5–0.98
Erythrosin	492	517	10^8	0.01

Table 1 Properties of fluorescent probes used in FIA and IFMA.

Lanthanide ion	Ligand*	Excitation max. (nm)	Emission max. (nm)	Decay time (µs)	Relative fluorescence†
Sm^{3+}	b-NTA	340	600,643	65	1.5
Sm^{3+}	PTA	295	600,643	60	0.3
Eu^{3+}	b-NTA	340	613	714	100.0
Eu^{3+}	PTA	295	613	925	36.0
Tb^{3+}	FTA	295	490,543	96	8.0
Dy^{3+}	FTA	295	573	approx. 1	0.2
Nd^{3+}	BTA	800	1,060	1,350	–

* β-NTA, β-naphthoyltrifluoroacetone, PTA, pivaloyltrifluoroacetone, BTA, benzoyltrifluoroacetone.
† At emission maximum, compared to Eu^{3+}/ b-NTA fluorescence.

Table 2 Fluorescent properties of some lanthanide chelates. Reproduced from Hemmilä (1985a) with permission.

to bilirubin, NADH, proteins and other fluorescent species decays rapidly with a half-life of less than 50 ns. The much longer-lived fluorescence of the europium ion is measured during a time window (e.g. 400–800 µs) chosen so that there is minimal interference from background fluorescence. The whole cycle is repeated, allowing the acquisition of multiple readings during the conventional counting time of 1 s per sample.

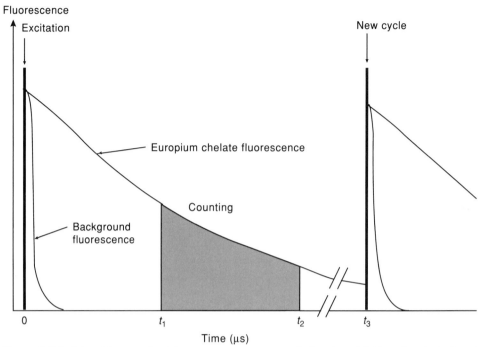

Figure 2 Principle of time-resolved fluorescence measurement. A pulse of light at the start of each cycle excites fluorescence. Measurement of the europium chelate fluorescence is delayed until background fluorescence has decayed (t_1–t_2). After a recovery period the cycle is repeated (t_3).

Theoretical Detection Limits of Fluorescent Probes

Although the majority of early immunoassay and immunoradiometric assay techniques used ^{125}I as the label, this is no longer the case, and it is by no means the ideal tracer. The signal provided by ^{125}I represents only one detectable event per second per 7.5×10^6 molecules (Ekins, 1985) so that only 0.000013% of the tracer is seen within a counting time of 1 s.

Theoretical predictions and practical experience have shown that radioisotope labels, when used in competitive radioimmunoassays, do not permit analysis of analyte levels below 10^{-14} mol l^{-1} or approximately 10^{10} molecules per litre (Ekins, 1985). Noncompetitive immunoradiometric assays can detect analyte levels approximately one order of magnitude lower.

Fluorescent tracers have the potential to provide many photons of emitted light per molecule because the cycle of excitation and fluorescence can be repeated many times for a single molecule during the measurement period. Conventional fluorescent-labelled immunoassay techniques are restricted to detection limits in the range of 10^{-9} to 10^{-10} mol l^{-1} (10^{15} to 10^{14} molecules per litre) because of high background readings associated with light scattering and fluorescence by the sample, reagents and cuvettes, and because of other interfering factors (see below). The use of fluorescence and other high-specific-activity tracers together with non-competitive immunometric assay systems could theoretically yield methods capable of detecting fewer than 10^6 molecules per litre (Jackson and Ekins, 1986). In practice, these very low detection limits have yet to be achieved, although time-resolved fluorescence measurements with IFMA assays have yielded detection limits similar to or slightly lower than those for corresponding IRMA systems.

Limitations on the Use of Conventional Fluorescence Probes

Interference from light scattering, background fluorescence and quenching can reduce the potential sensitivity of fluorescence measurement by factors of between 100 and over 1,000 (Wieder, 1978; Soini and Hemmilä, 1979).

Light Scattering

Light scattering causes high background readings from solutions containing proteins or small colloidal particles, as found in serum samples, for example. The problem is worse for fluorophores with a narrow Stokes's shift and for solid-phase fluorescence measurements in IFMA assays. Scattering can arise from dissolved molecules, particles or solid phases (Rayleigh, Raman and Tyndall scattering). Excitation and emission wavelengths are the same for Rayleigh and Tyndall scattering. Raman scattering shows a shift of approximately 50 nm.

Background Fluorescence

This can arise from sample, reagents and cuvettes. Serum has a high background fluorescence over a wide wavelength range of approximately 300–600 nm. Components in serum that contribute to this effect are serum proteins, which give a high background with short wavelength excitation (280 nm excitation and 320–350 nm emission), and NADH and bilirubin (300–360 nm excitation, 430–470 nm emission).

This interference can be reduced by pretreatment of serum with proteolytic enzymes, oxidising or denaturing agents (Ullman and Khana, 1981). The use of immobilised antiserum has the advantages of allowing simple washing and separation steps to remove serum components from the assay system.

Quenching

Fluorescent probes may be influenced strongly by relatively minor changes in their environment. Changes in pH, polarity (solvent effects), oxidation state (dissolved oxygen) and the proximity of quenching or absorbing groups can cause enhancement or quenching of the signal and influence the emission wavelength. Nonspecific binding of the fluorophore to serum proteins can quench the signal, and molecules such as bilirubin and haemoglobin present in serum samples can absorb excitation and/or emission light energies. The presence of two fluorophore molecules in close proximity can cause self-quenching if there is overlap between excitation and emission energies (the 'inner filter' effect) (Brand and Witholt, 1967).

Desirable Properties for Fluorescent Probes

Fluorescent probes for use with immunoassay techniques should have a high fluorescent intensity, giving a signal easily distinguishable from background. To achieve this, the probe must have a high molar absorptivity ($>10^4$) with as high a quantum yield as possible in the assay buffer system. For heterogeneous (separation) assays the binding of the probe to antibody or antigen should not adversely affect its properties. Light scattering and shorter wavelength background fluorescence can be reduced by using fluorophores with emission wavelengths greater than 500 nm and with Stokes's shifts of over 50 nm (Soini and Hemmilä, 1979). The probe must possess a suitable functional group (for example, carboxylic acid, organic or aliphatic amine, hydroxyl, or sulphonic acid residue) for covalent coupling to antibodies or antigens. Reaction intermediates that have been used for linkage include esters (carbodiimide or mixed anhydride linkage), acid anhydrides, acid chlorides, diazonium salts, isocyanates, isothiocyanates, triazinyl compounds, maleimides and N-hydroxysuccinimides. The introduction of hydrophilic linkages (peptides, sugars or amino sugars) has been used to overcome problems of insolubility of conjugates due to hydrophobicity of the fluorescent probe and/or antigen (Tsay et al., 1980).

The fluorophores that have been most widely used before the introduction of time-resolved fluorescence techniques are fluorescein, rhodamine and umbelliferone derivatives. All these probes have limitations; fluorescein and rhodamine have Stokes's shifts of only 28 and 35 nm, and umbelliferones have a lower quantum yield and relatively short emission wavelengths (Table 1).

HETEROGENEOUS FIA METHODS

Applications

The use of fluorescence techniques in immunoassay has been the subject of several reviews (Nakamura, 1979; O'Donell and Suffin, 1979; Maggio, 1980; Landon and Kamel, 1981; Quattrone et al., 1981; Smith et al., 1981; Visor and Shulman, 1981; Sidki and Landon, 1985; Hemmilä 1991). The main innovations in the development of reliable assay systems have involved the use of fluorophores, solid-phase antisera and convenient separation systems to improve 'signal-to-noise' ratios.

Bailey et al. (1983) used Lucifer Yellow VS, a vinyl sulphone dye which binds under mild alkaline conditions to amino and sulphydryl groups on proteins, to develop a FIA for albumin. This fluorophore has the advantages of a wide Stokes's shift of 110 nm and a relatively long emission wavelength of 540 nm (Table 1). The method used polyethylene glycol (PEG) precipitation of bound fluorophore and automated fluorometry on supernatants and could detect albumin levels above 4 mg l^{-1}.

The linking of antibodies to polyacrylamide beads with low fluorescent and light-scattering properties has helped the development of FIAs for triiodothyronine (T$_3$), thyroxine (T$_4$), theophylline and 11-deoxy cortisol (Currey et al., 1979; Chan et al., 1981; Watanabe et al., 1982). Following the immunoassay incubation, beads were separated, supernatants decanted and the beads resuspended in assay buffer before automated fluorometry. For T$_4$ and T$_3$, detection limits were 3 and 0.3 nmol l^{-1}, respectively, and both methods showed good correlation with the corresponding RIA procedures. Interassay precisions (percentage coefficient of variation, CV%) ranged from 4.5 to 10% (T$_4$) and from 3.6 to 7.5% (T$_3$).

One of the most successful and convenient approaches has been to use magnetisable cellulose to produce solid-phase antibodies. After separation and washing, bound fluorophore can be eluted and measured. This procedure has been used to develop a range of FIAs for drugs, steroids and proteins (Sidki and Landon, 1985) with detection limits going down to 10^{-9} to 10^{-10} mol l^{-1}. A cortisol assay using this principle could detect approximately 10–20 nmol l^{-1} with interassay precisions of 4.1–10.3% (Pourfarzaneh et al., 1980), and a progesterone protocol measured down to approximately 1–2 nmol l^{-1} with interassay precisions of 7.5–25.2% (Allman et al., 1981). In both these examples the FIA performance was similar to that for corresponding RIAs.

The FIAX™system (International Diagnostic Technology Inc.) represented an interesting development in FIA technology. The assay system uses antigen or antibody bound to a cellulose acetate/nitrate or polymethyl methacrylate disc attached to a plastic dipstick ('stiq'). For the quantification of immunoglobulins, for example, antigen in the standard or test is incubated with excess fluorescein-labelled antibody. A solid-phase antigen-coated 'stiq' is then introduced to remove excess labelled antibody. After a wash step, fluorescence measurements on the 'stiq' are performed using a surface-reflectance fluorometer, and correct positioning of the 'stiq' in the light path is aided by use of a removable precision viewing stage. Interassay precisions of between 6 and 8% were achieved for these immunoglobulin assays (Wang *et al.*, 1980). Drugs such as tobramycin and gentamicin can be measured by competition with hapten tracer labelled with fluoroscein isothiocyanate (FITC) for a limited amount of antibody immobilised on the 'stiq'; intra-assay precisions of less than 10% and good correlation with RIA and enzyme immunoassay were reported (Tsay *et al.*, 1980; Tsay and Palmer, 1981). Fluorescence determinations could be performed at a rate of 4 s per sample with this system.

The application of conventional fluorescence probes to two-site assays has been limited to a small number of proteins and polypeptides. The use of solid phases such as Sepharose (for pregnancy-specific β_1-glycoprotein (PSβ_1G) (Sykes and Chard, 1980)), polyacrylamide or aminostyrene beads (for C-reactive protein (Siboo and Kulisek, 1978), and alphafetoprotein (AFP) (Reimer *et al.*, 1978)) or magnetisable beads (for human placental lactogen (HPL) (Viinikka *et al.*, 1981)) has permitted the development of some IFMAs but these have not all performed as well as radioisotope-labelled assays. The performance of an IFMA for HPL for example, was satisfactory in terms of interassay precision (less than 10%), detection limit (0.02 mg l^{-1}) and correlation with RIA results (Viinikka *et al.*, 1981), whereas a two-site assay for PSβ_1G was found to give high results and poor precision relative to RIA (Sykes and Chard, 1980).

In addition to their relative lack of sensitivity, the requirement for sequential fluorescence readings on batches of samples limits the convenience of these systems unless the fluorometry can be automated.

Time-resolved Fluorescence Assays

Several reviews have covered the use of time-resolved fluorescence in immunoassay (Hemmilä *et al.*, 1984, 1985a, 1988, 1991; Kuo *et al.*, 1985; Lövgren *et al.*, 1985; Barnard *et al.*, 1988; Diamandis, 1988; Diamandis and Christopoulos, 1990; Gudgin Dickson *et al.*, 1995). The europium ion (Eu^{3+}) in aqueous solution is surrounded by 8 or 9 water molecules in an inner hydration sphere (Diamandis, 1988). In this state the europium ion is only very weakly fluorescent. Exclusion of these water molecules by organic ligands greatly enhances the Eu^{3+} fluorescence. Two different systems have been developed to adapt Eu^{3+} fluorescence to immunoassay systems.

The first time-resolved FIA and IFMA system to be developed commercially was the DELFIA system (dissociation-enhanced lanthanide fluorescence immunoassay; Wallac OY, Turku, Finland) (Soini and Kojola, 1983). DELFIA methods use antibody or antigen labelled with a stable europium chelate. In this form the europium ion has only weak fluorescence. On completion of the immunoassay or immunometric assay, the europium is released from the hydrophilic chelator into a highly lipophilic environment containing a β-diketone chelator which enhances the fluorescence of the europium ion.

Very recently, Lövgren *et al.* (1996) have described one-step dry-reagent time-resolved fluoroimmunoassays for human chorionic gonadotrophin, AFP and progesterone using fluorescent lanthanide chelates. The methods can be completed in 15 minutes and do not require the addition of enhancement solution.

Diamandis and colleagues have developed an alternative system which is based on time-resolved fluorescence measurement in the solid phase and uses biotinylated antibodies labelled with streptavidin-europium chelator reagent. The system has not gained widespread acceptance in routine clinical chemistry laboratories although a considerable number of assay methods using this system have been published (Diamandis, 1988; Diamandis and Christopoulos, 1990; Gudgin Dickson *et al.*, 1995).

The DELFIA System

DELFIA uses a microtitre plate format, but each plate is divided into 8 horizontal strips of 12 wells each. A plastic frame allows a variable number of strips to be inserted. Readings are performed on a Wallac 1232 or 1234 time-resolved fluorometer and the system includes a plate shaker, plate washer and reagent pipettors. Data reduction can be done on the fluorometer or with the 'Multi-calc' system on an IBM-compatible personal computer.

Assay Principle

The requirements for the components of this assay technique are: first, a stable europium chelator reagent which can be used to label proteins, but which will release europium rapidly into the enhancer reagent at acid pH. For europium, the bifunctional reagent N^1-(p-isothiocyanato-benzyl)-diethylene triamine tetra-acetic acid-Eu^{3+} (N^1-ITC-benzyl DTTA Eu^{3+}) is the most suitable labelling reagent (Figure 3). Reagents for europium (or samarium) labelling are available from Wallac UK Ltd. Incubation of an excess of this reagent with antibodies and other proteins at alkaline pH allows the incorporation of up to 20 Eu^{3+} atoms per molecule, linked through free amino groups on the protein. The second requirement is for a β-diketone in the enhancer reagent which has high absorptivity and which can also give the most efficient energy transfer to the lanthanide ion energy levels in order to produce maximum fluorescence. This is achieved by using a molecule with a triplet state energy just above the lowest emissive energy of the rare earth ion. Reagents therefore need to be tailored to individual lanthanides. The incorporation of fluorinated groups into the β-diketone pushes the keto-enol equilibrium in the direction of the enol form, making the ligand a stronger chelator

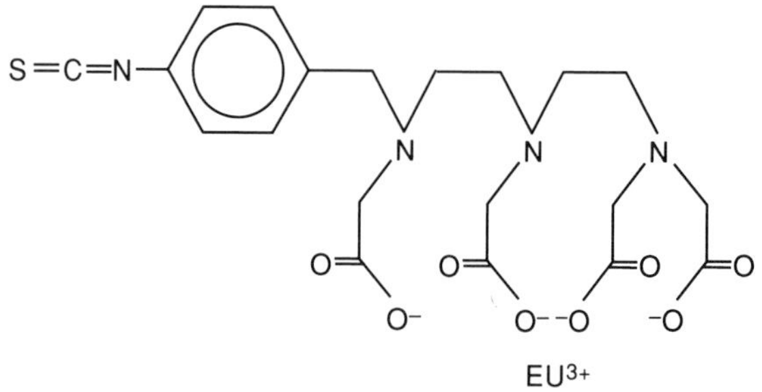

Figure 3 Structure of N^1-(p-isothiocyanato-benzyl)-diethylene triamine tetra-acetic acid-Eu^{3+} (N^1-ITC-benzyl DTTA Eu^{3+}).

at acid pH. For Eu^{3+} and Sm^{3+}, an aromatic β-diketone, which has a lower energy for the excited triplet state provides the optimum reagent (Hemmilä *et al.*, 1984; Bador *et al.*, 1987). Aliphatic fluorinated β-diketones with a higher excited triplet state energy are more suitable for Tb^{3+} and Dy^{3+} (Hemmilä, 1985b).

The final step in the DELFIA assay involves dissociation of the lanthanide ion from protein binding and the incorporation into micellar structures with enhancement solution. This is achieved using a reagent consisting of β-naphthyl trifluoroacetone (15 μmol l^{-1}), tri-octylphosphine oxide (50 μmol l^{-1}) and Triton X–100 (1 g l^{-1}) in acetate-phthalate buffer (0.1 mol l^{-1}, pH 3.2).

Fluorescence Measurement

The Wallac time-resolved fluorometer will read microtitre-format strips or plates. The light source used is a xenon flash tube which produces light pulses of duration of 0.5 μs at 1 ms intervals. Excitation and emission wavelengths for europium are 340 nm and 613 nm, respectively. The fluorescence signal is monitored between 400 and 800 μs following excitation (Figure 2), and the samples are counted for 1 s giving 1,000 readings per sample.

Assay Protocols

For the two-site IFMA assays, one-step or two-step procedures can be used, depending on whether or not addition of Eu^{3+}-labelled detection antibody is delayed until after removal of the sample. Two-step assays, by removing the sample and washing before addition of detection antibody avoid potential 'antigen excess' problems and are preferable for measurement of analytes such as serum β-human chorionic gonadotrophin (β-hCG) or serum AFP in situations where very high levels may be encountered.

The measurement of 'haptens' such as steroids and drugs relies upon competitive assays using either immobilised hapten-protein conjugates and labelled antibody, or immobilised antibody with labelled antigen. Steroid labels can be prepared from poly-L-lysine-steroid conjugates which can then be labelled with N^1-ITC-benzyl DTTA Eu^{3+}. Recently, improved steroid labels have been prepared by direct linkage of the europium chelate to steroid alkoxime derivatives (Mikola *et al.*, 1993).

Potential for In-house Assay Development

The DELFIA system can be used for in-house immunoassays. Antibodies, protein or hapten-protein conjugates can be labelled with N^1-ITC-benzyl DTTA Eu^{3+} to provide tracers for the DELFIA system (Wallac, 1992). The method involves 'de-salting' of antibody on a small Sephadex G50 column and incubation with a 20–100 molar excess of reagent in bicarbonate buffer (pH 8.5–9.8) overnight at room temperature. Reagents containing amino groups or azides should be avoided. The conjugate can be purified on a small Sephadex G50 column although gel filtration on a larger Sepharose 6B column may be necessary to separate aggregates. Purified conjugates can be stored in Tris-HCL buffer, pH 7.5, containing 1 g l^{-1} purified bovine serum albumin (BSA). It is important that the BSA used has been stripped of heavy metal contaminants (for example, by incubation with diethylene triamine penta-acetic acid (DTPA) and then purification of the BSA to remove complexing agents). Failure do this may result in exchange between europium in the tracer and lanthanide impurities in the BSA, resulting in loss of label activity.

The level of incorporation of the chelate can be calculated from fluorescence measurements calibrated against europium chloride standards in enhancement solution and from protein absorbance readings at 280 nm with correction for the absorbance due to the europium chelate.

An alternative Eu^{3+} chelator, DTPA anhydride, has been used to label a progesterone horseradish peroxidase conjugate for use in a progesterone FIA (Dechaud et al., 1988). However, in our laboratory DTPA anhydride labelling gives lower incorporation and less satisfactory tracers than N^1-ITC-benzyl DTTA Eu^{3+}.

The incorporation of europium into the detection antibody can be increased by biotinylation and linkage to europium-labelled streptavidin. This approach has the potential for reducing detection limits; for example, it has enabled us to develop an intact insulin assay with a detection limit in serum of 0.05 mU l^{-1} (Donovan and Wood, 1993).

Assay Optimisation

Microtitre wells can be coated with antibody or antigen-protein conjugates by incubation overnight at room temperature with 100–200 µl protein at concentrations ranging from 1 to 10 mg l^{-1} in Tris-HCl, phosphate or bicarbonate buffers at alkaline pH. Nonspecific binding effects can be minimised by blocking with BSA solution.

The concentration of reagents will depend on the antibodies or hapten-protein conjugates used and on the measuring range required. As a rough guide, a concentration of labelled antibody of 50 ng per well is a useful concentration to start optimisation studies (Wallac, 1992).

For nonextraction assays of steroids that are protein-bound, suitable displacement reagents must be incorporated into the incubation: for example, dilute trichloroacetic acid has been used in progesterone and cortisol FIAs (Dechaud et al., 1988; Diamandis et al., 1988).

Applications of Time-resolved Fluorescence Assays

The methods that have been developed with DELFIA technology cover a wide range of peptide, protein, steroid and drug assays. Assay times of 2–4 h are typical and in general between-assay imprecision (CV%) of 10% or less can be achieved over much of the dose-response range.

Where comparative data are available, the detection limits for time-resolved fluorescence assays compare favourably with those for similar methods using ^{125}I or alternative nonradio-isotopic tracers. A study from 1988 looked at second generation two-site assays for thyroid-stimulating hormone (thyrotrophin; TSH), and showed that the detection limits of 0.02–0.03 mU l^{-1} for the IFMA was better than that achieved for enzyme immunoassay (0.1 mU l^{-1}) or enhanced luminescence immunoassay (Amerlite™ system; 0.04 mU l^{-1}) and was as good as the most sensitive IRMAs (detection limits ranging from 0.02 to 0.25 mU l^{-1}) (Diamandis, 1988).

Limitations of Time-resolved Fluorescence Immunoassay Techniques

Although methods generally perform well, the additional enhancement step necessary with the DELFIA assays must contribute to the overall assay imprecision. The correct setting of the plate-shaker is vital to ensure good mixing but avoid splashing, particularly for the enhancement stage. Contamination of enhancement reagent with Eu^{3+} in the environment is a possibility, and particular care must be taken if laboratories are using high levels of Eu^{3+} for in-house label preparation.

Time/cost Considerations

The DELFIA system offers a viable alternative to ^{125}I-labelled immunometric and immunoassays. Incubation times and assay imprecision are similar to established ^{125}I-labelled methods, while detection limits are equivalent or lower. The use of the microtitre strip format is convenient and the facility to use multiples of single strips allows small assay batches to be processed quickly. In our laboratory we have found the DELFIA system valuable for the provision of a rapid turnaround service for serum β-hCG and AFP tumour markers.

Reagent costs are similar to or slightly more expensive than equivalent ^{125}I-labelled methods, and are generally the same as costs for assays using alternative enzyme or luminescence labels. Although assay imprecision for duplicate analysis is acceptable, cost saving by analysis in single wells needs very careful justification (Raggatt, 1989).

Time-resolved fluorescence methods are more convenient than many conventional ^{125}I-labelled assay systems, and this will be an important deciding factor in adopting them, particularly if older gamma-counters need replacement with newer equipment.

Multianalyte DELFIA Technology

The fluorescence emission wavelengths from alternative lanthanide chelates (Table 2) are sufficiently different to be able to discriminate between them using appropriate filters (Barnard *et al.*, 1988). This observation has been successfully exploited in the development of a separation IFMA for the simultaneous measurement of follicle stimulating hormone (FSH) and luteinising hormone (LH) in serum (Hemmilä *et al.*, 1987).

To help the development of dual and triple assays, there is a research fluorometer (Wallac 1234) that can measure up to three different lanthanides (europium, samarium and terbium) with the use of simple emission filters. DELFIA kits have been developed for dual assays of AFP and free β-subunit of human chorionic gonadotrophin (fβ-hCG) and for free and total prostate-specific antigen (PSA).

The simultaneous assay of AFP and fβ-hCG uses detection antibodies labelled with europium and samarium, respectively. The fluorescent signal for the AFP assay was approximately 50 times that of the fβ-hCG assay because of the greater fluorescence intensity of the europium chelate, but for both methods the detection limits were low (0.1 kU l^{-1} for AFP and 0.2 IU l^{-1} for fβ-hCG), and between-batch imprecision was less than 5% over the clinically relevant assay ranges (Petersson *et al.*, 1993).

A dual-analyte assay for total PSA and for PSA complexed with α_1-antichymotrypsin (ACT) has been described (Leinonen *et al.*, 1993; Mitrunen *et al.*, 1995), and more recently a DELFIA kit for the simultaneous assay of free and total PSA has been developed. The

DELFIA assay uses a capture antibody that binds both free and ACT-complexed PSA. Detection is achieved by the use of a europium-labelled antibody specific for free PSA and a samarium-labelled antibody that binds to both free and complexed PSA. Between-assay imprecisions for free and total PSA were less than 5% and less than 9%, respectively, over the assay ranges. At present the free:total PSA ratios are being assessed in the hope of increasing the ability to discriminate between patients with carcinoma of the prostate and benign prostatic hyperplasia.

In-house development of multiple analyte methods is also possible. For example, Barnard has described a novel time-resolved fluorescence immunoassay for the simultaneous measurement of oestrone-3-glucuronide (EG), pregnanediol-3-glucuronide (PG) and luteinising hormone (LH) in samples of early morning urine using three different lanthanide chelates as labels to monitor ovarian function in women (Barnard *et al.*, 1994). The assay involves the passive immobilisation of three antibodies (i.e. monoclonal antibody to PG-BSA; monoclonal anti-idiotypic antibody to anti-EG-BSA antibody; and monoclonal anti-LH capture antibody) to the walls of polystyrene microtitre wells and the addition of buffer containing three labelled reactants (i.e. europium-labelled PG; samarium-labelled antibody to EG; and terbium-labelled antibody to LH). After incubation for 3 h on a shaker at room temperature, the plate is washed and enhancement solution added to each well.

Europium and samarium fluorescence is measured using a plate fluorometer with appropriate emission filters. Subsequently, an enhancement additive containing an alternative β-diketone is added (*see* Table 2), and terbium fluorescence is measured. The method demonstrates appropriate sensitivity and precision (CVs less than 10%) across the relevant working ranges for each hormonal parameter. The technique has been applied to serial early morning urine samples collected from women with normal menstrual cycles, from those undergoing ovarian stimulation with gonadotrophins and from those presenting with symptoms of premenstrual syndrome.

Under certain colloidal conditions and in the presence of another lanthanide or yttrium it is possible to enhance the fluorescence intensity of β-diketone chelates of europium or samarium. This particular type of energy transfer phenomenon has been termed cofluorescence, and has been used by Xu and colleagues (1992) to develop single and multianalyte assays using up to four lanthanides, namely europium, samarium, terbium and dysprosium. Yttrium cofluorescence enhancement has been used to reduce the detection limit and imprecision from an in-house TSH IFMA (McConway and Beastall, 1994).

A novel multianalyte stick assay that measures LH, FSH, hCG and prolactin has been described (Kakabakos *et al.*, 1992). Capture antibodies were coated onto microtitre plate wells, and then the well bottoms were cut out and stuck to a plastic stick which was then incubated with the sample, biotinylated detection antibodies and streptavidin labelled with a europium chelate. The strips were dried and the solid-phase fluorescence of wells was measured on a Cyberfluor time-resolved fluorometer.

Noncompetitive Immunofluorometric Methods for Steroids

All immunoassay techniques can be divided into two basic types, competitive and noncompetitive, typified by radioimmunoassay (RIA) and immunoradiometric assay (IRMA), respectively. The advantages of the noncompetitive approach have been well documented and include greater sensitivity, precision and working range of analyte (Jackson and Ekins, 1986).

Noncompetitive technology has focused on the development of two-site assays for the measurement of compounds with more than one antigenic determinant (epitope). By definition, the two-site assay is unsuitable for the measurement of steroids and other haptens, although it is probable that a small molecule may possess more than one epitope. Invariably, the cleft nature of the antigen-binding site of one specific immunoglobulin will preclude, by steric hindrance, the binding of a second antibody that might recognise an alternative epitope. Consequently, noncompetitive technologies have not yet been applied successfully to the measurement of small molecules on a routine basis.

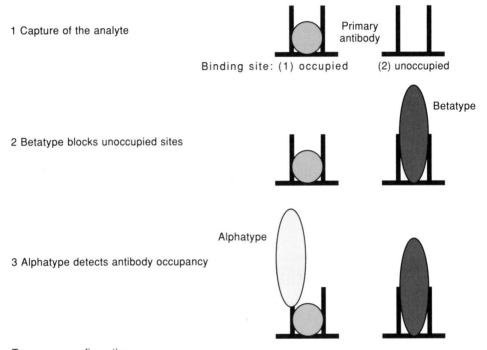

1 Capture of the analyte

Primary antibody

Binding site: (1) occupied   (2) unoccupied

2 Betatype blocks unoccupied sites

Betatype

Alphatype

3 Alphatype detects antibody occupancy

Two assay configurations:
1 Immobilised primary antibody and labelled alphatype
2 Immobilised alphatype and labelled primary antibody

Figure 4 The principle of steroid idiometric assay.

Ekins (1985) has suggested that the fundamental difference between competitive and noncompetitive procedures is based upon the detection of antibody occupancy. For example, the use of a labelled (or immobilised) antigen in a competitive immunoassay is to detect those antibody-binding sites that are not occupied by the analyte in the standard or sample. Alternatively, a labelled antibody can be used in a noncompetitive immunometric assay to detect the presence of the captured analyte (i.e. occupied antibody-binding sites). Accordingly, the development of a noncompetitive assay for the measurement of steroids primarily requires a method for detecting antibody occupancy.

It is quite straightforward to devise various schemes that are not based on the conventional two-site approach which require the availability of spatially separate and distinct epitopes on the surface of the antigen. For example, the identification and application of anti-idiotypes or anti-allotypes that bind to the antibody only when the antigen is bound would enable the development of a simple and possibly universal noncompetitive technology. Theoretically, reagent binding could be due to: (1) direct antigen-antibody recognition; or (2) binding to epitopes exposed by conformational changes in the tertiary structure of the immunoglobulin (constant or variable regions) after antigen binding.

Barnard and Kohen (1990) described three time-resolved fluorescence monoclonal antibody screening assays for the identification and production of the two types of anti-idiotypic antibody that recognise epitopes of the variable regions of the heavy and light chains of the primary immunoglobulin molecule. The anti-idiotypes were of two types: (1) betatypes, which recognise the binding site of the antibody (paratope) and compete with the antigen for binding; and (2) alphatypes, which recognise the framework region of the variable region of the antibody and which are not sensitive to the presence or absence of the antigen.

The availability of these reagents enabled the conception of a novel approach for the detection of antibody-occupancy, which has been termed idiometric assay. The method is applicable to the measurement of small and large molecules and is typified by a noncompetitive immunofluorometric assay for the determination of oestradiol in serum (Barnard and Kohen, 1990). In principle, the method can be adapted for the measurement of free steroid in serum and in samples of saliva taken daily throughout the menstrual cycle. The principle of a steroid idiometric assay is shown in Figure 4.

In addition, Altamirano-Bustamante et al. (1991) have described a competitive fluorescence immunoassay using the betatype labelled with europium. The method demonstrated appropriate sensitivity and good precision over the working range of the assay. The use of a labelled anti-idiotype provides an alternative approach to competitive technology when it proves difficult to label the hapten. This approach is not unique to the use of fluorophore labels and other labels can be used (Self, 1989; Mares et al., 1995).

HOMOGENEOUS FLUOROIMMUNOASSAY

In the early 1970s it was perceived that it would not be possible to develop nonseparation technology using radioisotopic labels and this was a major motivating factor behind the original development of these simple methods of nonisotopic immunoassays. Alternative nonradioisotopic homogeneous procedures have evolved to use a variety of labels. Of these, the use of enzymes (Curtiss and Patel, 1978; Engvall, 1980), chemiluminophores (Campbell et al., 1985) and fluorophores (Ullman et al., 1980) have been the most successful. The reasons for this include: (1) the ability to differentiate between the signal obtained from the free and antibody-bound fractions; (2) the chemistry required in coupling the label to the immunoreactant; (3) the stability of the labelled reagent; (4) the degree of interference from endogenous compounds; and (5) the sensitivity of detection.

The major characteristic of a homogeneous immunoassay is the modulation of the specific signal either by enhancement or quenching when the labelled reactant binds to its partner (e.g. an antibody where a labelled antigen is used). In particular, homogeneous FIAs are assays in which the antibody-binding reaction significantly alters the fluorescence properties of the label so that it is possible to monitor the extent of the binding reaction at any time from the homogeneous reaction mixture.

So far, the most serious limitation to the widespread application of nonseparation technology has been an inferior sensitivity when compared to the equivalent separation methodology. In addition, homogeneous assays are extremely vulnerable to matrix variations. In particular, the application of homogeneous fluorescence immunoassays for the measurement of analytes in untreated biological material is complicated by problems associated with the presence of endogenous fluorescent compounds and other species that quench the fluorescence of the labelled probe. For example, serum and other components of biological origin contain many fluorescent compounds that can contribute to a significant background fluorescence. These compounds include proteins, cofactors (e.g. NADH), porphyrins and drugs. The extent of this background contribution will depend on the exact excitation and emission wavelengths used. The high absorptivity demonstrated by haemolytic and icteric samples is a significant case in point. To complicate the matter further, binding of the fluorescent probe to serum proteins (e.g. albumin) may lead to significant fluorescence quenching effects. Also, serum and plasma contain components such as lipoproteins and immune complexes, which may lead to serious problems associated with light scattering. In general, interferences from endogenous substances may be minimised by sample dilution. Alternatively, various sample pretreatments such as protein precipitation, analyte extraction, treatment with proteases or various chemicals have been advocated (Ullman *et al.*, 1980).

In spite of these difficulties, several types of homogeneous immunoassay using fluorescence detection have been developed and successfully exploited. The vast majority of these procedures are competitive and have been developed for the measurement of low molecular mass analytes and haptens. The limitations on assay sensitivity imposed by a competitive design, together with the need to pretreat or dilute the sample to avoid matrix effects has led to assays that can rarely detect analytes in less than nanomolar concentrations.

The basic types of nonseparation or homogeneous fluorescence technology can be categorised as follows: (1) fluorescence polarisation immunoassays; (2) release fluoroimmunoassays; (3) fluorescence modulation immunoassays, which includes both enhancement and quenching phenomena; and (4) fluorescence energy transfer immunoassays. Most categories contain methods that employ conventional fluorophores such as fluorescein and rhodamine derivatives. These labels display a short-lived or prompt fluorescence (of nanosecond duration). Other methods use labels such as the lanthanide chelates that demonstrate a longer fluorescence decay time (microsecond duration) in association with time-resolution fluorescence measurement.

Fluorescence Polarisation Immunoassay (FPIA)

As described previously, when a molecule absorbs light, an electron is promoted to a higher unoccupied orbital. Subsequently this absorbed energy is rapidly dissipated by vibrational relaxation, by internal conversion and by light emission. This excitation and emission cycle is accompanied and facilitated by the establishment of intramolecular electronic processes termed oscillating dipoles, which have a defined planar orientation. Under normal circumstances, the orientation of these oscillating dipoles is of no consequence. Nevertheless, if polarised light is used to excite the molecules, this energy will be absorbed most efficiently by those molecules possessing oscillating dipoles that are parallel to the plane of the polarised light (Dandliker *et al.*, 1980; Rhys Williams, 1988).

Moreover, the degree of polarisation of the emitted light depends on the lifetime of the excited state and the rotational motion of the molecule. In particular, in solution, molecules are not static but in a constant state of Brownian motion. Consequently, molecular rotation will decrease the degree of emission polarisation. The extent of this rotation depends on a number of factors, which include: (1) molecular volume (size and shape); (2) solvent viscosity;

and (3) solvent temperature. For example, an aqueous solution containing low molecular mass fluorescent molecules will show minimal emission polarisation at room temperature. Nevertheless, cooling the solution or increasing its viscosity will lead to a concomitant increase in fluorescence polarisation. In particular, the Brownian motion of larger molecules or molecular complexes (e.g. antigen-antibody complexes) is reduced. Consequently, the molecular orientation of the oscillating dipoles in these complexes are partially preserved with the resulting fluorescence exhibiting an increase in the degree of polarisation (Dandliker *et al.*, 1980; Rhys Williams, 1988).

For example, large molecules (e.g. antibodies) have rotational times of approximately 10 to 100 ns. In contrast, small molecules (e.g. haptens) have rotational times of less than 1 ns. The necessary alteration in molecular volume brought about when a hapten binds to its antibody gives a practical limit for the size of antigen, which should be below 20,000 M_r. Furthermore, the fluorescence lifetime of the fluorophore must be longer than the rotational time of the labelled antigen but shorter than the rotational time of the antigen-antibody complex. Fluorescein, which has a fluorescence lifetime of 4.5 ns, is an ideal candidate.

The other labels employed have been rhodamine and dimethyl aminonaphthalene sulphonic acid derivatives, which exhibit a high fluorescence intensity not lost on coupling to the antigen. Ideally, excitation and emission wavelength maxima should be chosen to avoid sample fluorescence and light scattering. For larger antigens, fluorochromes with somewhat longer decay times such as Lucifer yellow, dansyl and umbelliferone derivatives have been tried but with much less success (Dandliker *et al.*, 1980; Urios and Cittanova, 1990).

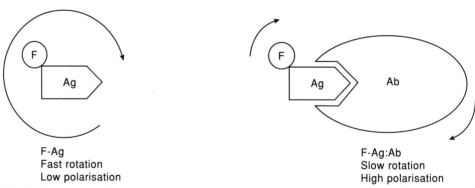

F-Ag
Fast rotation
Low polarisation

F-Ag:Ab
Slow rotation
High polarisation

Figure 5 The principle of fluorescence polarisation immunoassay. Ag, antigen; Ab, antibody; F, fluorescent label.

The basic principle of fluorescence polarisation immunoassay (FPIA) is shown in Figure 5. The first methods were described by Dandliker and Feigen (1961), who studied the interaction of fluorescein-labelled penicillin, ovalbumin and oestrone with specific binding proteins or receptors. Since 1976, Professor Landon's research group at St Bartholomew's Hospital, London have developed many FPIAs. Moreover, they simplified the technology by using one-step, one-reagent methods based on antibodies pre-equilibrated with FITC-labelled antigens (Colbert *et al.*, 1984, 1986).

A conventional method involves mixing samples with the fluorescent-labelled antigen followed by addition of the specific antibody. Subsequently the degree of polarisation, which is inversely proportional to the concentration of the authentic analyte, is measured. In other words, as the concentration of the analyte increases in the sample or standard, the more the labelled antigen remains free in solution, leading to a reduction in the level of fluorescence polarisation. Reaction times are typically between 3 and 15 min.

Widespread clinical application of competitive FPIA, however, only began in the early 1980s when Abbott introduced the TD_x series of automated instruments. More recently, other reagent and instrument manufacturers, such as Roche Diagnostics, CANAM Diagnostics, Innotron and Source Scientific Systems have led to an increasing proliferation of the technology. Several manufacturers are producing FPIA kits that are intended to be used either with the existing Abbott TD_x system or with the manufacturer's own instrument, such as the Roche FPIA, developed for the company's Cobas Bio and Cobas Fara automated systems.

One of the main limitations of FPIA is the effect of serum proteins, which is to compromise profoundly the methods that demand good sensitivity in the nanomolar range (Porter *et al.*, 1984). In addition, other workers have reported interference in a thyroxine FPIA by mildly haemolysed samples (Symons and Vining, 1985). Interferences in samples from patients with renal failure have also been reported for FPIAs for the measurement of phenytoin and theophylline (MacGregor *et al.*, 1978; Lu-Steffes *et al.*, 1982). Moreover, samples from uraemic patients contain higher concentrations of endogenous fluorophores, which contribute to a raised background fluorescence and can affect certain methods (Shaykh *et al.*, 1985).

To avoid the problem of low-affinity binding properties of albumin and other serum proteins that increase the level of polarisation nonspecifically, the sample is diluted or pretreated using chaotropic ions, proteolytic enzymes, protein-precipitating reagents or solvents. Reagent packs generally contain a pretreatment solution in addition to the specific antiserum and the fluorescein-labelled antigen. The instruments perform the required dilutions, record blank values and measure emission polarisation. The technology is used widely for therapeutic drug monitoring (Jolley *et al.*, 1981a) and for the screening of drugs of abuse (Jolley *et al.*, 1981b; Colbert *et al.*, 1985). Procedures have also been developed for the measurement of some hormones (e.g. oestriol, cortisol) and even for a few proteins (Spencer *et al.*, 1973; Kobayashi *et al.*, 1979; Grossman, 1983; Gonzalez-Buitrago *et al.*, 1988).

In general, FPIAs demonstrate excellent precision and reproducibility. Day-to-day coefficients of variations are typically in the range of 4 to 7% for analyte concentrations in the micromolar range. In addition, the reagents are stable for at least 6 months and calibration curve stability exceeds 6 weeks in many cases.

Release Fluoroimmunoassay (RFIA)

Release fluoroimmunoassay (RFIA) is based on the use of a nonfluorescent-labelled antigen conjugated through ester or glycosidic bonds to a potential fluorophore (e.g. at position 7 of a coumarin derivative). Hydrolysis of the bond leads to the release of a fluorescent product. RFIAs are essentially of two types. The first type has been described as antibody-enhanced hydrolysis using conjugates possessing ester bonds. The binding of the labelled antigen to its specific antibody brings the ester bond close to chemically reactive amino acid residues which catalyse the hydrolysis of the bond. Exploiting this phenomenon of catalytic antibodies, Kohen *et al.* (1979, 1980) have described nonseparation FIAs for the measurement of 17-α-hydroxyprogesterone and testosterone using conjugates linked via an ester or thioether bond to umbelliferone.

The second and more common type of RFIA is enzyme-hydrolysed antibody-protected FIA, more commonly called substrate-labelled FIA (SL-FIA; *see* Chapter 15). This procedure involves the hydrolysis of glycosidic linkages by additional enzymes, which are used in excess in

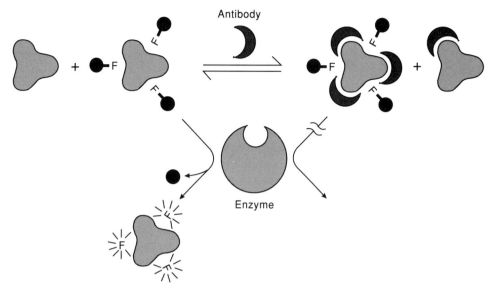

Antibody

Enzyme

Figure 6 The principle of substrate-labelled fluoroimmunoassay. F, fluorescent label.

the system. In addition, the tracer is an antigen labelled with a fluorogenic substrate. The binding of the conjugate to the antibody, which are both used in limited concentration, sterically hinders the hydrolytic action of the enzyme so that only the free fraction is hydrolysed and contributes to the signal.

Substrate-labelled FIA was originally developed by Burd *et al.* (1977) using umbelliferone-labelled biotin and fluorescein-labelled dinitrophenol as tracers labelled through ester bonds. Because of background interferences (including antibody-enhanced hydrolysis), subsequent applications have been developed using β-galactosidase with antigens labelled with umbelliferone galactoside (Boguslaski *et al.*, 1980), which is a more stable linkage less prone to spontaneous release. The hydrolysis of the conjugate leads to a shift in the absorptivity of the conjugate from 343 to 403 nm resulting in minimal background fluorescence. The principle of SL-FIA is illustrated in Figure 6.

The analyte in the sample or standard competes with the substrate-labelled hapten conjugate for binding to the specific antibody. As the concentration of the authentic compound increases, more substrate-labelled analyte remains free in solution to act as a substrate for β-galactosidase. The conjugate that is bound to the antibody is not available to the enzyme. Consequently, the fluorescent signal that represents the free fraction is directly proportional to the concentration of the analyte in the standard or sample. The antibody that is chosen for the method must possess the appropriate specificity and affinity to ensure the efficient protection of the labelled antigen. In addition, the antibody must be used in sufficient concentration to bind at least 80% of the labelled antigen in the absence of competing analyte. Consequently, potential assay sensitivity is reduced. Nevertheless, SL-FIAs can be operated kinetically, which can lead to increased precision with the advantage of in-built blank correction.

Ames (Ames Division, Miles Laboratories, now Bayer Diagnostics, Elkhart, USA) commercialised the SL-FIA technique primarily developed for therapeutic drug monitoring together with the company's dedicated filter SL-FIA fluorometer (Fluorostat®). In addition, a rapid dry-reagent strip procedure was also developed based on the SL-FIA principle (Greenquist *et al.*, 1981). Variations of the basic technology have been described. For example, Li and Burd (1981) used flavine mononucleotide as a fluorogenic substrate (coupled to theophylline via an AMP linker), together with pyrophosphatase. Moreover, Dean *et al.* (1983) developed a dual-label SL-FIA procedure using β-galactosyl-coumarin-labelled phenobarbital and 4-methylcoumarin-phosphodiester-labelled phenytoin. The application of two enzymes, β-galactosidase and phosphodiesterase, released labels that could be measured simultaneously with appropriate filters.

Fluorescence Modulation Immunoassay (FMIA)

In general, most fluorescent labels are very sensitive to many different environmental changes which include: (1) polarity; (2) dielectric strength; (3) hydrogen bonding; (4) pH; (5) rotational freedom; (6) viscosity; and (7) the close proximity of energy-donating or energy-accepting groups and quenching atoms or absorbing groups. Any or all of these factors may have a profound effect on the fluorescent properties of the label such as wavelength, quantum yield or decay time. Monitoring these changes may permit the development of nonseparation fluorescence modulation immunoassays (FMIAs).

Nevertheless, despite these real phenomena, FMIAs have not been widely used. The reason for this may well be due to the unpredictable nature of these changes which are invariably dependent on a specific antibody. As a variation to this theme, FMIAs have been developed using antibodies directed against the fluorophores as additional signal-modulating components. These indirect quenching FIAs attracted much attention in the 1970s and early 1980s (Watt and Voss, 1977; Nargessi and Landon, 1981).

Fluorescence Enhancement Immunoassays

Two basic approaches have been used in the development of fluorescence enhancement immunoassays. The first approach uses a fluorescent probe that is extremely sensitive to changes in environment causing a significant increase in fluorescence quantum yield when the probe is bound to a protein (e.g. as in a specific antibody-binding reaction). Examples of these probes include dansyl derivatives, 8-anilino-1-naphthalene sulphonic acid (ANS) and *N*-(3-pyrene)-maleimide (Lipurdy, 1979). Note that although fluorescein is generally quenched when bound to antibodies, enhancement effects have been reported and assay systems have been developed for the measurement of various haptens including thyroxine (Smith, 1977). In this last example, the fluorescence from fluorescein-labelled thyroxine is quenched by the presence of four iodine atoms. When the labelled probe binds to the specific antibody this quenching is partially reversed. This phenomenon is the basis for the second type of fluorescence enhancement immunoassay, which is based on the ability of the antibody to alleviate quenching caused by the presence of heavy atoms built into the fluorescent antigen conjugate.

Fluorescence-quenching Immunoassays

Shaw *et al.* (1977) reported the first fluorescence-quenching immunoassay in which fluorescein-labelled gentamicin fluorescence was quenched when it bound to anti-gentamicin antibodies. Several direct quenching immunoassays have been developed using this principle, including cortisol (Kobayashi *et al.*, 1980).

A more robust approach to quenching immunoassay has been termed indirect quenching FIA (IQ-FIA). The principle of this method is illustrated in Figure 7. This approach involves the use of anti-fluor antibodies (e.g. anti-fluorescein) which act as a signal modulator. Fluor-

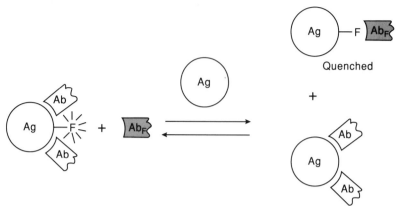

Figure 7 The principle of an indirect quenching fluorescence immunoassay. Ag, antigen; Ab, antibody; F, fluorescent label.

escein fluorescence is profoundly quenched (approximately 90%) when a labelled probe is bound to anti-fluorescein antibodies (Micheel *et al.*, 1988). In general, IQ-FIAs are sequential; the primary binding reaction between analyte and specific antibodies is allowed to proceed to completion prior to the addition of anti-fluorescein. The binding of this modulating antibody leads to fluorescence quenching of the free-labelled antigen which is not protected by the specific anti-hapten antibody. This indirect quenching approach has been given alternative names such as fluorescence protection immunoassay (Zuk *et al.*, 1979) and alternative binding FIA(Hassan *et al.*, 1982).

In general, IQ-FIAs are most appropriate for large molecules such as albumin, IgG and HPL (Nargessi and Landon, 1981). Nevertheless variations have been developed for the measurement of small molecules (e.g. haptens). For example, anti-analyte and anti-fluorescein antibodies have been linked together and used in a competitive alternative-binding assay for thyroxine (Hassan *et al.*, 1982). A major impediment to the use of all these methods, however, is the necessity to apply a blank correction for each sample.

Time-resolved Fluoroimmunoassay

As we have already described, the use of lanthanide chelates and time-resolved fluorescence immunoassay offers many potential advantages, including reduced interference from fluorophores present in biological materials and assay components. As a consequence, assay sensitivity can be improved dramatically. Lanthanide chelates, however, are extremely sensitive to the environment. In addition, the DELFIA principle involves the use of basically nonfluorescent probes. Before measurement, however, an enhancement solution is added that causes the release of the lanthanide, such as europium, into solution. The presence of detergent and fatty acid derivatives in the enhancement solution allows for the development of a microenvironment (micelle) in which water is excluded and europium is chelated to a β-diketone. Under these conditions, the lanthanide-β-diketone chelate is strongly fluorescent and is protected from quenching processes.

In order to develop nonseparation FIAs exploiting the advantages of time-resolved fluorescence, it has been necessary to develop a different type of lanthanide chelate that is fluorescent in aqueous solution and does not require the addition of enhancement reagent. For example, Hemmilä *et al.* (1988) have described an assay for thyroxine in which a fluorescent europium chelate was coupled to thyroxine. The concentration of BSA and detergents compared to assay buffer was critical to maximise the fluorescence of the labelled antigen. When the lanthanide-thyroxine conjugate was bound to antibody, fluorescence was profoundly quenched. Consequently, the fluorescence measured reflected the concentration of the labelled probe that remained free in solution.

Based on this principle, Barnard *et al.* (1989a,b) described the use of a novel fluorescent oestrone-3-glucuronyl-europium derivative to develop a simple, rapid and precise homogeneous time-resolved FIA for the measurement of urinary oestrone-3-glucuronide, a major metabolite of serum oestradiol. In terms of specificity and accuracy, the characteristics of the 15-min nonseparation assay were comparable to both a separation FIA and a RIA.

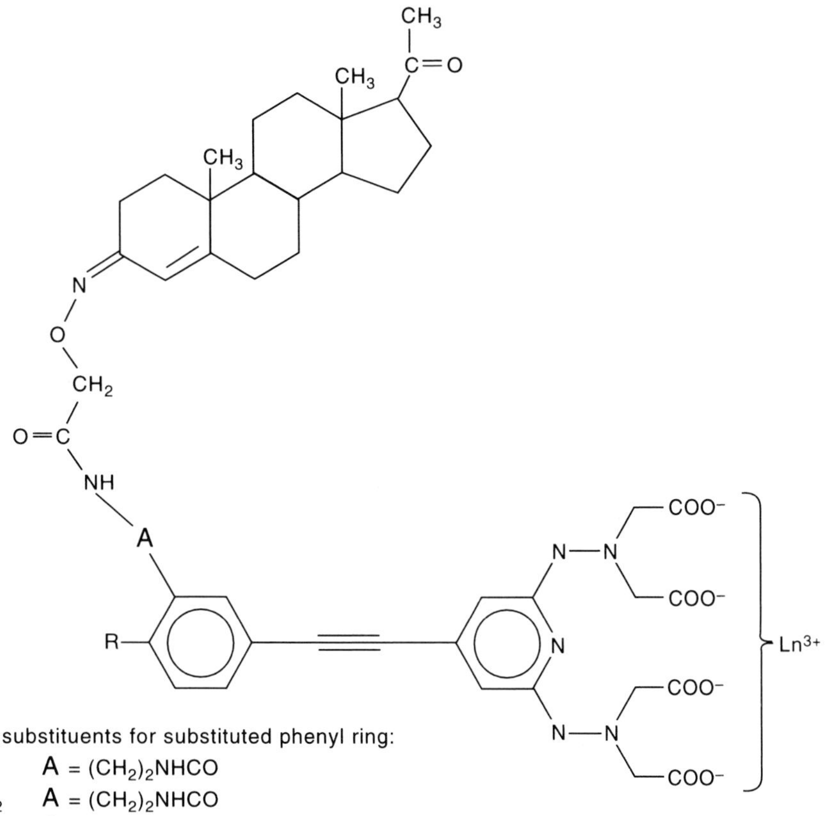

Sample substituents for substituted phenyl ring:
R = OH   A = (CH$_2$)$_2$NHCO
R = NH$_2$ A = (CH$_2$)$_2$NHCO
R = H   A = CH$_2$

Figure 8 Examples of fluorescent lanthanide-labelled progesterone derivatives. (From Mikola *et al.* (1995) with permission).

Considerable effort has gone into the synthesis of a fluorescent lanthanide chelate that has increased fluorescence quantum yields. For example, Mikola *et al.* (1995) have described the synthesis of labels containing substituted 4-(arylethynyl)-pyridine as the chromogenic moiety and iminobis (acetic acid) groups as the chelating part of the fluorescent probes. They reported that derivatives containing the para-amino-substituted phenyl ring demonstrated strong dependence on environmental changes. The structure of a fluorescent lanthanide-labelled progesterone is shown in Figure 8.

Various other schemes leading to the development of homogeneous time-resolved FIAs using lanthanide chelates have been described (Wieder and Hale, 1987). The methods involve such things as the formation of mixed-ligand chelates, ligand exchange, intraligand quenching, and different energy transfer routes.

The principle of time-resolution minimises the problems that affect most other nonseparation methods, which are subject to nonspecific interference from factors in biological materials, assay buffers, reagents and plastics. Consequently, with the synthesis of novel lanthanide chelates with increased quantum yields of fluorescence in the aqueous phase, we can envisage a gradual switch from separation to nonseparation methodology for the fully automated measurement of the majority of common analytes by time-resolved fluorescence assay.

Fluorescence Excitation Transfer Immunoassay (FETI)

The principle of fluorescence excitation transfer immunoassays (FETIs) involves the use of two different labels coupled to various components of the assay system. For example, a fluorescent probe may be conjugated to an antigen whereas an energy-accepting or energy-quenching group may be coupled to an antibody. When the two labels come close (e.g. upon antigen-antibody binding) energy transfer takes place between the two groups. Such dipole-dipole energy transfer depends, however, on the wavelength of emitted fluorescence from the donor being appropriate to excite the acceptor molecule. Other important features include the fluorescent quantum yield of the donor and the extinction coefficient of the acceptor molecule at the donor emission wavelength. In addition, the proximity of the donor and acceptor molecules profoundly affects the efficiency of the process. The rate of transfer is inversely proportional to the sixth power of the distance between the molecules and energy can be transferred efficiently across distances of about 10 nm or less. The principle of FETI is shown in Figure 9.

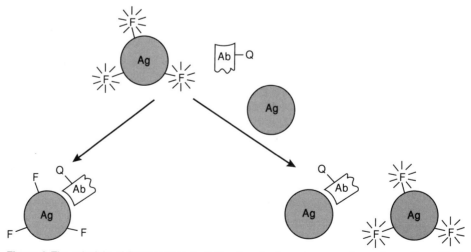

Figure 9 The principle of fluorescence excitation transfer immunoassay. Ag, antigen; Ab, antibody; F, donor fluorescent label; Q, acceptor fluorescent label.

Fluorescence excitation transfer immunoassay was first described by Ullman *et al.* (1976), when a fluorescein-labelled morphine was used as the energy donor for rhodamine-labelled antibodies with high specific activity. The technology was further developed by the Syva Corporation (Calvin *et al.*, 1986a, b) and marketed with the company's automated Syva Advance fluorometer. There have been many FETI applications developed using different fluorescein derivatives (e.g. carboxyfluorescein, FITC and various methoxy- and chloro-substituted fluoresceins) as the donor fluors and 4′,5′-dimethoxy-6-carboxy-fluorescein as the nonfluorescent acceptor. This acceptor molecule works well because it has good spectral overlapping with fluorescein but practically no fluorescence of its own, resulting in low background signals (Khana and Ullman, 1980).

It is possible to perform FETIs as end-point determinations (sequential addition of reagents) or kinetically (simultaneous addition of reagents). The sequential protocol offers the highest sensitivity but a separate blank measurement is needed to account for the fluorescence from endogenous materials. In the kinetic protocol, all three assay reagents are mixed simultaneously and the change in fluorescence intensity is monitored over a short time period. This approach is less sensitive but has the advantage of improved precision and compensation for endogenous fluorescence.

It can be argued that the greatest sensitivity will be achieved by monitoring fluorescence at the emission wavelength of the acceptor molecule (with the greatest Stokes's shift); in practice, however, it is the quenching of the donor molecule that is monitored because, in many cases, the excitation of the donor also results in some direct excitation of the acceptor molecule (because of overlap of excitation spectra) resulting in a high background. In the case of a fluorescent donor label being coupled to the antigen and an energy quencher being coupled to the antibody, the fluorescence intensity of the donor is reduced when the labelled antigen and labelled antibody combine. Accordingly, increasing the concentration of the analyte in the sample or standard leads to an increase in the concentration of the labelled antigen in solution. This in turn leads to a reduction in quenching and an increase in the measured fluorescence that is directly proportional to the concentration of the analyte in the sample.

To get the donor and acceptor dye molecules appropriately close after the binding reaction, it is necessary to label the antibody as close to the binding site as possible. Nevertheless, epitope- or site-directed labelling is technically difficult. In general, empirical labelling experiments are performed with any given batch of antiserum to produce a reagent that will perform satisfactorily. Over-labelling of antibody with an acceptor molecule (e.g. rhodamine) can lead to the precipitation of the conjugate, loss of immunoreactivity and increased background fluorescence. In addition, it is important to use affinity-purified antibody preparations to minimise the labelling of nonspecific proteins which would contribute to background fluorescence.

The choice of fluorescent donor molecule should take into account quantum yield, the excitation wavelength and the Stokes's shift together with any change in these characteristics that may occur on coupling. For example, Ullman and Khana (1981) have studied various fluoresceins that illustrate the variations that can be achieved with different substituents. Besides fluorescein and rhodamine, a number of alternative labels have also been tested in the homogeneous FETIs which include: (1) phycoerythrin; (2) pyrene; (3) Texas red; (4) Lucifer yellow; (5) quinacrine; (6) eosin; (7) fluorescamine; (8) squaric acid; and (9) gallocyanine (Miller *et al.*, 1980; Bailey *et al.*, 1984). In particular, the choice of an excitation wavelength greater than 490 nm together with a large Stokes's shift minimises problems caused by sample interference.

Methods have been described for haptens and proteins with a lower limit of detection between 1 and 10 nmol l^{-1}. In an evaluation of FETIs for individual serum proteins and haptens, various workers have demonstrated excellent precision and good correlation with existing methods and no significant interference from either gross haemolysis or gross lipaemia. In addition, the reagents were stable for at least three months when reconstituted (Calvin *et al.*, 1986a, b).

Time-resolved Fluorescence Excitation Transfer Immunoassays

Wieder and Hale (1987) have patented a time-resolved fluorescence excitation transfer immunoassay based on the use of lanthanide chelate labels for the measurement of theophylline. The fluorescence of the lanthanide chelate-labelled antigen was quenched when close to an organic fluorochrome or heavy metal atom. In another patent, Stavrianopoulos *et al.* (1987) have described a time-resolved FETI based on the use of complement.

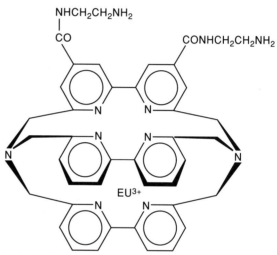

Figure 10 Example of a lanthanide cryptate.

More recently, Mathis and co-workers (1993) have developed time-resolved FETIs based on the use of lanthanide cryptates as donor molecules. The lanthanide cryptates used in this time-resolved amplified cryptic (TRACE) system are formed by the inclusion of the lanthanide ion into the cavity of a macropolycyclic ligand containing 2,2'-bipyridine groups as light absorbers. The structure of this compound is shown in Figure 10.

The energy acceptor molecule is allophycocyanin (APC), a phycobiliprotein of relative molecular mass (M_r) 105K. The choice of this molecule was for the following reasons: (1) a high molar absorptivity at the cryptate emission wavelength, which allows for a high transfer efficiency quoted as 75% over a distance of 7.5 nm; (2) APC fluorescence emission in a spectral range where the cryptate signal is insignificant; (3) an emission that is not quenched in the presence of serum; and (4) a high quantum yield.

A dedicated instrument has been designed ('Kryptor'; CIS Biointernational) that uses laser excitation at 337 nm and the time-resolved measurement of fluorescence at 620 nm (reference signal) and 665 nm (specific amplified signal). The measurement of prolactin has been used as a model system, where one monoclonal antibody was labelled with the europium cryptate and the other monoclonal (having a different epitope specificity) labelled with APC. The signal that is generated has two components, a long-lived fluorescence from the complex and a short-lived fluorescence from the free APC-labelled antibody. After the excitation pulse, the signal is measured at 665 nm after a delay of 10–100 µs, which eliminates the contribution of the fluorescence from the free APC label. For each standard and sample, the fluorescence ratio at 650 nm to 620 nm is calculated. The detection limit of the method is quoted as 0.3 µg l^{-1}, which compares very well with heterogeneous assay systems.

Other Homogeneous Fluorescence Immunoassays

Homogeneous Fluorescence Immunoassays Using Liposomes

Liposomes are vesicles made from phospholipids, cholesterol and fatty acids. A research group led by Kinsky (1974) was the first to show that liposomes could be used to carry the components for detection, such as enzymes, substrates and, in particular, fluorophores. Liposomes can be disrupted by complement lysis using suitable animal serum as the source of complement. This results in the release of their contents and, in this way, considerable signal amplification can be achieved. In addition, the use of liposomes allows for the development of homogeneous procedures.

In particular, nonseparation complement-mediated liposome-lysis FIAs have been developed and have been called microcapsule immunoassays (MCIA) (Rokugawa *et al.*, 1988; Fiechtner *et al.*, 1989). In addition, haptens can be linked to a cytolysin such as mellitin (Gerber *et al.*, 1990). The conjugate that is not bound to specific anti-hapten antibody remains effective in disrupting liposomes that have been loaded with fluorophore.

The stability of the liposomes is a critical factor in the development of such methods. If the liposome is 'leaky', it will result in very high background readings. Liposome stability is greatly affected by the choice of appropriate components, preparation method and sizes. In particular, the hydrophilicity of the fluorophore has a major effect on the rate of leakage (Fiechtner *et al.*, 1989).

Despite this difficulty of stability, the use of liposomes has the potential to solve the continuing problems of homogeneous FIAs: signal, sensitivity and the suitability for both large and small molecules. Although there has not been widespread use of liposome immunoassays, a model commercial system is available. Becton Dickinson have developed the Q Test which involves the use of liposomes loaded with rhodamine sulphate with a visual detection of the end-point (Gerber *et al.*, 1990).

Phase-resolved Fluorometry

In addition to fluorescence intensity, fluorescence decay time can also change during the immunoreaction. For example, using phase-resolved fluorometry, McGown (1988) demonstrated that fluorescence decay time was altered when fluorescein-labelled phenobarbital and Texas red-labelled albumin bound to their respective antibodies. Although these changes were extremely small (picoseconds) they were sufficient for the development of a quantitative assay. In addition, Soini *et al.* (1986) have patented a general technique that uses decay time differences in the development of a phase- and time-resolved homogeneous time-resolved FIA for the measurement of insulin.

Solvent Perturbation FIAs

Solvent perturbation techniques have been developed based on the use of modulating reagents that can enhance or quench the fluorescence from an appropriate labelled antigen (Halfman, 1987). For example, detergents (e.g. sodium dodecyl sulphate (SDS)) quench fluorescence and methods have been reported for the measurement of gentamicin and amphetamines using fluorescein as a label (Halfman *et al.*, 1985; Halfman and Jay, 1986).

Pseudohomogeneous FIAs

A true homogeneous assay does not involve any intervention by the operator in the physical separation of the antibody-bound and free fraction. Nevertheless, there are many FIAs that involve the use of solid-phase reagents but still do not require any operator intervention to separate the respective fractions. In these methods, however, fluorescence is measured from only one of the fractions. These methods have been termed 'space-resolved FIAs' (Hemmilä, 1991). A specific example of this principle is the use of magnetic particles that can be pulled to the side of a cuvette before the measurement of fluorescence in the free fraction.

In addition, several assays based on the use of microbeads and flow cytometry have been reported (Saunders *et al.*, 1985). In the flow cytometer, the bead used as a solid phase triggers the detection of the fluorescence of the bound label as it passes through the capillary. Alternative procedures have also been devised that discriminate between slow-moving particle and fast-moving nonparticle fluorescence by analysing signal fluctuations (Elings *et al.*, 1981).

Immunosensors

Various immunosensors have been described using fluorescence detection in association with fibre optics or solid surfaces. For example, Kronick and Little (1975) described a morphine biosensor method performed on quartz slides and using evanescent waves to excite fluorescent molecules in very close proximity to the reflecting surface. (*See* Chapter 20 for a discussion of optical sensors.)

SENSITIVITY AND CHOICE OF TRACER SYSTEM

In their review, Diamandis and Christopoulos (1990) have summarised the detection limits achieved with different nonradioisotopic labelling methods. Detection limits for alternative tracer assay systems are in the range 10^{-10} to 10^{-11} mol l^{-1} for conventional enzyme labels, 10^{-9} to 10^{-10} mol l^{-1} for conventional fluorophores, 10^{-9} to 10^{-10} mol l^{-1} for luminol and isoluminol chemiluminescence and 10^{-11} to 10^{-12} mol l^{-1} for acridinium ester chemiluminescence. The lowest detection limits, in the range 10^{-12} to 10^{-13} mol l^{-1}, can be achieved with europium chelate time-resolved fluorescence, enzyme label with fluorogenic or chemiluminogenic substrates, and enzyme recycling systems.

The comparison of immunoassay sensitivity between methods using different labels is not straightforward. Invariably the characteristics of the antibodies used together with the assay configuration will profoundly affect the actual sensitivity realised. For example, Kricka (1994) has compiled assay sensitivities obtained for the measurement of TSH in serum. The most sensitive TSH immunoassay reported so far (detection limit 0.0002 mIU l^{-1}) involves the use of two fluorescent labels (Texas red and fluorescein) and confocal microscopic detection

(Ekins, 1993). Madersbacker *et al.* (1993) have compared assays for the measurement of FSH using the same monoclonal antibodies with different labels. The results showed that the time-resolved procedure gave both the greatest sensitivity (2 ng l^{-1}) and the widest assay working range (2–160,000 ng l^{-1}).

If one considers competitive procedures for the measurement of small molecules, the limit of detection is rarely a feature of the label's detectability. If good quality antibodies are available, immunoassays with detection limits of <100 fg per tube may be obtained using either ^{125}I, enzymes, chemiluminophores or europium chelates as labels.

Of the systems that offer greatest sensitivity, time-resolved fluorescence offers the advantages of a rapid counting procedure with very high counting precision. Fluorescence readings can be repeated if necessary because label measurement is nondestructive. For the measurement of enzyme labels an additional incubation step is required, and reagents for this may be relatively expensive. Chemiluminescence assays offer a rapid throughput for samples if they are automated, but reanalysis is not possible if problems occur with the luminescence determination. Time-resolved fluorescence labels therefore have a clear advantages over other non-radioisotopic labels for use in routine diagnostic limited-reagent and excess-reagent immunoassay methods.

CONCLUSIONS

Fluoroimmunoassays and immunofluorometric assays using conventional fluorescence probes are insensitive and have not gained widespread acceptance.

Time-resolved heterogeneous fluorescence immunoassay systems offer a practical alternative to ^{125}I-labelled methods. Assay incubation times, imprecision and costs are similar to conventional assays, while detection limits may be slightly better and convenience is increased. Time-resolved fluorescence systems are the methods of choice as alternatives to radioisotopically labelled methods, offering convenience, low detection limits, good counting precision and the facility to transfer existing in-house methods to the new tracer and to develop new in-house time-resolved fluorescence assays.

Fluorescence polarisation technology has provided extremely successful homogeneous FIAs for therapeutic drug monitoring and the assay of drugs of abuse. Nevertheless, the quest for greater sensitivity remains. At the present time, the full potential of these methods cannot be realised. This is largely due to interference from endogenous fluorophores that contribute to an increased background signal and also to the presence of molecules in biological fluids that absorb light and thereby quench fluorescent signals. The solution to these difficulties may lie in the hands of the photochemist who is seeking to synthesise new fluorescent probes with ever-increasing quantum yields that can be protected from deleterious interference from endogenous compounds. In the meantime homogeneous fluoroimmunoassays provide a useful means of assaying small molecules in the micromolar concentration range.

A specific area that might see a breakthrough is the increasing development and application of time-resolution and quench correction in fluorescence measurement. There is no question that heterogeneous assays using the lanthanide chelates have provided a fluorescence technology with exquisite sensitivity to rival and supersede procedures using radioisotopes. It is tempting to speculate that it will soon be possible to develop single- and multilabel non-separation time-resolved FIAs with similar success.

Acknowledgements

We are grateful to Wallac UK Ltd and Dr I. Hemmilä, Wallac OY, Turku, Finland for help with information on DELFIA assay systems.

REFERENCES

Allman, B. L., Short, F. & James, V. H. T. (1981) Fluroimmunoassay of progesterone in human serum or plasma. *Clin. Chem.* **27**, 1176–1182.

Altamirano-Bustamante, A., Barnard, G. & Kohen, F. (1991) Direct time-resolved fluorescence immunoassay for serum estradiol based on the idiotypic anti-idiotypic approach. *Immunol. Meth.* **138**, 95–101.

Bador, R., Dechaud, H., Claustrat, F. *et al.* (1987) Europium and samarium as labels in time-resolved fluorometric assay of follitropin. *Clin. Chem.* **33**, 48–51.

Bailey, M. P., Rocks, B. F. & Riley, C. (1983) Use of Lucifer Yellow VS as a label in fluorescent immunoassays illustrated by the determination of albumin in serum. *Ann. Clin. Biochem.* **20**, 213–216.

Bailey, M. P., Rocks, B. F. & Riley, C. (1984) Homogeneous fluoroimmunoassay using Lucifer Yellow VS: Determination of albumin in plasma. *Ann. Clin. Biochem.* **21**, 59–64.

Barnard, G., Beazley, C. & Kohen, F. (1994) Monitoring ovarian function by a simultaneous time-resolved fluorescence immunoassay of three urinary metabolites. *J. Endocrinol.* **140**, 42.

Barnard, G. & Kohen, F. (1990) Idiometric assay: A non-competitive immunoassay for small molecules typified by the measurement of serum estradiol. *Clin. Chem.* **36**, 1945–1950.

Barnard, G., Kohen, F., Mikola, H. *et al.* (1989a) The measurement of estrone-3-glucuronide by a rapid nonseparation time-resolved fluoroimmunoassay. *Clin. Chem.* **35**, 555–559.

Barnard, G., O'Reilly, C. P., Dennis, K. *et al.* (1989b) A nonseparation, time-resolved fluoroimmunoassay to monitor ovarian function and predict potential fertility in women. *Fertil. Steril.* **52**, 60–65.

Barnard, G. J. R., Williams, J. L., Paton, A. C. *et al.* (1988) Time-resolved fluoroimmunoassay. In: *Complementary Immunoassays* (ed. Collins, W. P.) pp. 149–167 (John Wiley & Sons, Chichester).

Boguslaski, R. C., Li, J. L., Benovic, T. T. *et al.* (1980) Substrate labeled homogeneous fluorescent immunoassay. In: *Immunoassays: Clinical Laboratory Techniques for the 1980s* (eds Nakamura, R. M., Dito, W. R. & Tucker, E. S.) pp. 187–198 (Alan R. Liss, New York).

Brand, L. & Witholt, B. (1967) Fluorescence measurements. *Meth. Enzymol.* **11**, 776–787.

Burd, J. F., Carrico, R. S., Fetter, M. C. *et al.* (1977) Specific protein ligand binding reactions monitored by enzymatic hydrolysis of fluorescent dye conjugates. *Anal. Biochem.* **77**, 56–67.

Calvin, J., Burling, K., Blow, C. *et al.* (1986a) Evaluation of fluorescence excitation transfer immunoassay for measurement of specific proteins. *J. Immunol. Meth.* **86**, 249–256.

Calvin, J., Burling, K., Campbell, R. S. *et al.* (1986b) Evaluation of fluorescence excitation transfer immunoassay for the measurement of plasma cortisol. *J. Auto. Chem.* 8, 80–84.

Campbell, A. K., Roberts, P. A. & Patel A. (1985) Chemiluminescence energy transfer: A technique for homogeneous immunoassay. In: *Alternative Immunoassays* (ed. Collins, W. P.) pp. 153–183 (John Wiley & Sons, Chichester).

Chan, R. L., Krause, L. M. & Sweet, R. V. (1981) Fluorescent immunoassay for theophylline. *Clin. Chem.* 27, 1085–1091.

Colbert, D. L., Gallacher, G. & Mainwaring Burton, R. W. (1985) Single reagent polarisation fluoroimmunoassay for amphetamine in urine. *Clin. Chem.* 31, 1193–1195.

Colbert, D. L., Smith, D. J., Landon, J. *et al.* (1986) Single reagent polarisation fluoroimmunoassay for the cocaine metabolite benzoylecgonine in urine. *Ann. Clin. Biochem.* 23, 37–41.

Colbert, D. L., Smith, D. S. & Sidki, A. M. (1984) Single reagent polarisation fluoroimmunoassay for barbiturates in urine. *Clin. Chem.* 30, 1765–1769.

Coons, A. B., Creech, H. J. & Jones, R. N. (1941) Immunological properties of an antibody containing a fluorescent group. *Proc. Soc. Exp. Biol. Med.* 47, 200–202.

Curry, R. E., Heitzman, H., Riege, D. H. *et al.* (1979) A system approach to fluorescent immunoassay, general principles and representative applications. *Clin. Chem.* 25, 1591–1595.

Curtiss, E. G. & Patel, J. A. (1978) Enzyme multiplied immunoassays: A review. *CRC Crit. Rev. Clin. Lab. Sci.* 9, 303–318.

Dandliker, W. B. & Feigen, G. A. (1961) Quantification of the antigen-antibody reaction by polarisation of fluorescence. *Biochem. Biophys. Res. Commun.* 5, 299–304.

Dandliker, W. B., Hsu, M. L. & Vanderlaran, W. P. (1980) Fluorescence polarisation immuno/receptor assays. In: *Immunoassays: Clinical Laboratory Techniques for the 1980s* (eds Nakamura, R. M., Dito, W. R. & Tucker, E. S.) pp. 65–88 (Alan R. Liss, New York).

Dean, K. J., Thompson, S. G., Burd, J. F. *et al.* (1983) Simultaneous determination of phenytoin and phenobarbital in serum or plasma by substrate-labelled fluorescent immunoassay. *Clin. Chem.* 29, 1051–1056.

Dechaud, H., Bador, R., Claustrat, F. *et al.* (1988) New approach to competitive lanthanide immunoassay: Time-resolved fluoroimmunoassay of progesterone with labelled analyte. *Clin. Chem.* 34, 501–504.

Diamandis, E. (1988) Immunoassays with time-resolved fluorescence spectroscopy: Principles and applications. *Clin. Biochem.* 21, 139–150.

Diamandis, E. P., Bhayana, V., Conway, K. *et al.* (1988) Time-resolved fluoroimmunoassay of cortisol in serum with a europium chelate as label. *Clin. Biochem.* 21, 291–296.

Diamandis, E. P. & Christopoulos, T. K. (1990) Europium chelate labels in time-resolved fluorescence immunoassays and DNA hybridisation assays. *Anal. Chem.* 62, 1149A–1157A.

Donovan, S. J. & Wood, P. J. (1993) Development and evaluation of a two-site immunofluorometric assay for 'intact' insulin. *J. Endocrin.* 137 (suppl.), 97.

Ekins, R. (1985) Current concepts and future developments. In: *Alternative Immunoassays.* (ed. Collins, W. P.) pp. 219–237 (John Wiley & Sons, Chichester).

Ekins, R. (1993) Multianalyte testing. *Clin. Chem.* 39, 369–370.

Elings, V. B., Nicoli, D. F. & Briggs, J. (1981) Fluorescence fluctuation immunoassay. *Meth. Enzymol.* 92, 458–472.

Engvall, E. (1980) Enzyme immunoassay, ELISA and EMIT. *Meth. Enzymologica* **70**, 419–439.

Fiechtner, M., Wong, M., Bieniarz, C. *et al.* (1989) Hydrophilic fluorescein derivatives: Useful reagents for liposome immunolytic assays. *Anal. Biochem.* **180**, 140–146.

Gerber, M. A., Randolph, M. F. & DeMeo, K. K. (1990) Liposome immunoassay for rapid identification of group A streptococci directly from throat swabs. *J. Clin. Microbiol.* **28**, 1463–1464.

Gonzalez-Buitrago, M., Cava, F., Gomez del Campo, A. *et al.* (1988) Clinical evaluation of a fluorescence polarisation immunoassay for quantifying C-reactive protein. *Clin. Chem.* **34**, 595–596.

Greenquist, A. C., Walter, B. & Li, T. M. (1981) Homogeneous fluorescent immunoassay with dry reagents. *Clin. Chem.* **27**, 1614–1617.

Grossman, S. H. (1983) A fluorescence polarisation immunoassay for brain creatine kinase. *Clin. Chem.* **29** (abstract), 1194.

Gudgin Dickson, E. F., Pollak, A. & Diamandis, E. P. (1995) Time-resolved detection of lanthanide luminescence for ultrasensitive bioanalytical assays. *J. Photochem. Photobiol.* **27**, 3–19.

Halfman, C. J. (1987) Homogeneous fluorescence ligand binding assay based upon preferential alteration of the respective intensities of bound and free label by solvent components. *US Patent* No. 4,640,898.

Halfman, C. J. & Jay, D. W. (1986) Homogeneous, micelle quenching fluoroimmunoassay for detection of amphetamine in urine. *Clin. Chem.* **32**, 1677–1681.

Halfman, C. J., Wong, F. C. L. & Jay D. W. (1985) Solvent perturbation fluorescence immunoassay technique. *Anal. Chem.* **57**, 1928–1930.

Hassan, M., Landon, J. & Smith, D. S. (1982) A novel non-separation fluoroimmunoassay for thyroxine. *J. Immunoassay* **3**, 1–15.

Hemmilä, I. (1985a) Fluoroimmunoassays and immunofluorometric assays. *Clin. Chem.* **31**, 359–370.

Hemmilä, I. (1985b) Time-resolved fluorometric determination of terbium in aqueous solution. *Anal. Chem.* **57**, 1676–1681.

Hemmilä, I. (1988) Lanthanides as probes for time-resolved fluorometric immunoassays. *Scand. J. Clin. Lab. Invest.* **48**, 389–400.

Hemmilä, I. (1991) *Applications of Fluorescence in Immunoassays* (John Wiley & Sons, New York).

Hemmilä, I., Holtinen, S., Pettersen, K. *et al.* (1987) Double-label time-resolved immunofluorometry of lutropin and follitropin in serum. *Clin. Chem.* **33**, 2281–2283.

Hemmilä, I., Malminen, O., Mikola, H. *et al.* (1988) Homogeneous time resolved fluoroimmunoassay of thyroxin in serum. *Clin. Chem.* **34**, 2320–2322.

Hemmilä, I., Mukkala, V.-M., Dakubu, S. *et al.* (1984) Europium as a label in time-resolved immunofluorometric assay. *Anal. Biochem.* **137**, 335–343.

Jackson, T. M. & Ekins, R. P. (1986) Theoretical limitations on immunoassay sensitivity. *J. Immunol. Meth.* **87**, 13–20.

Jolley, M. E., Stroupe, S. D. & Schwenzer, K. S. (1981a) Fluorescence polarisation immunoassays I. Monitoring aminoglycoside antibiotics in serum and plasma. *Clin. Chem.* **27**, 1190–1197.

Jolley, M. E., Stroupe, S. J., Schwenzer, K. S. *et al.* (1981b) Fluorescence polarisation immunoassay III. An automated system for therapeutic drug determination. *Clin. Chem.* **27**, 1575–1579.

Kakabakos, S. E., Christopoulos, T. K. & Diamandis, E. P. (1992) Multianalyte immunoassay based on spatially distinct fluorescent areas quantified by laser-excited solid-phase time-resolved fluorometry. *Clin. Chem.* **38**, 338–342.

Khana, P. L. & Ullman, E. F. (1980) 4′,5′-Dimethoxy-6-carboxy fluorescein. A novel dipole-dipole coupled fluorescence excitation transfer acceptor for fluoroimmunoassay. *Anal. Biochem.* **108**, 156–157.

Kinsky, S. C. (1974) Preparation of liposomes and a spectrophotometric assay for release of trapped glucose marker. *Meth. Enzymol.* **32**, 501–513.

Kobayashi, Y., Amitani, K., Watanabe, F. *et al.* (1979) Fluorescence polarisation immunoassay for cortisol. *Clin. Chim. Acta* **73**, 241–247.

Kobayashi, Y., Tsubota, N., Miyai, K. *et al.* (1980) Fluorescence quenching immunoassay of serum cortisol. *Steroids* **36**, 177–183.

Kohen, F., Hollander, Z., Burd, J. F. *et al.* (1979) Assay based on antibody-enhanced hydrolysis of a steroid umbelliferone conjugate. *FEBS Lett.* **100**, 137–140.

Kohen, F., Kim, J. B., Barnard, G. *et al.* (1980) Antibody-enhanced hydrolysis of steroid esters. *Biochim. Biophys. Acta* **629**, 328–337.

Kricka, L. J. (1994) Selected strategies for improving sensitivity and reliability of immunoassays. *Clin. Chem.* **40**, 347–357.

Kronick, M. N. & Little, W. A. (1975) A new immunoassay based on fluorescence excitation by internal reflection spectroscopy. *J. Immunol. Meth.* **8**, 235–242.

Kuo, J. E., Milby, K. H., Hinsberg, W. D. *et al.* (1985) Direct measurement of antigens in serum by time-resolved fluoroimmunoassay. *Clin. Chem.* **31**, 50–53.

Landon, J. & Kamel, R. S. (1981) Immunoassays employing reactants labelled with a fluorophore. In: *Immunoassays for the 80s* (eds Voller, A., Bartlett, A. & Bidwell, D.) pp. 91–112 (MTP Press, Lancaster).

Leinonen, J., Lovgren, T., Vornanen, T. *et al.* (1993) Double-label time-resolved immunofluorometric assay of prostate-specific antigen and of its complex with α_1-antichymotrypsin. *Clin. Chem.* **39**, 2098–2103.

Li, T. M. & Burd, J. F. (1981) Enzymatic hydrolysis of intramolecular complexes for monitoring theophylline in homogeneous competitive protein-binding reactions. *Biochem. Biophys. Res. Commun.* **103**, 1157–1165.

Lipurdy, R. P. (1979) Antibody induced fluorescence enhancement of a N-(3-pyrene) maleimide conjugate of rabbit anti-human immunoglobulin G. Quantitation of human IgG. *J. Immunol. Meth.* **28**, 233–242.

Lövgren, T., Hemmilä, I., Pettersson, K. *et al.* (1985) Time-resolved fluorometry in immunoassay. In: *Alternative Immunoassays* (ed. Collins, W. P.) pp. 203–217 (John Wiley & Sons, Chichester).

Lövgren, T., Meriö, L., Mitrunen, K., *et al.* (1996) One step all-in-one dry reagent immunoassays with fluorescent europium chelate label and time-resolved fluorometry. *Clin. Chem.* **42**, 1196–1201.

Lu-Steffes, M., Pittluck, G. W., Jolley, M. E. *et al.* (1982) Fluorescence polarisation immunoassay IV. Determination of phenytoin and phenobarbitol in human serum and plasma. *Clin. Chem.* **28**, 2278–2282.

MacGregor, A. R., Crookall Greening, J. O., Landon, J. *et al.* (1978) Polarisation fluoroimmunoassay of phenytoin. *Clin. Chim. Acta* **83**, 161–166.

Madersbacker, S., Shu-Cren, T., Scwarz, S. *et al.* (1993) Time-resolved immunofluorometry and other frequently used immunoassay types for follicle stimulating hormone compared by using identical monoclonal antibodies. *Clin. Chem.* **39**, 14335–14339.

Maggio, E. T. (1980) Recent advances in heterogeneous fluorescence immunoassays. In: *Immunoassays: Clinical Laboratory Techniques for the 1980s* (eds Nakamura, R. M., Dito, W. R. & Tucher, E. S.) pp. 1–12 (Alan R. Liss, New York).

Mares, A., DeBower, J., Osller, J. *et al.* (1995) A direct non-competitive idiometric enzyme immunoassay for serum oestradiol. *J. Immunol. Meth.* **181**, 83–90.

Mathis, G. (1993) Rare earth cryptates and homogeneous fluoroimmunoassay with human sera. *Clin. Chem.* **39**, 1953–1959.

McConway, M. G. & Beastall, G. H. (1994) Cofluorescence enhancement improves immunofluorimetric assay minimum detection limit. *Ann. Clin. Biochem.* **31**, 576–578.

McGown, L. B. (1988) Phase-resolved fluoroimmunoassay. In: *Non-isotopic Immunoassay* (ed. Ngo, T. T.) pp. 93–105 (Plenum Press, New York).

Micheel, B., Jantscheff, P., Bottger, V. *et al.* (1988) The production and radioimmunoassay application of monoclonal antibodies to fluorescein isothiocyanate. *J. Immunol. Meth.* **111**, 89–94.

Mikola, H., Sundell, A.-C. & Hanninen, E. (1993) Labeling of estradiol and testosterone alkyloxime derivatives with a europium chelate for time-resolved fluoroimmunoassays. *Steroids* **58**, 330–334.

Mikola, H., Takalo, H. & Hemmilä, I. (1995) Syntheses and properties of luminescent lanthanide chelate labels and labeled haptenic antigens for homogeneous immunoassays. *Bioconj. Chem.* **6**, 235–241.

Miller, J. N., Lim, C. S. & Bridges, J. N. (1980) Fluorescamine and fluorescein as labels in energy transfer immunoassay. *Analyst* **105**, 91–126.

Mitrunen, K., Pettersson, K., Püronen, T., *et al.* (1995) Dual-label one-step immunoassay for simultaneous measurement of free and total prostate-specific antigen concentrations and ratios in serum. *Clin. Chem.* **41**, 1115–1120.

Nakamura, R. M. (1979) Recent advances in immunochemical fluorescent analytical methods. *Lab. Res. Meth. Biol. Med.* **3**, 211–226.

Nargessi, R. D. & Landon, J. (1981) Indirect quenching fluoroimmunoassay. *Meth. Enzymol.* **74**, 60–79.

O'Donell, C. M. & Suffin, S. C. (1979) Fluorescence immunoassays. *Anal. Chem.* **51**, 33–40.

Pettersson, K., Alfthan, H., Stenman, U.-H. *et al.* (1993) Simultaneous assay of α-fetoprotein and free β-subunit of human chorionic gonadotropin by dual-label time-resolved immunofluorometric assay. *Clin. Chem.* **39**, 2084–2089.

Porter, W. H., Hanver, V. M. & Bush, B. A. (1984) Effect of protein concentration on the determination of digoxin in serum by fluorescence polarisation immunoassay. *Clin. Chem.* **30**, 1826–1829.

Pourfarzaneh, M., While, G. W., Landon, J. *et al.* (1980) Cortisol directly determined in serum by fluoroimmunoassay with magnetizable solid-phase. *Clin. Chem.* **26**, 730–736

Quattrone, A. J., O'Donnell, C. M., McBride, J. *et al.* (1981) An update of approaches toward the fluorescence immunoassay of drugs. *J. Anal. Toxicol.* **5**, 245–248.

Raggatt, P. R. (1989) Duplicates or singletons?: An analysis of the need for replication in immunoassay and a computer program to calculate the distribution of outliers, error rate and the precision profile from assay duplicates. *Ann. Clin. Biochem.* **26**, 26–37.

Reimer, C. B., Phillips, D. J., Black, C. M. *et al.* (1978) Standardisation of ligand binding assays for alpha-fetoprotein. In: *Immunofluorescence and Related Staining Techniques* (eds Knapp, W., Holubar, K. & Wick, G.) pp. 189–197 (Elsevier/North Holland, Amsterdam).

Rhys Williams, A. T. (1988) Fluorescence polarisation immunoassay. In: *Complementary Immunoassays* (ed. Collins, W. P.) pp. 135–147 (John Wiley & Sons, Chichester).

Rokugawa, K., Takiguchi, Y., Ishimori, Y. *et al.* (1988) Microcapsule immunoassay. *Clin. Chem.* 34 (abstract), 1164.

Saunders, G. C., Jett, J. H. & Martin, J. C. (1985) Amplified flow cytometric separation-free fluorescence immunoassays. *Clin. Chem.* 31, 2020–2023.

Self, C. H. (1989) Determination method, use and components. *Patent Corporation Treaty Publication* No. WO89/05453.

Shaw, E. J., Watson, R. A. A., Landon, J. *et al.* (1977) Estimation of serum gentamicin by quenching fluoroimmunoassay. *J. Clin. Pathol.* 30, 526–531.

Shaykh, M., Bazilinski, N., McCaul, D. S. *et al.* (1985) Fluorescent substances in uremic and normal serum. *Clin. Chem.* 31, 1988–1992.

Siboo, R. & Kulisek, E. A. (1978) A fluorescence immunoassay for the quantitation of C-reactive protein. *J. Immunol. Meth.* 23, 59–66.

Sidki, A. M. & Landon, J. (1985) Fluoroimmunoassays and phosphoro- immunoassays. In: *Alternative Immunoassays* (ed. Collins, W. P.) pp. 185–201 (John Wiley & Sons, Chichester).

Smith, D. J (1977) Enhancement fluoroimmunoassay of thyroxine. *FEBS Lett.* 77, 25–27.

Smith, D. S., Al-Hakiem, M. H. H. & Landon, J. (1981) A review of fluoroimmunoassays and immunofluorometric assay. *Ann. Clin. Biochem.* 18, 253–274.

Soini, E. & Hemmilä, J. (1979) Fluoroimmunoassay: Present status and key problems. *Clin. Chem.* 25, 353–361.

Soini, E. & Kojola, H. (1983) Time-resolved fluorometer for lanthanide chelates: a new generation of non-isotopic immunoassays. *Clin. Chem.* 29, 65–68.

Soini, E., Hemmilä, I. & Lovgren, T. (1986) Method for quantitative determination of a bispecific affinity reaction. *US Patent* No. 4,587,223.

Spencer, R. D., Toledo, F. B., Williams, B. T. *et al.* (1973) Design construction and two applications for an automated flow cell polarisation fluorometer with digital readout: enzyme inhibitor (anti-trypsin) assay and antigen antibody (insulin–insulin antiserum) assay. *Clin. Chem.* 19, 838–844.

Stavrianopoulos, J., Rabbani, E., Abrams, S. B. *et al.* (1987) Analyte detection by means of energy transfer. *Eur. Patent Appl.* No. 242,527.

Sykes, A. & Chard, T. (1980) Two-site immunofluorometric assay for pregnancy-specific β_1-glycoprotein (SP$_1$). *Clin. Chem.* 26, 1224–1229.

Symons, R. G. & Vining, R. F. (1985) An evaluation of a fluorescence polarisation immunoassay of thyroxine and thyroxine uptake. *Clin. Chem.* 31, 1342–1348.

Tsay, Y.-G. & Palmer, R. J. (1981) A solid-phase fluoroimmunoassay of tobramycin. *Clin. Chim. Acta* 109, 151–158.

Tsay, Y.-G., Wilson, L. & Keef, E. (1980) Quantitation of serum gentamicin concentration by solid phase immunofluorescence method. *Clin. Chem.* 26, 1610–1615.

Ullman, E. & Khana, P. L. (1981) Fluorescence excitation transfer immunoassay. *Meth. Enzymol.* 74, 28–60.

Ullman, E. F., Ballet, N. F., Brinkley, J. M. *et al.* (1980) Homogeneous fluorescence immunoassays. In: *Immunoassays: Clinical Laboratory Techniques for the 1980s* (eds Nakamura, R. M., Dito, W. R. & Tucker, E. S.) pp. 13–43 (Alan R. Liss, New York).

Ullman, E. F., Schwarzberg, M. & Rubenstein, K. E. (1976) Fluorescence excitation transfer immunoassays. A general method for determination of antigens. *J. Biol. Chem.* **251**, 4172–4178.

Urios, P. & Cittanova, N. (1990) Adaptation of fluorescence polarisation immunoassay to the assay of macromolecules. *Anal. Biochem.* **185**, 308–312.

Viinikka, L., Landon, J. & Pourfarzaneh, M. (1981) A two-site immunofluorometric assay for human placental lactogen. *Clin. Chim. Acta* **114**, 1–9.

Visor, G. C. & Schulman, S. G. (1981) Fluorescence immunoassay: Literature survey. *J. Pharm. Sci.* **70**, 469–475.

Wallac (1992) *Europium Chelate Labelling* Wallac information booklet (obtainable from Wallac UK Ltd, Milton Keynes).

Wang, R., Merrill, B. & Maggio, E. T. (1980) A simplified solid-phase immunofluorescence assay for measurement of serum immunoglobulins. *Clin. Chim. Acta* **102**, 169–177.

Watanabe, F., Tsubota, N., Kobayashi, Y. *et al.* (1982) Solid-phase fluoroimmunoassay for 11-deoxy-cortisol in serum using 21-amino-17-hydroxy-progesterone. *Steroids* **40**, 393–399.

Watt, R. M. & Voss, E. W. (1977) Mechanism of quenching of fluorescein by anti-fluorescein IgG-antibodies. *Immunochemistry* **14**, 533–541.

Wieder, I. (1978) Background rejection in fluorescence immunoassay. In: *Proc. 6th Int. Conf. Immunofluorescence and Related Staining Techniques* (eds Knapp, W., Holubar, K. & Wick, G.) pp. 67–80 (Elsevier, Vienna).

Wieder, I. & Hale, R. L. (1987) Homogeneous fluoroassay method employing fluorescent background rejection and water-soluble rare earth metal chelate fluorophores. *PCT Int. Patent Appl.* No. WO87/07955.

Xu, Y.-Y., Hemmilä, I. & Lovgren, T. (1992) Co-fluorescence effect in time-resolved fluoroimmunoassays: A review. *Analyst* **117**, 1061–1069.

Zuk, R. F., Rowley, G. L. & Ullman, E. F. (1979) Fluorescence protection immunoassay: A new homogeneous assay technique. *Clin. Chem.* **29**, 155–160.

Chapter 17

Chemiluminescence Immunoassay

Ian Weeks

INTRODUCTION

In simple terms, chemiluminescence describes the emission of light that occurs as a result of certain chemical reactions. Such reactions involve the production of large amounts of energy which is lost in the form of photons when the electronically excited product molecules relax to their stable ground state. This type of luminescence is frequently confused with fluorescence and phosphorescence, both of which also involve emission of light as a result of the relaxation of excited states. However, in the latter two cases, the excited states are populated by prior absorption of light which causes the electronic excitation of ground-state molecules. In fluorescence, the emission occurs during a radiative transition between states of the same multiplicity whereas phosphorescence involves emission as a result of a transition between states of different multiplicities. These latter transitions are said to be 'spin forbidden' and generally give rise to longer emissions than fluorescent processes. Because chemiluminescence does not involve initial absorption of light, measurements of chemiluminescence emission are made against a lower background than is possible with conventional fluorescence measurements, thus potentially allowing greater sensitivities of detection. The Jablonski diagram below (Figure 1) shows some typical photochemical and photophysical processes and illustrates the differences between the various forms of luminescence described above. The light-emitting processes are represented by the straight, downward-pointing arrows and can originate from

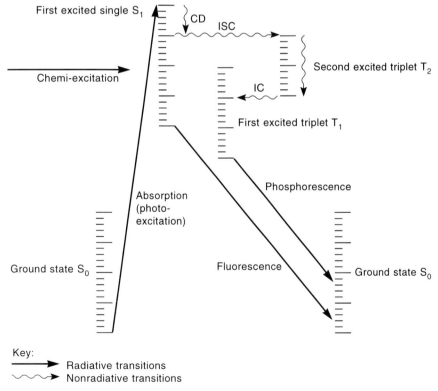

Figure 1 Jablonski diagram representing some typical photochemical and photophysical processes. Radiative transitions are represented by straight arrows. Nonradiative transitions are represented as intersystem crossing (ISC), internal conversion (IC) and collisional deactivation (CD).

singlet or triplet states. In photoluminescence these are termed fluorescence and phosphorescence, respectively. It can be seen that various electronic states may also be reached by non-radiative (i.e. dark) processes as well as by radiative pathways. These dark processes may be intersystem crossing (ISC), internal conversion (IC) or collisional deactivation (CD).

The following criteria must be fulfilled for a chemical reaction to exhibit chemiluminescence.

1   It must provide sufficient energy to produce a molecule in an electronically excited state.

2   The reaction product must be capable of excitation to an electronically excited state: not all molecules have electronic energy levels that can be populated from the energy produced by the reaction.

3   The reaction rate must be sufficiently high, particularly for the production of intense chemiluminescence.

4   The reaction coordinates must favour production of excited states: unless the potential energy surfaces permit the efficient population of electronically excited states, then excess energy will be lost as heat.

The efficiency of light emission from a chemiluminescent molecule is expressed as the chemiluminescence quantum yield, ϕ_{CL}, which describes the number of moles of photons emitted per mole of reactant. For example, a quantum yield of 1 (or 100%) means that every reactant molecule gives rise to a photon. ϕ_{CL} is a function of three more fundamental parameters such that

$$\phi_{CL} = \phi_C \phi_E \phi_F$$

where ϕ_C is the chemical yield of the primary excited molecule, ϕ_E is the fraction of such molecules that are produced in an excited state and ϕ_F is the fluorescence quantum yield of the product molecule.

Chemiluminescent reactions can occur in the solid, liquid and gas phases, although those of relevance to this chapter are oxidation reactions which occur in the liquid phase. Dioxetane and dioxetanone molecules have been implicated as key intermediates in many chemiluminescent reactions of this type and several stabilised dioxetanes have been used as the basis of chemiluminescent detection methods for immunoassay. Table 1 shows approximate decomposition energies for dioxetanes and related species and it can be seen that this type of structure is capable of supplying sufficient excitation energy, assuming appropriate energy channelling. Emission of blue light, for example, corresponds to an energy of approximately 300 kJ mol^{-1}.

There are many natural examples of chemiluminescence. The blue emission of will-o'-the-wisp is a 'cool flame' often observed in the oxidation of hydrocarbons, in this case marsh gas (mainly methane). Most examples are seen in the form of bioluminescence, which is the term used to describe the chemiluminescence of certain organisms. Early studies by Robert Boyle (1668a, b) involved comparison of the glow of burning coal (incandescence) with the 'cold

Reaction		Decomposition energy (kJ mol^{-1})
$\begin{array}{c} O-O \\ \mid\ \ \mid \\ H_2C-CH_2 \end{array}$	$\rightarrow 2CH_2O$	−827
$\begin{array}{c} O-O \\ \mid\ \ \mid \\ H_2C-C=O \end{array}$	$\rightarrow CH_2O + CO_2$	−773
$\begin{array}{c} O-O \\ \mid\ \ \mid \\ O=C-C=O \end{array}$	$\rightarrow 2CO_2$	−554

Table 1 Typical decomposition energies for cyclic oxygen intermediates.

light' of 'shining wood' (the bioluminescence of a particular fungus). He also demonstrated that oxygen was required for bioluminescence (this was not formally established at this stage because oxygen was not discovered until 1774). The chemical nature of bioluminescence was demonstrated by Dubois between 1885 and 1887 (Dubois, 1885, 1887) in which he extracted various materials from luminous beetles and bivalve molluscs and found that these materials could be mixed *in vitro* to yield light emission. Moreover, he established that certain components were heat stable and others were heat labile, and he termed these components luciferin and luciferase, respectively. The best-known bioluminescent system is that of the firefly in which an enzyme (luciferase) catalyses the oxidation of a specific substrate (luciferin) in the

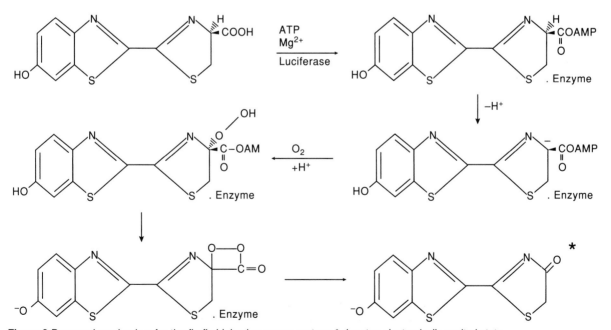

Figure 2 Proposed mechanism for the firefly bioluminescence system; * denotes electronically excited state.

presence of adenosine triphosphate (ATP). This process has been extensively studied *in vitro* (McElroy, 1947) (Figure 2), has a high quantum yield (~88%) and gives rise to an emission at approximately 540 nm.

Another well characterised bioluminescent system is found in certain marine bacteria (McElroy *et al.*, 1953). This involves a luciferase and an oxidoreductase in the presence of NAD/NADH, and the oxidation of a long-chain aldehyde.

Both of these systems have been used to demonstrate bioluminescence immunoassay in which the appropriate enzyme has been used to produce a label conjugate (DeLuca, 1982; Wannlund *et al.*, 1982). For example, firefly luciferase was used to produce an antigen conjugate in an immunoassay for methotrexate with a detection limit of 50 fmol.

Some bioluminescent organisms possess calcium-dependent photoproteins that contain a complex that has all the elements necessary for bioluminescence and that is triggered by the binding of calcium (Shimomura *et al.*, 1962). The best-known photoproteins are those present in the luminous jellyfish *Obelia* and *Aequorea*. The coelenterate luciferin, coelenterazine, can be synthesised (Inoue *et al.*, 1975) together with various analogues. Recent advances in molecular biology now also allow the protein component of the photoprotein to be biosynthesised (e.g. apo-aequorin) (Prasher *et al.*, 1985).

Several systems have been described in which the recombinant aequorin has been used as an immunoassay label where the final measurement is achieved by addition of calcium ions to facilitate light emission (Smith *et al.*, 1991).

There are numerous other examples of bioluminescence on land (e.g. beetles, earthworms, fungi and bacteria) and particularly in the sea (e.g. molluscs, deep-sea fish and jellyfish). Many of these organisms also contain molecules capable of causing wavelength shifts in the emission from the chemiluminescent system, e.g. green fluorescent protein. Such colour changes can be achieved by both inter- and intramolecular energy transfer. Several immunoassay systems based on the use of bioluminescent reactions *in vitro* have been described, although none have been used on a routine basis. Undoubtedly one problem has been the need to extract the various components from the organisms in sufficient quantity and purity to make the routine use of these materials feasible. However, recent advances in molecular biology have now made it possible to biosynthesise these materials and even to modify their characteristics (Wood *et al.*, 1989). The ready availability of bioluminescent enzymes that have been modified in the desired way may enable these systems to be more effectively used as immunoassay end points.

There are many chemical reactions that can exhibit chemiluminescence, although relatively few are associated with intense emission. The first observations of intense chemiluminescence from a synthetic organic compound were described by Radziszewski (1877) and were produced when oxygen was passed through an alkaline ethanolic solution of lophine (2,4,5-triphenylimidazole). The most widely known chemiluminescent compound is luminol (5-amino-2,3-dihydrophthalazine-1,4-dione) whose chemiluminescent properties were reported by Albrecht (1928). Shortly after this, Gleu and Petsch (1935) described the properties of an acridinium salt (lucigenin). Subsequently, the use of acridinium salts as immunoassay labels was described (Weeks *et al.*, 1982, 1983), and these labels have become the most successfully used direct chemiluminescent labels, forming the basis of several commercial immunoassay systems (Figure 3). Many people are familiar with the commercially available 'light sticks' that are used for emergency lighting, signalling and entertainment. The chemiluminescent process here is based on the bis-oxalate ester which reacts with hydrogen peroxide in organic solvents (Rauhut *et al.*, 1967). The emission is also dependent on the presence of a fluorescent acceptor molecule and the wavelength of the emission is dependent on the nature of the

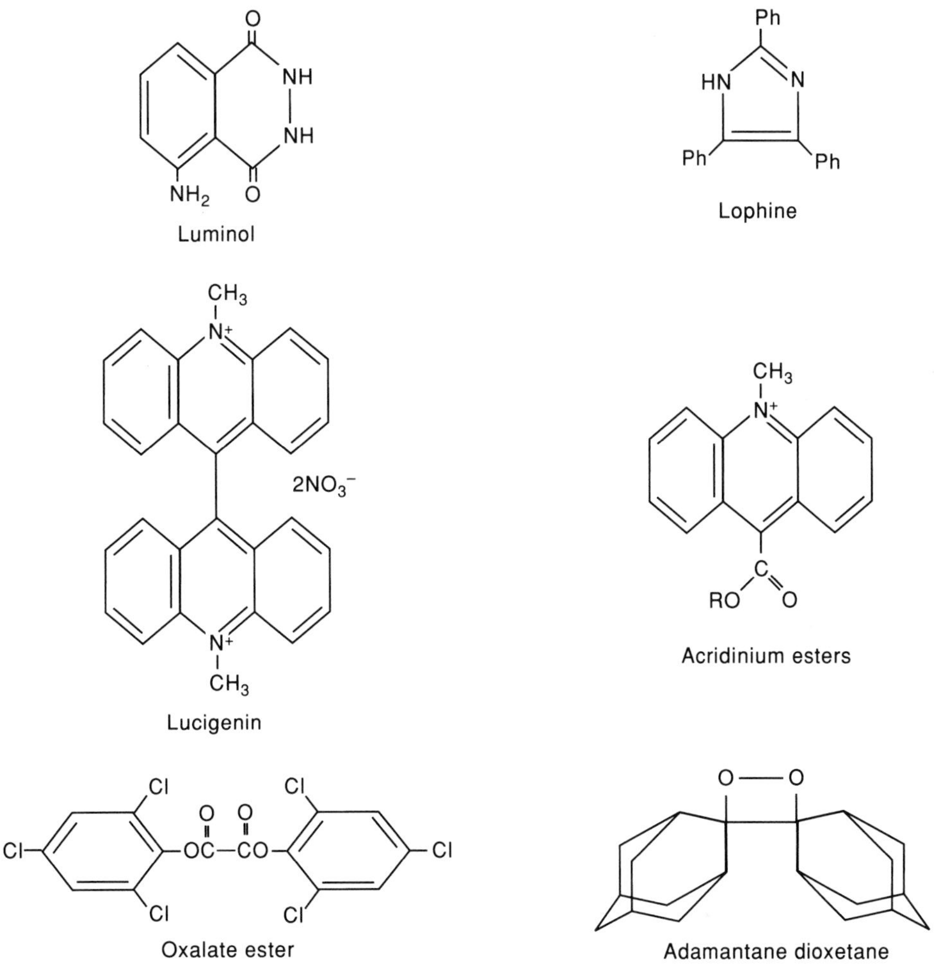

Figure 3 Examples of some chemiluminescent compounds.

acceptor. For example, fluorescein yields a green-yellow emission whereas rhodamine B gives rise to red chemiluminescence.

Chemiluminescence can also be initiated by methods other than those that involve the simple admixture of chemicals. Certain stabilised dioxetanes, for example, react when heated to form electronically excited states which then give rise to light emission (Hummelen *et al.*, 1986). This process is known as thermochemiluminescence. Certain other stabilised dioxetanes can be chemically modified by the simple chemical cleavage of stabilising groups to yield dioxetanes which then spontaneously undergo chemiluminescent reactions (Schaap *et al.*, 1987). Certain chelates of ruthenium can also be induced to emit light by electrochemical oxidation/reduction of the various oxidation states (Tokel and Bard, 1972; Faulkner and Bard, 1976; Tachikawa and Faulkner, 1984). This is an example of electrogenerated chemiluminescence. More recently, this type of approach has been used as an immunoassay end point (Blackburn *et al.*, 1991; Hoyle, 1994; Hoyle *et al.*, 1996) by using an appropriate ruthenium chelate, such as ruthenium(II) tris(bipyridyl), as a label, and a magnetisable particle separation system. Here the immunoassay mixture is drawn through a flow cell which permits isolation of bound label on an electrode. Application of an alternating voltage in the presence of the electron donor, tripropylamine, causes reduction of Ru(III) (formed by initial oxidation of the Ru(II) label at the electrode surface) to Ru(II) in its excited state, which relaxes to its ground state with emission of light at 620 nm.

The quantum yield of the reactions of these various synthetic chemiluminescent molecules is poor by comparison with the natural bioluminescent emission of the firefly. This is particularly so in aqueous media where the majority of chemiluminescent reactions exhibit quantum yields below 10%.

LIGHT MEASUREMENT

The emission of photons can be detected and quantified with great sensitivity. There are many ways of doing this depending on the level of sensitivity and sophistication required (Berthold, 1990). The most widely used detector is the photomultiplier tube (PMT) found in most luminometers. These devices can be used in either a current-measuring or photon-counting mode. The former can be used where high sensitivity is not required; however, it is generally accepted that the latter mode provides greater sensitivity and long-term stability. There is a wide range of parameters that need to be considered in the selection of a PMT for a particular purpose, including spectral response, gain and dynamic range. The first of these is determined by the chemiluminescent system being monitored. As an illustration, the most widely used acridinium ester and luminol systems emit at approximately 430 nm (blue light) whereas the firefly reaction emits a green-yellow light. Other systems, for example the peroxyoxalate reaction with rhodamine, are capable of emitting red light. Different types of PMTs exhibit different sensitivities to different wavelengths and it is therefore important to select the tube with the optimum spectral response for maximum sensitivity. Blue emissions are sensitively measured using photomultiplier tubes with bialkali or rubidium-bialkali photocathodes. Such tubes typically have quantum efficiencies of approximately 25% in the range 400–450 nm.

Where it is desired to detect very low photon fluxes, high gain is required to provide maximum sensitivity. The sensitivity is limited by the dark response of the system and it is thus desirable to achieve this high gain with minimum instrument background. Greater sensitivities can be obtained by cooling the photocathode because reduction of the photocathode temperature to 6 °C typically results in a fourfold reduction in background.

Luminometers can operate over a wide dynamic range, which typically may be as high as 10^6. In photon counting systems the upper end of this range is limited by the instrument dead-time which is typically 20 ns. The upper end may be extended in a number of ways, for example by the introduction of a neutral-density filter between the photon source and the detector.

In the interests of portability, robustness and lower cost, small luminometers have been developed using photodiodes as detectors. These do not offer the same level of performance as the PMT instruments but are appropriate where high sensitivity is not a requirement.

The ultimate in simplicity and portability is probably the use of photographic film to detect and record chemiluminescence emission (Kricka and Thorpe, 1986). The disadvantages are that this method is neither sensitive nor quantitative but is nevertheless suitable for specific applications. There have been several descriptions of the use of camera luminometers using instant film. Photographic detection is desirable where two-dimensional imaging is required, such as in the analysis of western blots using chemiluminescent end points.

In recent years there has been substantial interest in the development of imaging luminometers based on the use of charge-coupled devices (CCD) (Hooper and Ansorge, 1991). These solid-state detectors have been widely used in astrophysics for imaging purposes and are now being used in the two-dimensional imaging and quantification of bioluminescence and chemiluminescence. The detector consists of an array of light-sensing elements (typically 512 × 512 pixels) which, together with the appropriate optics and microprocessor, is capable of displaying the image on a monitor and quantifying the intensity of light emission from any given area of the image. The technique can be used in a macroscopic or microscopic mode for various objects such as microtitre plates, petri dishes, gels and blots. The most sensitive devices are either cryogenically cooled or ambient temperature intensified CCDs.

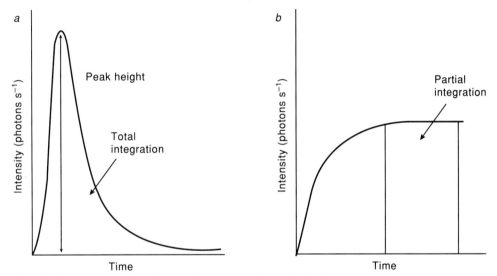

Figure 4 Typical profiles of *a*, short-lived and *b*, long-lived chemiluminescent reactions.

Whatever the mode of detection, the overall luminometer design depends on the chemistry of the chemiluminescent system. Where the chemiluminescent reaction is rapid (Figure 4), the sample cuvette or microwell must be next to the detector (or optically coupled via a fibre-optic link) when the reaction is initiated. Suitable luminometers with built-in reagent systems are routinely available. The simple luminometers measure one tube at a time and typically accept 12 × 75 mm immunoassay tubes. Other luminometers are available with automatic sample changers and, more recently, microtitre plate luminometers have become available. Luminometers for immunoassay purposes often carry the appropriate software on board to be able to perform data reduction of standards and samples. Luminometer systems have now also been built into random-access immunoassay analysers where chemiluminescence is used as the end point.

DESIGN OF CHEMILUMINESCENT IMMUNOASSAYS

There are numerous ways of configuring chemiluminescent immunoassays but only the general principles and the most widely used approaches will be described here.

Irrespective of the specific chemiluminescent system to be used, the main distinction between the various methods is whether the primary chemiluminescent emitter itself (or its precursor) is coupled to the antigen or antibody, or whether another component of what is normally a multicomponent system, is used as the label. The latter can be a cofactor or catalyst or even a molecule capable of converting a nonchemiluminescent precursor to a chemiluminescent, or potentially chemiluminescent species. For the sake of convenience, these various possibilities can be termed direct or indirect chemiluminescent systems, respectively.

There are a number of requirements for the configuration of direct chemiluminescence immunoassays.

1   The functional groups of the molecule to be labelled and the chemiluminescent molecule must permit covalent coupling.

2   The chemical procedures used to facilitate coupling should be sufficiently mild so as not to be deleterious to the molecules to be coupled.

3   Any chemical modifications should not greatly decrease the quantum yield of the chemiluminescent molecule.

4   The immunochemical activity of the molecule to be labelled should not be affected.

The approach to coupling chemiluminescent molecules to the required ligand obviously depends on the nature of the two species. Where both species are small molecules, then conventional synthetic organic chemistry can be used. However, when one or both are more complex molecules, such as proteins, then the range of chemistries that can be used is more limited because of the restricted chemical and physical environments within which such complex molecules can remain functional. The types of methods that can be used are well established and are essentially those that are used for producing small molecule-protein conjugates or protein-protein conjugates. Table 2 gives examples of the types of chemistry that are often considered for these purposes.

Early work involved the use of luminol as the chemiluminescent label and showed that there was a substantial loss of chemiluminescent activity caused by the structural changes in the molecule when it was chemically modified to facilitate covalent coupling. An example of this was the preparation of labelled antibodies by Simpson *et al.* (1979) who reported losses of chemiluminescent activity of greater than 90% during coupling reactions involving the formation of diazo compounds (diazotisation) of the luminol amine group. Such losses could be reduced to a certain extent by employing isoluminol derivatives (Schroeder *et al.*, 1978). These were used for the production of labelled steroid molecules (Kim *et al.*, 1982; Pazzagli *et al.*, 1983) and labelled antibodies (Schroeder *et al.*, 1981). However, low specific activity was still a feature of these early labelled molecules. Improvements were obtained by careful optimisation of the chemiluminescent systems. In particular, naphthalhydrazides were found to be effective as labels (Wood *et al.*, 1986). A feature of luminol and other phthalhydrazides is their requirement for a 'catalyst' to facilitate chemiluminescence in aqueous solutions. A wide range of chemical species can perform this function, from simple transition metal cations to more complex molecules such as horseradish peroxidase. The effectiveness of these 'catalysts'

Hapten functional group	Coupling reagent/ procedure	Protein functional group
(a) General reagents		
COOH	Mixed anhydride	NH$_2$
	Carbodiimide	NH$_2$
	Via *N*-hydroxysuccinimide	NH$_2$
	Via carbonyldiimidazole	NH$_2$
NH$_2$ (arom.)	Diazonium salt	Histidine
		Tyrosine
		Tryptophan
	Via isocyanate	NH$_2$
NH$_2$ (aliph.)	Carbodiimide	COOH
	Diisocyanate	NH$_2$
	Glutaraldehyde	NH$_2$
OH	Via succinic anhydride etc. to yield COOH, then as above	
OH (vicinal)	Via dialdehydes (periodate oxidation)	NH$_2$
C=O	*O*-(carboxymethyl)hydroxylamine to yield COOH, then as above	
CHO	Schiff base formation	NH$_2$
(b) Dedicated homobifunctional reagents		
NH$_2$	Difluorodinitrobenzene	NH$_2$
	Bis(imidoesters), bis(isothiocyanates), bis(succinimidyl esters)	NH$_2$
(c) Heterobifunctional reagents		
NH$_2$/SH	Maleimide/succinimidyl ester	NH$_2$/SH
	Photoaffinity crosslinkers	Various

Table 2 Examples of conjugation methods.

varies greatly and it was found that microperoxidase and haemin (Wood *et al.*, 1986) were particularly useful. Many assays based on these systems have been reported in the literature.

Acridinium salts, such as lucigenin, have no catalytic requirement and exhibit chemiluminescence in the presence of alkaline hydrogen peroxide. Acridinium esters were found to be effective chemiluminescent labels though early results were disappointing. The design and synthesis of stable compounds specifically for the spontaneous labelling of ligands (e.g. Figure 5) enabled high-specificity chemiluminescence activities to be obtained without loss of quantum yield.

It was proposed that the dissociative nature of these reactions enabled the chemiluminescent molecule to be coupled in such a way that the emitting species, *N*-methyl acridone,

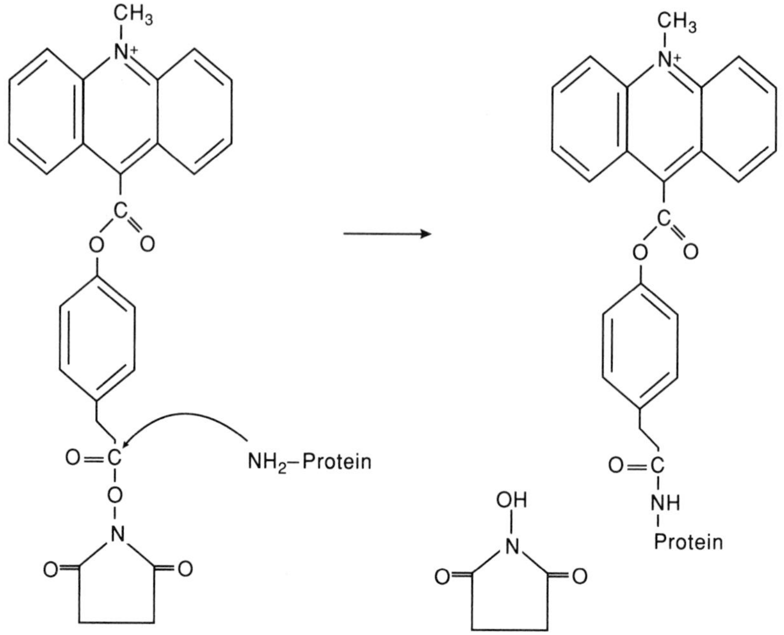

Figure 5 Structure of an acridinium salt used for labelling proteins which contains the chemiluminescent moiety joined to a *N*-succinimidyl ester group which is capable of reacting with amino groups to form stable amide bonds.

was dissociated from the rest of the labelled molecule before emission. The result of this is that any quenching effects due to the microenvironment of the labelled species would be minimised (Figure 6).

This approach has been widely used in a variety of applications and has demonstrated the ability to yield extremely sensitive immunoassay systems. As long ago as 1984, the combination of acridinium labels and high-affinity monoclonal antibodies demonstrated the dramatic improvements in assay sensitivity that could be achieved using this approach in an assay for thyroid-stimulating hormone (thyrotropin; TSH) (Weeks *et al.*, 1984). It was clear that such labels were able to yield sensitivities of detection at least 10 times lower than the other immunoassay methods then available. Chemiluminescent labels based on acridinium salts have been the most successful of the direct chemiluminescent labels and are able to yield sensitive, robust assays yet retain the advantages of the use of simple reagents. These labels have formed the basis of the Magic Lite and ACS:180 immunoassay systems marketed by Ciba Corning Diagnostics. Acridinium salts undergo a chemiluminescent reaction that is proposed to consist of a concerted multiple-bond cleavage mechanism. This proceeds via a dioxetanone intermediate and results in the formation of an electronically excited molecule of *N*-methylacridone which emits photons on relaxing to its ground state (Figure 6). The use of labelled reagents based on these substances means that after the normal immunochemical reactions and separation step, the isolated immune complexes are simply quantified by putting the reaction tube or microtitre plate into a luminometer capable of simultaneous reagent injection and intensity measurement. There is no requirement for further reagent additions and incubations after the washing procedure, which greatly speeds up and simplifies the assay protocol relative to enzyme-based methods.

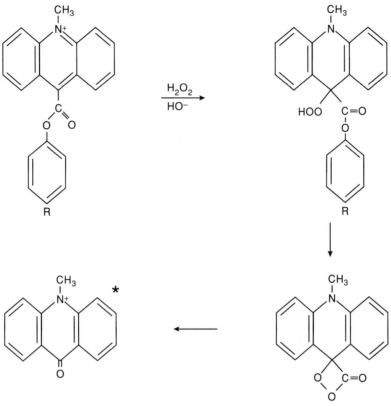

Figure 6 Proposed mechanism of the chemiluminescent reaction of acridinium salts; * Electronically excited state.

Indirect chemiluminescence immunoassays were among the first demonstrations of the use of chemiluminescent end points. One of the earliest examples of this was a chemiluminescent immunoassay for hepatitis B surface antigen which was developed using haematin as a label (Posch *et al.*, 1973). Thus haematin-labelled antigen could be quantified by the measurement of the intensity of light emitted upon addition of excess luminol. Another example involved the use of antigens and antibodies labelled with horseradish peroxidase (HRP) (Olsson *et al.*, 1979). Although such reagents had previously been used widely as the basis of enzyme color-imetric end points, here use was made of the ability of HRP to act as a catalyst of luminol chemiluminescence. In fact, HRP is a relatively poor catalyst of the luminol reaction and this limited the utility of such a method. However, it was found some years later that certain phe-nolic molecules were capable of 'enhancing' the chemiluminescent emission from this system to such a degree that the emission was sufficiently intense to make it suitable for use in a wide variety of immunoassay applications (Whitehead *et al.*, 1983). This particular method formed the basis of the Amerlite immunoassay system (Johnson and Johnson Clinical Dia-gnostics, Amersham, UK). Although the exact mechanism is not fully established, this system has proved to be particularly effective in the visualisation of western blots and in demonstra-ting the ability to use simpler detectors such as photodiodes and photographic film. This can be done because the emission consists of a glow that can be initiated before exposure to the

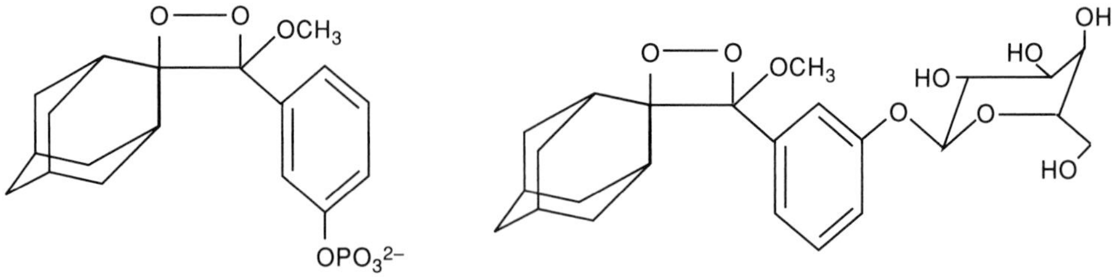

Figure 7 Two examples of stabilised dioxetanes that undergo spontaneous chemiluminescence following removal of the stabilising phosphate and galactose groups.

detector. The signal is reported to reach a peak after 2 minutes, following which it gradually decays over a period of 20 minutes.

Another widely established chemiluminescent enzyme system is based on the use of stabilised dioxetane substrates (Bronstein *et al.*, 1989). Dioxetanes are intermediates in several chemiluminescent reactions and it is possible to synthesise stabilised dioxetanes that do not spontaneously undergo a chemiluminescent reaction. Stabilising moieties have principally been phosphate and β-galactose moieties. When exposed to the relevant enzyme (in this case alkaline phosphatase and β-galactosidase, respectively), the dioxetane is destabilised and spontaneously undergoes a chemiluminescent reaction (Figure 7). The most widely used stable dioxetane has been 3,4-methoxyspiro(1,2-dioxetane-3,2'-tricyclo[3.3.1.1.3,7]decan)-4-yl phenyl phosphate (AMPPD). This molecule forms the basis of the DPC Immulite system (Diagnostics Products Corporation, Los Angeles, USA). It was also found that certain polymeric fluorescent molecules could be particularly useful in changing the wavelength of emission and 'amplifying' the chemiluminescent emission. Both of these enzyme-based chemiluminescent systems yield relatively long-lived emissions and have thus been found particularly useful in the photographic detection of gels and blots both in immunochemistry and oligonucleotide probe hybridisation techniques. The AMPPD emission has a relatively long delay before reaching constant light emission (<10 min) although more recent work (Bronstein *et al.*, 1991) has demonstrated that various chemical substitutions on the molecule can improve these characteristics.

There are many other methods of performing indirect chemiluminescent immunoassays, most of which are enzyme-mediated. Although many of these are elegant methods, they have not always found routine acceptance because of their complexity and lack of robustness. Further examples of indirect chemiluminescent immunoassays are given in Table 3.

Enzyme label	Substrate	Description	Reference
Glucose oxidase	Sucrose	Hydrogen peroxide product reacts with bis-oxalate ester	Arakawa *et al.*, 1985
Xanthine oxidase	Hypoxanthine	Superoxide anion produced converted to hydroxyl radicals used to initiate luminol reaction	Jansen *et al.*, 1989
Alkaline phosphatase	Luciferin phosphate	Dephosphorylated luciferin	Miska and Geiger, 1989

Table 3 Some examples of enzyme-mediated chemiluminescent systems.

HOMOGENEOUS IMMUNOASSAYS

In common with other sensitive immunoassays, the methods described above rely on physical separation of immune complexes before quantification of the label. However, as with other nonradioactive label systems, such as fluorescence or colorimetric enzyme end points, it is possible to configure chemiluminescence immunoassays in such a way that they do not require the prior separation of immune complexes. Although such chemiluminescent systems are not routinely used, the possibility of such systems have been demonstrated on the basis of intensity changes (Schroeder *et al.*, 1976; Kohen *et al.*, 1979) and energy-transfer chemiluminescence (Campbell and Patel, 1983). The former was first demonstrated in a competitive protein binding reaction for biotin. It was found that the intensity of chemiluminescent emission from a biotin-isoluminol conjugate increased up to 10-fold when bound to avidin and thus addition of analyte biotin to the system resulted in competition for avidin binding sites and subsequent reduction of light-emission intensity that was proportional to the amount of analyte biotin present.

A further demonstration of this principle was reported in a homogeneous chemiluminescent immunoassay for progesterone. It was shown that the degree of enhancement was dependent on the chemical structure of the chemiluminescent-steroid conjugate used and also upon the antiserum used. Indeed quenching rather than enhancement was also seen in certain circumstances. The degree of change was also different depending upon which part of the intensity-time profile was used for measurement. Clearly the variability of this phenomenon makes it difficult to base practical assays on such systems. In the case of energy-transfer chemiluminescent immunoassay, the antigen-antibody binding partners were labelled with a chemiluminescent molecule and a fluorescent molecule, respectively. The emission of light from such an immune complex is of a wavelength corresponding to the emission wavelength of the fluorophore. This is because the energy of the chemiluminescent reaction is transferred by the Förster mechanism to the fluorophore. Energy transfer of this type occurs when the donor and acceptor are within approximately 5 nm of each other and when the emission spectrum of the chemiluminescent emitter overlaps with the absorption spectrum of the fluorophore. When analyte antigen binds to the fluorescent-labelled antibody, the chemiluminescent-labelled antigen is displaced from the immune complex and, because no energy transfer can occur, the emission corresponds to the wavelength of the chemiluminescent emitter. Thus the ratio of the intensities of the chemiluminescence emission and the energy-transfer emission from the fluorophore is a measure of the amount of analyte antigen present in the system. Emissions of different wavelength can be measured independently by two photomultiplier tubes fitted with the appropriate optical filters.

Immunoassays generally may be subject to the effects of a number of variables on the immunochemical reaction or its components. Such variables may be, for example, pH, ionic strength, protein concentration, presence or absence of certain ions or presence of detergents or other materials exogenous to the analytical sample. In the case of radioimmunoassay using ^{125}I, for example, the label itself is not subject to interferences. However, any label based on chemical or optical properties of a molecule is potentially less robust than a radioisotope label. Thus it is possible that such assays may be subject to interference at the level of the label itself as well as at the level of the immunochemical reaction. However, the success of several routinely used chemiluminescent systems suggests that methods can be engineered to be free from possible interferences on the end point.

SUMMARY

Since the first demonstration of chemiluminescence immunoassay over 20 years ago, many different systems have been described, although relatively few have stood the test of time and been put to routine use (Kricka, 1994). There are still many analytical requirements that may possibly be met by immunoassays with chemiluminescent end points. For example, extra sensitivity of detection is always a useful feature because, as well as providing greater analytical sensitivity, it can often be traded off for greater assay speed or robustness. The development of chemiluminescent systems with greater quantum yields or the successful use of higher quantum yield bioluminescent systems would go some way to achieving this provided that it is not achieved at the expense of simplicity or robustness. Extremes of sensitivity have often been demonstrated but have been limited in practical use by excessive complexity or lack of robustness. Chemiluminescence immunoassay (Weeks, 1992) has now established its place as a valuable diagnostic tool both in manual and automated systems and there is no doubt that its advantages over conventional immunoassay end points will see its use continue to develop both in clinical and nonclinical arenas.

REFERENCES

Albrecht, H. O. (1928) Chemiluminescence of aminophthalic hydrazide. *Z. Phys. Chem.* **136**, 321–330.

Arakawa, H., Maeda, M. & Tsuji, A. (1985) Chemiluminescent enzyme immunoassay for thyroxine with use of glucose oxidase and a bis(2,4,6-trichlorophenyl)oxalate-fluorescent dye system. *Clin. Chem.* **31**, 430–434.

Berthold, F. (1990) Instrumentation for chemiluminescence immunoassays. In: *Luminescence Immunoassay and Molecular Applications* (eds Van Dyke, K. & Van Dyke, R.) pp. 11–25 (CRC Press, Boca Raton).

Blackburn, G. F., Shah, H. P., Kenten, J. H. *et al.* (1991) Electrochemiluminescence detection for development of immunoassays and DNA probe assays for clinical diagnostics. *Clin. Chem.* **37**, pp. 1534–1539.

Boyle, R. (1668a) *Phil. Trans. R. Soc. (London)* **2**, 211.

Boyle, R. (1668b) *Phil. Trans. R. Soc. (London)* **2**, 215.

Bronstein, I., Juo, R. R., Voyta, J. C. *et al.* (1991) Novel chemiluminescent adamantyl-1,2-dioxetane enzyme substrates. In: *Bioluminescence and Chemiluminescence: Current Status* (eds Stanley, P. E. & Kricka, L. J.) pp. 73–82 (John Wiley & Sons, Chichester).

Bronstein, I., Voyta, J. C., Thorpe, G. H. G. *et al.* (1989) Chemiluminescent assay of alkaline phosphatase applied in an ultrasensitive enzyme immunoassay of thyrotropin. *Clin. Chem.* **35**, 1441–1446.

Campbell, A. K. & Patel, A. (1983) A homogeneous immunoassay for cyclic nucleotides based on chemiluminescence energy transfer. *Biochem. J.* **216**, 185–194.

DeLuca, M. (1982) Bioluminescent assays of clinically important compounds. In: *Luminescent Assays: Perspectives in Endocrinology and Clinical Chemistry* (eds Serio, M. & Pazzagli, M.) pp. 115–123 (Raven Press, New York).

Dubois, R. (1885) *C. R. Séances Soc. Biol. Paris (Ser. 8)* **2**, 559.

Dubois, R. (1887) *C. R. Séances Soc. Biol. Paris (Ser. 8)* **3**, 564.

Faulkner, L. R. & Bard, A. J. (1976) Techniques of electrogenerated chemiluminescence. In: *Electroanalytical Chemistry* Vol. 10 (ed. Bard, A. J.) pp. 1–95 (Marcel Dekker, New York).

Gleu, K. & Petsch, W. (1935) Chemiluminescence of the dimethylbiacridylium salts *Angew. Chem.* **48**, 57–59.

Hooper, C. E. & Ansorge, R. E. (1991) Quantitative photon imaging in the life sciences using intensified CCD cameras. In: *Bioluminescence and Chemiluminescence: Current Status* (eds Stanley, P. E. & Kricka, L. J.) pp. 337–344 (John Wiley & Sons, Chichester).

Hoyle, N. R. (1994) The application of electrochemiluminescence to immunoassay-based analyte measurement. In: *Bioluminescence and Chemiluminescence: Fundamentals and Applied Aspects* (eds Campbell, A. K., Kricka, L. J. & Stanley, P. E.) pp. 28–31 (John Wiley & Sons, Chichester).

Hoyle, N. R., Eckert, B., Kraiss, S. (1996) Electrochemiluminescence: leading edge technology for automated immunoassay analyte detection. *Clin. Chem.* **42**, 157.

Hummelen, J. C., Luider, T. M. & Wynberg, H. (1986) Stable 1,2-dioxetanes as labels for thermochemiluminescent immunoassay. *Meth. Enzymol.* **133**, 531–557.

Inoue, S., Sugiura, S., Kakoi, H. *et al.* (1975) Squid bioluminescence II. Isolation from Watasenia scintillans and synthesis of 2-(*p*-hydroxybenzyl)-6-(*p*-hydroxyphenyl)-3,7-dihydroimidazo[1,2-a]pyrazin-3-one. *Chem. Lett.* 141–144.

Jansen, E. H. J. M., van den Berg, R. H. & Zomer, G. (1989) Characteristics and detection principles of a new enzyme label producing a long-term chemiluminescent signal. *J. Biolum. Chemilum.* **4**, 129–135.

Kim, J. B., Barnard, G. J., Collins, W. P. *et al.* (1982) Measurement of plasma 17β-estradiol by solid-phase chemiluminescent immunoassay. *Clin. Chem.* **28**, 1120–1124.

Kohen, F., Pazzagli, M., Kim, J. B. *et al.* (1979) An assay procedure for plasma progesterone based on antibody-enhanced chemiluminescence. *FEBS Lett.* **104**, 201–205.

Kricka, L. J. (1994) Selected strategies for improving sensitivity and reliability of immunoassays. *Clin. Chem.* **40**, 347–357.

Kricka L. J. & Thorpe, G. H. G. (1986) Photographic detection of chemiluminescent and bioluminescent reactions. *Meth. Enzymol.* **133**, 404–420.

McElroy, W. D. (1947) The energy source for bioluminescence in an isolated system. *Proc. Natl Acad. Sci. USA* **33**, 342–345.

McElroy, W. D., Hastings, J. W., Sonnenfeld, V. *et al.* (1953) The requirement of riboflavine phosphate for bacterial luminescence. *Science*, **118**, 385–386.

Miska, W. & Geiger, R. (1989) Luciferin derivatives in bioluminescence-enhanced enzyme immunoassays. *J. Biolum. Chemilum.* **4**, 119–128.

Olsson, T., Brunius, G., Carlsson, H. E. *et al.* (1979) Luminescence immunoassay (LIA): A solid-phase immunoassay monitored by chemiluminescence. *J. Immunol. Meth.* **25**, 127–135.

Pazzagli, M., Messeri, G., Caldini, A. L. *et al.* (1983) Preparation and evaluation of steroid chemiluminescent tracers. *J. Steroid Biochem.* **19**, 407–412.

Posch, N. A., Wells, A. F. & Tenoso, H. J. (1973) Detection of hepatitis in blood. *PB-224875* (National Technical Information Service, USA).

Prasher, D., McCann, R. O. & Cormier, M. J. (1985) Cloning and expression of the cDNA for Aequorin, a bioluminescent calcium-binding protein. *Biochem. Biophys. Res. Commun.* **126**, 1259–1268.

Radziszewski, B. (1877) *Ber. Dtsch. Chem. Ges.* **10**, 70.

Rauhut, M. M., Bollyky, L. J., Roberts, B. G. *et al.* (1967) Chemiluminescence from reactions of electronegatively substituted aryl oxalates with hydrogen peroxide and fluorescent compounds. *J. Amer. Chem. Soc.* **89**, 6515–6522.

Schaap. A. P., Sandison, M. D. & Handley, R. S. (1987) Chemical and enzymatic triggering of 1,2-dioxetanes 2:2 fluoride-induced chemiluminescence from tert-butyldimethylsilyloxy-substituted dioxetanes. *Tetrahedron Lett.* **28**, 1159.

Schroeder, H. R., Boguslaski, R. C., Carrico, R. J. *et al.* (1978) Monitoring specific protein binding reactions with chemiluminescence. *Meth. Enzymol.* **57**, 424–445.

Schroeder, H. R., Carrico, R. J., Boguslaski, R. C. *et al.* (1976) Competitive protein binding assay for biotin monitored by chemiluminescence. *Anal. Chem.* **48**, 1933–1937.

Schroeder, H. R., Hines, C. M., Osborne, D. D. *et al.* (1981) Immunochemiluminometric assay for hepatitis B surface antigen. *Clin. Chem.* **27**, 1378–1384.

Shimomura, O., Johnson, F. H. & Saiga, Y. (1962) Extraction, purification, and properties of aequorin, a bioluminescent protein from the luminous hydromedusan, Aequorea. *J. Cell. Comp. Physiol.* **59**, 223–239.

Simpson, J. S. A., Campbell, A. K., Ryall, M. E. T. *et al.* (1979) A stable chemiluminescent labelled antibody for immunological assays. *Nature* **279**, 646–647.

Smith, D. F., Stults, N. L., Rivera, H. *et al.* (1991) Applications of recombinant bioluminescent proteins in diagnostic assays. In: *Bioluminescence and Chemiluminescence: Current Status* (eds Stanley, P. E. & Kricka, L. J.) pp. 529–532 (John Wiley & Sons, Chichester).

Tachikawa, H. & Faulkner, L. R. (1984) Photoelectrochemistry and electrochemiluminescence. In: *Laboratory Techniques in Electroanalytical Chemistry* (eds Kissinger, P. T. & Heineman, W. R.) pp. 637–674 (Marcel Dekker, New York).

Tokel, E. & Bard, A. J. (1972) Electrogenerated chemiluminescence IX: Electrochemistry and emission from systems containing tris(2,2'-bipyridine)ruthenium(II) dichloride. *J. Amer. Chem. Soc.* **94**, 2862.

Wannlund, J., Egghart, H. & DeLuca, M. (1982) Bioluminescent immunoassays: A model system for detection of compounds at the attomole level. In: *Luminescent Assays: Perspectives in Endocrinology and Clinical Chemistry* (eds Serio, M. & Pazzagli, M.) pp. 125–128 (Raven Press, New York).

Weeks, I. (1992) Chemiluminescence immunoassay. In: *Comprehensive Analytical Chemistry* Vol. 29 (ed. Svehla, G.) (Elsevier Science, Amsterdam).

Weeks, I., Beheshti, I., McCapra, F. *et al.* (1983) Acridinium esters as high specific activity labels in immunoassay. *Clin. Chem.* **29**, 1474–1479.

Weeks, I., McCapra, F., Campbell, A. K. *et al.* (1982) Immunoassays using chemiluminescent labelled antibodies. In: *Immunoassays for Clinical Chemistry* (eds Hunter, W. M. & Corrie, J. E. T.) pp. 525–530 (Churchill Livingstone, Edinburgh).

Weeks, I., Sturgess, M., Siddle, K. *et al.* (1984) A high sensitivity immunochemiluminometric assay for human thyrotropin. *Clin. Endocrinol.* **20**, 489–495.

Whitehead, T. P., Thorpe, G. H. G., Carter, T. J. N. *et al.* (1983) Enhanced luminescence procedure for sensitive determination of peroxidase-labelled conjugates in immunoassay. *Nature* **305**, 158–159.

Wood, W. G., Braun, J. & Hantke, U. (1986) Luminescence immunoassays for haptens and proteins. *Meth. Enzymol.* **133**, 354–365.

Wood, K. V., Lam, Y. A., McElroy, W. D. *et al.* (1989) Bioluminescent click beetles revisited. *J. Biolum. Chemilum.* **4**, 31–39.

Chapter 18

Light-scattering Immunoassay

Christopher P. Price and David J. Newman

INTRODUCTION

Light-scattering immunoassays are based on the reaction between antigen and antibody to produce an aggregate or agglutinate large enough to scatter light to a greater degree than the constituents of the reaction. The use of agglutination as an analytical technique was first explored in the early 1920s for the detection of tubercle bacilli (Freund, 1925) and colloidal particles were also described at this time for use in immunoassays (Loeb, 1922–23). Monitoring of the antigen-antibody reaction by measurement of light scattering was described in the 1930s (Libby, 1938). Thus the basic concepts of light-scattering immunoassay have been around for over half a century but advances in our knowledge of the reaction mechanisms, the quality of the reagents and sophistication of the equipment have led to a much wider application of the technique than might have originally been envisaged. Indeed, optical techniques such as ellipsometry and surface plasmon resonance now enable direct monitoring of the antigen-antibody binding reaction without the need for aggregate formation.

The underlying principle of a light-scattering immunoassay is that polyvalent antigens react with divalent antibodies to form a large complex, the antibody effectively forming a bridge between antigen molecules. Under appropriate reaction conditions for a protein antigen this will lead to the formation of a precipitate (Tengerdy, 1967; Marrack and Richards, 1971; Buffone *et al.*, 1975b; Price *et al.*, 1983); this will depend on the colloidal stability of the constituents, as well as their size and relative proportions, as will be discussed in greater detail later. Haptens are monovalent and consequently will not form an aggregate unless coupled to a core protein or particle to form a multivalent structure.

The characteristics of the antigen and the antibody, the reaction conditions, the stoichiometry of the components and the configuration of the optical system all play a part in the light scattering signal produced and thus the performance of the assay. Each of these aspects, and how they interplay to produce a robust immunoassay technology with wide application, will be described here.

LIGHT-SCATTERING THEORY

Although many early students and philosophers developed ideas on the scattering of light, it was Lord Rayleigh who developed theories on the scattering of light by small particles (Strutt, 1871a,b). He proposed that, in the case of a particle less than 0.05 λ in its greatest dimension when it is illuminated by monochromatic light of intensity (I_0) and wavelength (λ), oscillating dipoles are set up in the particle which serve as secondary sources of emission. The intensity of scattered light ($i_\varnothing$) at an angle ($\varnothing$) from the direction of the incident light is given by the formula:

$$i_\varnothing = \frac{I_0 8 \Pi^4 N \alpha^2 (1 + \cos^2 \varnothing)}{r^2 \lambda^4}$$

Where r is the distance from the particle to the detector face, N the number of particles per unit volume and α the degree to which the molecule can be molecularly polarised (i.e. the

445

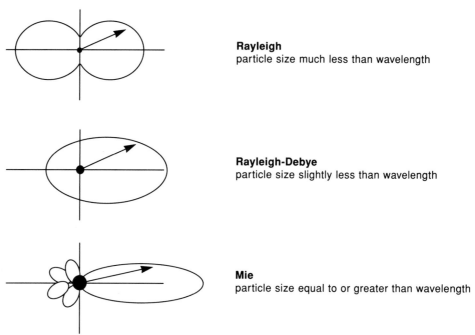

Rayleigh
particle size much less than wavelength

Rayleigh-Debye
particle size slightly less than wavelength

Mie
particle size equal to or greater than wavelength

Figure 1 Light-scattering intensity distribution around a point scattering source at different ratios of particle size:wavelength.

measure of the degree to which the electron cloud of a molecule is displaced when acted upon by an electric field).

Thus, for a particle, small compared to the wavelength of the incident light, the intensity of scattered light is proportional to $1/\lambda^4$. In addition, the angular distribution of scattered light is symmetrical about 90° as, at this angle, the $\cos^2\emptyset$ term approaches zero. There are equal amounts of light scattered backwards and forwards, the overlap envelope of distribution being dumbbell in shape (Figure 1). Under these conditions the ratio of light scattered forward to light scattered backward at any pair of supplementary angles centred on 90°, known as the dissymmetry ratio, equals unity for such small particles. It should also be noted that these considerations only apply if the distribution of particles is large enough (i.e. a dilute solution) to allow independent scattering. If the sources of scattered light are close together, destructive light scattering will occur with an apparent reduction in light detected at a given angle: if the sources are close together and regularly shaped, as in a crystal, then there will be a regular phase relationship between the reradiated waves and almost complete destructive interference with no light scattering detected.

The ideas on scattering of light by larger particles were developed by Debye (1915) and Mie (1908) in the early 1900s. They postulated that if the particle is larger than 0.05 λ it cannot be considered as a point source and destructive interference between light originating from different sites on the particle will occur. The envelope of scattered light intensity will then become asymmetrical with more light being scattered forwards than backwards, the proportion of forward scatter increasing with particle size (Figure 1). The larger particle should then be considered as multiple point sources in which the interaction between the sources is important. This reasoning led Mie to introduce refractive index into the considerations, pointing out that an increase in the refractive index of the particle results in an increase in light scattering. (For a more detailed description of theories on light scattering by large particles, *see* Tanford, 1961; Van Holde, 1971; Mayer-Arendt, 1989.) But note that as the size of particles increases, the intensity of light scattered decreases and eventually becomes independent of wavelength (which is why clouds are white).

The practical implications of the relationship between the intensity of scattered light, wavelength and particle size can be summarised as follows: (1) in the case of a protein antigen-antibody complex with a typical size of 50–100 nm (equivalent to 5–10 antibody molecules in a complex) and a wavelength of incident light of 340 nm or thereabouts, Rayleigh's scatter theory applies and monitoring at a 90° angle will provide a similar sensitivity to other angles; however (2), in the case of a larger complex, e.g. where antibody has been labelled with latex particles, Mie's theory applies and greater sensitivity can be achieved with forward angle scatter detection.

REACTION MONITORING

Early agglutination assays (done either in tubes or on slides with reagents labelled with latex particles) depended on visual inspection to provide a semiquantitative result. The assays described were with either antigen or antibody bound to bacteria (Gaechtgens, 1906), erythrocytes (Boyden, 1951) or latex particles (Singer and Plotz, 1956) in excess of 500 nm in diameter to enable visual detection of aggregation. More recently, the use of coloured latex particles has been adopted to facilitate detection of immunocomplex formation, a principle adopted in some immunochromatographic devices (*see* Chapter 22), albeit not based on light scattering.

Agglutination or immune complex formation can also be employed in gel matrices for the quantification of proteins using immunodiffusion and electroimmunoassay with visualisation enhanced by the use of polyethylene glycol (PEG), a variety of protein stains, enzyme-labelled second antibody complex or the use of gold sol (colloidal solution) particles (Urdal *et al.*, 1992).

Nephelometry

Traditionally the light scattering of a solution would be monitored using nephelometry. Nephelometry is the technique for measuring the light-scattering species in solution by means of the light intensity at an angle away from the incident light passing through the sample. The discussion of theory (above) indicates that the choice of angle will influence the sensitivity of detection, with the forward angle offering greater potential sensitivity particularly for larger scattering species. However, the choice of angle will have a major impact on the design of the instrument; in particular the use of a forward angle will require the differentiation of forward scattered light from the incident beam. Additionally, in the case of clinical applications, where samples may require both colorimetric and immunological assays, it would be desirable to have both assays on the same analyser; in this context an optical pathway that enables forward scatter and transmission measurement would be difficult to achieve. Attempts to integrate transmission and light-scattering measurement have therefore used 90° scatter, as in the case of centrifugal analysis (Tiffany, 1994). However, dedicated immunoassay systems using forward light scatter have been very successful (Anderson and Sternberg, 1978; Vuorinen *et al.*, 1988; van Rijn *et al.*, 1991).

The sensitivity of any nephelometric system can be adjusted to specific assay requirements by appropriate setting of the sensitivity of the detector. This situation is exactly analogous to fluorescence measurement in which the response of the detector is adjusted to the amount of light to be detected (often referred to as increasing the gain to improve the sensitivity of detection). This amplification has to take into account the increased noise of the signal that will result if sensitivity beyond the limits of the system are sought. The 'scale of amplification' is achieved by setting the zero and 100% limits of the fluorometer (or nephelometer) using appropriate solutions of fluorescence or scattering species; however, choice of too dilute a solution to set the 100% scale expansion may increase the noise of the signal and thereby reduce the precision of measurement. The sensitivity of nephelometric monitoring also depends on the intensity of the light source, with the highest sensitivity being achieved using a laser (Kusnetz and Mansberg, 1978). On a very practical note, it must be remembered that in all nephelometric methods the sensitivity of a method may be compromised by the presence of a high background light-scattering species in the reagents (possibly as a contaminant, e.g. dust particles or an integral component of the reagent, such as latex particles) or in the sample, e.g. lipoproteins. Reflection and scatter from components of the optical system may also contribute to the background signal.

Turbidimetry

Turbidimetry is the measurement of light-scattering species in solution by means of a decrease in intensity of the incident beam after it has passed through the solution. The light energy is reduced by absorption, reflection and scatter; however, the light energy measured may also include a small proportion of light scattered along the axis of the incident beam, i.e. forward light scatter.

Turbidimetric measurements can be made with a spectrophotometer and the signal will be a function of several factors, including monochromator wavelength, spectral bandwidth, stray light, cuvette path length and geometry, light source and detector stability (Maclin *et al.*, 1973). There is no doubt that the increased popularity of turbidimetric methods over the last three decades is due in large part to the improved performance of spectrophotometers acting as turbidimeters; many of these have been automated photometric analysers. Centrifugal analysers and other discrete analysers in which either the reaction cuvettes or the optics are rotated while the other remains stationary, creating a regular scanning mode with respect to time, have also proved to be very precise turbidimeters (Buffone *et al.*, 1975b; Finley *et al.*, 1979; Hills and Tiffany, 1980; Price *et al.*, 1983; Ng *et al.*, 1985; Shahangian *et al.*, 1992; Whicher *et al.*, 1992).

Turbidimetry versus Nephelometry

Nephelometry is a technique that is best performed with dilute solutions (in which absorption and reflection are minimal). Under these conditions, the relationship between particles and scattered light intensity is almost linear over a wide range of concentrations. However, at higher particle concentrations, nephelometry may suffer a loss of sensitivity due to destructive light scattering where the scattering is confined and dissipated in the body of the liquid. As indicated earlier, the sensitivity of nephelometric detection can be enhanced by reducing the light scattering of the reference solution; however, this will eventually result in a reduced signal-to-noise ratio because of the instability of the detection of low levels of scattered light.

By contrast, turbidimetry requires a relatively higher density of particles to achieve a measurable and precise signal. Furthermore, it only obeys Beer's law over a limited range of concentrations. However, turbidimetry is more tolerant of high concentrations of light-scattering species. It is, as stressed earlier, the high quality of the photometric system that enables precise measurement of very small changes in turbidity/transmitted light against a higher background scatter.

Signal and Aggregate/Particle Size

As pointed out earlier, the amount of light scattered shows an inverse relationship to the wavelength of the incident light and there are three important points to remember when designing a light-scattering assay. The optimum wavelength for turbidimetric monitoring (and nephelometric monitoring to a lesser extent) increases with the size of the immune complex. Thus, for monitoring of protein antigen-antibody complex formation, a wavelength of 340 nm (or less) is preferred, partly because it will enable detection of the early stages of complex formation more quickly. Nephelometry appears to be more sensitive to smaller particles than turbidimetry, apparent from the more rapid kinetics in a reaction mixture monitored by both nephelometry and turbidimetry (Whicher *et al.*, 1982); destructive light scattering may occur as larger complexes form and an apparent plateau is reached in the signal, produced more quickly than in the case of turbidimetry (Buffone *et al.*, 1975b; Hills and Tiffany, 1980). Thus, Deverill and Lock (1983), using photon correlation spectroscopy, showed that immune complex size was still increasing when a plateau had been reached in the nephelometric signal. It should therefore be remembered that a plateau in the signal, particularly using nephelometry – and thus also the equivalence point – is influenced by optical as well as reagent considerations and is only therefore applicable to that set of reagents and sample conditions, and the optical characteristics of the monitoring system used.

Kinetic versus End Point Monitoring

Given that an instrument is capable of gathering light-intensity data at precise time intervals after the initiation of the reaction, it is widely accepted that kinetic monitoring techniques offer advantages over end point procedures (Pardue *et al.*, 1974). The major benefit of kinetic monitoring, given that it is possible to take a reading immediately after initiation of the reaction (less than 5 s), is effectively the ability to take both a reagent and a sample blank reading. If there is a delay in taking this reading, sensitivity will be reduced; it is thus important when optimising your reaction conditions to choose a reaction rate that enables this early blank reading (*see* later discussion). It should also be noted that there is a sample volume (for turbidimetry and nephelometry) above which an increase in light scattering will be seen in the absence of antiserum (Price and Spencer, 1981). This is due to the increasing influence of endogenous light scattering species and the nonspecific precipitation of proteins at a high sample fraction; the degree of precipitation will depend to a certain extent on the reaction conditions, e.g. pH, ionic strength, buffer type and detergent concentration. In addition, the presence of paraprotein or increased levels of lipoprotein may lead to an increase in light scattering, particularly after the addition of PEG. These problems may be overcome by preincubation of the sample with PEG before the addition of antiserum. An alternative is to pretreat the sample with PEG (Hellsing and Enstrom, 1977) and to analyse the supernatant. Recognising that a nonspecific development of light scattering may be possible in the absence of antiserum, it is still worthwhile considering the use of a method that employs collection of two data readings, the first being immediately after mixing because it will deliver improved method precision.

Although a kinetic mode for reaction monitoring may involve only two data points, with the second chosen near to the apparent end point of the reaction, the choice of read points can influence the apparent accuracy when differences in reaction kinetics between sample and calibrator exist; this may lead to significant changes in the calibration curve for different data collection periods (Muller-Mathesius and Opper, 1980; Shahangian *et al.*, 1992). In general, the use of the second data collection point near the apparent end point will minimise the influence of sample-to-sample variations in reaction kinetics. However, in the case of immunoglobulin assays, the presence of a paraprotein may result in inaccurate quantification because the monoclonal protein epitopes do not match those of the antiserum in the same way as the normal polyclonal antigen population (Whicher, 1979; Whicher *et al.*, 1982, 1984; Price *et al.*, 1983).

An alternative approach to reaction monitoring is that described by Anderson and Sternberg (1978) who used continuous monitoring of the reaction to show that the peak rate of change of light scatter was related to antigen concentration. Assays could be optimised in such a way that the peak rate was reached in less than 40 s, the relationship of peak rate to antigen concentration being similar to that of the Heidelberger-Kendall curve (see later discussion). Clearly, the use of peak rate measurement enables a faster sample throughput; however, the dependence on a true rate measurement requires careful control of reaction conditions, e.g. mixing and reaction temperature.

Detection Limit

The sensitivity of the method and the lowest detectable concentration achievable will depend on the ability of the antisera to generate sufficient immune complex (bridging) of optimal size for the monitoring technique being employed. The performance will also depend on the optical characteristics of the photometric systems, primarily in terms of pure optical performance, and the speed with which the first data point can be collected and the accuracy of timing of data collection. As indicated earlier, most nephelometric systems cannot handle an early blank reading without extending reaction times and consequently a separate blank is required, compromising overall precision. Whicher *et al* (1982) reported detection limits for several proteins using two turbidimetric systems without particle enhancement, ranging between 50 and 100 ng protein per cuvette (approximately 1–2 mg l^{-1} in the sample). These figures are very comparable with the 100–200 ng protein per cuvette predicted for forward angle nephelometry (Anderson and Sternberg, 1978). Review of the performance of several nephelometric assay systems indicate a range of detection limits between 1.0 and 350 ng of protein per cuvette (Whicher *et al.*, 1982), with the lower figures reported for laser nephelometers; in practice this does not appear to have yielded any great advantage because of the need for a higher sample dilution. There are very few opportunities to compare directly the sensitivity and lower limit of detection of turbidimetric and nephelometric assays, mainly because most comparisons have used different photometric systems. However, there has been a direct

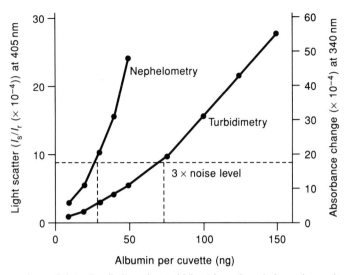

Figure 2 Comparison of detection limits using turbidimetric and nephelometric monitoring on the same analytical platform. I_s, Intensity of sample scattered light; I_r, intensity of reference scattered light.

comparison using common reagents with a turbidimetric and 90° nephelometric assay in a centrifugal analyser in which the reaction cuvette, pipetting systems and so on were common to both techniques. This has shown that the lower limit of detection (defined as three times the standard deviation (SD) of the baseline) for the nephelometric mode is about one third that of the turbidimetric mode (Figure 2). However, the advent of latex particle labels (see later discussion) and the fact that the sensitivity of nephelometry is often compromised by high blank values (Price *et al.*, 1983) limits any real benefits of nephelometry.

Particle Counting

Immunoassay techniques that employ particle counting recognise latex particles that are not agglutinated (unagglutinated). The reagent antigen or antibody is coupled to latex particles and then forms immunocomplexes with the sample antibody or antigen, respectively; the number of unagglutinated particles is thus inversely proportional to the analyte concentration.

A particle counter is designed to recognise a narrow range of particle size ensuring that agglutinated particles are not detected (Masson *et al.*, 1981; Wilkins *et al.*, 1988a). The particles are detected by either a change in electrical resistance or in light scattering. In the former, the passage of particles through a cell leads to an increase in resistance; however, the size of the aperture governs the sensitivity of the methods and attempts to increase the sensitivity can result in blockage of the aperture. In the case of light scattering, it has already been pointed out that the degree of light scattering depends on the size of the particle; the lens that collects the light and directs it to the photodetector is masked to limit the passage of light scattered outside a certain angular range. In this way, single particles can be differentiated from agglutinated particles. Thus, in the case of 600 nm particles, scattering from any particles smaller than 600 nm or larger than 1,200 nm can be ignored electronically.

The counting of unagglutinated particles allows the design of limited (inhibition) and excess (immunometric) reagent assay formats; in the latter case there is no need to form an immune complex of a size that can itself be detected by conventional light scattering. In other words, it is a sensitive means of detecting dimers; thus it has been possible to develop an

451

immunometric assay for protein hormones such as thyroid-stimulating hormone (thyrotropin; TSH) (Wilkins *et al.*, 1988b).

Photon Correlation Spectroscopy (PCS)

Photon correlation spectroscopy (PCS) uses a multiangle laser nephelometer with a powerful computer (the correlator) to monitor the time-dependent fluctuation in light-scattering intensity resulting from the Brownian motion of the illuminated particles (Bloomfield, 1985). The correlator consists of a number of digital channels (e.g. 64), each measuring the photons produced from light fluctuations over different time spans (nano- to microseconds). For a short time, particles will not have moved a great distance and consequently the light fluctuations will be small: the initial and final positions of the particles are highly correlated. The shorter delay times will pick up the faster-moving (i.e. smaller) particles and the greater the delay time the larger the size of the particle monitored.

The correlator calculates the autocorrelation function which, for the Brownian motion of colloidal particles, is an exponential function decaying with time. Using Fourier transform analysis a diffusion constant can be calculated that can be directly related to particle size (assuming the viscosity of the solution is known). Changes in average particle size can then be used to monitor an immunoaggregation reaction. Multiple estimations are needed to perform accurate size determination but these can be automated. However, this does mean that PCS measurement is time-consuming and requires more sophisticated equipment than, for example, nephelometry or turbidimetry; on the other hand, several very sensitive assays have been described (von Schulthess *et al.*, 1976a,b) with sample detection limits in the low μg l^{-1} range claimed.

Photothermal Spectroscopy (PS)

Photothermal spectroscopy (PS) is a sensitive spectroscopic technique applied more recently to immunoassay. In the technique of photothermal beam deflection (PBD) spectroscopy, the formation of a complex between antibody-coated latex (0.9 μm) or glass (50 μm) beads, antibody-coated colloidal gold particles (20 nm) and an antigen is monitored. The glass or latex particles act as a capture vehicle but also by virtue of their curvature amplify the PBD signal. The colloidal gold particle essentially forms a sandwich with the larger particle and absorbs the excitation beam (e.g. from an argon laser) thereby generating heat. It is the generation of this heat that creates a temperature gradient around the larger particle, deflecting the probe beam (e.g. from a helium neon laser) in proportion to the amount of colloidal gold – and thus antigen – captured. The colloidal gold in solution is not detected and hence this provides a homogeneous assay format. A sensitivity of detection of 10.7 amol IgE using latex beads and 0.25 μg l^{-1} for α-fetoprotein using glass beads has been described (Tu *et al.*, 1993; Sakaskita *et al.*, 1995).

Surface-effect Monitoring

There are a variety of techniques that use the principles of reagent design for light-scattering immunoassays but that are based on optical surface-effect monitoring. These include ellipso-

Monitoring system	Analyte	Sample	Concentration	Molar	Reference
Turbidimetry: nonenhanced	Human placental lactogen	Serum	1.6 mg l⁻¹	5.5×10^{-8}	Price and Spencer (1981)
Turbidimetry: latex particle-enhanced	Retinol-binding protein	Urine	25 µg l⁻¹	12×10^{-9}	Thakkar *et al.* (1991a)
Turbidimetry: gold sol particle-enhanced	Choriogonadotrophin	Serum	50 µg l⁻¹	1.6×10^{-10}	Leuvering *et al.* (1981)
Nephelometry: nonenhanced	Immunoglobulin M	CSF	6.1 mg l⁻¹	6.3×10^{-9}	Salden *et al.* (1988)
Nephelometry: latex particle-enhanced	Myoglogin	Serum	6.1 µg l⁻¹	3.4×10^{-10}	Delange *et al.* (1990)
Rate nephelometry	Immunoglobulin M	CSF	11.1 mg l⁻¹	1.1×10^{-9}	Salden *et al.* (1988)
Particle counting	C-reactive protein	Serum	1.0 µg l⁻¹	0.9×10^{-11}	Collet-Cassart *et al.* (1983)
Photon correlation spectroscopy	Immunoglobulin A	Serum	5.1 ng l⁻¹	3.0×10^{-14}	von Schulthess *et al.* (1976)
Photothermal spectroscopy	Immunoglobulin E	Serum	2.1 pg l⁻¹	1.1×10^{-17}	Tu *et al.* (1993)
Ellipsometry	Albumin	Serum	1.7 µg l⁻¹	2.5×10^{-9}	Morgan *et al.* (1996)
Surface plasmon resonance	β₂-Microglobulin	Serum	18.9 µg l⁻¹	1.6×10^{-9}	Morgan *et al.* (1996)

Table 1 A comparison of some detection limits quoted for light-scattering immunoassays using a range of monitoring techniques. These do not necessarily represent the lowest detectable amount for techniques using serum samples, as a dilution is often involved. CSF, Cerebrospinal fluid.

metry (Mondenius and Mosbach, 1988) and surface plasmon resonance spectroscopy (Mayo and Hallock, 1989). These techniques are discussed in more detail in Chapter 22 and are also reviewed with other immunosensor techniques (Morgan *et al.*, 1996).

A comparison of detection limits for these monitoring techniques for the measurement of proteins in biological samples, i.e. serum, plasma, cerebrospinal fluid or urine, is shown in Table 1.

IMMUNE COMPLEX FORMATION

The reaction between a haptenic antigen and its complementary antibody (both in solution) will only generate a couplet; this cannot readily be detected directly by any physical means, let alone by light scattering designed for the purposes of quantifying hapten in free solution. However, a protein antigen, which can be considered as multivalent with possibly multiple copies of the same epitope as well as different and distinct epitopes, can produce a large immune complex comprising several antigen and antibody molecules.

Thus, a polyvalent antigen will react with its 'complementary' antibodies to yield a complex that will precipitate: the immunoprecipitin reaction (Heidelberger and Kendall, 1935a). The general form of the relationship between antigen concentration and antibody precipitated is shown in Figure 3; the abscissa could equally be denoted as light-scattering signal. This is

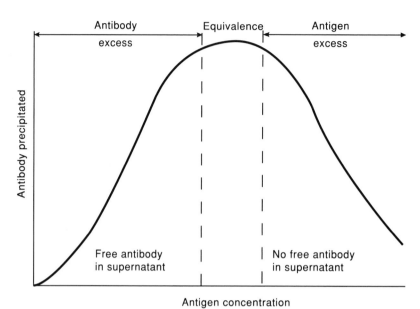

Figure 3 Heidelberger–Kendall curve for an immunoprecipitin reaction.

often referred to as the Heidelberger-Kendall curve. The first stage of the reaction involves binding of antigen to antibody initially on a 1:1 basis; in the presence of an excess of bivalent antibody molecules, 'bridging' occurs between polyvalent antigen molecules, and a lattice complex results (Heidelberger and Kendall, 1935b; Davies *et al.*, 1990). Clearly, the opportunity for bridging will depend on the availability of free binding sites, epitopes on the antigen and the concentration of antibody available. The high molecular mass lattice that results subsequently aggregates to form a precipitate (Marrack and Richards, 1971; Anderson and Sternberg, 1978); although there is good evidence to support bridging, it should be recognised that other factors may also promote the aggregation of the antigen-antibody complex at any stage in its development, e.g. colloidal instability; furthermore, certain reaction conditions may increase the rate of aggregate formation (Nakamura *et al.*, 1992; Thompson *et al.*, 1997).

There are three distinct elements of the immunoprecipitin curve. The first region, in which the antigen concentration increases, is one of antibody excess when the immune complexes are small, with some bridging. The second region, 'equivalence', represents an optimum ratio of antibody bridging in relation to antigen concentration, i.e. more antigen molecules to bind both 'arms' of the antibody; this is the point of maximum lattice, and thus precipitate, formation. In the third region, antigen excess, there is, in effect, a reduced supply of 'bridging' antibody molecules which, at an extreme, leads to two antigen molecules to every antibody and the maximum size of complex formed will be a triplet. This triplet may not be large enough to scatter light and, as a consequence of this antigen excess, the apparent light-scattering signal will be less than at the point of equivalence. These ideas have been supported by studies of the size of complexes at different antigen concentrations using zonal centrifugation (Moller and Steensgaard, 1979). One of the important consequences of these observations is that there are two possible antigen concentrations that will generate the same apparent light-scattering signal: one when there is antibody excess and the other when there is antigen excess.

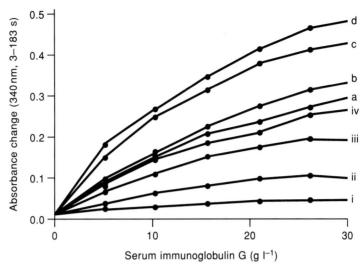

Figure 4 Calibration curves for the measurement of serum immunoglobulin G using a panel of monoclonal antibodies (MAb); i to iv, MAb A with increasing amounts of MAb B; a to d, condition iv with increasing amounts of MAb C.

The rate of reaction between the antigen and antibody, particularly the initial phase, depends upon the molar ratio of antigen to antibody (Tengerdy, 1967). The rate of reaction will also be influenced by the match of antibodies in the population to the determinants and the frequency of those determinants on the antigen. This is illustrated by observing the influence of the addition of monoclonal antibodies to the calibration curve of a protein such as immunoglobulin G (Figure 4). The rate of reaction and the shape of the immunoprecipitin curve will also be determined by the titre of the antibody, the amount of antibody preparation added, the affinity of antibody for antigen and the nature of the reaction environment, e.g. pH and ionic strength of the buffer. The titre of the antiserum can also be viewed as the concentration of antibody molecules determining how much antiserum is required to achieve equivalence. However, it must be borne in mind that, as pointed out earlier, the assessment of the equivalence point will depend on the means of monitoring the light scattering.

Polyclonal Antisera

The affinity and paratope density (or avidity) of an antibody for a specific antigen will be reflected in the rate of reaction, and differences in avidity can have a major influence on the kinetics of a reaction as well as the sensitivity of that reaction (Nimmo *et al.*, 1984). The early part of the reaction will involve the most avid among the population of antibodies; this may favour one particular isoform of an antigen. This may improve the specificity of a method as in the case of an assay for pregnancy-specific β_1-glycoprotein (Anthony *et al.*, 1980), but also may lead to apparent inaccuracies when one antigen isoform predominates in a mixture, as in the case of a monoclonal myeloma immunoglobulin (Whicher *et al.*, 1984) or in the case of haptoglobin phenotypes (van Rijn *et al.*, 1987).

Monoclonal Antibodies

The affinity (or avidity) of a monoclonal antibody is clearly less complicated as it represents a single species. The use of a monoclonal antibody in an immunoaggregation reaction is more dependent on the frequency of the complementary epitope on the antigen. Consequently, the affinity is defined by the characteristics of the antibody when a single species is present; when a cocktail of antibodies is used, the 'apparent affinity' will be determined by the relative proportions of the constituent antibodies and can be tailored by the appropriate choice of antibodies. Differences between monoclonal antibodies are revealed by the rate of aggregate formation and the equivalence point for a given antibody concentration and set of reaction conditions (Maynard *et al.*, 1986). It has also been shown that some monoclonal antibodies will bind simultaneously and cooperatively (i.e. to enhance the rate of reaction and to increase the equivalence point) (Ehrlich *et al.*, 1982; Moyle *et al.*, 1983) whereas others will not (Maynard *et al.*, 1986). Differences in the detection and quantification of paraproteins by assays based on monoclonal antibodies are also a reflection of the frequency of the antigen epitope complementary to the antibody (Jefferis *et al.*, 1985; Maynard *et al.*, 1986).

Antigen-Antibody Binding Energy

The affinity (or avidity) of an antibody will depend on the complementarity of the amino acid sequences between epitope and paratope (*see* Chapter 2 and Sutton, 1993; Wilson and Stanfield, 1994). The reaction between antigen and antibody is regarded as having two phases; the first phase or primary reaction is rapid, specific and reversible. Furthermore, the first stage of the reaction involves the overcoming of the inherent repulsion between two (protein) molecules partly brought about by the layer of water molecules on the surface of the protein. This reaction involves hydrophobic and electrostatic interactions, the latter between oppositely charged amino acids of the epitope- and paratope-binding domains (Jacobsen and Steensgaard, 1979; Davies *et al.*, 1990 and *see* Chapter 2); thus, altering the reaction pH and destroying the charge differences can reduce the rate of reaction. There may be some weak van der Waals bonding as well. These interactions represent the specific element of the reaction although not the total binding energy. The balance of forces depends on the nature of the interacting molecules; altering the pH and ionic strength will alter the balance between electrostatic attraction/repulsion, where an increasing ionic strength tends to reduce charge effects by compressing the ionic radii. The van der Waals forces operate over a variety of distances but are strongest at close range, depending on the 'goodness of fit' between epitope and paratope. Hydrophobic forces are generally more important to the secondary phase of the interaction which involves the 'squeezing out' of water molecules from the binding site (van Oss, 1994, 1995). This secondary stabilisation can involve interactions between residues outside the main binding site. After the secondary interaction, crosslinking or bridging continues to occur, resulting in immune aggregate formation. In the cases where the 'one-on-one' antigen-antibody reaction can usually be disrupted they become increasingly difficult to dissociate once an aggregate begins to form (van Oss *et al.*, 1979).

In the case of a protein antigen it is not always possible to dissociate epitope-paratope interactions from protein-protein interactions, and the same forces will be responsible for direct protein-protein and protein-solid-phase interactions. The reduced number of potentially reactive groups on a hapten may suggest to the reader that an irreversible reaction and non-specific hapten-protein interactions are less likely; in the latter case this is clearly not true

(Newman and Price, 1996). These considerations become extremely important when reagent antigen or antibody is coupled to a particle, resulting in the possibilty of nonspecific interactions with the surface particle.

The colloidal stability of proteins and particles must also be taken into account. Macromolecules and particles exist in suspension (as a monomeric dispersion) by virtue of the net repulsive forces (usually due to negative charges) on the surface of the species. As the net repulsive force tends to zero the suspension of macromolecules or particles agglutinate (Absolom and van Oss, 1986). There will also be agglutination if a net positively charged species, e.g. a protein, is mixed with negatively charged species.

Buffers and Ionic Species

Levison *et al.* (1970), using three antigen-antibody systems, have shown that the primary reaction is markedly influenced by the nature of the ionic medium. Furthermore, the reaction rate is influenced by the ions of the Hofmeister series such that ions that promote macromolecular unfolding inhibit immunoprecipitate formation whereas those that inhibit unfolding promote immunoprecipitate formation. The series and its influence can be summarised as follows:

$$SCN^-, ClO_4^-, NO_3^-, Br^-, Cl^-, F^-, SO_4^{2-}, HPO_3^-, PO_4^{3-}$$

Chaotropic $\qquad\qquad$ Antichaotropic

$\longleftarrow$ Promote macromolecular unfolding $\longrightarrow$

$\longrightarrow$ Promote immunoprecipitate formation $\longrightarrow$

Thus, at one extreme thiocyanate will inhibit immunoprecipitate formation whereas phosphate will promote it (Anderson and Sternberg, 1978). There is also a cationic series (Creighton, 1984) described by Hofmeister as follows:

$$NH_4^+, K^+, Na^+, Li^+, Mg^{2+}, Ca^{2+}$$

Chaotropic $\qquad\qquad$ Antichaotropic

The influence of cations is less clear and slightly contradictory; it has been shown that calcium and magnesium ions will slow immunoprecipitate formation (Price and Spencer, 1981). On the other hand, it has been suggested that some antigen-antibody interactions between like-charged amino acids may take place through calcium bridging (van Oss, 1995). It has also been shown, in immunonephelometric methods at least, that the reaction rate is faster with sodium than potassium salts (Killingsworth and Savory, 1973). Clearly, the reaction pH will also influence the rate of aggregate formation, although the rate of reaction is fairly consistent over the pH range 6–8; differences outside this range are likely to be due to the poor solubility of the proteins. Reduction of the reaction pH will lead to some proteins having a net positive charge (those with a p*I* above the reaction pH) leading to agglutination with negatively charged protein or particles.

The ionic strength of the reaction environment can also have a profound effect on the rate of the antigen-antibody reaction. As the ionic strength increases, the depth of the electrical double layer that forms around a charged molecule is compressed, reducing the distance over which repulsive forces that keep molecules apart can act. This, in effect, leads to the promotion of aggregation; however, the reduction in charge will also influence the electrostatic attraction between oppositely charged species, which may then reduce specific binding. In practice, the effect may vary from system to system depending on the charge of the antibody and antigen. This increase in ionic strength can be used to minimise nonspecific interactions; however, further increases in ionic strength may inhibit the antigen-antibody reaction.

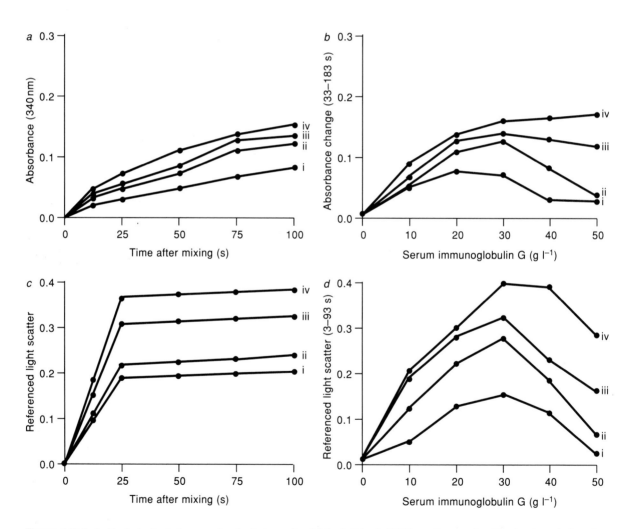

Figure 5 Data to illustrate the influence of polyethylene glycol (i-iv=1-4% w/v PEG) on the reaction kinetics (*a* and *c*) and on the calibration curve (*b* and *d*) for turbidimetric monitoring (i and ii) and 90° nephelometry (iii and iv), using the same analytical platform.

Influence of Polymers

A variety of polymers have been shown to influence the solubility of proteins, possibly by exclusion of water from the reaction microenvironment. The availability of techniques such as atomic force microscopy (Ducker *et al.*, 1991) and other surface techniques (Israelachivili, 1991) has enabled the study of intermolecular and interparticular forces. It has been shown for several particulate species that the forces between two charged species are repulsive at large distances but decrease at short distances and become attractive as van der Waals forces take over. However, there is a repulsive force component caused by water molecules in a hydration layer; it is argued that the water molecules are squeezed out as the molecules bind (Israelachivili and Wennerstrom, 1996). Thus, any means of assisting the removal of water will enhance the rate of binding (or complex formation in the case of the antigen-antibody reaction). Hellsing (1978) showed that nonionic polymers such as polyethylene glycol (1) enhanced the rate of the immunoaggregation reaction, (2) increased the light-scattering signal, and (3) extended the antigen concentration at which equivalence occurred. These points are illustrated in data from the optimisation of an assay for immunoglobulin G, which also shows the differing effects that may be seen for turbidimetric and nephelometric monitoring (Figure 5). Most of the work has been done with the dextrans and polyethylene glycols (PEG), with PEG 6000 being the most commonly used. In fact, the effect is a factor of both concentration and size, with higher concentrations of smaller dextrans having a similar effect to lower concentrations of larger polymers; in practice, however, the smaller polymers are more manageable because of their greater solubility. In this respect, it is important to note that batch-to-batch variation of polymer may influence method performance. It is also important to note, in the context of the effect of polymers on kinetics (by influencing the rate of aggregate formation), that the effect at a given concentration will depend on the means used to detect light scatter.

The action of PEG, apart from removing the hydration layer, may be considered to be the effective increase of the concentration of antigen and antibody, or simply protein concentration. It is not surprising, therefore, that the addition of PEG can also induce nonspecific aggregation of large proteins and lipoproteins, either again by removing the hydration shell or effectively increasing the protein concentration beyond its solubility level. As pointed out earlier, this can lead to blank reactions which can be overcome by preincubating the sample with PEG or using a PEG pretreatment step (Hellsing and Enstrom, 1977; Whicher and Blow, 1980; Ervin *et al.*, 1986).

Temperature

Although not conventionally considered to be temperature-dependent, the antigen-antibody reaction rate will obviously vary with reaction temperature. In one study of a range of antisera used in a turbidimetric assay format, Price and Spencer (1980) demonstrated considerable variation in temperature dependency of reaction rates between antisera. It has been demonstrated that increasing the reaction temperature will decrease the equilibrium constant (Tengerdy, 1967; van Oss, 1992) because molecules move more quickly; however, a light-scattering assay is not an equilibrium reaction, although it is correct to say that the rate of association will increase with temperature.

DIRECT NONENHANCED LIGHT-SCATTERING ASSAY

Direct measurement of analyte concentration by detection of imunoaggregate formation is only possible for multivalent antigens; modifications to facilitate the measurement of haptens will be discussed in a later section, Particle Enhanced Immunoassay. For the measurement of protein analytes, the choice of turbidimetric or nephelometric monitoring may depend on the availability of equipment and the degree of automation sought. Although there are no major reasons for choosing between nephelometry or turbidimetry, especially considering that the use of latex particle enhancement allows turbidimetry to achieve the higher sensitivity that can be achieved by nephelometry, it may be more practical to consider turbidimetry because the methods can be integrated with enzyme and colorimetric assays into a single photometric platform. Having said this, the overall impression from the literature is that turbidimetric methods offer slightly better precision.

Optimisation of Assays

	Analytical range	Lowest detectable amount	Units
Albumin (serum)	10–60	5.0	g l^{-1}
Albumin (urine)	5–1,000	2.0	mg l^{-1}
C-reactive protein (serum)	5–200	2.0	mg l^{-1}
β_2-microglobulin (serum)	0.5–12	0.2	mg l^{-1}
Cystatin C (serum)	0.5–12	0.2	mg l^{-1}
Immunoglobulin G (serum)	0.1–30	0.05	g l^{-1}
Immunoglobulin A (serum)	0.05–15	0.02	g l^{-1}
Immunoglobulin M (serum)	0.05–8	0.02	g l^{-1}
Prealbumin (serum)	50–450	5.0	mg l^{-1}

Table 2 Typical analytical specification for a range of specific protein assays; the analytical range is that concentration range encompassed within a total coefficient of variation of less than 10%.

There have been several reviews of light-scattering immunoassays that describe the major features of assay optimisation for both turbidimetry and nephelometry (Buffone *et al.*, 1975a; Anderson and Sternberg, 1978; Spencer and Price, 1979; Deverill, 1980; Whicher and Blow, 1980; Whicher *et al.*, 1982; Price *et al.*, 1983; Price and Newman, 1993, 1995). The specifications for the assays, irrespective of the instrumentation, are derived from the desired analytical range and the imprecision requirements at key clinical decision levels. Examples of typical analytical specifications for several protein assays are given in Table 2 and show in some cases the need for a wide concentration range while also maintaining low imprecision in the lower quartile (or below) of the range. By contrast, in other cases imprecision requirements are spread more evenly across a limited normal and pathological concentration range.

Instrumentation

The major instrument considerations that must be borne in mind during optimisation include the range and precision of liquid dispensing (for both sample and reagent), the range of best optical performance and the earliest time at which an initial optical reading can be made. The latter point, as mentioned earlier, determines whether a two-point pseudokinetic method can be developed and what level of signal may have to be sacrificed if an immediate reading after reagent addition cannot be made. In the case of a nephelometric assay it will be necessary to set the range (scale expansion) of the nephelometer by appropriate choice of a light-scattering reference solution (Hills and Tiffany, 1980).

Buffer Conditions

In general, development of a direct turbidimetric or nephelometric method is based on the use of a phosphate buffer (100 mmol l^{-1}, pH 7.4) as a starting point. The rate of immune aggregate formation will then primarily depend on the antiserum and the choice of PEG concentration. The choice of antiserum will determine the analytical range of the assay that is possible, a reflection of the equivalence point for that antiserum. In the case of turbidimetry, one general aim is to have achieved the maximum and plateau signal in less than 10 minutes; although PEG complements the antiserum in achieving adequate signal and range, care must be taken to ensure that the reaction rate is not too fast to negate the opportunity for an early blank reading. However, in the case of nephelometry it will probably be necessary to give up the option of an early sample blank reading as the PEG enhances the rate of reaction too much. It must also be remembered that the addition of PEG will increase the risk of non-specific precipitation of other proteins such as immunoglobulin M (Chambers *et al.*, 1987b) and at extreme cases even the protein of interest (e.g. PEG concentration greater than 4% will cause the precipitation of immunoglobulin M) (Spencer and Price, 1979; Deverill, 1980).

As indicated earlier, most method optimisations begin with a phosphate buffer at pH 7.4 and indeed this is probably the buffer of choice for most immunoaggregation reactions. The addition of chloride ions or an increase in the ionic strength appears to have rather variable effects and is probably antiserum dependent. The addition of complexing agents (e.g. EDTA) may be helpful for removing interfering cations if the sample fraction is high, although in itself it is a strategy to be avoided for obvious reasons (Price and Spencer, 1981). The addition of detergents in direct immunoaggregation reactions does not appear to have become particularly popular although it has been suggested that detergents may help to minimise endogenous light scattering (which is of greater importance in nephelometric assays). In this context, it has been suggested that the inclusion of borate ions in a reagent or buffer cocktail may help to minimise nonspecific aggregation (Zdunek and Weber, 1988); this may lead to the use of a higher reaction pH which may compromise the overall rate of reaction although this procedure has proved effective in some cases (Medcalf *et al.*, 1990).

Antiserum

Although the final choice of antiserum may be empirical (*see* Chapter 6) it will essentially depend on the titre and avidity. This information may be provided by the manufacturer but it may not be entirely reliable, the parameters having been devised in a different analytical system. Variations in the characteristics of antisera may lead to significant differences in the performance of the assay, e.g. calibration curve shape (Figure 6). The use of a cocktail of

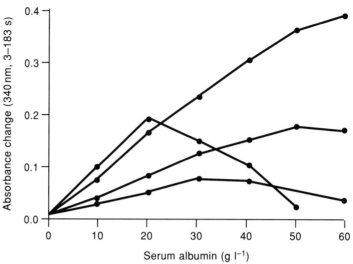

Figure 6 Data to illustrate the variation in performance of a turbidimetric assay for serum albumin using different sources of polyclonal antisera.

monoclonal antibodies illustrates the effects of altering the proportion of each antibody in the cocktail (Figure 4). Although it is possible to use single monoclonal antibodies or cocktails in direct immunoturbidimetric assays, there are few examples in the literature; in broad terms the approach to optimisation and the reaction conditions themselves will be similar for monoclonal and polyclonal reagents although the reaction kinetics may differ (Deverill and Reeves, 1980; Ehrlich *et al.*, 1982; Maynard *et al.*, 1986).

Assay Performance

Detection Limit

Direct immunoaggregation assays without any signal enhancement have been described for a range of proteins at concentrations of between 2 mg l^{-1} and 50 g l^{-1} using both turbidimetry and nephelometry. At the lower analyte concentration (2–100 mg l^{-1}), with turbidimetric monitoring it is necessary to undertake some form of pretreatment (Hellsing and Enstrom, 1977; Ervin *et al.*, 1986); however, it is more appropriate to consider the use of latex particle labelling for these lower analyte concentrations. Pretreatment protocols in the past have included PEG as indicated earlier (Hellsing and Enstrom, 1977), protamine sulphate (Wood *et al.*, 1978), dextran sulphate and calcium chloride (Kallner, 1977) or Arklone P (Whicher and Blow, 1980). Endogenous light scattering may give more problems with nephelometric methods and care needs to be taken with the preparation both of samples and of reagents.

Mean IgG (g l⁻¹)	Coefficient of variation (%)	
	Turbidimetry (0–180 s)	Nephelometry (0–111 s)
3.1	2.74	4.67
10.7	1.85	4.17
23.4	1.90	4.30

Table 3 Comparison of the relative imprecision of turbidimetric and nephelometric immunoassays obtained on the same analyser platform.

Imprecision

The imprecision of turbidimetric and nephelometric methods is very comparable with the expectation of within-run coefficients of variation of less than 3–4%, day-to-day being less than 6–8%. Where it has been possible to make direct comparison, turbidimetric monitoring appears to be the more precise (Table 3).

Accuracy

The accuracy of methods will depend in part on the specificity of the antiserum chosen and the calibration material. Although the choice of antiserum affects accuracy, particularly when there is more than one variant of the analyte of interest (Whicher, 1979; Whicher *et al.*, 1984; van Rijn *et al.*, 1987), the major influence on accuracy of results is the calibration material (Chambers *et al.*, 1984; Bullock *et al.*, 1990). The problems of producing primary reference materials for protein analytes is discussed in Reimer and Madison (1976) and Chambers *et al.* (1987a); however, a successful initiative has been completed for the production of an international reference material that traces analyte levels back to primary reference preparations (CRM 470) (Whicher *et al.*, 1994).

Antigen Excess Detection

As was pointed out earlier, in a direct light-scattering assay monitoring immunoaggregate formation as the antigen concentration increases beyond the equivalence point, small immune complexes are formed and consequently the signal diminishes. Thus, in a direct assay a particular signal of change may equate to an antigen concentration in antibody excess or, beyond the equivalence point, in antigen excess. It is therefore extremely important to ensure that an assay is set up in such a way that antigen excess cannot exist, or that an additional step is added to determine whether this situation has been reached. The potential problem must be recognised for any protein analyte in which there is a wide pathological range, e.g. serum C-reactive protein, immunoglobulins and urine albumin.

In the early continuous-flow nephelometric immunoassays antigen excess was recognised from a change in the peak shape (Richie, 1978). It has also been suggested by several authors that monitoring of the rate of immunoaggregate formation can facilitate the recognition of antigen excess because of the change in apparent reaction kinetics (Van Munster *et al.*, 1977; Spencer and Price, 1979; Deverill, 1980; Skoug and Pardue, 1986, 1988). Hills and Tiffany (1980) found this approach more successful for 90° nephelometry than turbidimetry, although they did not recommend the technique. It must be recognised that the kinetics of immunoaggregate formation are very dependent on the individual antiserum preparation and consequently discrimination where it exists may not be maintained when batches of antiserum change.

Alternative approaches to the detection of antigen excess include: (1) repeat of the assay on a dilute sample; (2) addition of a further aliquot of antigen or antibody; and (3) the choice of an inhibition-format assay (see Assay Format below). In the second category, addition of more sample when the assay is already in antigen excess will not influence the signal; if the system is in antibody excess then addition of more antigen will result in an increase in signal. On the other hand, if more antibody is added to a system in antigen excess there will be an increase in signal; in antibody excess there will be no increase in signal. The latter approach is clearly more costly; indeed, any method that involves a further step is more costly and so it is preferable to design assays that are able to avoid antigen excess. However, the peak-rate monitoring technique with continuous reaction monitoring will allow early detection of antigen excess and additional antigen or antibody can be added quickly, reducing overall machine time.

PARTICLE-ENHANCED IMMUNOASSAY

The benefits of a particle-enhanced approach are twofold: (1) the enhancement of the sensitivity of the method by increasing the relative light-scattering signal; and (2) the opportunity to use an alternative assay format, in particular introducing the opportunity to measure haptens and avoiding the difficulty of antigen excess.

Assay Format

There are three formats of particle-enhanced light scattering and each has its own strengths and weaknesses. Indeed, it should also be recognised that, in certain circumstances (where less sensitivity is required), it is possible to use a protein rather than a particle core, e.g. albumin and ferritin (Finley *et al.*, 1981; Wu *et al.*, 1982); however, these protein core alternatives are considered here to illustrate an immunoinhibition format with a nonparticle core. The first format, however, is an immunoaggregation assay analogous to the direct approach described earlier but in which the antiserum is coupled to particles (Figure 7*a*). This approach can be used with turbidimetric or nephelometric monitoring and is applicable to polyvalent antigens, e.g. proteins or microorganisms. The second format involves the coupling of pure antigen to the particles; the addition of antiserum will lead to immunoaggregate formation (Figure 7*b*). Quantification of analyte in the sample is achieved by determining the degree of inhibition of the immunoaggregate formation when free sample analyte is added. This approach is applicable to mono- and polyvalent antigens, i.e. haptens and proteins. The third format is really an extension of the second in which the antibody is also coupled to particles as well as the antigens (Figure 7*c*); this is a dual-particle format and can be applied to both mono- and polyvalent antigens.

In addition to the enhancement of the signal that can be achieved by using a particle label, it is worth stressing the two unique features of the immunoinhibition format. First, it enables the quantification of hapten with light-scattering detection. Second, it avoids the possibility of

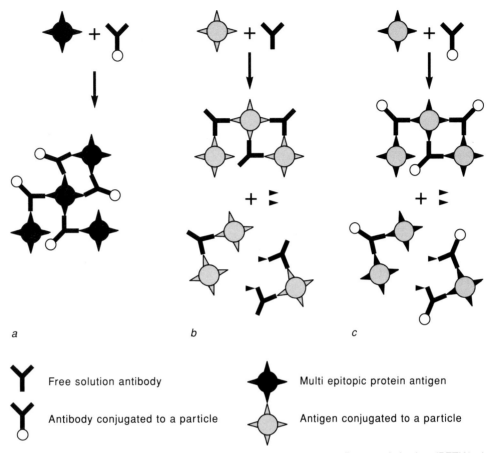

a   b   c

Y   Free solution antibody   ◆ Multi epitopic protein antigen

Y   Antibody conjugated to a particle   ✦ Antigen conjugated to a particle

Figure 7 Possible formats for particle-enhanced immunoassays. *a*, direct agglutination (PETIA); *b*, antigen-coated particle, inhibition of aggregation (PETINIA); *c*, dual-particle assay.

antigen excess, as described earlier, and consequently the likelihood of misrepresentation of high analyte concentrations (Pauli *et al.*, 1987; Thakkar *et al.*, 1997).

The first two formats can be considered as analogous to antibody reagent excess and limited antibody reagent, respectively, and therefore basic considerations applicable to immunoradiometric assay (IRMA) and radioimmunoassay (RIA) methods apply. Thus, the addition of an excess of antiserum in a direct immunoaggregation assay will extend the calibration range, and to a degree will improve the sensitivity at lower analyte concentrations. But in the immunoinhibition format the reagent antigen and antibody concentrations should be reduced as much as possible to achieve maximum sensitivity. However, this trend has to be compromised sufficiently to enable the light scattering at zero analyte concentration (i.e. maximum aggregate formation) to be detected and for there to be sufficient signal to be modulated at antigen concentrations within the analytical range. In this respect, it is also possible to consider the immunoinhibition format as lying entirely within the antigen excess region depicted in Figure 3.

Types of Particles

A variety of particles has been described for use in quantitative immunoassay including erythrocytes (Coombs *et al.*, 1987), metal sols (Leuvering *et al.*, 1980; Cais, 1983; Weetall and Gaigalas, 1992) and latex particles (Grange *et al.*, 1977; Cambiaso *et al.*, 1977; Galvin *et al.*, 1983; Newman *et al.*, 1992). Erythrocytes have generally been used in qualitative and semi-quantitative assays.

Metal Sols

Gold, silver, silver iodide, selenium, ferrofluid and barium sulphate sols (colloidal solutions) have all been described, although gold sols have been the most popular for immunoassay applications (Gribnau *et al.*, 1986). The main advantages of gold sols are their high refractive index and ease of preparation. The sol particles are produced by a controlled reduction of an aqueous solution of tetrachloroauric acid. Strong reducing agents, such as white phosphorus, citrate-tannic acid or sodium borohydride, induce larger numbers of nuclei than weaker reducing agents and this results in smaller particles. Particles can be produced to give uniform sizes between about 5 and 60 nm; they can be stored in dark bottles at 4 °C for at least 6 months.

Latex Particles

The use of latex particles in light-scattering immunoassay has proved to be very popular over the past 15 years as knowledge and experience of the synthesis of robust, well defined particles has developed.

The synthesis of latex particles follows one of three main principles: (1) emulsion polymerisation; (2) suspension polymerisation; and (3) swollen emulsion polymerisation. Emulsion polymerisation is the process most often used for smaller particles (40–100 nm) and involves the generation of a detergent micelle into which is introduced a monomer and a polymerisation initiator, e.g. persulphate. The average particle size is controlled by the detergent concentration, the amount of monomer, initiator, rate of mixing and temperature. Multiple polymerisation steps can also be introduced to increase the size of particles or to introduce an alternative shell (Litchfield *et al.*, 1984; Kapmeyer *et al.*, 1988).

Core and Surface Chemistry

The refractive index of the particle influences the degree of light scatter and it has been suggested that the use of a polyvinylnaphthalene core will enhance sensitivity of detection over the more conventional polystyrene (Litchfield *et al.*, 1984); the refractive index of polyvinylnaphthalene is 1.682 compared to 1.591 for polystyrene when measured at 569 nm; water has a value of 1.333. In addition, the choice of an appropriate monomer can enable the introduction of active groups on the particle surface, e.g. -COOH (acrylic acid), -NH$_2$ (acrylamide), epoxide (glycidyl methacrylate) (Molday *et al.*, 1975) or chloromethyl (vinylbenzylchloride) (Craig *et al.*, 1983; Crane, 1987). The reader is referred to Galvin (1983), Newman *et al.* (1992) and Griffin *et al.* (1994) for more information on coupling chemistry.

Size and Density

The discussion above on light-scattering theory and practical observations with turbidimetric and nephelometric assays highlights the importance of particle size on the level of light scattering measured at any particular angle. In addition, it is best to use latex particles with a narrow size distribution because it is considered that the maximum light scattering occurs when a single particle combines with another to form a dimer, hence the importance of a monodispersed species. The smaller particles will also have the benefit of providing the largest surface area (relative to volume) and thus the potential for higher antibody loading (but see later discussion); in this respect, protein loading will in itself obviously increase the size of the particle (a monolayer of immunoglobulin G increasing the diameter by approximately 10 nm). There are examples where large particles have been used, however, with infrared monitoring of the scattering (Sorin *et al.*, 1989). The size of the particle may be determined by either electron microscopy or photon correlation spectroscopy, the latter being more convenient for determination after coupling of ligand.

The density of the particle is determined by the selection of monomer and the size of particle produced; clearly, smaller and neutral-density particles offer the benefit of greater movement in the liquid phase while also minimising the degree of flocculation, thereby negating the need for constant mixing of the reagent to maintain homogeneity.

Surface Charge and Zeta Potential

The surface charge plays an important part in the characteristics of an assay. It is determined by the nature of the surface chemistry, unreacted monomer, the nature of protein or other ligand coupled to the particle and detergent as well as the nature of the reaction buffer. In broad terms, neutral particles will self-aggregate whereas highly charged particles will remain dispersed because of repulsion between particles; however, too great a charge may result in no aggregation in the presence of sample analyte because the binding energy of the antigen–antibody reaction is too low to overcome the repulsion. Note that some serum proteins may be positively charged at neutral pH, which could lead to nonspecific aggregation (Serra *et al.*, 1992; Hidalgo-Alvarez and Galisteo-Gonzalez, 1995). It is therefore important to choose an appropriate reaction pH and ensure that surface charge measurements are made under the conditions of the assay.

A measure of the net surface charge is the zeta potential, which is the potential at the surface of shear or the slipping plane (Hidalgo-Alvarez, 1991). It can be measured by applying an electric field across a capillary containing the sample; the electrical field causes the particles to move to the oppositely charged electrode with a velocity termed the electrophoretic mobility, which is related to the zeta potential.

Reagent Optimisation

The broad guidance on optimisation of reagents and reaction parameters for nonenhanced turbidimetric and nephelometric assays are applicable to particle-enhanced assays. However, it is important to recognise that the characteristics of the final particle reagent, e.g. size and surface charge, will have a major influence on the final performance of the reagent.

Particle Reagents

The major factors that influence method performance include: (1) reagent antibody or antigen loading on the particle; (2) the use of passive adsorption versus covalent coupling; (3) the use of a spacer molecule when coupling a hapten; and (4) the blocking of remaining active groups and free surface on the particle.

Particle Loading

In the case of an antibody particle reagent for a direct aggregation assay, experience has shown there is an optimum level of protein loading to achieve the best results (i.e. maximum signal change). As the protein is loaded the overall size increases and multiple protein layers may be introduced. It is evident that the colloidal stability of the particle decreases with increased protein loading; the practical implications of this are twofold: (1) a nonspecific aggregation may occur when sample is added; and (2) the particle becomes highly susceptible to self-aggregation when PEG is added. Clearly, overloading may also lead to steric hindrance and less availability of binding sites. These points notwithstanding, the choice of loading will be determined by the performance of the reagent with particular respect to the initial scattering of the reagent (i.e. the number of particles per assay), the analytical range required and the signal change per unit of analyte while also ensuring that antigen excess does not occur. It is also likely that overloading of particles will result in poor batch-to-batch coupling reproducibility (and thus assay performance).

In the case of an inhibition assay where the antigen is coupled to the particle, as indicated earlier, sensitivity is related to antigen concentration: the lower the loading the greater the sensitivity. However, sufficient antigen has to be loaded to ensure a measurable level of aggregate formation. It is then important to block the remaining bare surface of the particle with, for example, bovine serum albumin or detergent.

Coupling Technique

The majority of early particle-based assays used adsorption of protein. Passive adsorption is probably a hydrophobic interaction but is also pH dependent. This may make it more prone to inhibition by detergent and leeching of reagent constituents with time. It is also thought that passive adsorption may lead to suboptimal orientation of antibody molecules rendering them inaccessible for immunoaggregation (Spitznagel and Clark, 1993). There is an increasing awareness that modification of the antibody can also improve functionality when using passive absorption techniques (Davies *et al.*, 1994; Davies *et al.*, 1995).

Coupling through carboxyl, amino or chloromethyl groups has been used for proteins and haptens whereas the epoxide group has been reserved for haptens because the process requires heating to $70\,°C$. The carbodiimide (CDI) coupling chemistry is commonly used with carboxylated particles (Galvin, 1983) and involves the production of acylurea groups, which readily react with amino groups on the protein or hapten; in the case of coupling of protein a two-stage process will ensure that crosslinking of the protein is avoided. Glutaraldehyde may be used with particles modified at their amino group, with activation of particles as the first step and removal of excess coupling agent before coupling to protein (Quash *et al.*, 1978). Note that there are examples of specific coupling chemistries designed to minimise interference from, for example, rheumatoid factor (Limet *et al.*, 1979). It has also been suggested that universal coupling systems, particularly for antibodies, may be helpful, e.g. protein A or G (Goding, 1978) or streptavidin (Kohe *et al.*, 1988). It may be argued that use of protein A or G may improve the orientation of antibody molecules with respect to the particle surface improving the yield of viable antibody by virtue of universal attachment through the Fc region; however, there is little data to support this idea. In all cases it is important to block remaining reactive groups after coupling.

In the case of haptens coupled to particles, it may be considered helpful to link the hapten through a spacer molecule to limit the steric interference from the particle surface and thus making the hapten more available for the antibody (Corrie *et al.*, 1980; Litchfield *et al.*, 1984). The spacer molecules are often repeat lengths of amino acids. However, if the chain length is too long, additional problems may arise in the case of hydrophobic haptens (e.g. thyroxine and digoxin) because the hapten can interact with the surface. As in the case of proteins, it is important to block unreacted groups and bare surface, perhaps here bearing in mind that large blocking molecules may hinder access to the hapten, even if this is a detergent, as they can have long chain lengths.

Reaction Conditions

As has already been suggested, the particle reagent should be optimised to minimise the attraction between particles by ensuring sufficient electrostatic repulsion (reflected by the negative zeta potential) while ensuring that antigen-antibody attractive forces are not swamped. It is also important to ensure that the ionic strength is adjusted so that nonspecific aggregation is avoided (Newman *et al.*, 1992).

The addition of a ballast protein such as human or bovine serum albumin may also enhance particle reagent stability (Galvin, 1983; Newman *et al.*, 1992)), as can the use of ionic detergents. However, it is worth reiterating the caution of not loading too much protein as it may lead to a large increase in the size of particle, be difficult to synthesise reproducibly because of the multiple protein layers and also promote colloidal instability. In this case the use of an affinity-purified antibody preparation will result in the minimum protein (not antibody) being loaded, giving the greatest flexibility for adding ballast protein while maintaining good colloidal stability (Newman *et al.*, 1992). On the other hand, we have noticed that in the development of two assays for protein antigen using a high sample fraction, addition of ballast protein led to a reduction of immunoaggregate formation.

It has been shown that some particle reagents are more stable in glycine-based buffers although these in themselves are not good for promoting immunoaggregate formation (Masson *et al.*, 1981; Galvin, 1983). The optimal pH range for particle-enhanced assays lies between 6.5 and 7.5 although in some cases a higher pH has been chosen to reduce nonspecific aggregation (Medcalf *et al.*, 1990). The use of a lower pH will invariably lead to a net positive charge on the serum proteins relative to the particle and immediate onset of nonspecific aggregation; note that nonspecific aggregation is invariably seen as a very rapid increase in light scattering. An alternative approach to reducing nonspecific aggregation is to choose a buffer from the Hofmeister series referred to earlier. This observation serves to emphasise the point that with a particle reagent the electrostatic interactions between antibody particle reagent and antigen may be particle-particle or particle-protein or protein-protein and it is therefore vital to recognise the need to consider the chemistry of particle surface interactions as well as the antigen-antibody interactions.

In this respect the effect of PEG on particle-based assays is also more complex than with nonenhanced assays; PEG may induce nonspecific aggregation of particles alone and most definitely will induce nonspecific aggregation of particles with a heavy protein loading. It is therefore best, as with nonenhanced assays but for different reasons, to consider the effects of antibody concentration (i.e. loading) and PEG concentration as complementary.

Finally, in terms of assay configuration, surfactants such as Tween and SDS may also enhance particle reagent stability and minimise nonspecific aggregation. However, an excess amount of detergent (possibly above 0.5% depending upon respective critical micelle concentration) may inhibit the immunoaggregate formation.

Thus, the design of direct particle-enhanced immunoaggregation assays is similar to that described for nonenhanced methods for proteins. The concern about antigen excess remains although it may be possible to flag high levels by setting the top calibrator significantly below the equivalence point (as with nonenhanced assays); an example is the case of a C-reactive protein assay where the top calibrator was set at 120 mg l^{-1}, equivalence being at 250 mg l^{-1}, and the signal equivalent to 120 mg l^{-1} was not reached in antigen excess until 600 mg l^{-1}, giving a good safety margin (Price *et al.*, 1987). If extreme caution is required then an inhibition format can be used to negate any risk of antigen excess; it might be argued that this style of assay also requires less antibody reagent but it does require pure antigen to couple onto the particles (Pauli *et al.*, 1987; Thakkar *et al.*, 1997).

A novel development in the field of particle-labelled agglutination is the use of an ultrasonic standing wave to enhance the rate of aggregation. Particles suspended in an ultrasonic standing wave (not sufficient to induce cavitation or acoustic streaming) rapidly concentrate at positions of potential energy minima in the field. The concentrated particles also experience sound-induced particle-particle interactions, the extent of these effects being dependent on the size, density and compressibility of the particles (Coakley *et al.*, 1989; Jepras *et al.*, 1989; Grundy *et al.*, 1993, 1995). Grundy *et al.* (1995) found a decrease in reaction time of between 14- and 50-fold compared with conventional microbiological agglutination systems, although it was not clear whether the assays had been optimised to achieve maximum reaction rates. Although Grundy *et al.* (1993) found no difference in the specificity or sensitivity of the assays, Jepras *et al.* (1989) used ultrasound to enhance the rate of agglutination of *Legionella pneumophila* with diluted antiserum and found that agglutination occurred with an antibody 512 times more dilute; the authors were able to detect by eye a twofold lower concentration of cells; detection of agglutination was 100 times quicker using the ultrasound device with a capillary reaction tube than the conventional microtitre well approach. These early data suggest interesting possibilities for reducing reaction times and possibly lower detection limits, particularly for microbiological assays and other dual-particle assays which may be of particular advantage for assays used at the point of care. However, it is likely that the sensitivity gain will only be achieved using larger (>1 μm) particles because the smaller submicrometre particles are already moving under Brownian motion. The choice may be between the needs of the detector (large particles offering more light scattering) and the desired rate of reaction.

Assay Performance

There is now a wide range of particle-enhanced assays described in the literature, the majority using a range of latex particles (Table 4). It is now possible to expect within-run imprecision figures between 2 and 5% depending on the signal change, with day-to-day figures typically less than 8%. The lower limit of detection for an assay of a protein in serum is around 80 μg l^{-1} for turbidimetric assays with figures around 1.0 nmol l^{-1} for haptens (Galvin *et al.*, 1983; Jaggon and Price, 1987; Simo *et al.*, 1994). Lower detection limits are achievable for proteins

Proteins

Albumin (S, U, *)	Fibrinogen (P)
α_1-Microglobulin (U, *)	Fibrin degradation products (P)
β_2-Microglobulin (S, *)	Ferritin (S, *)
C-reactive protein (S, *)	Sex hormone-binding globulin (S, *)
Cystatin C (S, *)	Thyroxine-binding globulin (S)
Immunoglobulin G, A, M (S, *)	Prealbumin (S, *)
Light chains (U, *)	Rheumatoid factor (S)
α_1-Antitrypsin (S)	TSH (S,*)
Haptoglobulin (S)	Prolactin (S, *)
α_1-Acid glycoprotein (S)	α-fetoprotein (S, *)
α_1-Antichymotrypsin (S)	Carcinoembryonic antigen (S, *)
Antithrombin III (S)	Myoglobin (S, *)

Haptens

Theophylline	Gentamicin
Digoxin	Tobramicin
Phenobarbital	Drugs of abuse
Phenytoin	Thyroxine

Table 4 Summary of the range of light-scattering immunoassays available; * assays using latex particle labels with a diluted sample; S, serum; U, urine; P, plasma.

in urine, partly because a larger sample volume can be tolerated, an example being an assay for retinol-binding protein with a detection limit of 25 μg l^{-1} equivalent to 1 nmol l^{-1} (Thakkar *et al.*, 1991a). Similar performance has been demonstrated for assays labelled with a gold sol for constituents in urine (Leuvering *et al.*, 1980) but there have been problems using this technology for analytes in serum because of significant problems with nonspecific aggregation (Gribnau *et al.*, 1986). The limits of detection for particle-counting assays are comparable or even better than those for particle-labelled turbidimetric and nephelometric assays (Galvin *et al.*, 1983), albeit the reaction times are longer.

The relative merits of turbidimetry and nephelometry follow similar arguments to those used earlier with nonenhanced assays. However, there is some evidence to suggest that nephelometric assay systems may be able to deliver an additional order of magnitude of sensitivity with detection limits down to 6 μg l^{-1} (Borque *et al.*, 1991); certainly comparison of turbidimetric and nephelometric particle-enhanced assays for the same analyte indicate that sample dilution is required for the latter technique which, while reducing the likelihood of interference, also points to a lower potential detection limit. Such an example is the measurement of serum cystatin C which uses a 2.0% sample fraction for a turbidimetric approach (Newman *et al.*, 1995) and a sample fraction of 0.375% for a nephelometric system (Finney *et al.*, 1997).

Accuracy, as in nonenhanced assays, is closely linked to the choice of calibrant. However, in the case of particle-enhanced assays there is more potential for nonspecific aggregation; an often-quoted problem with latex particle-based assays is interference due to rheumatoid factor binding to the Fc portion of immunoglobulins. It can be overcome by the use of Fab fragments instead of whole immunoglobulin (Limet *et al.*, 1979; Larsson and Sjööquist, 1988). Alternative approaches include the use of a high pH buffer, heat pretreatment of the sample or preincubation with a protease; in the case of the DuPont aca analyser, which enables containment of volatile reagent in packs, dithiothreitol is used as an inhibitor (Schwartz *et al.*, 1988).

APPLICATIONS

Light-scattering assays have been described for a wide range of analytes including proteins, haptens and whole cells; some examples are given in Table 4. The hapten assays have involved the inhibition format with generation of a multivalent antigen using either latex particles or proteins such as albumin or ferritin. The assays are mainly for therapeutic drugs, drugs of abuse or hormones with detection limits in the nanomolar range, as exemplified by digoxin and thyroxine (Galvin *et al.*, 1983; Jaggon and Price, 1987), and use turbidimetric monitoring.

The protein assays use either turbidimetric or nephelometric monitoring, the former technique enabling assays to be integrated into routine clinical chemistry analytical platforms. The advantage of this is illustrated by the integration of the measurement of C-reactive protein into the neonatal profile which minimises sample wastage and maximises turnaround time in addition to the benefits of the analytical performance. A further example is the recently described turbidimetric assays for haemoglobin A1c (Holownia *et al.*, 1997) enabling the analyte to be measured quickly with the same analyser used for other related analytes such as glucose and cholesterol. In this respect, it is worth pointing out that light-scattering assays have also been developed for point-of-care application in disposable cartridge devices, a reflection of the robust nature and simplicity of the technology (Klotz, 1993; Pope *et al.*, 1993; see also chapter 22).

SUMMARY AND CONCLUSIONS

Light-scattering immunoassay is an extremely robust analytical technology that can be used on most spectrophotometric systems or with dedicated nephelometers. Improvements in the production of antisera and particles have enabled the production of a wide range of robust methods and stabilisation of reagents with covalent coupling of components to particles which help to produce more stable calibration (Price *et al.*, 1987; Medcalf *et al.*, 1990; Thakkar *et al.*, 1991b). Thus, calibration curves have remained stable for longer than 6 months.

This reagent technology has now been applied to alternative analytical systems including biosensors such as surface plasmon resonance (Severs and Schasfoort, 1993) and also encapsulated in disposable cartridge devices to use away from the laboratory environment. This latter application is perhaps the best witness to the reliability of the technique.

REFERENCES

Absolom, D. R. & van Oss, C. J. (1986) The nature of the antigen-antibody bond and the factors affecting its association and dissociation. *CRC Crit. Rev. Immunol.* **6**, 1–46.

Anderson, R. J. & Sternberg, J. C. (1978) A rate nephelometer for immunoprecipitin measurement of specific serum proteins. In: *Automated Immunoanalysis* Vol. 2 (ed. Ritchie, R. F.) pp. 410–469 (Marcel Dekker, New York).

Anthony, F., Spencer, K., Mason, P. *et al.* (1980) The variable influence of an α component in pregnancy plasma on four different assay systems for the measurement of pregnancy-specific β_1-glycoprotein. *Clin. Chim. Acta* **105**, 287–295.

Bloomfield, V. A. (1985) Biological applications. In: *Dynamic Light Scattering: Applications of Photon Correlation Spectroscopy* (ed. Pecora, R.) pp. 363–416 (Plenum Press, New York).

Borque, L., Rus, A. & Ruiz, R. (1991) Quantitative automated latex nephelometric immunoassay for determination of myoglobin in human serum. *J. Clin. Lab. Anal.* **5**, 175–179.

Boyden, S. V. (1951) The adsorption of proteins on erythrocytes treated with tannic acid and subsequent haemagglutination by antiprotein sera. *J. Exp. Med.* **93**, 107–120.

Buffone, G. J., Savory, J., Cross, R. E. *et al.* (1975a) Evaluation of light scattering as an approach to the measurement of specific proteins with the centrifugal analyser: I, Methodology. *Clin. Chem.* **21**, 1731–1734.

Buffone, G. J., Savory, J. & Hermans, J. (1975b) Evaluation of kinetic light scattering as an approach to the measurement of specific proteins with the centrifugal fast analyser: Theoretical considerations. *Clin. Chem.* **21**, 1735–1746.

Bullock, D. G., Dumont, G. & Vassault, A. (1990) Immunochemical assays of serum proteins: A European external quality assessment survey and the effects of calibration procedures on interlaboratory agreement. *Clin. Chim. Acta* **187**, 21–36.

Cais, M. (1983) Metalloimmunoassay: Principles and practice. *Meth. Enzymol.* **92**, 445–458.

Cambiaso, C. L., Leek, A. E., De Steenwinkel, F. *et al.* (1977) Particle counting immunoassay (PACIA): A general method for the determination of antibodies, antigens and haptens. *J. Immunol. Meth.* **18**, 33–44.

Chambers, R. E., Bullock, D. G. & Whicher, J. T. (1987a) Improved between laboratory agreement for specific protein assays in serum following introduction of a common reference preparation (SPS-01) demonstrated in an external quality assessment scheme. *Clin. Chim. Acta* **164**, 189–200.

Chambers, R. E., Whicher, J. T. & Bullock, D. G. (1984) External quality assessment of immunoassays for specific proteins in serum: 18 months' experience in the United Kingdom. *Ann. Clin. Biochem.* **21**, 246–253.

Chambers, R. E., Whicher, J. T., Perry, D. E. *et al.* (1987b) Over estimation of immunoglobulins in the presence of rheumatoid factor by kinetic immunonephelometry and rapid immunoturbidimetry. *Ann. Clin. Biochem.* **24**, 520–524.

Coakley, W. T., Bardsley, D. W., Grundy, M. A. *et al.* (1989) Cell manipulation in ultrasonic standing wave fields. *J. Chem. Tech. Biotechnol.* **44**, 43–62.

Collet-Cassart, D., Mareschal, J. C., Sindic, C. J. M. *et al.* (1983) Automated particle-counting immunoassay of C-reactive protein and its application to serum, cord serum, and cerebrospinal fluid samples. *Clin. Chem.* **29**, 1127–1131.

Coombs, R. R. A., Scott, M. L. & Cranage, M. P. (1987) Assays using red cell-labelled antibodies. *J. Immunol. Meth.* **101**, 1–14.

Corrie, J. E. T., Hunter, W. M. & MacPherson, J. S. (1980) ^{125}I- labelled radioligands in steroid radioimmunoassay: The question of 'bridge recognition'. *J. Endocrinol.* **87**, 8–9.

Craig, A. R., Frey, W. A., Leflar, C. C. *et al.* (1983) Covalently bonded high refractive index particle reagents and their use in light scattering immunoassays. *US Patent* No. 4,401,765.

Crane, J. E. (1987) Latex agglutination immunoassays. *Am. Biotech. Lab.* **5**, 34–41.

Creighton, T. E. (1984) *Proteins: Structures and Molecular Principles* (W. H. Freeman and Co., New York).

Davies, D. R., Padlan, E. A. & Sheriff, S. (1990) Antibody-antigen complexes. *Ann. Rev. Biochem.* **59**, 439–473.

Davies, J., Dawkes, A. C. & Haymes, A. G. (1994) A scanning tunnelling microscopy comparison of passive antibody adsorption and biotinylated antibody linkage to streptavidin on microtiter wells. *J. Immunol. Meth.* **167**, 263–269.

Davies, J., Dawkes, A. C., Haymes, A. G. *et al.* (1995) Scanning tunnelling microscopy and dynamic constant angle studies of the effects of partial denaturation on immunoassay solid phase antibody. *J. Immunol. Meth.* **186**, 111–123.

Debye, P. (1915) Zerstreuung von Röntgerstrahlen. *Ann. Physik.* **46**, 809–823.

Delange, J. R., Chapelle, J.-P. & Vanderschueren S. C. (1990) Quantitative nephelometric assay for determining myoglobin evaluated. *Clin. Chem.* **36**, 1675–1678.

Deverill, I. (1980) Kinetic measurement of the immunoprecipitin reaction using the centrifugal analyser. In: *Centrifugal Analysers in Clinical Chemistry* (eds Price, C. P. & Spencer, K.) pp. 109–124 (Praeger, Eastbourne).

Deverill, I. & Lock, R. J. (1983) Kinetics of the antigen:antibody reaction. *Ann. Clin. Biochem.* **20**, 224–226.

Deverill, I. & Reeves, W. G. (1980) Light scattering and absorption: Developments in immunology. *J. Immunol. Meth.* **38**, 191–204.

Ducker, W. A., Senden, T. J. & Pashley, R. M. (1991) Direct measurement of colloidal forces using an atomic force microscope. *Nature* **353**, 239–241.

Ehrlich, P. H., Moyle, W. R., Moustafa, Z. A. *et al.* (1982) Mixing two monoclonal antibodies yields enhanced affinity for antigen. *J. Immunol.* **128**, 2709–2713.

Ervin, P. E., Jansson, N. O. & Bergdahl, A. (1986) A turbidimetric immunochemical method for determination of serum β_2-microglobulin using a centrifugal analyser. *Clin. Chim. Acta* **155**, 151–156.

Finley, P. R., Dye, J. A., Williams, R. J. *et al.* (1981) Rate-nephelometric inhibition immunoassay of phenytoin and phenobarital. *Clin. Chem.* **27**, 405–409.

Finley, P. R., Williams, R. J., Lichti, D. A. *et al.* (1979) Immunochemical determination of human immunoglobulins: Use of kinetic turbidimetry and a 36-place centrifugal analyzer. *Clin. Chem.* **25**, 526–530.

Finney, H., Newman, D. J., Gruber, N. *et al.* (1997) Initial evaluation of cystatin C measurement by particle enhanced immunonephelometry on the Behring Nephelometer System (BNA, II). *Clin. Chem.* (accepted for publication).

Freund, J. (1925) Agglutination of tubercle bacilli. *Amer. Rev. Tuberc.* **12**, 124–141.

Gaechtgens, W. (1906) Beitrag zur Agglutinationstechnik. *München med. Wchnschr.* **53**, 135–141.

Galvin, J. P. (1983) Particle enhanced immunoassays: A review. In: *Diagnostic Immunology: Technology Assessment and Quality Assurance* (eds Nakamura, R. M. & Rippey, J. H.) pp. 18–30 (College of Pathologists, Skokie, Illinois).

Galvin, J. P., Looney, C. E., Leflar, C. C. *et al.* (1983) Particle enhanced photometric immunoassay systems. In: *Clinical Laboratory Assays: New Technology and Future Directions* Vol. 3 (eds Nakamura, R. M., Ditto, W. R. & Tucker, E. S.) pp. 73–95 (Masson Publishing, New York).

Goding, J. W. (1978) Use of staphylococcal protein A as an immunological reagent. *J. Immunol. Meth.* **20**, 241–253.

Grange, J., Roch, A. M. & Quash, G. A. (1977) Nephelometric assay of antigens and antibodies with latex particles. *J. Immunol. Meth.* **18**, 365–375.

Gribnau, T. C. J., Leuvering, J. H. W. & van Hell, H. (1986) Particle labelled immunoassays: A review. *J. Chromatogr.* **76**, 175–189.

Griffin, C., Sutor, J. & Shull, B. (1994) *Microparticle Reagent Optimization* (Seradyn Inc., Indianapolis).

Grundy, M. A., Barnes, R. A. & Coakley, W. T. (1995) Highly sensitive detection of fungal antigens by ultrasound enhanced latex agglutination. *J. Med. Vet. Mycol.* **33**, 201–203.

Grundy, M. A., Bolek, W. E., Coakley, W. T. *et al.* (1993) Rapid agglutination testing in an ultrasonic standing wave. *J. Immunol. Meth.* **165**, 47–57.

Heidelberger, M. & Kendall, F. (1935a) Quantitative theory of the precipitin reaction: Study of azoprotein-antibody system. *J. Exp. Med.* **62**, 467–483.

Heidelberger, M. & Kendall, F. (1935b) The precipitin reaction between Type III Pneumococcus polysaccharide and homologous antibody. *J. Exp. Med.* **61**, 563–591.

Hellsing, K. (1978) Enhancing effects of nonionic polymers on immunochemical reactions. In: *Automated Immunoanalysis* Vol. 1 (ed. Ritchie, R. F.) pp. 67–112 (Marcel Dekker, New York).

Hellsing, K. & Enstrom, H. (1977) Pre-treatment of serum samples for immunonephelometric analysis by precipitation with polyethylene glycol. *Scand. J. Clin. Lab. Invest.* **35**, 529–536.

Hidalgo-Alvarez, R. (1991) On the conversion of experimental electrokinetic data into double layer characteristics in solid–liquid interfaces. *Adv. Colloid. Interface Sci.* **34**, 217–241.

Hidalgo-Alvarez, R. & Galisteo-Gonzalez, F. (1995) The adsorption characteristics of immunoglobulins. *Hetero. Chem. Rev.* **2**, 249–268.

Hills, L. P. & Tiffany, T. O. (1980) Comparison of turbidimetric and light scattering measurements of immunoglobulins by use of a centrifugal analyser with absorbance and fluorescence/light scattering optics. *Clin. Chem.* **26**, 1459–1466.

Holownia, P., Bishop, E., Newman, D. J. *et al.* (1997) Adaptation and validation of a particle enhanced assay for percent glycated hemoglobin to a DuPont Dimension® analyser. *Clin. Chem.* **43**, 76–84.

Israelachvili, J. (1991) *Intermolecular and Surface Forces* 2nd edn (Academic Press, New York).

Israelachvili, J. & Wennerstrom, H. (1996) Role of hydration and water structure in biological and colloidal interactions. *Nature* **379**, 219–225.

Jacobsen, C. & Steensgaard, J. (1979) Evidence of a two stage nature of precipitin reactions. *Molec. Immunol.* **16**, 571–576.

Jaggon, R. & Price, C. P. (1987) Performance characteristics of a light scattering immunoassay for thyroxine on a discretionary analyser. *J. Auto. Chem.* **9**, 97–99.

Jefferis, R., Reimer, C. B., Skvaril, F. *et al.* (1985) Evaluation of monoclonal antibodies having specificity for human IgG subclasses: Results of an IVIS/WHO collaborative study. *Immunol. Lett.* **10**, 223–252.

Jepras, R. I., Clarke, D. J. & Coakley, W. T. (1989) Agglutination of *Legionella pneumophila* by antiserum is accelerated in an ultrasonic standing wave. *J. Immunol. Meth.* **120**, 201–205.

Kallner, A. (1977) Removal of background interference in nephelometric determination of serum proteins. *Clin. Chim. Acta* **80**, 293–297.

Kapmeyer, W. H., Pauly, H-E. & Tuengler, P. (1988) Automated nephelometric immunoassays with novel shell/core particles. *J. Clin. Lab. Anal.* **2**, 76–83.

Killingsworth, L. M. & Savory, J. (1973) Nephelometric studies of the precipitin reaction: A model system for specific protein measurements. *Clin. Chem.* **19**, 403–407.

Klotz, U. (1993) Comparison of theophyline blood measured by the standard TD$_x$ assay and a new patient-side immunoassay cartridge system. *Ther. Drug Monit.* **15**, 462–464.

Kohen, F., Amir-Zaltsman ,Y., Strasburger, C. J. *et al.* (1988) The avidin-biotin reaction in immunoassay. In *Complementary Immunoassays* (ed. Collins, W. P.) pp. 57–69 (John Wiley & Sons, Chichester).

Kusnetz, J. & Mansberg, H. P. (1978) Optical considerations: Nephelometry. In: *Automated Immunoanalysis* Vol. 1 (ed. Ritchie, R. F.) pp. 1–43 (Marcel Dekker, New York).

Larsson, A. & Sjööquist, J. (1988) False positive results in latex agglutination tests caused by rheumatoid factor. *Clin. Chem.* **34**, 767–768.

Leuvering, J. H. W., Thal, P. H. J. M., van der Waart, M. *et al.* (1980) Sol particle immunoassay (SPIA). *J. Immunoassay* **1**, 77–80.

Leuvering, J. H. W., Thal, P. J. H. M., van der Waart, M. *et al.* (1981) A sol particle agglutination assay for human chorionic-gonadotropin. *J. Immunol. Meth.* **45**,183–194.

Levison, S. A., Kierszenbaum, F. & Dandliker, W. B. (1970) Salt effects on antigen-antibody kinetics. *Biochemistry* **9**, 322–331.

Libby, R. L. (1938) A new and rapid quantitative technique for the determination of potency of types I and II antipneumococcal serum. *J. Immunol.* **34**, 269–279.

Limet, J. N., Moussebois, C. H., Cambiaso C. L. *et al.* (1979) Particle counting immunoassay: IV, The use of F(ab')$_2$ fragments and Ne-chloroacetyl lysine N-carboxy-anyhdride for their coupling to polystyrene latex particles. *J. Immunol. Meth.* **28**, 25–32.

Litchfield, W. J., Craig, A. R., Frey, W. A. *et al.* (1984) Novel shell/core particles for automated immunoassays. *Clin. Chem.* **30**, 1489–1493.

Loeb, J. (1922–1923) The influence of electrolytes on the cataphoretic charge of colloidal particles and the stability of their suspensions: I, Experiments with collodion particles. *J. Gen. Physiol.* **5**, 109–126.

Maclin, E., Rohlfing, D. & Ansour, M. (1973) Relationship between variables in instrument performance and results of kinetic enzyme assays: A system approach. *Clin. Chem.* **19**, 832–837.

Marrack, J. R. & Richards, C. B. (1971) Light scattering studies of the formation of aggregates in mixtures of antigen and antibody. *Immunolology* **20**, 1019–1040.

Masson, P. L., Cambiaso, C. L., Collet-Cassert, D. *et al.* (1981) Particle counting immunoassay (PACIA). *Meth. Enzymol.* **74**, 106–139.

Mayer-Arendt, J. R. (1989) *Introduction to Classical and Modern Optics* 3rd edn (Prentice Hall, Englewood Cliffs, New Jersey).

Maynard, Y., Scott, M. G., Nahm, M. H. *et al.* (1986) Turbidimetric assay of IgG with use of single monoclonal antibodies. *Clin. Chem.* **32**, 752–757.

Mayo, C. S. & Hallock, R. B. (1989) Immunoassay based on surface plasmon oscillation. *J. Immunol. Meth.* **120**, 105–114.

Medcalf, E. A., Newman, D. J., Gilboa, A. *et al.* (1990) A rapid and robust particle-enhanced turbidimetric immunoassay for serum β_2-microglobulin. *J. Immunol. Meth.* **129**, 97–103.

Mie, G. (1908) Beiträge zur Optik trüber Medien, Speziell kolloidaler Metallosungen. *Ann. Physik.* **25**, 344–377.

Molday, R. S., Dreyer, W. J., Rambaum, A. *et al.* (1975) New immunolatex spheres: Visual markers of antigen on lymphocytes for scanning electron microscopy. *J. Cell Biol.* **64**, 75–88.

Moller, N. P. H. & Steensgaard, J. (1979) Fc-mediated immune precipitation: II, Analysis of precipitating immune complexes by rate zonal ultracentrifugation. *Immunology* **38**, 641–648.

Mondenius, C. F. & Mosbach, K. (1988). Detection of biospecific interactions using amplified ellipsometry. *Anal. Biochem.* **170**, 68–72.

Morgan, C. L., Newman, D. J. & Price, C. P. (1996) Immunosensors: technology and opportunities in laboratory medicine. *Clin. Chem.* **42**, 193–209.

Moyle, W. R., Lin, C., Corson, R. L. *et al.* (1983) Quantitative explanation for increased affinity shown by mixtures of monoclonal antibodies: Importance of a circular complex. *Molec. Immunol.* **20**, 439–452.

Muller-Matthesius, R. & Opper, C. (1980) Influence of measurement time and reaction medium on kinetic immunoturbidimetric protein determination. *J. Clin. Chem. Clin. Biochem.* **18**, 501–508.

Nakamura, M., Ohshima, H. & Kondo, T. (1992) Aggregation behavior of antibody-carrying latex particles. *J. Colloid Interface Sci.* **154**, 393–399.

Newman, D. J. & Price, C. P. (1996) Molecular aspects of design of immunoassays for drugs. *Ther. Drug Monit.* **18**, 493–497.

Newman, D. J., Henneberry, H. & Price, C. P. (1992) Particle enhanced light scattering immunoassay. *Ann. Clin. Biochem.* **29**, 22–42.

Newman, D. J., Thakkar, H., Edwards, R. G. *et al.* (1995) Serum cystatin C measured by automated immunoassay: A more sensitive marker of changes in GFR than serum creatinine. *Kidney Int.* **47**, 312–318.

Ng, R. H., Altaffer, M. & Statland, B. E. (1985) Determinations of immunoglobulins G, A, and M in the Technicon RA-1000. *Clin. Chem.* **31**, 1554–1557.

Nimmo, G. R., Lew, A. M., Stanley, C. M. *et al.* (1984) Influence of antibody affinity on the performance of different assays. *J. Immunol. Meth.* **72**, 177–182.

Pardue, H. L., Hewitt, T. E. & Milano, M. J. (1974) Photometric errors in equilibrium and kinetic analyses based on absorption spectroscopy. *Clin. Chem.* **20**, 1028–1042.

Pauli, C., Bardelli, F., Tarli, P. *et al.* (1987) A simple latex agglutination test for urinary albumin screening. *Clin. Chim. Acta* **166**, 67–71.

Pope, R. M., Apps, J. M., Page, M. D. *et al.* (1993) A novel device for the rapid in-clinic measurement of haemoglobin A1c. *Diab. Med.* **10**, 260–263.

Price, C. P. & Newman, D. J. (1993) Precipitation and agglutination methods: 1, Turbidimetric and nephelometric immunoassay. In: *Methods of Immunological Analysis* (eds Masseyeff, R. F., Albert, W. H. & Staines, N. A.) pp. 134–158 (VCH, Weinheim).

Price, C. P. & Newman, D. J. (1995) Light scattering immunoassay. In: *Endocrinology and Metabolism In-service Training and Continuing Education* Vol. 13 pp. 293–302 (AACC, Washington DC).

Price, C. P. & Spencer, K. (1980) The measurement of specific proteins by kinetic immunoturbidimetry. *UV Spectrosc. Group Bull.* **8**, 29–37.

Price, C. P. & Spencer, K. (1981) Kinetic immunoturbidimetry of human choriomammotropin in serum. *Clin. Chem.* **27**, 882–887.

Price, C. P., Spencer, K. & Whicher, J. (1983) Light scattering immunoassay of specific proteins: A review. *Ann. Clin. Biochem.* **20**, 1–14.

Price, C. P., Trull, A. K., Berry, D. *et al.* (1987) Development and validation of a particle-enhanced immunoassay for C-reactive protein. *J. Immunol. Meth.* **99**, 205–211.

Quash, G., Roch, A-M., Niveleam, A. *et al.* (1978) The preparation of latex particles with covalently bound polymers, IgG and measles agglutinin and their use in viral agglutination test. *J. Immunol. Meth.* **22**, 165–174.

Reimer, C. B. & Maddison, S. E. (1976) Standardization of human immunoglobulin quantitation: a review of current status and problems. *Clin. Chem.* **22**, 577–582.

Ritchie, R. F. (1978) Automated precipitin analysis. In: *Automated Immunoanalysis* Vol.1 (ed. Ritchie, R. F.) pp. 45–66 (Marcel Dekker, New York).

Sakaskita, H., Tomita, A., Umeda, Y. *et al.* (1995) Homogeneous immunoassay using photothermal beam deflection spectroscopy. *Anal. Chem.* **67**, 1278–1282.

Salden, H. J. M., Bas, B. M., Hermans, I. T. H. *et al.* (1988) Analytical performance of three commercially available nephelometers compared for quantifying proteins in serum and cerebrospinal fluid. *Clin. Chem.* **34**, 1594–1596.

Schwartz., M. W., Schifreen, R. S., Gorman, E. G. *et al.* (1988) Development and performance of a fully automated method for assay of C-reactive protein in the aca discrete clinical analyzer. *Clin. Chem.* **34**, 1646–1649.

Serra, J., Puig, J., Martin, A. *et al.* (1992) On the absorption of IgG onto polystyrene particles: Electrophoretic mobility and critical coagulation concentration. *Colloid Polym. Sci.* **270**, 574–583.

Severs, A. H. & Schasfoort, R. B. M. (1993) Enhanced surface plasma resonance inhibition test (ESPRIT) using latex particles. *Biosens. Bioelect.* **8**, 365–370.

Shahangian, S., Agee, K. A. & Dickinson R. P. (1992) Concentration dependencies of immunoturbidimetric dose-response curves: Immunoturbidimetric titer and reactivity, and relevance to design of turbidimetric immunoassays. *Clin. Chem.* **38**, 831–840.

Simo, J. M., Joven, J., Clivillée, X. *et al.* (1994) Automated latex agglutination immunoassay of serum ferritin with a centrifugal analyzer. *Clin. Chem.* **40**, 625–629.

Singer, J. M. & Plotz, C. M. (1956) The latex fixation test: I, Application to the serologic diagnosis of rheumatoid arthritis. *Amer. J. Med.* **21**, 888–892.

Skoug, J. W. & Pardue, H. L. (1986) Evaluation of multipoint kinetic methods for immunoassays: Kinetic equilibrium quantitation of immunoglobulin G. *Anal. Chem.* **58**, 2306–2312.

Skoug, J. W. & Pardue, H. L. (1988) Kinetic turbidimetric methods for the immunochemical quantitation of immunoglobulins, including samples with excess antigen. *Clin. Chem.* **34**, 309–315.

Sorin, T., Ifutan, Y., Safok, K. et al. (1989) Development of an automated latex photometric immunoassay (LPIA) for detection of hepatitis B surface antigen (HB$_s$Ag). *Clin. Chem.* **35**, 1206.

Spencer, K. & Price, C. P. (1979) Kinetic immunoturbidimetry: the measurement of serum albumin. *Clin. Chim. Acta* **95**, 263–276.

Spitznagel, T. M. & Clark, D. S. (1993) Surface density and orientation effects on immobilized antibodies and fragments. *Biotechnology* **11**, 825–829.

Strutt, J. W. Rt. Hon. (Lord Rayleigh) (1871a) On the light from the sky, its polarization and colour. *Phil. Mag.* **41**, 107–120.

Strutt, J. W. Rt. Hon. (Lord Rayleigh) (1871b) On the scattering of light by small particles. *Phil. Mag.* **41**, 447–454.

Sutton, B. J. (1993) Molecular basis of antigen-antibody reactions: Structural aspects. In: *Methods of Immunological Analysis* (eds Masseyeff, R. F., Albert, W. H. & Stainess, N. A.) pp. 66–79 (VCH, Weinheim).

Tanford, C. (1961) *Light Scattering in Physical Chemistry of Macromolecules* (John Wiley & Sons, New York).

Tengerdy, R. P. O. (1967) Reaction kinetic studies of the antigen-antibody reaction. *J. Immunol.* **99**, 126–132.

Thakkar, H., Cornelius, J., Dronfield, D. M. et al. (1991a) Developement of a rapid latex enhanced turbidimetric assay for retinol binding protein. *Ann. Clin. Biochem.* **28**, 407–411.

Thakkar, H., Davey, C. L., Medcalf, E. A. et al. (1991b) Stabilisation of turbidimetric immunoassay by covalent coupling of antibody to latex particles. *Clin. Chem.* **37**, 1248–1251.

Thakkar, H., Newman, D. J., Holownia, P. et al. (1997) Development and validation of a particle turbidimetric inhibition assay for urine albumin on the DuPont aca® analyser. *Clin. Chem.* **43**, 109–113.

Thompson, J. C., Craig, A. R., Davey, C. L. et al. (1997) Kinetics and proposed mechanism of the reaction of an immuno-inhibition, particle-enhanced immunoassay. *Clin. Chem.* (submitted).

Tiffany, T. O. (1994) Fluorometry, nephelometry, and turbidimetry. In: *Tietz Textbook of Clinical Chemistry* 2nd edn (eds Burtis, C. A. & Ashwood, E. R.) pp. 132–158 (W. B. Saunders & Co., Philadelphia).

Tu, C. Y., Kitamori, T., Sanwada, T., et al. (1993) Ultrasensitive heterogeneous immunoassay using photothermal deflection spectroscopy. *Anal. Chem.* **65**, 3631–3635.

Urdal, P., Borch, S. M., Landaas, S. et al. (1992) Rapid immunometric measurement of C-reactive protein in whole blood. *Clin. Chem.* **38**, 580–584.

Van Holde, K. E. (1971) Scattering. In: *Physical Biochemistry* Vol. 9 (Prentice-Hall, Englewood Cliffs, NJ) pp. 209-234.

Van Munster, P. J. J., Hoelen, G. E. J. M., Samwell-Mantingh, M. et al. (1977) A turbidimetric immunoassay (TIA) with automated individual blank compensation. *Clin. Chim. Acta* **76**, 377–388.

van Oss, C. J. (1992) Antigen-antibody reactions. In: *Structure of Antigens* Vol. 1 (ed. Van Regenmortel, M. H. V.) pp. 99–125 (CRC Press, Boca Raton).

van Oss, C. J. (1994) Nature of specific ligand-receptor bonds, in particular the antigen-antibody bond. In: *Immunochemistry* (eds van Oss, C. J. & van Regenmortel, M. H. V.) pp. 581–614 (Marcel Dekker, New York).

van Oss, C. J. (1995) Hydrophobic, hydrophilic and other interactions in epitope-paratope binding. *Molec. Immunol.* **32**, 199–211.

van Oss, C. J., Absolom, D. E., Grossberg, A. L. *et al.* (1979) Repulsive van der Waals forces: I, Complete dissociation of antigen-antibody complexes by means of negative van der Waals forces. *Immunol. Commun.* **8**, 11–29.

van Rijn, H. J. M., Vanderwilt, W., Stroes, J. W. *et al.* (1987) Is the turbidimetric immunoassay of haptoglobin phenotype dependent? *Clin. Biochem.* **20**, 245–248.

van Rijn, J. L. M. L., van Landeghem, A. A. J. & Goldschmidt, H. M. J. (1991) Evaluation of a bench-top nephelometric immunoassay analyzer. *J. Clin. Lab. Anal.* **5**, 3–13.

von Schulthess, G. K., Cohen, R. J. & Benedek, G. B. (1976a) Laser light scattering immunoassay in the agglutination-inhibition mode for human chorionic gonadotropin (hCG) and human luteinising hormone (hLH). *Immunochemistry* **13**, 963–966.

von Schulthess, G. K., Cohen, R. J., Sakato, N. *et al.* (1976b) Laser light scattering spectroscopic immunoassay for mouse IgA. *Immunochemistry* **13**, 955–962.

Vuorinen, P. I., Soppi, E. T., Laine, S. T. *et al.* (1988) Evaluation of the new Behring nephelometer in the measurement of M proteins. *Amer. J. Clin. Path.* **92**, 93–96.

Weetall, H. H. & Gaigalas, A. K. (1992). Studies on antigen-antibody reactions using light scattering from antigen coated colloidal particles. *Anal. Lett.* **25**, 1039–1053.

Whicher, J. T. (1979) Problems encountered in immunochemical techniques: Methodology. In: *Immunochemistry in Clinical Laboratory Medicine* (eds Milford Ward, A. & Whicher, J. T.) pp. 51–61 (MTP Press, Lancaster, UK).

Whicher, J. T. & Blow, C. (1980) Formulation of optimal conditions for an immunonephelometric assay. *Ann. Clin. Biochem.* **17**, 170–177.

Whicher, J. T., Price, C. P. & Spencer, K. (1982) Immunonephelometric and immunoturbidimetric assays for proteins. *CRC Crit. Rev. Clin. Lab. Sci.* **18**, 213–260.

Whicher, J. T., Ritchie, R. F., Johnson, A. M. *et al.* (1994) New international reference preparation for proteins in human serum (RPPHS). *Clin. Chem.* **40**, 934–938.

Whicher, J. T., Warren, C. & Chambers, R. E. (1984) Immunochemical assays for immunoglobins. *Ann. Clin. Biochem.* **21**, 78–91.

Wilkins, T. A., Brouwers, G., Mareschall, J. C. *et al.* (1988a) Immunoassay by particle counting. In: *Complementary Immunoassays* (ed. Collins W. P.) pp. 227–240 (John Wiley & Sons, Chichester).

Wilkins, T. A., Brouwers, G. & Mareschall, J. C. (1988b) High sensitivity, homogeneous particle based immunoassay for thryrotropin (Multipact). *Clin. Chem.* **34**, 1749–1752.

Wilson, I. A. & Stanfield, R. L. (1994) Antibody-antigen interactions: New structures and new conformational changes. *Curr. Opin. Struct. Biol.* **4**, 857–867.

Wood, P. J., Cockett, D. & Mason, P. (1978) A rapid and inexpensive laser nephelometric assay for plasma pregnancy specific β_1-glycoprotein levels. *Clin. Chim. Acta* **90**, 87–91.

Wu, J. W., Hoskin, S., Riebe, S. M. *et al.* (1982) Quantitation of haptens by homogeneous immunoprecipitation: 1, Automated analysis of gentamicin in serum. *Clin. Chem.* **28**, 659–661.

Zdunek, D. & Weber, F. (1988) Process for eliminating non-specific turbidity. *European Patent* No. 0,301,554.

Chapter 19

Electrochemical Immunoassay

Paul Treloar, John Kane and Pankaj Vadgama

INTRODUCTION

Electrochemistry offers a convenient route to the detection of a wide range of organic and inorganic species. It offers substantially simplified transduction mechanisms that rely on the direct intrinsic redox behaviour either of an analyte species or of some reporter molecule. Instrumentation can also be considerably simpler than, say, for spectrophotometric analysis, with the measurement of either a simple current or a voltage charge. Potentially, a direct, analyte-responsive probe can be made that demands the minimum in sample preparation and is capable of operating in optically opaque media, readily miniaturisable and ultimately amenable to mass fabrication. Although these are essentially the proposed advantages of biosensors generally (Vadgama and Crump, 1992), they have actually been realised in only a few cases. Even here there have been major practical issues to be addressed. With electrochemical devices, the voltage window for measurement in a biological fluid is frequently narrow and careful sample extraction or chromatographic separation may be required. Also, as an interfacial technique demanding direct sample contact, electrochemistry is highly vulnerable to surface-active sample colloids leading to passivation or poisoning of the detector surface. Despite these drawbacks, increasing effort has been applied to the integration of electrochemical detection with immunorecognition. In this way it is commonly hoped to avoid the conventional drawbacks of immunoassay using radioisotopes, complex reaction cascades or cumbersome assay protocols.

Although in many instances the most notable aspect of the electro/immuno system is its level of scientific innovation rather than the degree of practical or commercial success achieved, the likelihood is that with refinement of selectivity and biocompatibility the measurement strategies to be described in this chapter will ultimately form the basis for future, viable immunosensors. An immediate challenge, before practical analysis is considered, is the best way in which a binding event between antigen and antibody can be sensitively detected. Differences in ionic binding, dipole interfacial charge etc. have proved insufficient to allow reliable transduction. Usually, therefore, some mode of labelling protocol has proved to be necessary and how well this has 'mapped' onto electrochemical sensors will also be discussed here.

Specifically, in this chapter we will outline the principles of electrochemical detection and discuss some of the labels that have been exploited in assay development; examples will be given, and the potential of electrochemical labels in the future development of true, integrated immunosensor devices discussed.

Some basic background issues are worth considering at this stage. The use of nonisotopic labels in immunoassay has increased dramatically in the past decade. The properties of enzymes as well as fluorescent and luminescent compounds have been thoroughly explored. Despite offering many potential advantages, electrochemically active labels and enzyme reaction products have hardly been explored. Because a nonoptical detection system is used it is possible to detect signal from the label in the presence of whole blood samples. Amperometric detection, say, not only offers a much wider dynamic range but is capable of a level of sensitivity, if not selectivity, that compares very favourably with conventional spectrophotometry (Thompson *et al.*, 1991). A major new practical strategy for improving selectivity has been the exploitation of selective membranes to separate the reactant from the electrochemical transducer (hitherto responses to electrochemically active interferent species in biological samples at unmodified electrodes were too high and too unpredictable). Homogeneous immunoassay then becomes feasible having reduced the background response (Christie *et al.*, 1992).

Also, simplified immunoassay is possible by exploiting *in situ* membrane separation of bound from free antigen prior to detection.

ELECTROCHEMICAL DETECTION STRATEGIES

Amperometric Detection

When an electrochemical cell consisting of two electrodes is immersed in an electrolyte, an interfacial potential is generated at each electrode that can lead to a net potential difference between the two electrodes and a resultant flow of current through the external circuit. In amperometric detection an external potential is actually applied to drive the electrochemical reaction at the electrode surface in a desired direction and the resulting current is then measured and used to quantify the rate of that surface reaction.

The simplest electrochemical redox reaction takes the form:

$$R \rightarrow O + ne^-$$

where R is a reduced species which may be oxidised to species O with the loss of n electrons (e^-). For this reaction to occur three processes must take place: species R must be supplied to the electrode from bulk solution; electron transfer must occur to convert R into O; species O must be removed from the electrode into the bulk solution. An electrochemical reaction therefore has both mass transfer and electron transport elements.

The basic electrochemical process is described by the Nernst equation:

$$E = E° - \frac{RT}{nF} \ln \frac{[R]c}{[O]_c}$$

where E is the potential of the electrode; $E°$ the standard potential of the O/R reaction; R the gas constant; T the temperature; n the number of electrons; F the charge of a mole of electrons; [O] and [R] the surface concentrations of O and R. When the external applied potential is made more or less positive it can be seen from the Nernst equation that the ratio of [R]/[O] must become smaller or larger so the equilibrium state of the reaction must be shifted with an electrochemical redox reaction possible in either direction for a reversible process. In either case the Faradaic current flow (resulting from electrochemical oxidation or reduction) can be readily measured. However, mass transport of the species to and from the electrode is a complicating feature that requires control, e.g. by forced convection of the solution (hydrodynamic control), if current flow is to be reproducible.

In the initial assessment of an electrochemical reaction the current response to a range of potentials can be measured and a voltammogram (or hydrodynamic voltammogram if

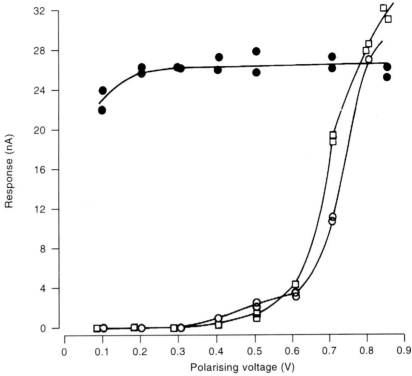

Figure 1 Effect of varying polarising voltage (against Ag/AgCl) on current responses to various phenolic species: (●) 4-aminophenol; (○) phenol; (□) phenolphthalein; all 0.01 M solutions in stirred AMP buffer at pH 10.4.

performed in the presence of a constantly stirred solution) constructed by plotting current against voltage (Figure 1). Voltammograms can be simply regarded as the electrochemical equivalent of the spectrum obtained in spectroscopy. They comprise a region of anodic current where R is oxidised to O and a region of cathodic current where O is reduced to R. Limiting values occur for both currents when the species is reacting at a maximum rate at the electrode surface with mass transport to the electrode limiting any increase in reaction rate at higher voltages.

An example of a simple electrochemical cell which can be used to monitor amperometric reactions is given in Figure 2. This cell consists of a 2 mm platinum working electrode with an outer 12 mm diameter silver-silver chloride ring pseudo-reference electrode which provides a relatively stable potential while acting as a sink for electron flow. It can be connected to a potentiostat which supplies a variable potential to the cell and allows sensitive measurement of the current derived from the electrochemical reactions (e.g. ~30 pA given a background noise of 10 pA). After processing, the current output can be directed either to a chart recorder or into the serial port of a computer.

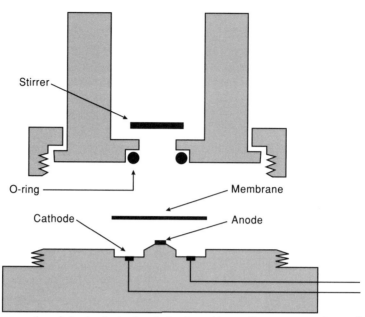

Figure 2 Cross-section of simple electrochemical cell used to monitor amperometric reactions.

Potentiometric Detection

This alternative technique relies on the measurement of the potential obtained when a species interacts at a sensor surface, either a membrane or an electrode, showing selective affinity for that species. An example of potentiometry is the ion-selective electrode as used in clinical chemistry laboratories. Binding of a charged species leads to an interfacial potential change that can be detected with negligible flow of current. Potentiometric detection thus offers the possibility of monitoring antigen-antibody reactions without the use of labels on the basis of a net electrical charge difference between a precoated antibody on the surface and the antigen-antibody complex. However, the swamping effects of nonspecific adsorption (mediated by electrostatic, hydrophobic and van der Waals interactions) generate a response that has usually precluded analysis in all but the simplest aqueous solution. A more promising approach has been the monitoring of an enzyme-catalysed reaction with potentiometric devices. However, the response obtained from a potentiometric device is logarithmically related to the concentration of measured species, and detection limits are poor, so limiting the dynamic range of measurement of potentiometric labels.

The advent of the solid-state ion selective field-effect transistor (ISFET) (Figure 3) has stimulated further research into potentiometric detection of antigen, e.g. via enzyme-catalysed reactions. In a basic field-effect transistor (FET) an interfacial charge over a p– (or n) type silicon substrate can modulate current flow between source and drain. The result is the conversion of a high-input impedance signal to one of low impedance with less likelihood of electrical noise. With an ion-sensing membrane incorporated in the gate area of the FET, membrane interaction with the ions in solution leads to a change in the charge field in the membrane, again altering the source/drain current. The current can be kept constant by adjusting the voltage drop. A common mode used to determine the response of the device is to measure the voltage adjustment required to normalise the current to a baseline value. These devices can be

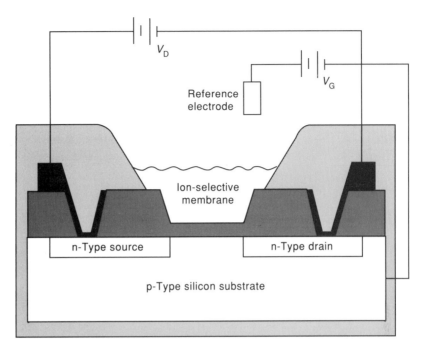

Figure 3 Ion-selective field-effect transistor (ISFET).

used in the detection of enzyme labels where an ionic species (i.e. H^+ ion) is generated or consumed. However, the need for control over sample pH and buffer capacity poses significant problems for practical substrate monitoring. Additionally, problems with stability and encapsulation of the microfabricated structure still need to be resolved before these devices achieve widespread practical usage. However, the use of microelectronic solid-state structures means that the actual sensing area can be very small and, with the added advantage of simple mass-production techniques, it is probable that this approach will become accepted in the development of enzyme-based immunoassays.

An alternative approach that avoids some of the encapsulation problems associated with ISFETS is the light-addressable potentiometric sensor (LAPS) for pH. The sensing surface of this device is an H^+ sensitive silicon nitride layer. An appropriate bias potential is applied to a silicon plate, which has its surface nitride layer exposed to solution (Figure 4). Illumination of this surface by means of a (modulated) light-emitting diode causes a current to flow, the amplitude of which is a function of the pH of the solution (Hafeman *et al.*, 1988). This device can be used as a detector in an immunoassay when combined with an enzyme label catalysing, for example a hydrolase reaction.

Conductimetric Detection

Ionic conductivity detectors can measure ionic solutes, without causing their degradation, in media of low background conductivity. The detection technique has a wide linear dynamic range (up to 6 orders of magnitude), a universal response to ionic species and, with micromachined devices, can perform measurements in small volumes of sample (0.5 μl). The de-

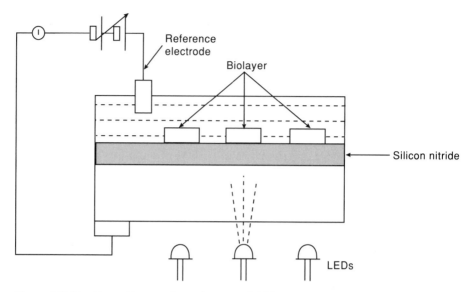

Figure 4 Light-addressable potentiometric sensor (LAPS) (from Hafeman *et al.*, 1988).

tector cell consists of two electrodes, usually made of platinum, to which is applied a constant alternating potential. The resulting frequency domain current is readily monitored and gives a measure of solution conductivity. The general principles underlying conductivity-based measurement of enzymatic reactions have been well established (Laurence, 1971) and a broad range of enzymes can now be measured with this technique. Although conductimetry itself cannot select for a particular ion, substrate selectivity is obtained through the specific nature of the enzyme reaction.

LABELS FOR ELECTROCHEMICAL IMMUNOASSAY

Electrochemistry as a detection system in immunoassay can be subdivided into three general areas:

1   Use of enzymes as amplification labels with the enzyme monitored by measurement of electroactive product/substrate.

2   Use of electroactive compounds as labels.

3   Techniques that do not use labels; direct monitoring of the antigen-antibody reaction without any label requirement.

A range of labels and enzyme-label reaction products that have been determined by electrochemical detection in immunoassays is surveyed in Table 1.

Measurement	Detection mode	Detection limit (M)	Reference
Electrochemically active labels			
Indium	DPASV	7.5×10^{-10}	Hayes *et al.*, 1994
Bismuth	DPASV	8.5×10^{-10}	Hayes *et al.*, 1994
Enzyme-labels			
Alkaline phosphatase	Square-wave voltammetry	2.8×10^{-14}	La Gal La Salle *et al.*, 1995
Alkaline phosphatase	FIA–EC	3.6×10^{-13}	Thompson *et al.*, 1991
Enzyme-label reaction product			
Phenol	LC–EC	0.4×10^{-12}	Tang *et al.*, 1988
4-Aminophenol	FIA–EC	7×10^{-9}	Thompson *et al.*, 1991
4-Aminophenol	FIA–EC	2.4×10^{-8}	Xu *et al.*, 1989
4-Aminophenol	LC–EC	0.2×10^{-12}	Tang *et al.*, 1988
NADH	FIA–EC	1×10^{-7}	Wehmayer *et al.*, 1983

Table 1 Comparison of electrochemically active labels and enzyme-labels used in immunoassays with electrochemical detection.

Enzyme Immunoassay with Electrochemical Detection

There have been problems in obtaining sufficient sensitivity in the detection with simple instrumentation of direct electrochemical labels. Thus, the majority of electrochemical immunoassay development has focused on the measurement of enzyme-labels by detection of electroactive products arising from enzyme catalysed reactions. Such assays have been developed using a diversity of enzyme-labels including catalase, glucose oxidase, glucose-6-phosphate dehydrogenase and alkaline phosphatase (Heineman and Halsall, 1985). Because of the inherent signal amplification obtained when using enzymes, much simpler instrumentation can be used and background effects are more readily overcome. Alkaline phosphatase has been frequently used because its broad substrate specificity and high turnover number ensure large signal amplification. Early work used the substrate phenyl phosphate which liberates electroactive phenol following enzymatic hydrolysis (Wehmeyer *et al.*, 1983; Doyle *et al.*, 1984). However, electrochemical oxidation of phenol requires relatively high polarising voltages (~ +800 mV against Ag/AgCl) (Tang *et al.*, 1988). Moreover, loss of electrode performance has been noted owing to polymerisation of phenolic radicals formed on the electrode surface during the oxidation process (Tang *et al.*, 1988). Alternative phenolic substrates have therefore been specifically synthesised to reduce the required polarising voltage and avoid electrode fouling (McNeil *et al.*, 1988; Tang *et al.*, 1988; Frew *et al.*, 1989; Christie *et al.*, 1992). Of these, 4-aminophenyl phosphate appears to be highly suitable because the reaction product, 4-aminophenol, oxidises readily at <+200 mV (against Ag/AgCl) without fouling of the electrode surface (Tang *et al.*, 1988) (Figure 5). At these low potentials, the level of background interference is also much reduced.

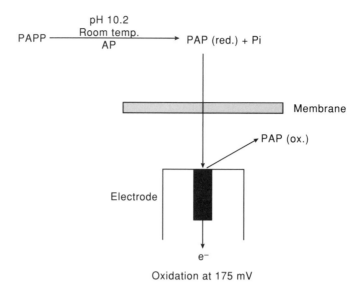

Figure 5 Reaction scheme for the electrochemical detection of alkaline phosphatase (AP). PAPP, 4-Aminophenol phosphate; PAP, 4-aminophenol.

A variety of instrumentation has been used in the electrochemical detection of enzymes. Earlier studies used liquid-chromatographic separation of the reaction product and the use of flow-injection systems (Heineman and Halsall, 1985; Jenkins *et al.*, 1991). Enzyme products have also been determined using simpler nonflow instrumentation. Here, glassy carbon has been used as an indicator electrode in a three-electrode cell (Cardosi *et al.*, 1989). Elsewhere, a screen-printed two-electrode cell for single use has also been used, incorporating a carbon-based working electrode (Frew *et al.*, 1989). We have found that a simple two-electrode device (Figure 2) can readily allow the kinetic determination of alkaline phosphatase using 4-aminophenyl phosphate as the enzyme substrate (Treloar *et al.*, 1994). By using a kinetic approach and measuring response slopes, reduced measurement times were achieved. Also the use of a membrane mounted over the polarised electrode allowed the enzyme reaction to be monitored without reduction of the response due to electrode surface fouling by enzyme protein.

NAD(P)$^+$-dependent dehydrogenases, particularly glucose-6-phosphate dehydrogenase (G6PDH), have been specifically targeted in immunoassay development; however, their exploitation in the development both of amperometric enzyme electrodes and in immunoassays remains rather rudimentary. This is despite the possibility of developing simplified (homogeneous) immunoassays by using a dehydrogenase eliminating the need to separate free from bound label (Eggers *et al.*, 1982). The neglect, in part, reflects the difficulty of the direct electrochemical measurement of NAD(P)H. Not only is a high overvoltage required for the electrode oxidation reaction (+0.75 V against Ag/AgCl), but passivation of the electrode surface occurs following adsorption of the oxidised cofactor (Eggers *et al.*, 1982). The net practical consequence is an obligatory pretreatment and conditioning of electrodes between measurements for reproducible detection and also a laborious sample pretreatment step.

To overcome some of these problems, redox mediators have been used to diminish the required overpotential and eliminate electrode fouling. Quinones (Jaegfeldt *et al.*, 1981), ferrocenes (Matsue *et al.*, 1991) and phenoxazine (Bremle *et al.*, 1991) mediators have been inves-

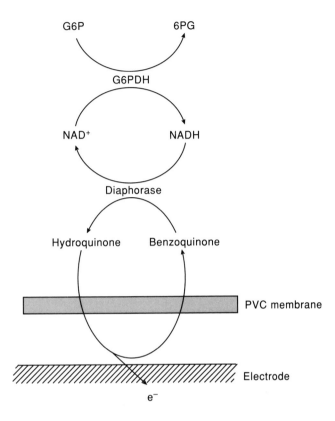

Figure 6 Reaction scheme for the electrochemical detection of glucose-6-phosphate dehydrogenase (G6PDH). G6P, Glucose-6-phosphate; 6PG, 6-phosphogluconate (from Treloar *et al.*, 1995).

tigated, all of which may facilitate the flow of electrons from cofactor to electrode at reduced operating voltages. It is possible to immobilise mediators, e.g. by simple adsorption to an electrode surface (Jaegfeldt *et al.*, 1981). They have also been covalently attached (Ueda *et al.*, 1982), entrapped in a polymeric support (Matsue *et al.*, 1991) and incorporated into the bulk of the electrode material (Bremle *et al.*, 1991). A further refinement possible in some cases is augmentation of the redox mediator reaction by inclusion of diaphorase (Miki *et al.*, 1989). We have recently described a system for the detection of G6PDH using diaphorase and 1, 4 benzoquinone as the redox mediator (Treloar *et al.*, 1995) (Figure 6). By covering the electrode with a highly lipophilic specially plasticised PVC membrane, responses to major ionic and polar interferents found in serum samples could be virtually eliminated. The lack of an interferent signal makes the system eminently suitable for use in detecting G6PDH in homogeneous immunoassay where the presence of a high background signal either with electrochemistry or with conventional spectrophotometric detection has precluded high-sensitivity assay development.

Glucose oxidase has also been exploited in immunoassay development. The enzyme catalyses the conversion of glucose to gluconic acid with reduction of oxygen to hydrogen peroxide:

$$\text{Glucose} + H_2O + O_2 \xrightarrow{\text{glucose oxidase}} \text{gluconic acid} + H_2O_2$$

In principle either the consumption of oxygen or the liberation of hydrogen peroxide can be monitored. Because of the high background, which is due to the intrinsic presence of oxygen in biological fluids, H_2O_2 detection has been most usually proposed, giving a low background current and resulting in more sensitive measurement, at least for glucose sensors.

A number of electrochemical detection strategies for glucose oxidase have now been described in which oxygen has been replaced by an alternative electron acceptor. The rationale for this strategy is that faster reaction rates can be obtained, the oxidation potential is lower and the detection system is less sensitive to the levels of oxygen in a sample. Examples of mediators that have been used include ferrocene (and its derivatives) and 1,4-benzoquinone (Cass *et al.*, 1984; Robinson *et al.*, 1986, 1988; Weetall and Hotaling, 1988). The reaction sequence for mediation using a ferrocenium derivative is shown below:

$$\text{Glucose} + 2FeCp_2R^+ \xrightarrow{\text{glucose oxidase}} \text{gluconic acid} + 2FeCp_2R$$

As the $FeCp_2R$ is formed in the enzymic reaction, it is reoxidised at the electrode surface to give $FeCp_2R^+$. However, these reagents have a number of disadvantages. The most important is that the polarising potentials required for oxidation (100–400 mV against Ag/Ag) are still too high and common compounds in biological fluids, e.g. ascorbic acid and uric acid, interfere with measurement by contributing to the response.

A number of approaches have been made in the electrochemical detection of peroxidase. The general reaction scheme for peroxidase detection is:

$$H_2O_2 + O_2 \text{ acceptor} + 2H^+ \xrightarrow{\text{peroxidase}} 2H_2O + \text{product}$$

Detectable oxygen acceptors that have been used in the reaction include hydroquinone, 1,2-phenylenediamine and pyrocatechol (Deasy *et al.*, 1994; Kalab and Skladal, 1995). In addition, direct electron transfer between the oxidised active-site of horseradish peroxidase and an activated carbon electrode has recently been used for immunoassay (McNeil *et al.*, 1995). One of the major problems in the sensitive electrochemical detection of peroxidase is the electroactivity of hydrogen peroxide itself and careful choice of operational potential is required to minimise background effects. This has resulted in limited use of this enzyme in electrochemical immunoassay development even though it is one of the most widely used labels in spectrophotometric enzyme immunoassay.

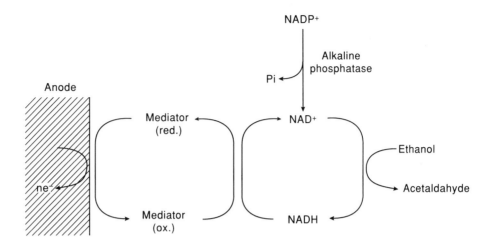

Figure 7 General reaction sheme for the electrochemical detection of alkaline phosphatase using a redox amplification step.

Amplification, using a product-cycling step, is a method for increasing the apparent activity of a given enzyme label and thereby potentially the speed and sensitivity of an enzyme immunoassay. Amplified systems for the electrochemical measurement of alkaline phosphatase have been described (Stanley *et al.*, 1987; McNeil and Spoors, 1988; Bates, 1989). An example of a general reaction scheme that can be used is given in (Figure 7).

Electroactive Compounds as Immunoassay Labels

For use as an immunoassay label, an electrochemically active compound has to possess suitable electrochemical properties, be stable in solution over a wide pH range and should be soluble in aqueous media. It is also desirable that the substance is naturally absent from biological fluids. Furthermore, it must allow highly selective electrochemical detection or possess chemical properties allowing selective membranes to be used at the measurement electrode.

Relatively little work has explored the use of directly electrochemically active labels in immunoassay, despite the availability of powerful differential pulse voltammetric techniques capable of high sensitivity. Pulse voltammetry, like time-resolved fluorometry, uses a delayed measurement after activation such that the desired signal can be separated from background effects. The potential is applied for 50 milliseconds and the resulting current is measured in the last few milliseconds of the pulse. This procedure allows the background current to decay before measurement of the signal due to the electroactive species, allowing concentrations as low as 10^{-8} mol l^{-1} to be determined. Typically, a dropping-mercury electrode is used where mercury is the polarised (working) electrode that provides a renewable electrode surface. Although this is likely to be an impractical detector for immunoassays in routine use, forms of pulse voltammetry can be performed using more practical solid electrodes and flow-through mercury electrode cells are becoming available. Differential pulse anode-stripping voltammetry (DPASV) has been used to measure metal ions and gives high sensitivity with detection limits as low as 10^{-10} mol l^{-1} (Doyle *et al.*, 1982). Commonly used ions include In^{3+},

Co^{2+} and Zn^{2+}, which can be coupled to proteins using chelating agents and released after the immunological reaction to enable detection (Doyle *et al.*, 1982). Detection involves a two-step process; the metal ion is first reduced to its metallic state by a constant negative potential at a stable hanging mercury-drop electrode. The metal dissolves in the liquid mercury and a pulsed positive potential is then applied to the mercury drop, oxidising the dissolved metal and stripping it from the mercury electrode. The current produced during the stripping step can be directly related to the concentration of metal in the sample as this determines the rate of initial metal ion uptake into the electrode under reducing conditions.

An alternative form of pulse voltammetry is differential pulse polarography (DPP) where a train of small pulses (5–100 mV) is applied, superimposed on a linear potential ramp, immediately prior to the end of a mercury-drop lifetime at a dropping-mercury electrode. The current resulting from the oxidation of an electroactive species is sampled just before pulse application and just before the end of the pulse. By subtracting the two current measurements, background effects can be eliminated and a sensitive measurement of the current due to the electroactive species obtained. Using this technique, Wehmeyer *et al.* (1982) developed an immunoassay for oestriol using a dinitro functional group as the electroactive label. When a solution of labelled oestriol was titrated with oestriol antibody the resulting polarograms showed a decrease in peak current on binding of antibody to labelled antigen which was then reversed by the addition of oestriol to the solution. The peak current attenuation was thought to be due to a restriction of access of the nitro group to the electrode surface following binding of the labelled antigen to antibody. Problems were encountered when the technique was applied to human serum samples as a large reduction of the response to the labelled antigen resulted, possibly the result of electrode poisoning, which made the assay unsuitable for use in this matrix.

It would obviously be advantageous if simple electrochemical techniques were developed that properly exploit the fundamental analytical convenience of electrochemistry. Direct, reliable detection of an electroactive label remains an important goal that would facilitate immunoassay development. Weber and Purdy (1979) used a ferrocene label with amperometric detection at a carbon electrode by flow-injection analysis in the development of an assay for morphine. The label could be detected at low polarising voltages and would have been subject to less interferent effects; however, no attempt was made to perform the reaction in a biological matrix. Furthermore the ferrocene label was photosensitive and needed to be shielded from light prior to measurement. Recently we have shown that fluorescein, in addition to its use as a fluorescent label, can be used as an electroactive label in an immunoassay (Treloar, 1993). With a competitive immunoassay format, superimposable standard curves for the assay of ephedrine were obtained using electrochemical and fluorescent detection, respectively. To obtain sensitive electrochemical measurement of the ephedrine fluorescein label in this study, a liquid-chromatographic separation had to be coupled with detection at a large surface area graphite electrode commonly used for electrochemical detection in high-performance liquid chromatography (HPLC). If the detection system were simplified the above approach would be especially advantageous because fluorescein conjugates of antigens and antibodies are readily available. Furthermore the fluorescent behaviour of the conjugates could be used for optimisation of an immunoassay prior to testing of an electrochemical detection system.

Ferrocyanide is readily detected as a redox species in solution, but when encapsulated within liposomes it serves as the basis for an amplified, direct electrochemical label assay. Kannuck *et al.* (1988) showed that complement lysis released ferrocyanide from liposomes. If such a release could be activated at antigen-sensitised liposomes, a viable immunosensor might be possible.

Techniques without Label

This concept was proposed in the early 1970s by Janata (1975) to measure polysaccharide, albeit with concanavalin A as a bioaffinity layer to confer specificity rather than an antibody. Concanavalin A was coupled to the surface of a PVC membrane coated on a platinum wire and the change in electrode potential on exposure of the sensor to polysaccharide was measured. A fundamental problem of specificity was found with this sensor in that although membrane potential change was demonstrated in the presence of polysaccharide this was also observed in background electrolyte.

An immunosensor measuring the binding of human chorionic gonadotrophin (hCG) to anti-hCG was developed by Yamamoto *et al.* (1978) which involved the immobilisation of antibody on the surface of a titanium wire electrode. A change in electrode potential was found on exposure of this sensor to the antigen. Unfortunately, sensitivity was limited as only small changes in potential were observed; furthermore the specificity of the system was not investigated. A variety of innovative methods have also been more recently explored exploiting amperometric and conductimetric detection. These will be discussed later in this chapter.

SPECIFIC IMMUNOASSAY SYSTEMS

Enzyme Label Immunoassays

Flow Analysis

One attractive approach to the development of an electrochemical immunoassay is simply to exploit a conventional immunoassay protocol, replacing the enzyme substrate with one designed to yield an electrochemically active product; this allows ready substitution of conventional (spectrophotometric) detectors with an electrode. In tandem with this strategy, frequently adopted over the past 15 years, has been the use of flow-through electrochemical (EC) detectors in flow-injection analysis (FIA) or liquid chromatography (LC) (Heineman and Halsall, 1985). Although both techniques require instrumentation to control sample flow, stable background and sensitive detection are important advantages.

In a competitive immunoassay for phenytoin with a glucose-6-phosphate dehydrogenase label, LC–EC proved advantageous over FIA–EC (Wehmeyer *et al.*, 1983). With the former, low detection limits for the NADH product (1×10^{-7} mol l^{-1}) were achieved by the separation of the NADH peak from the currents associated with the sample matrix. This was effected by column retention of NADH producing a 30 s separation. In addition, a 121-fold dilution of the assay mixture prior to injection together with the use of a C-18 reversed-phase column prevented gradual fouling of the electrode surface by protein adsorption. Thus, 80–100 injections were made before column regeneration was required. In a similar LC–EC immunoassay, but using a column switching technique, less dilution of the immunoassay solution was required (Wright *et al.*, 1986). The NADH zone was 'heart-cut' from the chromatographic profile to avoid earlier eluting macromolecular passivators and later eluting electrochemically active interferents (e.g. uric acid). Liquid chromatography thus increases detection sensitivity and enables homogeneous immunoassay without interference by exploiting chromatographic separation of the indicator species. A number of drawbacks also result: notably a complex high-pressure system is required, and sample throughput inevitably is limited by retained signal peaks.

By contrast, FIA–EC is a low-pressure method without chromatographic separation and hence simpler with a more rapid throughput. Detection sensitivity is compromised because of the current spike produced after sample injection, a consequence of the mobile phase changing in composition because of the sample matrix. This non-Faradaic current spike is potential dependent, cannot be resolved from the analytical signal peak and occurs because of disruption of the capacitance at the electrode surface. Electrode operation at low bias potentials enables sensitivity to be significantly increased, facilitating wider use of FIA–EC in place of LC–EC.

A flow system can deliver reagents to an immobilised antibody as well as delivering the indicator species to the detector electrode. Boitieux *et al.* (1989) demonstrated a two-site sandwich immunoassay for α-fetoprotein (AFP). Here, the polypropylene membrane of a flow-through oxygen electrode was modified with the enzyme inhibitor *p*-aminophenylthio-β-D-galactopyranoside. First, antibody labelled with β-D-galactosidase was incubated with AFP and catalase-labelled antibody in a noncompetitive format. On subsequent introduction of the mixture to the flow cell, the β-D-galactosidase label bound to the electrode membrane so immobilising the two-site immunocomplex on the electrode surface. Contact with a mobile phase containing 40 mmol l^{-1} H_2O_2 resulted in production of O_2 by the second catalase label which was readily determined at the electrode. The measured signal was directly proportional to AFP concentration and the assay developed had a detection limit of ~0.5 µg l^{-1} AFP, inter-assay coefficient of variation (CV) of 2% and measurement time of 10 min. An important feature was the ability to regenerate the immunosensor surface by exposure to 0.1 mol l^{-1} borate buffer (pH 10) for 2 min, which released 99.2% of bound immunocomplex, enabling at least 30 measurements with the same membrane. Palmer *et al.* (1992) used an analogous approach where protein A immobilised onto controlled pore glass (CPG) upstream of the electrode was exploited. In the immunoassay, alkaline phosphatase-labelled drug (theophylline) and drug standard, mixed with antibody, were injected onto the immunoreactor. Antibody-complexed label bound to the CPG column, was separated from unbound, and substrate was then introduced via a second injection valve into the mobile phase with a 4-aminophenol product detected downstream at an amperometric (wall-jet) electrode. Despite the short exposure time of the reaction mixture within the immunoreactor (20 s), the assay had a detection limit of less than 25 µg l^{-1}, and gave a total assay time of 18 min. No separation step was required, and regeneration of the reactor with citric acid allowed up to 100 runs to be made before replacement.

By combining electrochemical immunoassay with a flow system, higher sensitivity and greater versatility is possible with some control over the need for conventional separation steps. Such systems could certainly be developed into laboratory assays, but further reduction in assay time and instrument complexity is probably needed for electrochemical immunoassay systems to compete with the latest generation of optical analysers. Although FIA is probably preferable to LC, even here relatively cumbersome instrumentation is involved.

Nonflow Analysis

Avoidance of flow has the advantage that it reduces instrumentation requirements. In particular, simple kinetic detection of an enzyme-label becomes possible. Electrochemical kinetic detection in alkaline phosphatase-label immunoassays has been demonstrated for thyroxine-binding globulin (TBG) and cortisol using noncompetitive and competitive hetero-geneous assay formats, respectively (Treloar *et al.*, 1994). Here, by following the current in-crease with time, alkaline phosphatase-label activity could be determined within 2 min and a predetection incubation step was avoided. Dose-response curves covered the relevant clinical ranges for TBG (31–1,000 μg l^{-1}) and cortisol (100–2,000 nmol l^{-1}), respectively. An important requirement was the use of a Cuprophan® (as used in haemodialysis membranes) or microporous polycarbonate membrane covering over the electrode to prevent fouling due to particulate solid phases. This form of solid phase is especially attractive for enhancing reac-tion kinetics, and electrochemical detection is not affected by the turbidity of the sample.

As well as preventing fouling of electrode surfaces, membranes may be exploited to en-hance detection selectivity and sensitivity. In one recent study (La Gal La Salle *et al.*, 1995), a glassy carbon electrode was modified with a polyanionic perfluorosulphonated Nafion poly-mer, and homogeneous, and heterogeneous immunoassay investigated for phenytoin using an alkaline phosphatase-label and the substrate 6-(*N*-ferrocenoylamino)-2,4-dimethylphenyl phosphate. This substrate was unusual in that both phosphate and phenol forms were elec-trochemically active, but only the phenolic product could pass through the Nafion film be-cause of the charge repulsion of the di-anionic phosphate. Normally, a reduction in detection sensitivity would be anticipated on interposing such a barrier membrane, particularly if the membrane has a high selectivity (Christie *et al.*, 1992). However, with Nafion, preconcentra-tion of product in the membrane phase can actually amplify response (La Gal La Salle *et al.*, 1995). Homogeneous immunoassay was possible here because of inhibition of enzyme activity after antibody binding. In serum, however, responses were attenuated, probably because of nonspecific interaction of the enzyme product with serum proteins and possibly some inhibi-tion of enzyme activity. With a separation step and serum matrix removed, a viable assay was obtained.

Membrane modification of electrodes under nonflow can enhance label detection and sim-plify assay protocols. However, in a conventional heterogeneous immunoassay, a separation is still necessary. The procedure has been simplified using a magnetic electrode (Robinson *et al.*, 1985). In a two-site model immunoassay for hCG, Robinson *et al.* used capture antibody coupled to a magnetic particulate solid phase. Urine samples containing hCG were incubated with glucose oxidase-labelled antibody and a fluorescein isothiocyanate (FITC)-labelled capture antibody. An anti-FITC magnetic particle suspension was added, then substrate solu-tion and mediator added. When the working electrode was placed in the cell, antibody-bound label was readily separated by drawing of the magnetic immunocomplex onto the electrode. The immunoassay gave a sensitivity of 150 U l^{-1} hCG and had a total assay time of 20 min.

Ultrasensitive Immunoassays

Heterogeneous immunoassays overcome problems of background interference by enabling antibody-bound label to be transferred into an interferent-free media. For electrochemical immunoassay, this is a special advantage because it is inherently a less selective technique. Furthermore, the levels of redox-active interferents (ascorbate, urate and cysteine) are con-siderably higher than those of the species likely to be measured. By combining a separation with a high label activity, a powerful strategy is created that can enhance immunoassay sensi-tivity.

One approach has been to amplify the levels using a substrate-recycling scheme (Figure 7). Thus, in the development of an immunoassay for prostatic acid phosphatase (PAP), Cardosi *et al.* (1989) used an alkaline phosphatase-label to convert $NADP^+$ to NAD^+ which in turn was catalytically cycled using alcohol dehydrogenase and diaphorase. In this case, the ferrocyanide product of the diaphorase reaction was determined at $+650$ mV (against Ag/AgCl) using a glassy carbon working electrode and measuring the amount of charge passed over 12 s. Some protein fouling of the electrode surface was possible and a degree of inhibition of the electrode reaction was noted, but this was not a serious drawback. The levels of PAP assayed were $0.3-100$ µg l^{-1}, which is a better dynamic range than commercially available spectrophotometric immunoassays can achieve. This reflects the problem of making absorbance measurement over a wide dynamic range with sufficient accuracy and precision.

In keeping with heterogeneous immunoassay design (irrespective of the detection system used) the efficiency of separation of bound from free label is critical when attempting to optimise immunoassay sensitivity, particularly with noncompetitive assays where nonspecific binding reduces assay sensitivity. Jenkins *et al.* (1988) optimised a two-site alkaline phosphatase-label immunoassay for mouse IgG using LC–EC and found that merely enhancing label activity increased the zero antigen response with no reduction in detection limit. Decreased background response with increasing primary antibody density suggested that hydrophobic (and possibly electrostatic) interaction of the protein conjugate with the underlying polystyrene solid phase was probably responsible. Tween 20 and bovine serum albumin (BSA) in the rinsing solution prior to measurement of enzyme activity allowed reduction in nonspecific adsorption of the enzyme conjugate by 96%. Consequently the immunoassay detection limit was lowered from 100 to 7.5 ng l^{-1} IgG, with extension of the working range by more than one order of magnitude. The detection limit for mouse IgG was subsequently lowered to 0.81 ng l^{-1} and a calibration curve linear over six orders of magnitude was produced (Xu *et al.*, 1989) by substituting phenyl phosphate with 4-aminophenyl phosphate as an enzyme substrate. This enabled electrode potential to be lowered from $+895$ to $+300$ mV (against Ag/AgCl) and, by using the same buffer for substrate incubation and mobile phase, the result was a significantly reduced interferent current spike due to the sample matrix.

Augmenting antigen-antibody binding kinetics has value in shortening assay time. A particulate solid phase can achieve this (Treloar *et al.*, 1994); however, an interesting alternative has been the use of a capillary-tube reaction vessel (Halsall and Heineman, 1990). This reduced the diffusional path-length to the capillary wall which supported the antibody. However, a special requirement emerges; that of minimising nonspecific binding, because the surface-to-volume ratio is considerably higher than in a conventional vessel. In addition, it was necessary to use Tween 20 and BSA blocking agents as well as the ion-pairing reagent pentane sulphone to block underivatised amino groups on the inner capillary surface. Assay time was 30 minutes where the phenol generated by alkaline phosphatase was determined by LC–EC. The detection limit was 5.6×10^{-20} moles IgG in serum and a linear range over four orders of magnitude was obtained with the potential for further enhancement by replacing the substrate phenyl phosphate with 4-aminophenyl phosphate.

In the pursuit of ever lower detection limits, ultrasensitive immunoassay here as elsewhere depends critically upon antibodies with high binding affinity/specificity and skilful design of all aspects of the assay, including reduction of nonspecific binding. Although enzyme recycling systems may enhance label activity, significant attention must be given to the differing solution requirements of the multiple enzymes used in such a system (e.g. pH and ionic strength).

Simplified Immunoassays

The complexity of conventional immunoassay protocols can have an impact on laboratory analysis and in the time taken to generate results. It also poses a significant hurdle to development of immunoassays outside the laboratory. Homogeneous immunoassays overcome this drawback to some extent in that they avoid separation steps. The most common approaches to this use an enzyme-labelled hapten where activity is modulated by antibody binding. Although this simplifies the assay protocol, it is far more demanding of the electrochemical detection system, as enzyme activity must now be determined in the sample matrix. Certainly interference due to coloured, turbid samples is not an issue, but the redox-active compounds produce major spurious and variable electrode currents. More subtly, some low molecular mass species of undefined nature in plasma and blood (Desai *et al.*, 1993) may passivate the electrode surface and greatly attenuate response.

Glucose-6-phosphate dehydrogenase-label monitored by measurement of the reduced co-factor NADH has been widely exploited for homogeneous immunoassay. For electrochemical detection, signal attenuation caused by electrode fouling (both due to oxidation of NADH and protein adsorption) along with potential interference from electrochemically active species in serum had to be addressed (Wehmeyer *et al.*, 1983; Wright *et al.*, 1986).

Homogeneous immunoassay for theophylline in haemolysed, lipaemic and icteric sera, with G6PDH-label, normally difficult by spectrophotometric methods, has been demonstrated using FIA–EC (Yao *et al.*, 1993). Furthermore, a number of homogeneous immunoassays have now been reported for direct analysis of whole blood (Athey *et al.*, 1993; Yao *et al.*, 1995). One approach has been to exploit a platinised activated-carbon electrode, prepared by adsorption of colloidal platinum to large surface area carbon, to enable oxidation of NADH at low potentials (+150 mV against Ag/AgCl) (Athey *et al.*, 1993). The electrode surface was nominally protected from fouling (due to surface active components in solution) by a 0.05-μm pore-size polycarbonate membrane. After initiation of the immunoreaction, the current was recorded for 16 minutes, and enzyme activity determined from currents at 12 and 16 minutes, respectively; subtraction of a reagent blank proved necessary. The dose-response curve for theophylline covered the therapeutic range (10–20 mg l^{-1}) and gave good correlation (y = 0.9x – 1.01, r = 0.98, n = 12) between blood and plasma theophylline concentrations measured by amperometric and spectrophotometric immunoassay, respectively. The rate method avoids interference from redox-active components, but the apparent electrode stability is remarkable given its exposure to a final 1/20 dilution of whole blood. Possibly the protecting membrane afforded an adequate barrier, and electrode pretreatment with NAD$^+$ and BSA possibly reduced further electrode changes in the assay. A dehydrogenase-label immunoassay of whole blood samples has also used FIA–EC with the electron transfer coupling reagent 2,6-dichloroindophenol, DCIP) (Yao *et al.*, 1995). Detection of reduced DCIP following reaction with NADH avoids the high overpotentials and electrode fouling problems generally associated with direct electrochemical oxidation of the cofactor. Here endogenous interferents were also inhibited by *p*-hydroxymercuribenzoate.

To maintain electrode stability totally and to avoid sample manipulation steps a major approach has been to shield the electrode surface with a highly permselective, biocompatible membrane (Christie *et al.*, 1992). The membrane is tailored to allow high flux of the chosen indicator while potential fouling agents (e.g. proteins, cells or colloids) and interferents are prevented from contacting the electrode surface and so do not directly affect electrochemical detection (Treloar *et al.*, 1995). A modification of this detection system like that in Figure 6 has been used in the immunoassay of phenytoin. The redox indicator benzoquinone was replaced with naphthoquinone and its intrinsic high reaction rate with NADH avoided the requirement for diaphorase. Calibration covered the required clinical range for phenytoin (3.9–7.2×10^{-5} mol l^{-1}) in plasma samples. The potential for a dry-reagent immunoassay for undiluted whole blood measurement has been demonstrated, as this plasticised PVC-coated electrode shows practically no direct response to whole blood (<10 pA) even at 650 mV against Ag/AgCl, and no diminution in sensitivity even after 2 hours continuous exposure (response to 10 μmol l^{-1} hydroquinone constant at 17 nA). In a further step, glucose-6-phosphate dehydrogenase was stabilised using a polyelectrolyte/sugar system, impregnated into a cellulose matrix and dried. This was incorporated into a multilayer cellulose matrix containing requisite substrate, cofactor and redox indicator (Knowles, 1994). When this dry reagent electrode was exposed to aqueous solution, a calibration was produced for G6PDH which was linear to 600 U l^{-1}. This should form the basis of a future complete dry-reagent homogeneous immunoassay.

In a departure from the use of NADH-dependent dehydrogenase enzymes, Robinson *et al.* (1988) developed a homogeneous immunoassay for hCG, using modulation of glucose oxidase activity. This is distinct from other homogeneous immunoassays, which are used only to determine low molecular mass analytes, because a close interaction is required between antibody and enzyme-label to elicit a change in catalytic activity. Thus, anti-hCG was coimmobilised with glucose oxidase on a glassy carbon electrode. Binding of hCG to the antibody masked and modulated the activity of surface-immobilised glucose oxidase, determined using ferrocene. A sensitivity limit of 7 IU l^{-1} hCG was obtained in serum and the immunosensor could be reactivated by soaking in 50% ethylene glycol.

More recently, Suzawa *et al.* (1994) have used ferrocene-derivatised glucose oxidase to develop a homogeneous immunoassay for digoxin. Ferrocene carboxylic acid and digoxin were coupled to glucose oxidase to produce a labelled derivative of the drug. The oxidative glucose current of this labelled digoxin was proportional to the number of ferrocene molecules coupled to the glucose oxidase. In the presence or absence of anti-digoxin antibody, little change in enzyme activity was observed as determined by spectrophotometry. However, on repeating this experiment using cyclic voltammetry to detect enzyme activity by scanning from 0 to +0.5 V against Ag/AgCl, there was a difference between specific and nonspecific binding at the electrode. This suggested that electron transfer between labelled ferrocenes and the electrode was inhibited by specific antibody binding. The modulation observed in electrode current was relatively small and clearly requires enhancement, but gives an interesting future possibility for homogeneous immunoassay.

An elegant solution to the development of a homogeneous enzyme-immunoassay suitable for high molecular mass analytes has been demonstrated in an assay for hCG by Duan and Meyerhoff (1994). The innovative step here has been to use a gold-coated microporous nylon membrane to act both as an antibody solid phase and as a working electrode. Immobilisation of capture antibody involved producing a self-assembled monolayer of thioctic acid on the gold surface prior to covalent coupling of antibody. To enhance sensitivity, hCG and alkaline phosphatase-labelled anti-hCG antibodies were preincubated (30 minutes) in the presence of the electrode modified by the capture antibody. Unlike conventional sandwich immunoassays, a separation step was avoided by introducing the substrate 4-aminophenyl phosphate, through the inner side of the porous membrane. Thus, 4-aminophenol was detected immediately at the membrane-electrode (at +0.19 V against Ag/AgCl) because of the local accumulation of surface-complexed label and gave an overall response time of <1 minute. Most importantly, unbound label in bulk solution did not interfere with the response. A whole blood assay was demonstrated with a detection limit of 2.5 U l⁻¹ hCG, comparable to hetero-geneous immunoassays with multiple washing steps.

Electrochemical Label Immunoassays

If antigen is labelled with a functional group that is intrinsically electrochemically active, the need for substrate, cofactor, special incubation steps for an enzyme-label etc. may be avoided. A consequence of this, however, is the loss of biochemical (enzyme) signal amplification and hence increased demands on detection sensitivity. Early work demonstrated the utility of metal ion labels in the development of a competitive heterogeneous immunoassay for human serum albumin using indium ions (In^{3+}) which were released prior to detection (Doyle *et al.* 1982). More recently, there has been increasing interest in simultaneous multianalyte immunoassay (Ekins *et al.*, 1990). Two basic strategies here are (1) to use one labelling and detection system with an array of different spatially resolved detection zones (Ekins *et al.*, 1990) or (2) to use different labels in the same detection vessel which can be individually resolved to indicate specific analytes. Hayes *et al.* (1994) adopted the latter approach, using two different metal ion labels in a simultaneous dual-analyte immunoassay. Two model analytes human serum albumin (HSA) and (IgG), were targeted and bismuth and indium ion labels separately coupled to these proteins using the bifunctional chelating agent diethylenetriamine pentaacetic acid (DTPA). After performing competitive immunoassay, bound metal ions were released by acidification and detected by sensitive differential pulse anodic-stripping voltammetry (DPASV). To further enhance sensitivity, protein analytes were maximally derivatised with DPTA to maximise ion labelling (6 and 10 chelates per molecule for HSA and IgG, respectively). Calibration curves for HSA and IgG were generated and analysis for these proteins in serum samples correlated with results from nephelometry. Despite the sensitivity afforded using DPASV, the concentration of metal ions released into solution was close to the detection limits of the hanging mercury-drop electrode instrumentation. This increased imprecision, and the electrode potential used (−50 mV against Ag/AgCl), furthermore, required samples to be purged with argon to remove oxygen prior to analysis. Clearly, however, simultaneous detection of In^{3+} and Bi^{3+} is possible for dual-analyte immunoassay, and an increase in the number of analytes simultaneously detected is theoretically possible, e.g. by using additional metal ions such as gallium (Ga^{3+}) and thallium (Tl^{3+}).

Immunosensors without Labels

By far the simplest approach to electrochemical immunoassay is to exploit direct detection of antigen-antibody binding. Emons and Heineman (1990) adsorbed IgG on working electrodes and followed the effects of antibody on Faradaic reactions. Thus, they studied both reversible ($Fe(CN)_6^{3-}$–$Fe(CN)_6^{4-}$, hydroquinone-benzoquinone) and irreversible (phenol, NADH) reactions and found that IgG, in all cases, had some inhibitory effect. Interpretation was complex, but the main factors were related to mass transport, double layer and surface availability, as well as subtle reaction mechanism changes. IgG-coated electrodes could, apparently, be used for immunoassay, but any diminished sensitivity effect would depend on the redox system used and the electrode material. An interesting development is the work of Willner *et al.* (1994) who used dinitro-spiropyran antigen, to form a self-assembled antigen monolayer on an electrode surface, and a redox probe in solution to produce an amperometric response (Figure 8). Exposure of the electrode to dinitrophenyl antibody resulted in antibody binding

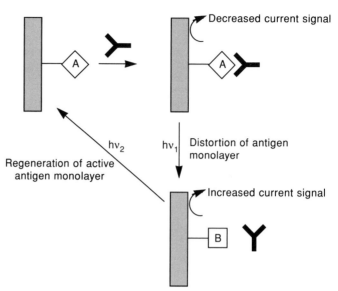

Figure 8 Detection strategy for an optically reversible electrochemical immunosensor (redrawn from Willner *et al.*, 1994).

to the monolayer which insulated the electrode towards the redox probe; hence electrode response was diminished. A particularly elegant strategy to enable sensor reuse used a photoisomerisable component in a self-assembled coated monolayer. Thus in one photoisomer state (A), antigen-antibody complex formation occurred and could be followed electrochemically through a change in electrode behaviour. However, antigen could be subsequently photoisomerised to an alternative state (B) which distorted the monolayer, reduced the antibody binding affinity and allowed antibody to be washed off. The monolayer was then regenerated by illumination at a second wavelength (hv_2).

Conductimetric detection systems are attracting increasing attention. An early approach involved using interdigitated copper electrodes coated with antigen (parylene) and the insulator silicon monoxide. A decrease in capacitance was observed when anti-parylene antibody was bound (Newman *et al.*, 1988); this was attributed to a dielectric constant change. Other work

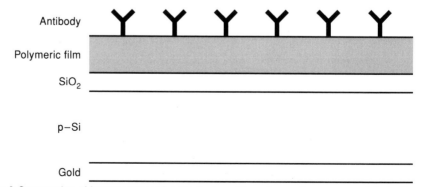

Figure 9 Construction of immunosensor for monitoring of impedance changes associated with antigen-antibody binding (redrawn from Souteyrand *et al.*, 1994).

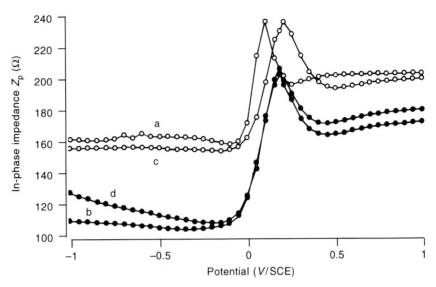

Figure 10 Modulation of in-phase impedance (Z_p) changes showing immunosensor response before exposure to antigen (a), after exposure to antigen (b), regeneration of sensor by rinsing in glycine buffer (c) and second exposure to antigen (d) (redrawn from Souteyrand *et al.*, 1994).

has shown that capacitance correlates with thickness of the dielectric layer (Bataillard *et al.*, 1988). Souteyrand *et al.* (1994) found that impedance changes provided a powerful tool in the fabrication of the immunosensor electrode. Here, deposition of heteropolysilsesquioxane polymer (Figure 9) facilitated antibody immobilisation and enhanced chemical continuity between the antibody layer and the Si/SiO$_2$ transducer. Impedance changes could be related to complexation of antigen with immobilised antibody and could be clearly discriminated from nonspecific adsorption. (Figure 10)

Sadik *et al.* (1994) used polypyrrole to immobilise antibody on an electrode surface. This conducting polymer was grown at the electrode surface from aqueous solution containing just the pyrrole monomer and antibody, incorporated as the counterion (anion) in the polymer structure. After exposure to thaumatin (antigen), cyclic voltammetry confirmed that no Faradaic current was produced upon immune complex formation. The immunoelectrode was then interrogated by AC voltammetry, and although this indicated antigen binding it was neither sensitive nor selective. FIA using a flow-through cell polarised at constant potential was subsequently used, although here broad tailing signals were found that were irreproducible, presumably due to the irreversible nature of the antigen-antibody reaction. Therefore pulsed potential waveforms were used, previously shown to be sensitive, reversible and rapid (Sadik and Wallace, 1993). Pulsing at negative potentials produced small signals, whereas signals increased with increasing positive voltage to a plateau at $> +0.6$ V at which point the polymer was overoxidised. A pulsed potential waveform ($E_1 = 0.00$ V, $E_2 = +0.4$ V against Ag/AgCl) was used that produced well defined (nontailing) reproducible responses, linear up to 120 parts per million (p.p.m.). A substantial finding was that pulsing control in the millisecond region enabled the interaction of antigen with the antibody-modified conducting polymer electrode to be made reversible, indicated by response reproducibility. Switching of applied potential is known to cause significant changes in the chemical properties of conducting polymers, even affecting antigen-antibody reactions (Wallace *et al.*, 1990). This electrochemical mode of inducing binding reversibility may simplify renewal of electrodes by comparison with chemical disruption of an immunocomplex. However, it is also likely to affect the sensitivity of the immunosensor by diminishing the binding affinity of the immobilised antibody; indeed major sensitivity differences were observed. Some interference was noted from simple anions, but responses were considerably lower than those to thaumatin antigen. Conductimetric immunosensors are at an early stage of development. They may ultimately allow measurement of antigen in real samples, and aside from this, could offer useful basic data to refine methods for antibody immobilisation.

Nikolelis *et al.* (1993) have achieved direct transduction of an immunological reaction using bilayer lipid membranes. Membranes were formed, using a monolayer folding technique, from dipalmitoyl phosphatidic acid and egg phosphatidyl choline with antibody to thyroxine incorporated. It was unlikely that the protein fully spanned the membrane to form a conductive pore, as transmembrane currents were transient. The antibody probably resided at the membrane-solution interface with Fab and Fc groups extending into the electrical double layer. With thyroxine antigen, responses were proportional to antigen concentration, but were not found in control experiments with nonselective protein. Currents were reproducible, had a duration of seconds and appeared to indicate some critical magnitude of surface charge leading to a transition in membrane structure. Current magnitude was consistent with capacitive charging events caused by ion concentration changes of the double layer. Responses were observed from 50 to 120 seconds; however, the current magnitudes (typically < 30 pA) demanded high-sensitivity detection equipment that needed to be isolated and grounded in a Faraday cage.

It has to be noted that the 'nonlabel' immunosensors described in this section were demonstrated by analysing simple solutions. It is likely that considerable work will be necessary to resolve responses due to specific antibody binding from those due to nonspecific surface interactions when sensors are exposed to biological sample matrices. A number of 'nonlabel' sensors based on evanescent wave optical detection have now been successfully developed; this required the minimising of nonspecific binding at the solution-sensor interface. It is possible that some of these strategies can be translated to electrochemical transducers alongside development of new biocompatible interfaces.

FUTURE DEVELOPMENTS

Electrode designs are increasing in their novelty and exploitation of technology. Niwa *et al.* (1993) investigated the use of an interdigitated array for detection of alkaline phosphatase via the product 4-aminophenol. This electrochemical cell had a number of interesting benefits including an ability to redox-cycle 4-aminophenol between the two finger sets of the electrode and hence amplify the signal magnitude. In addition, the sample volume was reduced to 800 nl and detection time to < 1 minute, increasing sample throughput. The electrode was fabricated from a silicon wafer using photolithography and dry-etching techniques. Further exploitation of silicon poses attractive possibilities for immunoassay development, particularly with the advance of silicon micromachining resulting in the development of micropumps liquidic circuits and microelectrode arrays (Van den Berg and Bergveld, 1995). With these building blocks, the development of micro-multianalyte immunoassays is conceivable.

It is clear that electrochemical detection offers certain 'niche' capabilities (identified in the introduction) and therefore has reasonable prospects of addressing future instrumentation requirements. Modification of electrode materials and exploitation of highly selective barrier membranes has already achieved high selectivity. Direct reliable performance in biological solutions is an inevitable next step, and commercialisation is likely to follow. Opportunities also exist for the development of ultrasensitive immunoassays, small volume immunoassays and simplified immunoassays. Commercial systems exploiting enzyme-based biosensor technology are now widely available (e.g. blood glucose analysers for use in or out of the laboratory) and provide some pointers to the way in which practical systems might emerge. The difficulty in interrogation of immune complex formation can be avoided with label signalling, and many of the basic fabrication designs have already been developed for enzyme electrodes. If one adds microfabrication methods that can optimise sample and reagent presentation, then the prospects are considerably enhanced. Once the sensing element can be made, the extremely simple current registering apparatus (potentiostat) for monitoring a response gives electrochemical detection an advantage that is unmatched by apparatus for any other type of technique.

REFERENCES

Athey, D., McNeil, C. J., Bailey, W. R. *et al.* (1993) Homogeneous amperometric immunoassay for theophylline in whole blood. *Biosens. Bioelectron.* **8**, 415–419.

Bataillard, P., Gardies, F., Jaffrezic-Renault, N. *et al.* (1988) Direct detection of immunospecies by capacitance measurements. *Anal. Chem.* **60**, 2374–2379.

Bates, P. C. (1989) Enzyme amplified immunoassays. *Ann. Biol. Clin.* **47**, 527–532.

Boitieux, J. L., Biron, M. P. & Thomas, D. (1989) Bioaffinity electrochemical sensor. Study of the reversibility of immunocomplexes. *Anal. Chim. Acta.* **222**, 235–246.

Bremle, G., Persson, B. & Gorton, L. (1991) Amperometric glucose electrode based on carbon paste, chemically modified with glucose dehydrogenase, nicotinamide-adenine dinucleotide and a phenoxaxine mediator, coated with poly (estersulphonic acid) cation exchanger. *Electroanalysis* **3**, 77–86.

Cardosi, M. F., Birch, S. W., Stanley, C. J. *et al.* (1989) An electrochemical immunoassay for prostatic acid phosphatase incorporating enzyme amplification. *Am. Biotechnol. Lab.* **7**, 50–58.

Cass, A. E. G., Davis, G., Francis, G. D., *et al.* (1984) Ferrocene mediated enzyme for amperometric determination of glucose. *Anal. Chem.* **56**, 667–671.

Christie, I. M., Treloar, P. H., Koochaki, Z. B. *et al.* (1992) Simplified measurement of serum alkaline phosphatase utilising electrochemical detection of 4-aminophenol. *Anal. Chim. Acta.* **257**, 21–28.

Christie, I. M., Treloar, P. H. & Vadgama, P. (1992) Plasticised poly(vinyl chloride) as a permselective barrier membrane for high-selectivity amperometric sensors and biosensors. *Anal. Chim. Acta.* **269**, 65–73.

Deasy, B., Dempsey, E., Smyth, M. R. *et al.* (1994) Development of an antibody based biosensor for the determination of 7 hydroxy coumarin (umbelliferone) using horseradish peroxidase labelled anti-7-hydroxy coumarin antibody. *Anal. Chim. Acta.* **294**, 219–297.

Desai, M. A., Ghosh, S., Crump, P. W. *et al.* (1993) Internal membranes and laminates for adaptation of amperometric enzyme electrodes to direct biofluid analysis. *Scand. J. Clin. Lab. Invest.* **53**, 53–60.

Doyle, M. J., Halsall, H. B., & Heineman, W. R. (1982). Heterogeneous immunoassay for serum proteins by differential pulse anode stripping voltametry. *Anal. Chem.* **54**, 2318–2322.

Doyle, M. J., Halsall, H. B. & Heineman, W. R. (1984). Enzyme linked immunoadsorbent assay with electrochemical detection for a1-acid glycoprotein. *Anal. Chem.* **56**, 2355–2360.

Duan, C. & Meyerhoff, M. E. (1994) Separation-free sandwich enzyme immunoassays using microporous solid gold electrodes and self-assembled monolayer/immobilised capture antibodies. *Anal. Chem.* **66**, 1369–1377.

Eggers, H. M., Halsall, H. B. & Heineman, W. R. (1982) Enzyme immunoassay with flow-amperometric detection of NADH. *Clin. Chem.* **28**, 1848–1851.

Ekins, R., Chu, F. & Biggart, E. (1990) Fluorescence spectroscopy and its application to a new generation of high sensitivity multi-microspot, multianalyte, immunoassay. *Clin. Chim. Acta.* **194**, 91–114.

Emons, H., & Heineman, W. R. (1990) Influence of bovine immunoglobulin G on faradaic reactions at electrodes. *Analyst* **115**, 895–897.

Frew, J. E., Foulds, N. C., Wilshere, J. M. *et al.* (1989) Measurement of alkaline phosphatase activity by electrochemical detection of phosphate esters: Application to amperometric enzyme immunoassay. *J. Electroanal. Chem.* **66**, 309–316.

Hafeman, D. G., Parce, J. W. & McConnell, H. M. (1988) Light-addressable potentiometric sensor for biochemical systems. *Science* **240**, 1182–1185.

Halsall, H. B. & Heineman, W. R. (1990) Electrochemical immunoassay: An ultrasensitive method. *J. Int. Fed. Clin. Chem.* **2**, 179–187.

Hayes, F. J., Halsall, H. B. & Heineman, W. R. (1994) Simultaneous immunoassay using electrochemical detection of metal ion labels. *Anal. Chem.* **66**, 1860–1865.

Heineman, W. R. & Halsall, H. B. (1985) Strategies for electrochemical immunoassay. *Anal. Chem.* **12**, 1321–1331

Jaegfeldt, H., Torstensson, A. B. C., Gorton, L. G. O. *et al.* (1981) Catalytic oxidation of reduced nicotinamide-adenine dinucleotide by graphite electrodes modified with adsorbed aromatics containing catechol functionalities. *Anal. Chem.* **53**, 1979–1982.

Janata, J. (1975) An Immunoelectrode. *J. Amer. Chem. Soc.* **97**, 2914–2916.

Jenkins, S. H., Halsall, H. B. & Heineman, W. R. (1991) Eclectic immunoassay: An immunochemical approach. *Adv. Biosens.* **1**, 171–189.

Jenkins, S. H., Heineman, W. R. & Halsall, H. B. (1988). Extending the detection limit of solid-phase electrochemical enzyme immunoassay to the attomole level. *Anal. Biochem.* **168**, 292–299.

Kalab, T. & Skladal, P. (1995) A disposable amperometric immunosensor for 1,2-dichlorophenoxyacetic acid. *Anal. Chim. Acta.* **304**, 361–368.

Kannuck, R. M., Bellama, J. M. & Durst, R. A. (1988) Measurement of a liposome released ferrocyanide by a dual function polymer modified electrode. *Anal. Chem.* **60**, 142–147.

Knowles, M. (1994) Development of a dry reagent format for amperometrically detected G6PDH for use in simplified homogeneous immunoassay. Thesis, University of Manchester.

La Gal La Salle, A., Limoges, B. & Degrand, C. (1995) Enzyme immunoassays with an electrochemical detection method using alkaline phosphatase and a perfluorosulfonated ionomer-modified electrode. Application to phenytoin assays. *Anal. Chem.* **67**, 1245–1253.

Laurence, A. J. (1971) Conductimetric enzyme assays. *Eur. J. Biochem.* **18**, 221–225.

Matsue, T., Kasai, N., Narumi, M. *et al.* (1991) Electron-transfer from NADH dehydrogenase to polypyrrole and its applicability to electrochemical oxidation of NADH. *J. Electroanal. Chem. Interfacial Electrochem.* **300**, 111–118.

McNeil, C. J., Atley, D. & Ho, W. O. (1995) Direct electron transfer bioelectronic interfaces: Application to clinical analysis. *Biosens. Bioelectron.* **10**, 75–83.

McNeil, C. J., Higgins, I. J. & Bannister, J. V. (1988) Amperometric determination of alkaline phosphatase activity: Application to enzyme immunoassay. *Biosensors* **3**, 199–209.

McNeil, C. J. & Spoors, J. A. (1988) Thermostable reduced nicotine adenine dinucleotide oxidase: Application to amperometric enzyme assay. *Anal. Chem.* **61**, 25–29.

Miki, K., Ikeda, T., Todoriki, S. *et al.* (1989) Bioelectrocatalysis at NAD-dependent dehydrogenase and diaphorase-modified carbon paste electrodes containing mediators. *Anal. Sci.* **5**, 269–274.

Newman, A. L., Hunter, K. W. & Stanbro, W. D. (1988) The capacitive affinity sensor: A new biosensor. *Proc. 2nd Int. Mt, Chemical Sensors* Bordeaux, France July 7–10.

Nikolelis, D. P., Manolis, G. T. & Krull, U. J. (1993) Direct electrochemical transduction of an immunological reaction by bilayer lipid membranes. *Anal. Chim. Acta.* **282**, 527–534.

Niwa, O., Xu, Y., Halsall, H. B. *et al.* (1993) Small-volume voltammetric detection of 4-aminophenol with interdigitated array electrodes and its application to electrochemical enzyme immunoassay. *Anal. Chem.* **65**, 1559–1563.

Palmer, D. A., Edmonds, T. E. & Seare, N. J. (1992) Flow injection electrochemical enzyme immunoassay for theophylline using a Protein A immunoreactor and *p*-aminophenyl phosphate-*p*-aminophenol as the detection system. *Analyst* **117**, 1679–1682.

Robinson, G. A., Cole, V. M. & Forrest, G. C. (1988) A homogeneous electrode based bioelectrochemical immunoassay for human chorionic gonadotrophin. *Biosensors* **3**, 147–160.

Robinson, G. A., Hill, H. A. O., Philo, R. D. *et al.* (1985) Bioelectrochemical enzyme immunoassay of human choriogonadotropin with magnetic electrodes. *Clin. Chem.* **31**, 1449–1452.

Robinson, G. A., Martinazzo, G. & Forrest, G. C. (1986) A homogenous bioelectrochemical immunoassay for thyroxine. *J. Immunoassay* **7**, 1–15.

Sadik, O. A., John, M. J., Wallace, G. G. *et al.* (1994) Pulsed amperometric detection of thaumatin using antibody-containing poly(pyrrole) electrodes. *Analyst* **119**, 1997–2000.

Sadik, O. A. & Wallace, G. G. (1993) Pulsed amperometric detection of proteins using antibody containing conducting polymers. *Anal. Chim. Acta.* **279**, 209–212.

Souteyrand, E., Martin, J. R. & Martelet, C. (1994) Direct detection of biomolecules by electrochemical impedance measurements. *Sens. Actuators B* **20**, 63–69.

Stanley, C. J., Ellis, D. H., Bates, D. L. *et al.* (1987) Enzyme amplified immunoassays. *J. Pharm. Biomed. Anal.* **5**, 811–820.

Suzawa, T., Ikariyama, Y. & Aizawa, M. (1994) Multilabeling of ferrocenes to a glucose oxidase-digoxin conjugate for the development of a homogeneous electroenzymatic immunoassay. *Anal. Chem.* **66**, 3889–3894.

Tang, H. T., Lunte, C. E., Halsall, H. B. *et al.* (1988) *p*-Aminophenol phosphate: An

507

improved substrate for electrochemical enzyme immunoassay. *Anal. Chim. Acta.* **214**, 187–195.

Thompson, R. Q., Barone, G. C. III, Halsall, H. B. *et al.* (1991) Comparison of methods for following alkaline phosphate catalysis: Spectrophotometry versus amperometric detection. *Anal. Biochem.* **192**, 90–95.

Treloar, P. H. (1993). Investigation of phenolic and enzyme labels in the development of simplified electrochemical immunoassays. Thesis, University of Manchester.

Treloar, P. H., Christie, I. M., Kane, J. W. *et al.* (1995) Mediated amperometric detection of glucose 6-phosphate dehydrogenase at a poly(vinyl chloride) covered electrode using 1,4 benzoquinone and diaphorase. *Electroanalysis* **7**, 216–220.

Treloar, P. H., Nkohkwo, A. T., Kane, J. W. *et al.* (1994) Electrochemical immunoassay: Simple kinetic detection of alkaline phosphatase enzyme labels in limited and excess reagent systems. *Electroanalysis* **6**, 561–566.

Ueda, C., Tse, D. C. S. & Kuwana, T. (1982) Stability of catechol modified carbon electrodes for electrocatalysis of dihydronicotinamide adenine dinucleotide and ascorbic acid. *Anal. Chem.* **54**, 850–856.

Vadgama, P., & Crump, P. W. (1992) Biosensors: Recent trends – A review. *Analyst* **117**, 1657–1670.

Van den Berg, A. & Bergveld, P. (eds) (1995) *Micro Total Analysis Systems* (Kluwer Academic Publishers, Dordrecht).

Wallace, G. G., Maxwell, K., Lewis, T. W. *et al.* (1990) New conducting polymer affinity chromatography stationary phases. *J. Liq. Chromatogr.* **13**, 3091–3110.

Weber, S. G. & Purdy, W. C. (1979) Homogenous voltametric assay: A preliminary study. *Anal. Lett.* **12**, 1–9.

Weetall, H. H. & Hotaling, T. (1988) A simple inexpensive disposable electrochemical sensor for clinical and immunoassay. *Biosensors* **3**, 57–63.

Wehmeyer, K. R., Doyle, M. J., Wright, D. S. *et al.* (1983) Liquid chromatography with electrochemical detection of phenol and NADH for enzyme immunoassay. *J. Liq. Chromatogr.* **6**, 2141–2156.

Wehmeyer, K. R., Halsall, H. B. & Heineman, W. R. (1982) Electrochemical investigation of hapten-antibody interactions by differential pulse polarography. *Clin. Chem.* **28**, 1968–1972.

Willner, I., Blonder, R. & Dagan, A. (1994) Application of photoisomerizable antigenic monolayer electrodes as reversible amperometric immunosensors. *J. Amer. Chem. Soc.* **116**, 9365–9366.

Wright, D. S., Halsall, H. B. & Heineman, W. R. (1986) Digoxin homogeneous enzyme immunoassay using a high-performance liquid chromatography column switching with amperometric detection. *Anal. Chem.* **58**, 2995–2998.

Xu, Y., Halsall, H. B. & Heineman, W. R. (1989) Solid-phase electrochemical enzyme immunoassay with attomole detection limit by flow injection analysis. *J. Pharm. Biomed. Anal.* **7**, 1301–1311.

Yamamoto, N., Nagasawa, Y., Sawai, M. *et al.* (1978) Potentiometric investigations of antigen-antibody and enzyme-enzyme inhibitor reactions using chemically modified metal electrodes. *J. Immunol. Meth.* **22**, 309–317.

Yao, H., Halsall, H. B., Heineman, W. R. *et al.* (1995) Electrochemical dehydrogenase-based homogeneous assays in whole blood. *Clin. Chem.* **41**, 591–598.

Yao, H., Jenkins, S. H., Pesce, A. J. *et al.* (1993) Electrochemical homogeneous enzyme immunoassay of theophylline in hemolysed, icteric, and lipemic samples. *Clin. Chem.* **39**, 1432–1434.

Chapter 20

Direct Immunosensors

Duncan R. Purvis, Denise Pollard–Knight and Christopher R. Lowe

INTRODUCTION

Antibodies belong to a group of complex glycoproteins, the immunoglobulins, that are produced as part of an intricate mechanism known as the immune response. Antibodies recognise and bind specific molecules (known as antigens), or parts of molecules (the antigenic site), which are usually proteins, whole microorganisms or cells, but in fact could be any type of molecule that elicits a specific immune response. This recognition and binding of antibodies to complementary antigens occurs with affinity constants ranging from 10^3 to 10^{14} l mol^{-1}.

The immune response results in a range of antibodies that are heterogeneous with respect to function and physiochemical properties. These 'polyclonal' antibodies can form large insoluble complexes with the antigen, but before they can be used as reagents for immunoassay systems the specific antibodies must be purified and analysed for affinity and crossreactivity with related antigens. The development of monoclonal antibodies made it possible to produce greater quantities of specific antibodies, with defined antigenic characteristics *in vitro*, for use in the development of clinically useful diagnostic immunoassays and immunosensors.

This important recognition system is exploited in immunosensors for detection and quantification of specific target molecules. There are three assay formats that can be used to quantify antibody/antigen concentrations in a range of sample types: competitive, noncompetitive (also known as the sandwich assay) and direct assays, in which the antibody is immobilised on a solid phase.

Competitive and noncompetitive assays require additional reagents, usually labelled, before the target concentration can be determined. In competitive assays, a known amount of labelled antigen competes for available binding sites with the sample antigen. Thus, the concentration of the target analyte (antigen or antibody) in the sample is determined from the ratio of labelled and unlabelled antigen bound to the antibody activated surface. Noncompetitive assays use a second antibody binding to the target already captured by the immobilised primary antibody. The second antibody may be labelled, for example, with an enzyme or a fluorescent molecule to aid detection and, therefore, quantification of the target molecule.

These types of immunoassay are all extensively described in other chapters of this book and therefore are only briefly covered here.

DIRECT IMMUNOSENSOR CONCEPT

In direct assays the antigen-antibody binding event itself is detected. This type of assay is dependent on achieving a high ratio of specific to nonspecific binding, because the binding of any molecule to the antibody or antigen sensor surface will cause a response. Because the binding event itself does not provide a significant signal, it is the physical or bulk effect which is detected via changes in the local density, dielectric constant or refractive index using electrical, gravimetric or optical transducers. A way of differentiating specific binding from nonspecific binding may be achieved by having a control surface identical to the sensor surface in all ways bar the presence of the specific binding molecule.

A transducer is designed to convert the detection of the binding event into an electronic signal which can easily be analysed (Figure 1). Immunosensors can detect the specific antigen-antibody binding events by coupling the immunochemical reaction to the surface of the transducer. This is generally achieved by immobilising the antibody, although the reverse format in which the antigen is immobilised is also exploited. Immunosensors have stimulated

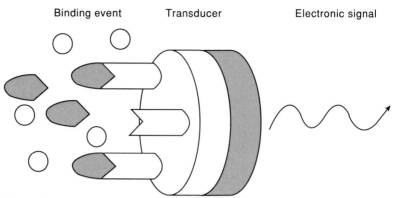

Figure 1 Schematic of an Immunosensor.

increasing interest over the past two decades because of their potential in clinical diagnostics and environmental monitoring. Regardless of the detection method or application the ideal system comprises the following:

1 Rapid detection and quantification within the required concentration range in 'real-time' (preferably seconds).

2 Transduction of the binding event directly, without the need for additional reagents.

3 Regeneration of the transducer surface, allowing multiple sequential analyses using the same device, or reproducible inexpensive disposable devices.

4 Detection of the binding event in 'real' unprocessed samples, such as urine, serum and blood.

There are very few current devices, if any, that satisfy all these criteria. However, this does not detract from their commercial potential or their increasing importance in the development of both the physical and biochemical aspects of sensor technology, as shown by the escalating number of research papers published each year. Today, commercial biosensors, specifically immunosensors, are a powerful tool for allowing scientists to monitor biospecific interactions in real-time and to derive information about binding kinetics, structure and function of molecules. The fields of application for these biosensors include monitoring of intrinsic and physical parameters of binding, ranging from simple tests for presence or absence to active concentration measurements and relative/comparative binding patterns, such as monoclonal antibody binding affinities, investigations of surface binding phenomena, epitope mapping and evaluation of kinetic constants.

TRANSDUCTION PRINCIPLES

A variety of electronic, acoustic and optical techniques have been used in the construction of immunosensors. These include field-effect transistors (FET devices) (Chandler *et al.*, 1990), amperometric biosensors, piezoelectric sensors (Kosslinger *et al.*, 1992), stopped flow spectrometry (Clarke, 1991; Noy *et al.*, 1992) solution depletion (Cornelius *et al.*, 1992), total internal reflection fluorescence techniques (TIRF) (Lok *et al.*, 1983a, b; Krull *et al.*, 1991; Noy *et al.*, 1992; Pearce *et al.*, 1992), ellipsometry (Eddowes, 1987; Jonsson *et al.*, 1988; Ruzgas *et al.*, 1992a, b; Martenson *et al.*, 1993) and surface plasmon resonance (Lok *et al.*, 1983b; Cullen *et al.*, 1987; Daniels *et al.*, 1988; Cullen and Lowe, 1990; Jonsson *et al.*, 1991, 1993; Karlsson *et al.*, 1991; Altschuh *et al.*, 1992; Karlsson, 1992). The key factors determining the rate of adsorption to the surface are the binding kinetics between the analyte and immobilised ligand and the diffusion of analyte to the surface of the sensor (Chaiken *et al.*, 1992).

Optical Sensors

Evanescent Waves

An evanescent wave is an electromagnetic field that decays exponentially away from the surface but propagates along the surface (Figure 2).

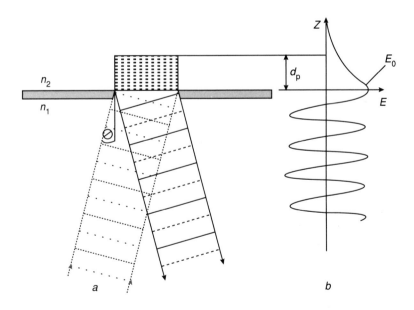

Figure 2 Generation of an evanescent wave at the interface between the transducer and the sample medium. a, Where the refractive index, $n_2 > n_1$ and Ø is larger than the critical angle $Ø_c$ at which refraction occurs, the evanescent wave is produced at the reflecting surface. b, as a, but showing the electric field amplitude E, on either side of the interface (Z, distance from the surface interface into the sample medium; d_p, the characteristic penetration depth of the evanescent wave) (Sutherland and Dähne, 1987).

When a beam of light is directed at an interface between two transparent media striking from the medium of higher refractive index ($n_2 > n_1$), total internal reflection occurs when the angle of reflection $\varnothing$ is larger than the critical angle $\varnothing_c$ (Sutherland and Dähne, 1987).

$$\varnothing_c = \sin^{-1}(n_2/n_1)$$

When this happens an evanescent wave of light energy is generated which penetrates a fraction of a wavelength beyond the reflecting medium into the rarer medium (n_2) (Figure 2). There is no net flow of energy into the nonabsorbing rarer medium, but there is an evanescent field in that medium. The electric field amplitude (E) is largest at the surface (E_0) and decays exponentially with distance (Z) from the surface. The depth of penetration (d_p) of the evanescent wave is defined as the distance at which the electric field amplitude falls to $\exp(^{-1})$ (approximately 36%) of its value at the surface, approximately 100 Å. The depth of penetration decreases with increasing $\varnothing$ and increases with closer index matching (i.e. as n_2/n_1 approaches 1), it is also a function of wavelength (when water acts as the low-index optical medium, the depth of penetration is approximately 100 nm at a wavelength of 500 nm). As soon as an absorbing or fluorescent molecule comes within the depth of penetration of the evanescent wave, there is a flow of energy across the reflecting surface to maintain the evanescent field. This transfer of energy results in a dip in reflectance, i.e. attenuation, and can be detected. This is called attenuated total reflection (ATR). With a fluorescent molecule the energy is absorbed at one wavelength and re-emitted at another wavelength which is fed back across the interface and detected by a detector placed either parallel to the interface or in-line with the primary light beam. This is called total internal reflection fluorescence (TIRF).

Surface Plasmon Resonance

Surface plasmon resonance (SPR)(Fontana *et al.*, 1990; Fägerstam *et al.*, 1992; Vancott *et al.*, 1992; Fägerstam and O'Shannessy, 1993) is a quantum optical-electrical phenomenon that arises from the interaction of light with a suitable metal or semiconductor surface. Under certain conditions, the photon's energy is transferred to packets of electrons called plasmons on the metal's surface. This energy transfer only occurs at a specific wavelength of light where the quantum energy carried by the photon exactly matches the quantum energy level of the plasmons. The resonance wavelength can be determined accurately by measuring the light reflected from the metal surface. At most wavelengths the metal acts as a mirror reflecting virtually all of the incident light. At the wavelength that excites the plasmons the incident light is almost completely absorbed. The wavelength that produces the maximum absorption is termed the resonance wavelength. Surface plasmon resonance can also be achieved by using a single wavelength but changing the angle at which the light strikes the metal surface. The maximum absorption occurs at a particular angle of incidence, i.e. changing the wavelength at a fixed angle is equivalent to changing the angle of a fixed wavelength.

Plasmons are a cloud of electrons but behave as if they were single charged particles. Part of their energy is expressed as oscillations in the plane of the metal surface which generates an electric field that extends about 100 nm above and below the metal surface, decaying exponentially as a function of distance. The interaction between the plasmon's electric field and the matter within the field determines the resonance wavelength or angle of incident light that resonates with the plasmon. Any change in the composition of the matter alters the wa-

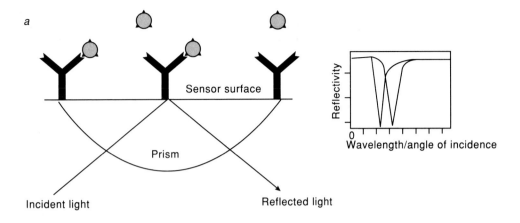

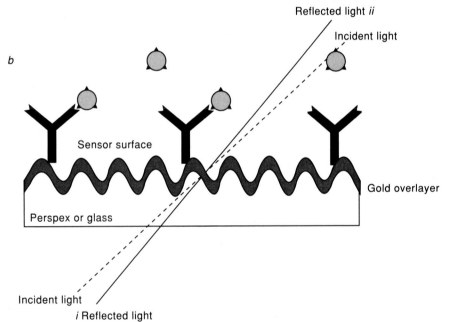

Figure 3 Two different coupling configurations of SPR devices. (a) prism, and (b) diffraction grating interrogated either from i) the back, or ii) the front, through the sample medium.

velength of light that resonates with the plasmon. The magnitude of the change in resonance wavelength or angle of incidence, the SPR shift, is directly and linearly proportional to the change in composition at the surface.

The SPR wavelength of resonance, or angle of incidence, is determined by three factors: the metal, the structure of the metal's surface and the nature of the medium in contact with the metal's surface (Cullen *et al.*, 1987; Cullen and Lowe, 1990; Lukosz, 1991; Sjolander and Urbaniczky, 1991; Meyer, 1992).

The resonance condition that allows energy transfer from photons to plasmons depends on the exact matching of both the energy and momentum of the photons and plasmons. For a flat metal surface there is no wavelength of light that satisfies this constraint because the momentum can never be matched. However, there are two simple methods to alter the momentum of photons in order to excite resonance: the use of (1) prisms and (2) diffraction gratings. The most common coupling method used is the prism, which enables coupling to occur when the angle of incidence exceeds the critical angle at which total internal reflection takes place, and in which the light is constrained to propagate along the face of the prism (Figure 3a). The alternative method for controlling the photon momentum involves the diffraction of light at the surface of a diffraction grating (Figure 3b). If the metal/dielectric surface is distorted in a periodic fashion, incident light is split into a series of beams reflected at a range of angles. This alters the direction of momentum and a portion is directed along the interface of the diffraction grating. Both techniques have been used to generate SPR-based immunosensors.

The metal must have conduction band electrons capable of resonating with light at a suitable wavelength, especially the visible and near-infrared parts of the spectrum, because optical components and detectors are readily available that are in this range of the spectrum. There are a few metals that satisfy this condition, namely silver, gold, copper, aluminium, sodium and indium. Two additional limitations reduce the practical choice to that of gold. The surface exposed to light must be pure metal, free from oxides, sulphides and other films formed by exposure to the atmosphere that would interfere with SPR. The metal must also be compatible with suitable immobilisation chemistries for attaching the binding molecules (antibodies or antigens) in an active state to the metal surface without impairing the resonance.

Surface plasmon resonance can therefore be exploited as a direct optical sensing technique that allows the real-time measurement of interfacial refractive index (dielectric) changes to be made at suitable metal or dielectric surfaces, typically gold or silver, without the use of labels or probes (Fontana *et al.*, 1990; Fägerstam *et al.*, 1992; Vancott *et al.*, 1992; Fägerstam and O'Shannessy, 1993). The excitation of surface plasmons at a metal/dielectric surface can be demonstrated by measuring the reflectivity of metallised diffraction gratings or prisms as a function of the incident angle of transverse magnetic (TM)-polarised light. Sharp reductions in reflectivity are seen, at a specific incident angle, that correspond to the excitation of surface plasmons, at the metal/aqueous interface as energy from the incident light beam is transferred to the metal surface to excite the surface plasmons which eventually decay as Joules heat in the metal (Cullen *et al.*, 1987; Cullen and Lowe, 1990; Lukosz, 1991; Sjolander and Urbaniczky, 1991; Meyer, 1992). Macromolecular complexes formed at the metal-liquid interface, result in a change in refractive index at the interface, perturbing and altering the propagation characteristics of the plasmons. Changes in these characteristics alter the incident angle at which a surface plasmon is excited, and can be detected and quantified.

The BIAcore™ (Biosensor, Sweden) comprises a surface plasmon resonance device, an integrated microfluidic cartridge and a sensor chip coated with a thin gold film. The sensor chip is held in contact with the prism by the microfluidic cartridge. Plane-polarised (transverse magnetic, TM) light from a near infrared light-emitting diodel (LED) is focused in a transverse wedge through a prism onto the side of the sensor chip opposite to the gold layer. The reflected light is monitored by a fixed two-dimensional array of light-sensitive diodes. Adsorption is monitored by following the shift of the SPR minimum caused by the increase in refractive index detected at the surface of the sensor chip. The sensor chip consists of a glass substrate and a 50-nm-thick gold film covered with a monolayer of long-chain hydroxylalkanethiols which serves both as a barrier to prevent adsorption of analytes to the gold surface and as a functionalised linker layer to which a matrix of carboxymethylated dextran is attached. The use of carboxymethylated dextran enables substances containing primary amine functions to be immobilised to the coated surface after activation with carbodiimide and *N*-

hydroxysuccinimide (Jonsson *et al.*, 1991; Fägerstam *et al.*, 1992; Fägerstam and O'Shannessy, 1993; Malmqvist, 1993).

Diffraction gratings are also used in many SPR sensors currently used for research (Cullen *et al.*, 1987; Cullen and Lowe, 1990; Lawrence *et al.*, 1996). The diffraction gratings are parallel sinusoidal grooves with a depth of around 10–70 nm and a pitch of 500–800 nm; they are either perspex replicas of a holographic 'master' grating etched into silica glass or, less commonly, silica glass gratings themselves, with a thin gold coating (50–200 nm). The majority are front illuminated through the sample and with the grooves of the diffraction grating oriented perpendicular to the plane of incidence (Figure 3*bii*). This arrangement ensures that the polarisation of the incident light is retained. The obvious disadvantage is that measurements are made through the bulk sample solution which changes refractive index at the beginning and end of sample addition. Illumination can be stimulated from the back of the grating through the perspex or glass, which significantly reduces the latter problem (Figure 3*bi*). In both cases the excitation of SPR is detected by measuring the minima in reflection at a certain angle of incidence with a fixed wavelength or the wavelength at a fixed angle of incidence. These change with any change of refractive index at the surface of the grating because of adsorption of biological material. However, if the grating is rotated so that the grooves lie at an angle between 0° and 90° with respect to the angle of incidence, the polarisation of the incident light is not conserved and the TM (p-polarised) light is converted to transverse electric (TE) (s-polarized) light (Lawrence *et al.*, 1996). This is observed by placing a polariser in front of the detector which allows only TE light through. Peak reflectivity is observed at the angle of incidence that excites SPR, superimposed against a near-zero background, providing a superior signal-to-noise ratio compared with other SPR systems. Adsorption can be measured by changes in the plasmon wavelength or plasmon angle.

SPRFiber Probe™ is a fibre-optic sensor based on surface plasmon resonance developed by EBI Sensors Inc. It is a SPR-based immunosensor constructed from a multimode optical fibre with a sensor at one end and connected at the other end to a light source and a detection system. The sensor end has a short length of exposed optical fibre core coated with a thin layer of gold (55 nm). The distal end has a 300-nm layer of silver acting as a mirror to return the light along the fibre to the detector. A white light source is sent down the fibre and the reflected light of a certain range of wavelengths is attenuated because of coupling of incident light to an SPR evanescent wave at the gold-surface interface. The dynamic range of the sensor is between 1.25 and 1.4 refractive index units. This range can be increased to between 1.0 and 1.4 by addition of an overcoat of zirconium oxide (18 nm), a high refractive index film. Using an optical fibre with a sapphire core further extends the range to 1.72 refractive index units. This allows the sensor to probe dynamic changes not only in water, but also in organic solvents and chemical soups (Jorgenson and Yee, 1994).

The Resonant Mirror

The IAsys™ system is based on an integrated optical chip called the resonant mirror (RM). The RM comprises a glass prism with the top surface coated with a low refractive index silica spacer layer which is in turn coated with a thinner high refractive index monomode waveguide of titania, hafnia or silicon nitride. This is then coated with the bioselective layer (Figure 4) [Davies *et al.*, 1994; George *et al.*, 1995; Yeung *et al.*, 1995].

Laser light (λ = 670 nm) is polarised to produce equal intensities of transverse electric and magnetic (TE and TM) components which are directed at the prism. The laser is repeatedly swept through an arc of specific angles, thus continuously changing the angle of incidence at

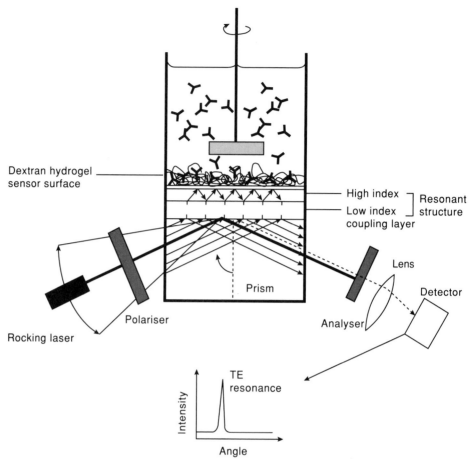

Figure 4 The resonant mirror cuvette system used in IAsys™.

which the light enters the prism. Some of the light entering the prism tunnels through the spacer where, at an angle unique to each polarisation (the resonant angle), it propagates by multiple internal reflections along the monomode waveguide. The light also tunnels back across the spacer to leave the prism. At the same time an evanescent wave is generated at the waveguide surface which penetrates about 100 nm into the sample. This wave detects surface binding events by detecting the changes in the refractive index which in turn change the resonance angle that is tracked by diode arrays. Both incident polarisations (TE and TM) can undergo resonance and could be simultaneously detected with the appropriate configuration. Monitoring both resonance angles would allow the determination of refractive index and thickness. However, because the resonance angles of the two modes are widely separated the instrument is optimised to track only the TE resonance [Davies *et al.*, 1994].

Surface plasmon resonance and resonant mirror devices are similar in that they both produce an evanescent wave at a discrete resonance angle. The SPR device results in more than double the resonance angle shift of RM devices but the resonance width is broader. They differ in two basic ways. First, there is no significant variation in the intensity of the reflected light with angle in the RM, but a phase shift occurs in some of the reflected light which is translated into an intensity peak at the resonant angle using phase optics. Second, in the RM, light propagating along the waveguide strikes the sample-waveguide interface many times, whereas in SPR there is a single point of interaction. This is because the excitation of an SPR only needs one strike for all the energy to be absorbed, whereas multiple strikes of photons producing an evanescent wave increase the attenuation of the light or ratio of phase-changed light.

Ellipsometry

Ellipsometry uses information obtained from the reflection of both TE and TM light at a thin film. Parallel and perpendicularly polarised light exhibit different reflectivities and phase shifts when reflected at monolayers or multilayers, depending on their dielectric properties (refractive index) and thickness or degree of coverage. Thus, ellipsometry allows the measurement of refractive index, and the thickness of the adsorbed layer. Ellipsometry is one of the most common methods for measuring thin films deposited on solid substrates and it is also one of the most sensitive methods. However, it is based on external rather than internal reflection techniques and would ideally need to be combined with either a single or multimode waveguide in order to measure thin biological films (Sutherland and Dähne, 1987; Brecht and Gauglitz, 1995). Ellipsometry is a complicated system to couple with an optical waveguide immunosensor and adds an extra layer of complexity to the system which gives no real benefits above other optical sensors. Published information on the use of ellipsometric biosensors is limited (Eddowes, 1987; Jonsson *et al.*, 1988; Ruzgas *et al.*, 1992a, b; Martenson *et al.*, 1993) and for this reason, will not be discussed further.

Other Waveguides

Waveguides work in a similar way to fibre optics but in a planar format. A monomode thin-film waveguide couples directly with the evanescent wave of a metal overlayer in contact with the sample medium and can be interrogated by measuring the change in transmission of the waveguide structure (Figure 5a). An example of a novel optical waveguide comprises a glass chip with two superimposed uniform diffractive gratings of different periodicities etched into the surface covered by a thin waveguiding layer of high refractive index TiO_2. The bidiffractive grating coupler serves as input and output ports for coupling and decoupling light to and from the waveguiding layer. The bioselective layer is immobilised at the surface of the waveguide and is probed by an evanescent wave emanating from the waveguide (Fattinger *et al.*, 1994). This method is being developed at Hoffmann La Roche.

A new planar waveguide immunosensor measures the changing refractive index contrast caused by adsorption at the bioselective sensor surface. Called the 'critical' sensor, the change in the effective refractive index contrast between a shielded surface and unshielded sensor surface is transduced to a shift in the critical reflection angle (Schipper *et al.*, 1996). Light is deflected when passing through an interface between two media with different refractive indices (N_1 and N_2). The critical angle for reflection is the angle above which light is totally internally reflected. This critical angle becomes a function of adsorption at one of the adjoining surfaces. The sensor can be tuned so that the incoming light strikes the interface between the shielded and unshielded areas in such a way that half the light is reflected (R) and half is transmitted (T). A change in the critical angle due to adsorption in the unshielded area results in a change in the difference between R and T, measured by photodiodes in the outcoupling holes (Figure 5b).

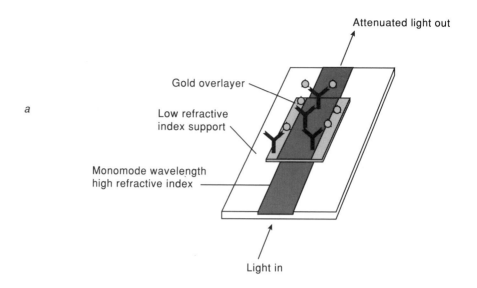

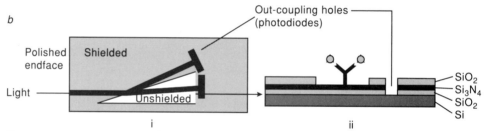

Figure 5 a, Thin film or slab waveguide with a gold overlayer. The bioselective surface is attached to the surface of the gold overlayer. b, The critical sensor waveguide i) top view, ii) cross section. The bioselective surface is attached to the unshielded section.

Interferometric Immunosensors

The thin-film waveguide difference interferometric affinity sensor measures the phase difference between two orthogonally polarised light beams (TE and TM) coupled in parallel to a waveguide. Changes of interfacial refractive index due to adsorption of analyte at the bioselective surface induce phase changes of the incoupled light beams. The phase difference between TE and TM light is proportional to the adsorption at the surface (Figure 6a). A similar device is termed the Mach-Zehnder interferometer where light is coupled and split into a dual-channel etched waveguide where one channel serves as a reference and the other channel binds analyte from solution. Phase changes produced by surface adsorption over the test channel are evident in the recombined beam due to interference patterns (Figure 6b) (Plowman *et al.*, 1996).

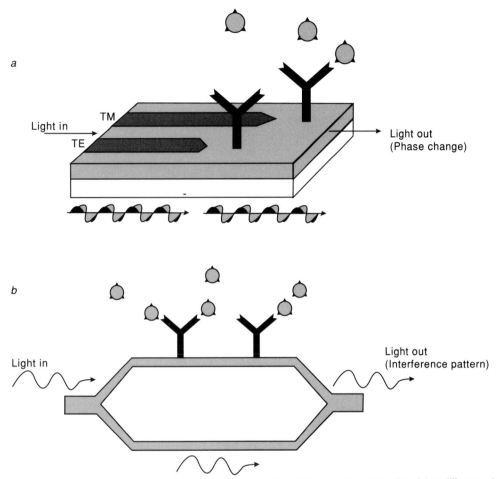

Figure 6 Two configurations of interferometric sensors. *a*, A differential interferometer measures the phase difference between TE and TM light. *b*, Mach-Zehnder interferometer measures the interference patterns generated when the light from a reference channel and a sensor channel are recombined.

Fluoroimmunosensors Based on Total Internal Reflection Fluorescence (TIRF)

Total internal reflection fluorescence (TIRF) systems usually involve competitive immunoassay formats where the unlabelled antigen competes with a fluorescently labelled antigen for binding to a surface-immobilised antibody, or sandwich assay formats where the second antibody is fluorescently labelled. The choice of fluorescent label has to be compatible with the light source and detector in relation to the excitation and emission wavelengths (for example, fluorescein λ_{max} 515 nm; rhodamine λ_{max} 550 nm). The intensity of the fluorescent signal is influenced by the extinction coefficient and quantum yield of the fluorophore. The binding of antigen to immobilised antibody is measured via interaction of fluorophore with an evanescent wave arising from a totally internally reflected light beam. The waveguide used may be an optical fibre, a prism or a planar waveguide (Domenici *et al.*, 1995). The formats are the same as for SPR devices: the prism and waveguide work by using TIR at their planar surfaces, whereas the function of the fibre is characterised by its cylindrical geometry and its abi-

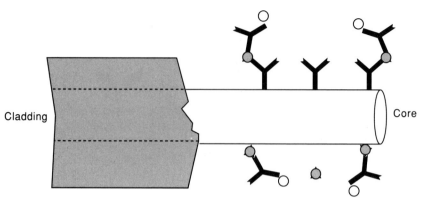

Figure 7 Basic fibre-optic sensor.

lity to collect the fluorescence emitted by the surface-adsorbed fluorophores by reflection or transmission modes.

In general, the fibre-optic system is the most sensitive method, both in theory and in practice (Domenici *et al.*, 1995). There are a variety of fibre-optic geometries used for TIRF sensors and at least two different detection systems (Auge *et al.*, 1994; Domenici *et al.*, 1995; Feldman *et al.*, 1995; Hale *et al.*, 1996). Multimode (Domenici *et al.*, 1995; Feldman *et al.*, 1995) or single-mode (Hale *et al.*, 1996) fibres can be used. The sensor area is a short piece of fibre stripped of cladding with the exposed core coated with immobilised antibody (Figure 7). This exposed piece of core can be at the distal end of the fibre and detection of the coupled fluorescence is performed by measuring the returning light reflected back up the fibre, or in the middle of the fibre between the light source and the detector. In either case, the core can be straight (Domenici *et al.*, 1995) or tapered (Feldman *et al.*, 1995; Hale *et al.*, 1996). An alternative method of detection is a charge-coupled device (CCD) camera which can monitor the emission wavelength of the fluorophores *in situ* (Plowman *et al* ., 1996). The advantage of tapered fibres over straight fibres is sensitivity. Because the fibre cladding is removed in the sensing region and the surrounding medium is usually of a lower refractive index than the cladding, tapering the core to a smaller diameter in the sensing region increases the light propagation angles to match the larger critical angle required for total internal reflection in the region where the cladding has been stripped. In addition, the magnitude of the exciting evanescent field and the subsequent fluorescent signal are enhanced by the taper. The light is conserved as it travels down the taper, as long as the taper is gradual and the fibre surface is smooth and free from excessive flaws. If the taper is too sharp or if there are excessive flaws on the surface, then there is leakage of light into the medium and the probe generates a signal originating from bulk fluorescence in solution, swamping any signal generated at the surface. A distal tapered optical fibre TIRF has shown a potential sensitivity for an antigen of 4 pmol l^{-1} (5 ng ml^{-1}) (Feldman *et al.*, 1995). Another example is a single-mode tapered optical fibre loop immunosensor (Hale *et al.*, 1996). An evanescent field is generated at the tapered loop and detects a two-step sandwich assay with the fluorescently labelled second antibody. Generated fluorescence is coupled back into the fibre and measured at the far end of the fibre. The loop was coated with an immobilised antigen cholera toxin B subunit-derived synthetic peptide, CTP_3, conjugated to BSA, and used to detect and bind IgG raised against cholera in serum and jejunal fluid samples. The sensitivity of this system was cited to be 75 pg ml^{-1} positive IgG ($\sim$60 fmol l^{-1}) (Hale *et al.*, 1996).

Another sensitive fluoroimmunosensor with reported femtomolar sensitivity is a dual-channel etched silicon oxynitride thin-film integrated optical waveguide (Plowman *et al.*, 1996). A thin layer of Si_2O_3N (1 μm) is deposited onto SiO_2 (quartz) wafers and subsequently etched to produce two parallel Si_2O_3N waveguide channels. A coupling prism is used to couple the light beam into the waveguide. The whole device is placed in a flow cell with sample and reference channels and detection of the emitted fluorescence carried out by a (CCD)-based spectrograph. The bioselective layer is immobilised to only one of the channels and conjugated cyanine 5 (red emitter) was used to detect binding. The high sensitivity of this device was attributed to the elimination of background emissions by using a red-emitting fluorescent label; the waveguides were intrinsically non-fluorescent and the propagation losses were minimal, thus reducing excitation of bulk fluoresence. Finally, the waveguides had a reflection density of approximately 500 reflections per cm at the sensing surface, providing extensive interaction between the incoupled light and the adsorbed fluorescent label (Plowman *et al.*, 1996).

Acoustic Sensors

Principles

Gravimetric devices directly measure changes in mass at the surface interface due to chemical or bioselective adsorption. Resonant systems, such as the quartz crystal microbalance (QCM) (Auge *et al.*, 1994; Bodnehöfer *et al.*, 1995), and acoustic systems, such as surface acoustic wave (SAW) devices (Gizelli *et al.*, 1991), are both examples of gravimetric sensors. When an alternating current is applied across the surface of a piezoelectric material, such as quartz, small mechanical deformations occur in the material. At a specific frequency, a mechanical or acoustic resonance is induced. As with the optical systems an evanescent wave extends into the region beyond the surface. The resonance frequency is modulated when a change in mass occurs at the surface of the crystal. The change in frequency is proportional to the mass adsorbed or released.

Bulk and Surface Acoustic Waves

Quartz crystal microbalances are bulk acoustic wave (BAW) devices and lose resolution in liquid media because of damping caused by viscous coupling between the crystal and the liquid. The sensitivity is limited by the thickness of the piezoelectric material, which cannot be reduced below certain values without affecting the durability of the device. An alternative device is the SAW device which uses interdigital transducers to couple electrical to acoustic energy and excite a wave known as a Rayleigh wave (Clark *et al.*, 1987; Gizelli *et al.*, 1992; Gizelli and Lowe, 1996). This wave is generated by one set of interdigitated electrodes, propagates across the crystal surface with very low penetration into the bulk and is detected by a second set of electrodes. Mass changes on the crystal surface alter the propagation characteristics and cause frequency changes in the wave. The disadvantage of these devices is that at frequencies above 10 MHz the presence of liquid results in signal loss. As a result, the devices have to be dried in order to determine the amount of mass deposited onto the surface. This drying step can be eliminated by using surface-guided shear-horizontally polarised waves (SH), which are not damped in water. SH waves are used in acoustic plate devices, which are thin plates of piezoelectric crystal forming acoustic waveguides, confining the waves near the surface (Gizelli *et al.*, 1992). These devices have been used for *in situ* detection of binding

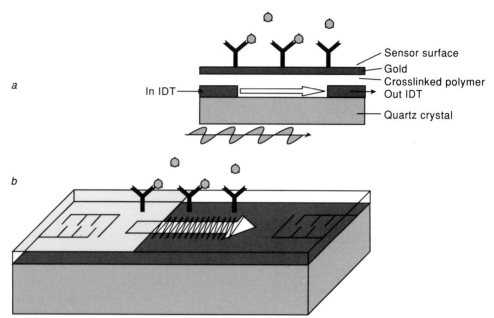

Sensor surface
Gold
Crosslinked polymer
Out IDT
Quartz crystal

In IDT

a

b

Figure 8 An example of an acoustic immunosensor. A Love Plate. *a*, Cross section, *b*, top view.

events at the surface in liquid. However, there is still some loss of acoustic energy because a wave reflection mechanism occurs and the energy is distributed between the top and bottom surfaces of the device and cannot be focused entirely on the sensing surface unless very thin plates are used, which compromises their durability.

Love Plates

Love plates comprise a surface-skimming bulk wave (SSBW) device which has a thin guiding overlayer (1–12 μm). The effect of this geometry is to convert the SSBW into a guided-surface SH wave, or Love wave, and thus concentrate the acoustic energy at the surface while maintaining 'workable' devices. The conversion to a surface SH wave can only occur if the overlayer has a lower shear acoustic velocity than the piezoelectric substrate (Stevenson *et al.*, 1993). The larger the difference between the two acoustic velocities, the greater the coupling to a Love wave and the higher the sensitivity. The overlayer is usually made of a metallic or dielectric material, with silica being the most popular, although greater sensitivity can be achieved using layers of up to 2-μm-thick polymethyl methacrylate (PMMA) and other polymeric materials (Stevenson *et al.*, 1992, 1993). The interrogation depth of the acoustic wave into the solution is about 50 nm and is independent of the thickness of the overlayer (Gizelli *et al.*, 1992). The surface of the PMMA layer can be subsequently coated with a thin layer of gold (5 nm) for immobilisation of the bioselective layer via thiolate or silane coupling (Figure 8).

Flow Sensors

Flow immunosensors, primarily developed by the Naval Research Laboratory (NRL) in Washington DC, comprise a cylinder slightly bigger than a pencil eraser packed with beads

(Pennisi, 1991). The beads are coated with antibodies and loaded with fluorescently labelled antigen. The sample is passed through the column, and any antigen present in the sample displaces the fluorescently labelled antigens which are subsequently detected downstream with a fluorometer. However, in the absence of antigen there is no displacement and the column can be reused, reducing cost. Beads have been coated with cocaine-specific antibodies and loaded with fluorescently labelled cocaine, and are used by the military as well as for roadside drug detection. This technology is very simple and easily adapted for monitoring pollutants in water, drug levels and blood chemistry in patients (Pennisi, 1991). The potential of this approach, as for all other immunosensors, is limited only by the versatility of antibodies and the imagination of the user. Recent efforts have been focused on the detection of opiates using immobilised anti-morphine antibodies and subsequent saturation with a fluorescently tagged antigen. Morphine has been detected to levels as low as 10 ng ml^{-1} within minutes of sample addition. Future work aims to develop detection systems for other drugs of abuse in urine and saliva.

TRANSDUCER SURFACES AND MATERIALS

Materials used as transducer surfaces include gold, silver, PMMA, polytetra-fluorethylene (PTFE), silica, quartz, metal oxides and silicon nitride. There are two principal methods of immobilisation for surface-effect immunosensors: physical adsorption at the solid surface or, preferably, covalent bonding for reactive support matrices. The method chosen can have a significant impact on the surface concentration of antigen/antibody and the biological activity of the immobilised molecules. Many of the immobilisation methods to a reactive support matrix originate from those developed for use in affinity chromatography (Lowe and Dean, 1974, 1979; Scouten, 1980; Dean *et al.*, 1985; Groman and Wilchek, 1987; Hermanson *et al.*, 1992). The bioselective layer has first to be immobilised to the transducer surface, which is generally a noble metal or a glass-like material. The specific binding molecule can be attached directly to the transducer surface or indirectly via linker layers and gel matrices. In general, a linker layer has to be bound, to reduce nonspecific binding to the sensor surface and to allow simpler immobilisation chemistries to be performed. The immobilisation methods are generally based on silane or thiol chemistry.

Thermochemical immobilisation reactions have been used extensively to immobilise biomolecules to the transducer surface of optical sensors. The gold surfaces of SPR sensors have been modified by exploiting the strong interaction between gold and sulphur. These interactions enable the formation of self-assembled monolayers (SAMs) of thiol- or disulphide-bearing molecules. In the BIAcore^{TM} sensor chip the gold surface is coated with a linker layer of 1, ϖ-hydroxyalkylthiols for subsequent attachment of functionalised dextran hydrogels (carboxymethyldextran) (Löfås *et al.*, 1995).

Inorganic waveguide materials, such as hafnia, TiO_2, TiO_2/SiO_2, Ta_2O_5 and Si_3N_4 are activated using an organic linker. Linker layers have been prepared by silanisation of the hydroxylated surfaces with short-chain and long-chain polyfunctional silanes (Gao *et al.*, 1995). These can be used for direct coupling to the bioselective component, as an intermediate for further spacers such as glutaraldehyde, or for a support matrix of functionalised dextrans.

The two main commercial sensors, BIAcore^{TM} and IAsys^{TM}, use a functionalised dextran hydrogel as the main support matrix. Immobilisation of ligands carrying a primary amine is performed by activation with a solution of carbodiimide and hydroxysuccinimide. Unreacted active carboxyl groups are then blocked with ethanolamine (Buckle *et al.*, 1993; Löfås *et al.*, 1995). Ligands carrying a reactive disulphide can be immobilised using 2-(2-pyridinyldithio)ethaneamine-HCl (PDEA). A hydrophobic surface (HPA) sensor chip and a streptavidin-coated (SA) sensor chip are available for BIAcore™. Bare surfaces of aminosilanes for direct attachment of the ligand are also provided with the IAsys™ sensor.

Photochemical methods can been used for immobilisation of ligands to 'inert' surfaces although this is not often used; for example, bovine serum albumin derivatised with aryldiazirines (T-BSA) was used as a photolinker polymer to immobilise F(ab')₂ fragments in a single-step photoreaction (Gao *et al.*, 1995). A mixture of F(ab')₂ fragments and T-BSA (1:4) was dried onto the surface of a transducer and irradiated with a light source to immobilise the F(ab')₂ fragments and T-BSA to the surface. T-BSA also suppressed nonspecific adsorption of proteins to the transducer surface.

The effectiveness and quality of the bioselective layers depend on mobility, accessibility and structure of the receptor and the spacer molecules. As a result a significant amount of research in the sensor field involves characterisation of the sensor layers and interfaces in order to optimise the sensor quality (Brecht and Gauglitz, 1995). There is still a considerable amount of practical work needed to improve schemes for ligand immobilisation, especially for oriented or site-specific immobilisation of antibodies. Recent work has shown that IgG molecules modified by carboxypeptidase-Y-catalysed cysteinylation, specifically at the carboxyl termini, can be immobilised on a gold substrate via metal-thiolate bonds (You *et al.*, 1995). The use of streptavidin-biotin binding has also been used for immobilisation of biotinylated antibodies. Streptavidin was first immobilised to the carboxymethyldextran coating of a sensor chip using the standard amine coupling method (Löfås *et al.*, 1995).

A new coating technique for SPR-based sensor surfaces using immunoactivated latex beads has been developed (Schasfoort *et al.*, 1994). Latex particles with blocking agents and immobilised ligands are preloaded onto the sensor in order to prepare a bioselective surface. The binding assay can then be performed. Surface as opposed to ligand regeneration can be performed using a flow- injection-based automated washing procedure using organic solvents. The sensor is then ready for the application of a new and different bioselective latex surface. Because the size of the latex bead is extremely large compared to the interrogation depth of the evanescent field, a single binding event is greatly enhanced by the presence of the bead, which produces a significant change in the SPR signal.

ANALYSIS OF ANTIGEN-ANTIBODY BINDING CURVES

The thickness of the adsorbed layer on a sensor surface can be calculated using the total shift in the resonance angle or phase following macromolecular deposition. For example, the change in the surface plasmon wave vector due to the deposition of a thin dielectric layer on a metal surface can be calculated using the first order expression obtained by Pockrand (Pockrand, 1978; Fontana *et al.*, 1990).

For the purposes of illustration, we will discuss the changes in refractive index but the principle also holds for phase shifts and interference. Refractive index changes on the sensor surface are monitored continuously, with a buffer defining the baseline level from which all responses are expressed. The relative response recorded is a combination of the refractive index components of the buffer, the immobilised ligand and the analyte (antigen or antibody) bound to the ligand. Because both the buffer and the ligand are constant the detector response to the resonance signal (R) measured by the reflection of light from the sensor surface at a fixed angle of incidence is directly proportional to the surface concentration of a bound analyte (antigen or antibody) ([PL]). Thus

$$Rc = [PL] \qquad (1)$$

The proportionality factor (c), relating response (R) to surface concentration ([PL]) is approximately the same for all proteins. This is a consequence of the fact that the refractive index increment for biomolecules with high protein and low lipid and carbohydrate content is essentially independent of molecular size and amino acid composition and is, therefore, constant. Deviations for high lipid or carbohydrate content are generally small, for example β_1-lipoprotein (35% lipid) has a refractive index about 8% lower than that of pure protein (Jonsson *et al.*, 1991; Karlsson *et al.*, 1991; Chaiken *et al.*, 1992).

The change in response (R) over time multiplied by the proportionality factor (c) is, therefore, equal to the change in concentration of the analyte ([PL]) bound to the immobilised ligand at the surface of the sensor.

$$\frac{d[Rc]}{dt} = \frac{d[PL]}{dt} \qquad (2)$$

A more complete description of kinetic analysis can be found in Chapter 5 of this book.

Considerations on the Limitations of Fitting Binding Curves

Mass Transport

When the association rate between an antibody and antigen is $\geq 1 \times 10^6$ l mol^{-1} s^{-1}, the measured binding rate may reflect the transport of analyte to the ligand rather than the kinetics of the interaction itself. In such cases, the binding rate is often constant during the initial phase of the interaction (Chaiken *et al.*, 1992). By increasing the flow or transport of the antigen/antibody to the sensor surface, the mass transport limitation can be eliminated. This is shown experimentally when there is no change in the binding rate with increasing flow because the diffusion layer is influenced by flow rate, whereas the intrinsic reaction rate is independent of flow. This can be illustrated by plotting d[PL]/dt versus [PL], i.e. the gradient (rate of binding) at each point against [PL]. If the binding curve is limited by mass transport, the initial points on the plot will be horizontal as the rate of binding is constant until the concentration of the ligands ([L]) is low enough to allow measurement of the association rate (Fägerstam *et al.*, 1992). The balance between mass transport and reaction rate is influenced by the concentration of immobilised ligand (Kooyman *et al.*, 1988; Chaiken *et al.*, 1992). For measurement of high-association rate constants, ($\geq 1 \times 10^6$ l mol^{-1}s^{-1}), either the amount of immobilised ligand should be very low, ($\leq 20 \times 10^{-15}$ mol mm^{-2}), or the flow rate correspondingly high (Karlsson *et al.*, 1991; Chaiken *et al.*, 1992). This is because at very low ligand concentrations the analyte availability will be greater than the demand and thus there will be no diffusion limitations.

In earlier publications, where data was analysed using Langmuirian-type assumptions and binding curves were fitted and analysed using a single exponential fit, authors appeared either not to recognise, or chose to ignore the presence of at least two association rates within their binding curves. Several explanations have purported to account for the double exponential binding curves observed when measuring real-time binding events. These include nonspecific adsorption (Fägerstam *et al.*, 1992), conformational differences (Debono *et al.*, 1992; Pearce *et al.*, 1992) or configurational changes, diffusion (either to the surface of the sensor or, in the case of BIAcore™ and IAsys™, through the dextran layer which may extend further than the effective interrogation depth of the SPR evanescent wave) (Debono *et al.*, 1992; Fägerstam *et al.*, 1992; Pearce *et al.*, 1992), background drift/change (Fägerstam *et al.*, 1992), and the presence of two or more populations of binding sites (Fontana *et al.*, 1990; Debono *et al.*, 1992), either at the surface or on the analyte (Edwards *et al.*, 1995). All these explanations are plausible, and in reality double exponential binding curves may result from a combination of those effects. Alternative explanations include the presence of two or more exponentials within the binding curve can be explained by the presence of two distinct populations of binding sites, or by a conformational change on binding. This phenomenon is universally observed and this may be indicative of another underlying parameter which may reflect the nature of surface interactions or steric considerations. Until these issues are resolved, determining the true values of the rate constants of macromolecules binding at surfaces will prove problematic.

When fitting a curve to a double exponential it is difficult to assign physical meanings to the parameter values obtained because there are several sets of exponentials that fit the binding curves equally well. For example, the addition of two smaller exponential rises give the same fit as a larger exponential rise added to an exponential fall. The fitting relies heavily on the initial estimates of the constants and floating points used. A large change in the value of one of the constants has little effect on the fit of the curve if all the other values are still floating. This is because the parameters are separate: they need to be linked in some way to enable a trend to be elucidated. A more robust and powerful method of analysis is global fitting, which can fit association, dissociation and steady-state phases of several binding curves at different concentrations of analyte in a single operation (Debono *et al.*, 1992). Global fitting is described in detail in Chapter 5 of this book.

An alternative method for fitting the multiexponential binding curves generated by biosensors is fractal analysis (Sadana and Beelaram, 1995). During immobilisation of the antibody or antigen to the transducer, surface irregularities inevitably occur and these may be characterised using Mandelbrot's non-Euclidean fractal geometry. Fractals are disordered systems which can be described as nonintegral dimensions. Based on the assumption that the surface irregularities show scale invariance, they can be described by a single number, the fractal dimension D_f. Antibodies are heterogeneous and their immobilisation on a surface would also result in some degree of heterogeneity created by different orientations and accessibility. This is a good example of a disordered system for which fractal analysis is appropriate. Fractal analysis may provide insights into the state of disorder or heterogeneity of the antigen-antibody complex at the biosensor surface. It may also provide a framework for comparing the different types of surfaces and immobilisation procedures under development and thereby provide a useful basis by which improvements in sensor surface design can be

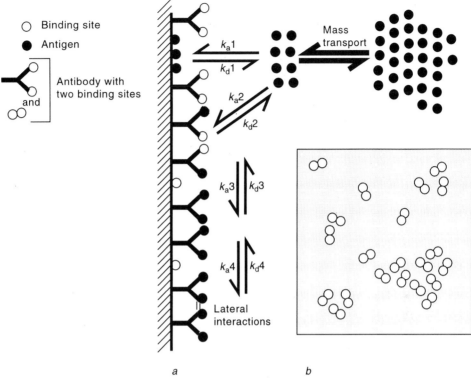

Figure 9 *a*, Illustration of the different association and dissociation events that could occur at the sensor surface. k_a and k_d are association and dissociation constants, respectively. *b*, Representation of the immobilisation irregularities that influence the environment, for example, crowding which may affect the kinetic parameters.

measured. Nonspecific binding may provide a major contribution to the multiexponential binding curves observed (Intersens Instruments, 1995). Nonspecific binding only due to the adsorption of unrelated material to the surface but also to any binding that is affected by steric hindrance, lateral interactions, different binding states or multiple antigens bound to the antibody. All of these interactions will have different association and dissociation rates (Figure 9) which will be represented in the binding curve. Most of these interactions can be minimised by using very low concentrations of immobilised antibody or antigen. At low concentrations the expected monoexponential binding curves are observed although they occur at the expense of signal resolution, and lie near the limits of sensitivity.

Fitting a curve only confirms that a model is consistent with the experimental data; it may not reveal what mechanisms are operating at the sensor surface. There will often be several alternative models that will fit the curve and thus generate a different set of apparent constants. Therefore, model fitting should be used to define a putative interaction regime and to identify further experiments that will test the validity of the model.

Furthermore, one must always remember that the rate constants and affinity constants derived from the analysis of binding data are apparent constants only, and are highly dependent on the conditions of the experiment and the methodology used to obtain the data (Fägerstam and O'Shannessy, 1993).

Determination of Kinetic Constants: Solid Phase versus Solution Phase

Kinetic constants determined by immunosensors in many cases do not mirror solution-based measurements. One of the sources of the difference is the retarded transport of material through the matrix that must occur before the binding event, compared to unimpeded free binding in solution. Other effects which may contribute include orientation, steric hindrance and nonspecific binding.

In general, there is substantial variation in the values of kinetic constants reported in the literature which may be attributable to the variable nature of biological materials, different measurement techniques and even sample preparation. For example, measurement of the binding affinity of iodinated antibodies to suspended erythrocytes has recently been shown to vary by almost an order of magnitude simply by varying the equilibration volume (Yeung *et al.*, 1995). In this sense, immunosensors provide a consistent, reproducible measure of affinity and rate constants, which is precisely what is required by the practical scientist.

Despite these reservations regarding true values for the rate constants, immunosensors provide a quick and simple analytical tool where the selection of an antibody with the quickest on-rate from a tested population is the criterion for success.

Effect of Immobilisation Chemistry/Supports on Kinetic Rate Constants: Bare Surface versus Hydrogel

IAsys[TM] has been used for comparative studies of human serum albumin (HSA) binding to anti-HSA antibodies immobilised on either an aminosilane activated surface or in carboxy-methyldextran (CMD) activated cuvettes, (Edwards *et al.*, 1995). The binding curves produced using CMD cuvettes had higher binding response and were characteristically biphasic. In aminosilane cuvettes, monophasic binding curves were observed with almost all the binding occuring within the first few seconds of sample addition. The two rate constants that can be extracted from a double exponential fit to the CMD data show that the faster of the two phases is comparable to the single phase observed in an aminosilane cuvette. When a CMD cuvette and decreased sample concentration (12 nM) is used, binding curves that fit a single exponential are generated.

These observations are interpreted by the authors to indicate that steric hindrance is associated with the double exponential binding curves, the first fast binding phase representing binding to easily accessible sites with a value that should be directly comparable to the situation in free solution. The slower binding rate may arise from restricted accessibility and/or steric constraints (Edwards *et al.*, 1995).

COMMERCIAL SENSORS

At present there are four companies with instruments on the market for detection of real-time binding of label-free intermolecular interactions (Hodgson, 1994). These are all based on optical devices: Artificial Sensor Instruments (ASI), Zurich, Switzerland with BIOS-1; Affinity Sensors Ltd (formerly Fisons Applied Sensor Technologies (FAST)), Bar Hill, Cambridge, UK with IAsys[TM] and IAsys[TM] Auto+; Pharmacia Biosensor AB, Uppsala, Sweden and Piscataway, New Jersey, USA with BIAcore 2000[TM], BIAcore[TM] and BIAlite[TM]; and Intersens Instruments

(Winthontlaan 200, 3526 KV Utrecht, The Netherlands) has a biosensor known as IBIS[TM] (Intersens Instruments, 1995) which is available in the Netherlands and will soon be available in England and Germany. A fifth company, Quantech Ltd, 1419 Energy Park Drive, St Paul, Minnesota, USA may have launched their SPR instrument, Lambda, by the time this book comes to print. The methods used in these commercial instruments are based on the behaviour of light at the boundaries of different refractive indices (Hodgson, 1994). As described previously beyond a critical angle, light will totally internally reflect at the interface of the sensor (high refractive index) and the biological solution (lower refractive index). When total internal reflection occurs, an evanescent wave (electromagnetic field) passes from the interface into the biological solution, where it decays exponentially over several hundred nanometres (Hodgson, 1994). The angle of incidence at which the evanescent wave is propagated is extremely sensitive to the refractive index of the adsorbed layers at the surface of the sensor. In the ASI BIOS-1 instrument, the sensor consists of a planar waveguide layer coating a glass or plastic diffraction grating. The waveguide film consists of various metal oxides depending on the required refractive index. The coupling between the incident laser light and the propagating evanescent wave is a resonance phenomenon that occurs at a precise angle of incidence, dependent on the refractive index at the surface. This device is called a resonance mirror.

Affinity Sensor's IAsys[TM] instrument is also a resonant mirror device. It also uses a waveguide, but uses a low index coupling layer on an integrated prism instead of a diffraction grating. The waveguide is prepared from dielectric materials such as zirconia, hafnia or silicon nitride which have high refractive indices. The IAsys[TM] uses a dual-channel vibro-stirred microcuvette as the transducer surface which comprises the low index coupling layer, high index resonant layer and the reactive sensor surface. The microcuvette sits on top of the prism and both cuvettes can be measured simultaneously (George *et al.*, 1995; Yeung *et al.*, 1995). The kinetic constants are calculated by fitting the individual binding curves using IAsys[TM] proprietary FASTfit[TM] software. FASTfit[TM] applies exponential curve fitting algorithms to both the binding and dissociation phases to abstract the best values for the association and dissociation constants.

In contrast, BIAlite[TM], BIAcore[TM] and BIAcore[TM] 2000 are SPR devices that use polarised light passing through a prism to excite an evanescent wave on a gold-coated sensor chip. The sensor chip is a glass slide with a thin layer of gold deposited on one side. The gold film is coated with a covalently bound hydrophilic dextran matrix which, when activated, enables covalent immobilisation of biomolecules. The chip assembly includes all the microfluidics to enable injection of the sample to the sensor surface and, depending on the chemistries used, can easily be regenerated for reuse. The BIAcore[TM] 2000 chips have multichannel microfluidics with four flow cells which can be measured simultaneously, allowing multiple analyte analysis. Low molecular mass analytes can be studied using BIAcore[TM] 2000 by immobilising four different ligand concentrations and comparing the interaction against a low background of signal-to-noise bulk refractive index changes. In addition, the BIAcore[TM] 2000 instrument is more sensitive and can detect analytes with a relative molecular mass as small as 200 (Pharmacia Biosensor AB, 1994); more information is available from http://www.Pharmacia.se/biosensor (Pharmacia Biosensor AB; internet address). Standard binding immunoassays, sandwich and competition immunoassays can all be performed easily and rapidly. Epitope mapping is simplified by running four analyses in a single injection, increasing throughput and decreasing sample consumption. Specificity, affinity and crossreactivity analyses can all be performed. In addition, sample recovery and fractionation is possible using a new recovery channel. This is used for collecting excess sample during injection, thereby saving expensive samples and reagents. The eluted sample can also be collected for subsequent analysis.

The IBIS™ (Intersens Instruments) is a modular and compact SPR sensor arranged in a similar manner to BIAcore™, with two configurations, either a four-cuvette or a flow system which can use Pharmacia's sensor chip in addition to their own IBIS™ wafers (Intersens Instruments, 1995).

Lambda™ (a sensor made by Quantech Ltd) is also an SPR device but is based on a gold-coated plastic diffraction grating. The grating is illuminated and read from the rear using a dual-beam SPR reader. Light from a single source illuminates two adjacent sites on the sensor, one of which is a reference site coated with nonreactive antibodies that are unable to bind the target analyte but are otherwise identical to the specific antibodies on the measurement site. The reader collects light reflected from both sites simultaneously and calculates the measurement shift which is automatically corrected for nonspecific binding by subtraction of the reference SPR shifts. In addition to the practical advantage of eliminating fluid exchanges and wash steps, simultaneous readings of the reference and measurement signals cancel out time-dependent and transient variations in the optics and electronics (further information from Quantech Ltd, http://www.biosensor.com). EBI Sensors Inc. (2333 West Crokett, Seattle, Washington 98199, USA, recently bought by Pharmacia Biosensor AB) are developing a fibre-optic SPR biosensor called SPR FiberProbe™, which enables remote sensing with the additional advantages of sensor multiplexing, dip-probe and *in situ* sensing. This sensor comprises a multimode optical fibre with a thin layer of gold deposited on a short piece of exposed optical fibre core, having undisclosed underlayer and overlayer films. At the distal end of the fibre there is a mirror that reflects the light back down the fibre for subsequent detection of the attenuated light at a specific frequency related to the binding events occurring at the surface of the sensor. The sensitivity of this instrument is lower than that of the previously described sensors.

Sensor	Mode of operation	Fluidics	Dynamic detection range
IAsys™	Resonant mirror waveguide (prism coupled)	Stirred cuvette	$10^{-3} - 10^{-12}$ mol l^{-1}
BIAcore™	SPR (prism coupled)	Microfluidics (flow)	$10^{-3} - 10^{-11}$ mol l^{-1}
BIOS-1™	Resonant mirror waveguide (grating coupled)	Flow-injection	$10^{-3} - 10^{-9}$ mol l^{-1}
Lambda™	SPR (grating coupled)	–	–
IBIS™	SPR (prism coupled)	Microfluidics (flow) and cuvette	–
SPR FiberProbe™	SPR fibre optic	Dip into sample	–

Table 1 A summary of the differences between immunosensors.

Table 1 summarises the differences between the commercially available sensors and those sensors soon to be available that can be used as immunosensors.

RELATIVE SENSITIVITIES OF THE IMMUNOSENSORS

Based on technical specifications, BIAcore™ has a dynamic concentration range for measurement of 10^{-3}–10^{-10} mol l^{-1}, and there is one report of detection for antibody binding of 10 pM (10^{-11} mol l^{-1}) (Davies *et al.*, 1994). Another report cites a measured affinity constant of 1.6×10^4 l mol^{-1} for a monoclonal antibody against maltose (Pharmacia Biosensor AB, 1996). IAsys™ has a dynamic range for concentration detection of 10^{-3}–10^{-12} mol l^{-1} (Clarke, 1991) and BIOS-1™ is reported to have lower sensitivity of around 1–10 nmol l^{-1} (10^{-9} mol l^{-1}) (Plowman *et al.*, 1996).

A differential interferometric affinity sensor has a detection limit of 200 fmol l^{-1} (10^{-13} mol l^{-1}), whereas a Mach-Zehnder interferometer has been reported to have a limit of 100 pmol l^{-1} (10^{-10} mol l^{-1}) (Plowman *et al.*, 1996). Using a fluoresently labelled analyte, the detection limit has been reduced to a few femtomoles (10^{-15} mol l^{-1}) by using an optical fibre tapered loop (Hale *et al.*, 1996) and a channel-etched thin film waveguide (Schipper *et al.*, 1996).

Acoustic Love plate immunosensors have an equivalent sensitivity to both IAsys™ and BIOS-1 optical systems with a detection limit of 10 µg ml^{-1} IgG (~8 nmol l^{-1}) (Gizelli *et al.*, 1991). Using acoustic sensors such as QCM (quartz crystal microbalance) and SAW (surface acoustic wave) devices, where the surface has to be dried before measuring, the detection limit is closer to 10 ng ml^{-1} for antibodies (~8 pmol l^{-1}) and 1 ng ml^{-1} for insulin (Gizelli and Lowe, 1996). However, there is still much work required in acoustic sensors to make them as reliable as optical systems and, they have yet to be developed into commercial systems with fluid and data handling and disposable, reproducible devices.

APPLICATIONS

Immunosensors can provide information on the kinetic interactions of antibodies and antigens more rapidly and simply than traditional methods such as radioimmunoassay, fluorescence spectroscopy, enzyme-linked immunosorbent assay (ELISA), equilibrium dialysis, stopped-flow photometry and chromatography. Their versatility, speed, ease of use and ability to use impure samples containing small amounts of analyte should facilitate their increasing acceptance to complement or even replace some of the traditional techniques.

Biological (bioanalytical) applications of surface plasmon resonance have been extensively explored by various groups (Liedberg *et al.*, 1983; ; Flanagan and Pantell, 1984; Cullen *et al.*, 1987; Daniels *et al.*, 1988; Kooyman *et al.*, 1988; Mayo and Hallock, 1989; Cullen and Lowe, 1990; Fontana *et al.*, 1990; Karlsson *et al.*, 1991; Vancott *et al.*, 1992). The main applications for SPR are detection of antigen-antibody interactions in the development of biosensors and immunosensors and epitope mapping of monoclonal antibodies (Johne *et al.*, 1993). Other applications include the surface plasmon microscope (Rothenhausler and Knoll, 1988; Hickel and Knoll, 1990) and surface plasmon immunoassay of dinitrophenyl and keyhole limpet haemocyanin antibodies in blood serum samples (Karlsson *et al.*, 1991).

Immunosensors provide kinetic information on the interaction of an antibody with its complementary antigen, which is likely to have clinical relevance in a number of conditions. It takes only a few seconds before it is apparent whether an analyte is present and a few minutes later reliable concentration data are available. In this section, specific examples of applications of immunosensors will be cited in order to illustrate the potential of such devices.

Specificity, affinity and rate of binding determine the suitability of an antibody for a particular application. Antibody design is a highly active research area. Aims of the antibody design are to improve affinity for the target molecule and to prepare chimeric antibodies (genetically grafting binding sites from antibodies of other species onto human antibodies) in order to eliminate immunorecognition and rejection. Antibody fragments have recently been prepared which demonstrate acceptable affinities. These are expected to have greater tissue penetrative power and hence enhanced therapeutic and diagnostic efficacy. Immunosensors can be used to determine the relative suitability of the antibody or fragment for a particular application.

IAsys™ has been used for the quantitative determination of the relative binding strengths and rate constants of Staphylococcal protein A (SpA) to different species and subclasses of immunoglobulins (Affinity Sensors, 1994a; Yeung *et al.*, 1995). SpA was first immobilised to the sensor surface, and the binding of different IgG species observed for 40 minutes. After washing with buffer, dissociation could also be observed. IgG was completely removed and the sensor surface regenerated ready for further applications of different IgG solutions at the same concentration. Thus, the relative binding strengths of each IgG were obtained using one sensor cuvette, by measuring the change in resonance angle after a constant time.

IAsys™ has also been used to measure the circulating levels of human anti-mouse antibodies (HAMA) in patients with neoplastic disease who had been treated with a murine monoclonal antibody (Fattinger *et al.*, 1994; Affinity Sensors, 1994d). Inhibition assays were performed and the degree of binding of HAMA to an immobilised human milk fat globule 1 (HMFG1) IgG was used to determine the epitopes recognised by HAMA. The average affinity of the polyclonal HAMA was also estimated using inhibition assays, with preincubation with a range of concentrations of free HMFG1. The estimated average dissociation equilibrium constant is given by the concentration required to block 50% of the binding of the antisera. It is possible to screen sera rapidly to determine if levels of circulating HAMA are low enough to consider continued antibody therapy. The specificity and average affinity of these antibodies was also measured. This application is of importance not only for tumour immunotherapy, but for the treatment of allograft rejection with anti-CD3 and other antibodies. The approach could be readily adaptable to any condition where the antigen is available: the qualitative information obtained on antibody affinity and kinetics may have important clinical implications.

Determination of antibody affinities is important in a number of circumstances. For example, measurement of the affinity of anti-viral antibodies against rubella, cytomegalovirus and human herpes virus-6 has been used to distinguish primary infections (which generate low-affinity antibodies) from secondary or chronic infection (which are associated with high-affinity antibodies). In addition, high-affinity autoantibodies are probably more pathogenic than their low-affinity counterparts. Evidence for this can be found in systemic lupus erythematosus and vasculitis, where levels of high-affinity antibodies against double-stranded DNA or nuclear antigens correlate more closely with disease activity than circulatory levels of low-affinity antibodies. Most clinical assays for measuring the affinity of antibodies in serum require the use of high concentrations of denaturing agents, such as urea or diethylamine, to inhibit the binding of so-called 'low-avidity' antibodies. Alternatively, in the case of anti-DNA antibodies, immune complexes formed between the antibodies and DNA are precipitated with polyethylene glycol (PEG assay) or ammonium sulphate (Farr assay). In the PEG assay, both high- and low-affinity antibodies are measured; the Farr assay detects only high-affinity antibodies. These assays, although clinically useful, are crude and nonquantitative, and it is likely that, as measurement of antibody affinity is simplified, correlations between antibody affinity and disease status will be found (George *et al.*, 1995).

Haptens (analytes of low molecular mass) cannot usually be detected in a direct binding immunoassay because the change in refractive index or thickness is too low. There are several techniques that the immunologists can use to amplify the signal, such as competitive inhibition or the use of enhancer particles. In order to detect haptens such as theophylline, a competitive inhibition assay format has been used. This involves competition between a theophylline–IgG conjugate and free theophylline in solution binding to an immobilised anti-theophylline antibody. An immobilised antibody such as anti-IgG binds an IgG macromolecule directly. Alternatively, further enhancement can be achieved by using a sandwich assay format for non-hapten antigens, where a third layer of anti-IgG is bound to an already captured antigen. This method significantly improves the sensitivity of immunoassays for macromolecules but not generally for haptens because of the lack of sufficient antigenic sites. An alternative method for enhancement of sensitivity is by the use of enhancer particles. Enhancer particles are around 5–100 nm in diameter and are prepared from materials having a refractive index greater than 2. Colloidal gold particles are an example of such a material and they can be easily attached to biomolecules. Detection of HSA bound to 30 nm gold particles showed a thousand-fold enhancement in sensitivity over detection of HSA free in solution, when binding to an immobilised anti-HSA antibody (Buckle *et al.*, 1993).

Immunosensors can also be applied to the detection of whole cells. *Staphylococcus aureus*, which expresses protein A at its surface, may be detected by binding to immobilised hIgG (Watts *et al.*, 1994). IgG is immobilised to a surface activated with aminosilane via a glutaraldehyde linker. The system could detect a cell concentration of 8×10^6 cells per ml. Sensitivity was increased to 8×10^3 cells per ml by using colloidal-gold-conjugated IgG in a sandwich assay format. The sandwich assay was demonstrated for *S. aureus* detection in milk. This approach could be used in the detection and the study of cell surface antigens and receptor proteins for cell types ranging from mammalian cells to bacteria and even viruses. For example, binding of cells carrying the cell surface expressed carcinoembryonic antigen (CEA) to surface-immobilised anti-CEA has been shown (Affinity Sensors Ltd, 1994c). CEA has been identified as one of the most useful tumour markers and was detected at concentrations of between 2×10^4 and 5×10^5 cells per ml. L cells expressing CEA typically showed response curves three times higher than those for L cells not expressing CEA.

Fermentation monitoring is another application readily accessible to immunosensors. Fermentation of microorganisms and cells for the production of recombinant proteins is of increasing importance especially in the biopharmaceutical industry. Rapid analysis or quantification of the bioproduct of interest during fermentation would be of considerable benefit by enabling fine-tuning of the bioprocess. Recombinant Fv fragments, derived from the monoclonal anti-hen egg lysozyme antibody D1.3, produced by periplasmic secretion in *Escherichia coli* fermentation broths have been monitored by IAsys™. To demonstrate the application of immunosensors for rapid fermentation monitoring, samples were removed from the broth and centrifuged (11,600*g* for 5 minutes) to remove particulates, and the supernatant was applied to the sensor surface for 3 minutes before surface regeneration. The data were analysed for concentration in two ways: absolute change in response after 3 minutes, and determination of the initial binding rate by linear regression after fitting data from the first 30 seconds. Both methods produced similar results, indicating that a 30-second assay time, in this case, is adequate for 'at line' monitoring (Affinity Sensors Ltd, 1994b).

Sensitivity enhancement of optical immunosensors can be achieved by the use of surface plasmon resonance fluoroimmunoassay, where the use of fluorescently labelled antigen is used either directly or in a competitive immunoassay format (Attridge *et al.*, 1991; Domenici *et al.*, 1995; Feldman *et al.*, 1995; Hale *et al.*, 1996; Plowman *et al.*, 1996).

OUTLOOK

It is evident that in the past five years significant progress has been made in both the understanding of immunosensors and their commercial exploitation. There are still many hurdles ahead before immunosensors fulfil the expectations of 10 years ago. Although researchers will continue to devise new sensing methods per se, many of the existing devices must be developed and improved upon by developments in associated technologies. For example, there is a significant amount of research needed to develop new surface chemistries, to design new fluidics/mechanisms to improve the transport of the antigen/antibody to the binding surface during association (and away from the surface during the measurement of dissociation rates), and to increase the sample throughput by using more rapid or multi analyte systems.

One of the major requirements is to develop immunosensors with the ability to monitor directly low concentrations of haptens/small molecules in the absence of labels. Further challenges include the need to understand more fully the interaction kinetics of antibodies and antigens on surfaces, and how these may be correlated with solution-based analyses especially where the final application of screened antibodies, for example, is in solution.

Finally, although there are some limitations in sensitivity, throughput and surface chemistries compared to conventional assay systems, the range of potential applications on the current devices is limited only by the imagination of the user and perhaps, based on current prices, by the size of their budget. Instrument costs will certainly be observed with interest as more systems are developed into products.

ACKNOWLEDGEMENTS

We gratefully acknowledge the assistance of Peter Lowe of Affinity Sensors in discussions on IAsys™ and immunosensors in general.

REFERENCES

Affinity Sensors Ltd. (1994a) Molecular Recognition: Species and subclass specificity of Staphylococcal protein A (SpA) for immunoglobulins. IAsys™ *Application Note 3.1.*

Affinity Sensors Ltd. (1994b) Fermentation monitoring: Recombinant antibody fragment quantification in fermentation broths. IAsys™ *Application Note 4.1.*

Affinity Sensors Ltd. (1994c) Receptor-Cell Interactions: Binding of L cells bearing the CEA antigen to an immobilized anti-CEA antibody. IAsys™ *Application Note 5.2.*

Affinity Sensors Ltd. (1994d) Clinical Analysis: Characterization of human anti-mouse antibodies (HAMA) in serum from a patient underoing radioimmunotherapy. IAsys™ *Application Note 6.1.*

Altschuh, D., Dubs, M. C., Weiss, E. *et al.* (1992) Determination of kinetic constants for the interaction between a monoclonal-antibody and peptides using surface-plasmon resonance. *Biochemistry*, **31**, 6298–6304.

Attridge, J. W., Daniels, P. B., Deacon, J. K. *et al.* (1991) Sensitivity enhancement of optical immunosensors by the use of a surface-plasmon resonance fluoroimmunoassay. *Biosens. Bioelectron.* **6**, 201–214.

Auge, J., Hauptman, P., Eichelbaum, F. *et al.* (1994) Quartz crystal microbalance sensor in liquids. *Sens. Actuators B* **19**, 518–522

Bodenhöfer, K., (1995) Comparison of mass sensitive devices for gas sensing: Bulk acoustic wave (BAW) and surface acoustic wave (SAW) transducers. In: *Proc. Transducers 95* **2**, 728–731

Brecht, A. & Gauglitz, G. (1995) Optical probes and transducers. *Biosens. Bioelectron.* **10**, 923–936.

Buckle, P. E., Davies, R. J., Kinning, T. *et al.* (1993) The resonant mirror: A novel optical sensor for direct sensing of biomolecular interactions Part II: Applications. *Biosens. Bioelectron.* **8**, 395–363.

Chaiken, I., Rose, S. & Karlsson, R. (1992) Quantitative-analysis of protein-interaction with ligands 2. Analysis of macromolecular interactions using immobilized ligands. *Anal. Biochem.* **201** 197–210.

Chandler G. K., Dodgson J. R. & Eddowes M. J. (1990) An isfet-based flow-injection analysis system for determination of urea: Experiment and theory. *Sens. Actuators. B-Chem.* **1**, 433–437.

Clark, D. J., Blake-Coleman, B. C. & Calder, M. R., (1987) Principles and potential of piezoelectric transducers and acoustical techniques. In: *Biosensors: Fundamentals and Applications* (eds Turner, A. P. F., Karube, I. & Wilso, G. S.) pp. 551–571 (Oxford Science Publications, Oxford)

Clarke, R. J. (1991) Binding and diffusion kinetics of the interaction of a hydrophobic potential-sensitive dye with lipid vesicles. *Biophys. Chem.* **39**, 91–106.

Cornelius R. M., Wojciechowski P. W. & Brash J. L., (1992) Measurement of protein adsorption-kinetics by an *in situ*, real-time, solution depletion technique. *J. Coll. Interf. Sci.* **150**, 121–133.

Cullen, D. C., Brown, R. G. W. & Lowe, C. R. (1987) Detection of immuno-complex formation via surface-plasmon resonance on gold-coated diffraction gratings. *Biosensors* **3**, 211–225.

Cullen, D. C. & Lowe, C. R. (1990) A direct surface-plasmon polariton immunosensor: Preliminary investigation of the nonspecific adsorption of serum components to the sensor interface. *Sens. Act. B-Chem.* **1**, 576–579.

Daniels, P. B., Deacon, J. K., Eddowes, M. *et al.* (1988) Surface-plasmon resonance applied to immunosensing. *Sens. Actuat.* **15**, 11–18.

Davies, R. J., Edwards, P. R. & Watts, H. J. (1994) The resonant mirror: A versatile tool for the study of biomolecular interactions. *Tech. Protein Chem.* V, 285–292.

Dean, P. D. G., Johnson, W. S. & Middle, F. A. (1985) *Affinity Chromatography: A Practical Approach* (IRL Press, Oxford).

Debono, R. F., Krull, U. J. & Rounaghi G. (1992) Concanavalin-A and polysaccharide on gold surfaces. Study using surface-plasmon resonance techniques. *ACS Symp. Ser.* **511**, 121–136.

Domenici, C., Schirone, A., Celebre, M. *et al.* (1995) Development of a TIRF immunosensor: Modelling the equilibrium behaviour of a competitive system. *Biosens. Bioelectron.* **10**, 371–378.

Eddowes, M. J. (1987) Direct immunochemical sensing: Basic chemical principles and fundamental limitations. *Biosensors* **3**, 1–15.

Edwards, P. R., Gill, A., Pollard-Knight, D. V. *et al.* (1995) Kinetics of protein-protein interactions at the surface of an optical biosensor. *Anal. Biochem.* **231**, 210–217.

Fägerstam, L. G., Frostellkarlsson, A., Karlsson, R. *et al.* (1992) Biospecific interaction analysis using surface-plasmon resonance detection applied to kinetic, binding-site and concentration analysis. *J. Chromatogr.* **597**, 397–410.

Fägerstam, L. G. & O'Shannessy, D. J. (1993) Surface plasmon resonance detection in affinity techniques. BIAcore. In: *Handbook of Affinity Chromatography* (ed. Kline, T.) pp. 229–252 (Marcel Dekker, New York).

Fattinger, Ch., Mangold, C., Heming, M. *et al.* (1994) Affinity sensing using ultracompact wave guiding films. In: *Biosensors 94 Abstracts* The Third World Congress on Biosensors (Elsevier Science, Oxford).

Feldman, S. F., Uzigiris, E. E., Penney, C. M. *et al.* (1995) Evanescent wave immunoprobe with high bivalent antibody activity. *Biosens. Bioelectron.* **10**, 423–434.

Flanagan, M. T. & Pantell, R. H. (1984) Surface-plasmon resonance and immunosensors. *Electron. Lett.* **20**, 968–970.

Fontana, E., Pantell, R. H. & Strober, S. (1990) Surface-plasmon immunoassay. *Appl. Optics* **29**, 4694–4704.

Gao, H., Sanger, M., Luginbul, R. *et al.* (1995) Immunosensing with photo-immobilised immunoreagents on planar optical waveguides. *Biosens. Bioelectron.* **10**, 317–328.

George, A. J. T., Danga, R., Gooden, C. S. R. *et al.* (1995) Quantitative and qualitative detection of serum antibodies using a resonant mirror biosensor. *Tumor Targeting* **1**, 245–250.

Gizelli, E., Goddard, N. J., Stevenson, A. C. *et al.* (1992) A Love plate biosensor utilising a polymer layer. *Sens. Actuators B* **6**, 131–137.

Gizelli, E. & Lowe, C. R. (1996) Immunosensors. *Curr. Opin. Biotechnol.* (in the press).

Gizelli, E., Stevenson, A. C., Goddard, N. J. *et al.* (1991) Surface skimming bulk waves: A novel approach to acoustic biosensors. In: *Proc. Int. Conf. Solid-state Sensors and Actuators*, San Francisco, pp. 690–692 (Associated Business Publishers, NSW).

Groman, E. V. & Wilchek, M. (1987) Recent developments in affinity-chromatography supports. *Trends Biotechnol.* **5**, 220–224.

Hale, Z. M., Payne, F. P., Marks, R. S. *et al.* (1996) The single mode tapered optical fibre loop immunosensor. *Biosens. Bioelectron.* **11**, 137–148.

Hermanson, G. T., Mallia, A. K. & Smith, P. K. (1992) *Pragmatic Affinity, Immobilised Affinity Ligand Techniques* (Academic Press, London).

Hickel, W. & Knoll, W. (1990) Surface-plasmon microscopy of lipid layers. *Thin Solid Films* **187**, 349–396.

Hodgson, J. (1994) Light, angles, action: Instruments for label-free, real-time monitoring of intermolecular interactions. *Bio/technology* **12**, 31–39.

Intersens Instruments (1995) *IBIS Announcement Sheet* (February 1995). More information obtained from: Intersens Instruments Tel: +31 33 472 6664.

Johne, B., Gadnell, M. & Hansen, K. (1993) Epitope mapping and binding-kinetics of monoclonal-antibodies studied by real-time biospecific interaction analysis using surface-plasmon resonance. *J. Immunol. Meth.* **160**, 191–198.

Jonsson, U., Fägerstam, L., Ivarsson, B. *et al.* (1991) Real-time biospecific interaction analysis using surface-plasmon resonance and a sensor chip technology. *Biotechniques* **11**, 620.

Jonsson, U., Fägerstam, L., Löfås, S. *et al.* (1993) Introducing a biosensor based technology for real-time biospecific interaction analysis. *Ann. Biol. Clin.* **51**, 19–26.

Jonsson, U., Malmqvist, M., Olofsson, G. *et al.* (1988) Surface immobilization techniques in combination with ellipsometry. *Meth. Enzymol.* **137**, 381–388.

Jorgenson, R. C. & Yee, S. S. (1994) Control of the dynamic range and sensitivity of a surface plasmon resonance based fiber optic sensor. *Sens. Actuatators.* **43**, 44–48.

Karlsson, R., (1992) Biospecific interaction analysis using surface-plasmon resonance detection: Mapping of binding-sites on igf-ii and kinetic-analysis of the interaction of igf-ii with igfbp-1 and the igf-ii receptor. *Fresenius J. Anal. Chem.* **343**, 100–101.

Karlsson, R., Michaelsson, A. & Mattsson, L. (1991) Kinetic-analysis of monoclonal antibody-antigen interactions with a new biosensor based analytical system. *J. Immunol. Meth.* **145**, 229–240.

Kooyman, R. P. H., Kolkman, H., Vangent, J. *et al.* (1988) Surface-plasmon resonance immunosensors: Sensitivity considerations. *Analytica Chim. Acta* **213**, 39–45.

Kosslinger, C., Drost, S., Aberl, F. *et al.* (1992) A quartz crystal biosensor for measurement in liquids. *Biosen. Bioelect.* **7**, 397–404.

Krull U. J., Debono R. F., Helluly A. *et al.* (1991) Applications of surface-plasmon resonance techniques: Imaging of chemically selective surfaces and amplification of fluorescence transduction techniques. *Abstr. Am. Chem. Soc.* **201**, 63.

Lawrence, C. R., Geddes, N. J., Furlong, D. N. *et al.* (1996) Surface plasmon resonance studies of immunoreactions utilizing disposable diffraction gratings. *Biosens. Bioelectron.* **11**, 389–400.

Liedberg, B., Nylander, C. & Lundstrom, I. (1983) Surface-plasmon resonance for gas-detection and biosensing. *Sens. Actuators* **4**, 299–304.

Löfås S., Johnson, B., Edstrom, A. *et al.* (1995) Methods for site controlled coupling to carboxymethyldextran surfaces in surface plasmon resonance sensors. *Biosens. Bioelectron.* **10**, 813–822.

Lok B. K., Cheng Y. L. & Robertson, C. R. (1983a) Total internal-reflection fluorescence: A technique for examining interactions of macromolecules with solid-surfaces. *J. Coll. Interf. Sci.* **91**, 87–103.

Lok B. K., Cheng Y. L. & Robertson C. R., (1983b) Protein adsorption on crosslinked polydimethylsiloxane using total internal-reflection fluorescence. *J. Coll. Interf. Sci.* **91**, 104–116.

Lowe, C. R. & Dean, P. D. G. (1974). *Affinity Chromatography* (John Wiley and Sons, London)

Lowe, C. R. & Dean, P. D. G. (1979). *Affinity Chromatography* (John Wiley and Sons, London)

Lukosz, W. (1991) Principles and sensitivities of integrated optical and surface-plasmon sensors for direct affinity sensing and immunosensing. *Biosens. Bioelectron.* **6**, 215–225.

Malmqvist, M. (1993) Biospecific interaction analysis using biosensor technology. *Nature* **361**, 186–187.

Markey, F. (1995) Interpreting kinetic data. *BIA J.* **2**, 118–119.

Martensson, J., Arwin, H., Lundstrom, I. *et al.* (1993) Adsorption of lactoperoxidase on hydrophilic and hydrophobic silicon dioxide surfaces: An ellipsometric study. *J. Coll. Interf. Sci.* **155**, 30–36.

Mayo, C. S. & Hallock, R. B. (1989) Immunoassay based on surface-plasmon oscillations. *J. Immunol. Meth.*, **120**, 105–114.

Meyer, E. (1992) Atomic force microscopy. *Prog. Surs. Sci.* **41**, 3–49.

Noy, N., Leonard, M. & Zakim, D. (1992) The kinetics of interactions of bilirubin with lipid bilayers and with serum-albumin. *Biophys. Chem.* **42**, 177–188.

Pearce K. H., Hiskey R. G. & Thompson N. L., (1992) Surface binding-kinetics of prothrombin fragment-1 on planar membranes measured by total internal-reflection fluorescence microscopy. *Biochemistry* **31**, 5983–5995.

Pennisi, E. (1991) Quirk in antibody action yields cheap assay. *Science News* **139**, 263.

Pharmacia Biosensor AB (1994). *BIAcore 2000 Announcement Notes.*

Pharmacia Biosensor AB (1996). *BIA J.* **3**, 6.

Plowman, T. E., Reichert, W. M., Peters, C. R. *et al.* (1996) Femtomolar sensitivity using a channel-etched thin film waveguide fluoroimmunosensor. *Biosens. Bioelectron.* **11**, 149–160.

Pockrand, I. (1978) Surface plasma oscillations at silver surfaces with thin transparent and absorbing coatings. *Surface Sci.* **72**, 577–588.

Quantech Ltd. Internet address. http://www.biosensor.com/

Rothenhausler, B. & Knoll, W. (1988) Surface-plasmon microscopy. *Nature*, **332**, 615–617.

Ruzgas, T. A., Razumas, V. J. & Kulys, J. J. (1992a). Ellipsometric immunosensors for the determination of gamma-interferon and human serum-albumin. *Biosen. Bioelectron* **7**, 305–308.

Ruzgas, T. A., Razumas, V. J. & Kulys, J. J. (1992b). Ellipsometric study of antigen-antibody interaction at the interface solid-solution. *Biofizika* **37**, 56–61.

Sadana, A. & Beelaram, A. M. (1995) Antigen-antibody diffusion-limited binding kinetics of biosensors: A fractal analysis. *Biosens. Bioelectron.* **10**, 301–316.

Sadana, A. & Chen, Z. (1996) Influence of non-specific binding on antigen-antibody binding kinetics for biosensor applications. *Biosens. Bioelectron.* **11**, 17–33.

Schasfoort, R. B. M., Severs, A. H. & van der Gaag, A. (1994) Coating of SPR based affinity sensors with immuno activated latex and regeneration strategies. In: *Biosensors 94 Abstracts* The Third World Congress on Biosensors (Elsevier Science, Oxford).

Schipper, E. F., Kooyman, R. P. H., Borreman, A. *et al.* (1996) The critical sensor: A new type of evanescent wave immunosensor. *Biosens. Bioelectron.* **11**, 295–304.

Scouten, W. H. (1980) Affinity chromatography. In: *Bioselective Adsorption on Inert Matrices* (John Wiley and Sons, New York).

Sjolander, S. & Urbaniczky, C. (1991) Integrated fluid handling-system for biomolecular interaction analysis. *Anal. Chem.* **63**, 2338–2345.

Stevenson, A. C., Gizelli, E., Goddard, N. J. *et al.* (1992). A novel Love-plate sensor utilising polymer overlayers. *Inst. Elect. Electron. Engrs Trans. Ultrasonics Ferroelect. Freq. Cont.* **39**, 657–659.

Stevenson, A. C., Gizelli, E., Goddard N. J. *et al.* (1993). Acoustic Love plate sensors: A theoretical model for the optimization of the surface mass sensitivity. *Sens. Actuators B* **13–14**, 639–637.

Sutherland, R. & Dähne, C. (1987) IRS devices for optical immunoassay. In: *Biosensors: Fundamentals and Applications* (eds Turner, A. P. F., Karube, I., & Wilson, G. S.) pp. 655–678 (Oxford Science Publications, Oxford).

Vancott, T. C., Loomis, L. D., Redfield, R. R. *et al.* (1992) Real-time biospecific interaction analysis of antibody reactivity to peptides from the envelope glycoprotein, gp160, of hiv–1. *J. Immunol. Meth.* **146**, 163–176.

Watts, H. J., Lowe, C. R. & Pollard-Knight, D. V. (1994) Optical biosensor for monitoring microbial cells. *Anal. Chem.* **66**, 2465–2470.

Yeung, D., Gill, A., Maule, C. H. *et al.* (1995) Detection and quantification of biomolecular interactions with optical biosensors. *Trends Anal. Chem.* **14**, 49–56.

You, H. X., Lin, S. & Lowe, C. R. (1995) A scanning tunneling microscope study of site specifically immobilised immunoglobulin G on gold. *Micron* **26**, 311–315.

Chapter 21

Single-layer and Multilayer Thin-film Immunoassays

Susan J. Danielson and David A. Hilborn

INTRODUCTION

Single-layer and multilayer immunoassays refer to devices that contain most or all of the reagents required to carry out a single immunoassay in a thin, unitised element (Berke, 1988). The dry-reagent chemistry technology utilised in these assays was first applied to traditional clinical chemistry analysis (Free *et al.*, 1957, 1960; Mazzaferri *et al.*, 1960; Curme *et al.*, 1978; Spayd *et al.*, 1978; Walter, 1983). Film-casting and lamination manufacturing techniques are typically used to prepare large areas of thin films which are subsequently cut into individual elements. The application of the unknown sample to the element rehydrates the dried reagents and initiates the immunoreactions needed for the measurement of the analyte. Sample application may be preceded by the addition of reagents to the sample or it may be followed by the addition of small volumes of other reagents to the element. After an incubation period the reaction product is measured, usually by either reflectance densitometry or front-face fluorometry.

CHARACTERISTICS OF SINGLE-LAYER AND MULTILAYER FILM IMMUNOASSAYS

There are several distinguishing characteristics of single-layer and multilayer immunoassays (also called thin-film immunoassays). One characteristic is that usually a single analyte concentration from a sample can be determined on one element. The elements are small (<1 mm thick and 1–5 cm^2 surface area). This permits many elements to be packaged together for the analysis of multiple samples, for calibration, and for quality control. These elements are dry (solvents used in the manufacturing process have been removed). Finally, very specific detection instrumentation is generally required to read optimally the result of an individual element.

It is the above characteristics that have caused the single- and multilayer immunoassays to be the almost exclusive domain of commercial producers of immunoassay systems. Because the elements are self-contained, they are useful only if they are produced in large, uniform quantities so that users are confident that the signal produced during calibration accurately represents the signals on elements to which unknown samples are applied. Precisely controlled specialised manufacturing processes are used to ensure reagents are incorporated into all elements in very accurate and precise amounts. Additionally, the engineering of specialised photometric instrumentation is only economically justifiable if large quantities of the elements are to be used.

For the same reasons, dry single- and multilayer immunoassays are ideal both for large volume users and for dispersed testing sites. The fact that each element contains most or all of the reagents in the exact amounts required for the determination of an analyte eliminates the need to prepare reagents and reduces the waste due to unused materials. Because the elements are dry, shelf-life is usually longer than for liquid reagents. Unitisation of the elements permits the design of instruments that can process large quantities of samples in either batch or random access mode, or the design of small instruments that can process single samples that can be used at dispersed test sites. These instruments incorporate the specific detection systems required to read the signal produced by each element and the data systems required for calibration, quality control and sample predictions. Because the elements can be used in large quantities, manufacturers are willing to invest in the manufacturing processes and instrumental design required to support use of this type of immunoassay. A disadvantage to the end-user is the inflexibility of these systems. It is difficult for users to change any features of the systems to meet their specific needs or to develop tests for analytes not covered by the manufacturer.

In this chapter we present the basic features of single- and multilayer immunoassays. Topics include descriptions of the functional 'zones' common to these immunoassays, the processes used to create these zones, some constraints on immunoassays in thin films, detection methods, and specific examples of the embodiment of these assays. Unique materials and processes that have enabled the successful adaptation of immunoassays to these elements are discussed. We are assuming that the reader is familiar with the basic characteristics of immunoassays (e.g. homogeneous and heterogeneous methods, competitive and sandwich mechanisms, enzyme-linked immunosorbent assay (ELISA), etc.) that have been covered in previous chapters.

FUNCTIONAL ZONES

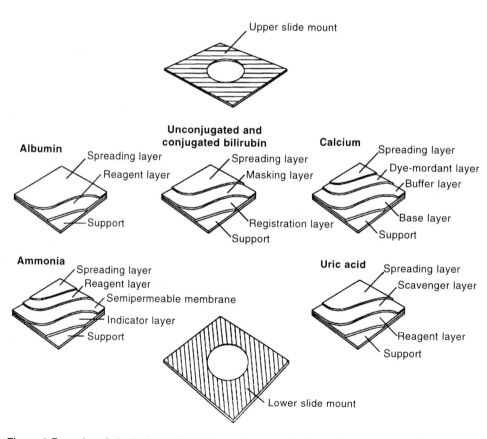

Figure 1 Examples of physical and chemical reaction layers that have been incorporated into Johnson & Johnson Clinical Diagnostics VITROS thin-film elements.

Single- and multilayer elements are small. Nevertheless, several distinct functional zones are contained within the thin vertical dimension (<1 mm) of most elements. These zones may be constructed out of individual layers or be combined into one layer during the manufacturing of an element. Although many specific functional names have been used to describe these zones (see Figure 1), for the purposes of this chapter the zones will be described as having either a support, an analytical, a reflective, or a spreading function (Walter, 1988).

Support Zone

The support zone provides structural integrity for the other zones. It is typically a thin film of transparent plastic (e.g. polyethylene terphthalate) through which the detection radiation passes undisturbed and on which the other layers are coated or laminated.

Analytical Zone

The analytical zone contains reagents required to convert the analyte in the sample into a signal that can be measured by the detection instrumentation. This zone may contain antibodies and labels as well as buffers, dyes, coupling enzymes, stabilising agents, and any other reagent necessary to convert the analyte into a readable signal. The analytical zone can be placed on the support layer by either lamination processes or by thin-film coating processes.

Several separate specialised layers may together constitute an analytical zone. Specialised layers that have been described include capture layers which contain immobilised immunomaterials capable of binding other immunoreagents, detection or registration layers which contain signal-generating reagents, and reagent layers which produce intermediates in amounts proportional to that analyte concentration which subsequently diffuse to the detection layer. There are radiation-blocking layers which limit the depth of penetration of probing radiation in the element. These layers may contain ferric oxide, carbon black, or light-absorbing pigments.

Reflective Zone

The function of the reflective layer is to reflect any detection radiation that is not adsorbed by the signal-generating chemistry to the detector. Elements are too opaque for convenient optical transmission detection. Instead, refectance densitometry and front-face fluorometry are commonly used as the detection methods. In both these methods the source of the probing radiation and the detector for the signal radiation are on the same side of the immunoassay element. The reflective layer is positioned within the element to maximise the amount of signal reaching the detector. Pigments, such as TiO_2 or $BaSO_4$, or metal foils have been used in these layers.

Spreading Zone

The uppermost zone (the zone farthest away from the support layer) is the spreading zone, which functions to ensure that a sample spreads quickly and uniformly into the element. The ideal spreading layer allows a sample to enter rapidly (seconds) and spread so that the ratio of applied sample volume to occupied volume is a constant. In this way, the element provides a result that is independent of the applied sample volume.

Single- and Multilayer Elements

In single-layer elements, all the functional zones are in one layer. For example, filter paper that has been saturated with solutions containing all the reagents necessary for analyte detection can contain all four functional zones. The sample is applied to the filter paper and spreads (spreading zone). All reactions occur within the filter paper void volume (analytical zone). Probing radiation is applied to the sample spot and is returned to the detector (reflective zone). The paper is strong enough not to need any additional structural support (support layer). With multilayer immunoassays, the designers of the element can choose to integrate or separate the various functional zones into as many or as few layers as is necessary to optimise the assay. This versatility has led to many different commercial incarnations of thin-film immunoassays (which will be discussed later).

THIN-FILM CHARACTERISTICS AND CONSTRAINTS

Although the basic mechanisms for immunoreactions in single- and multilayer immunoassays are the same as those in solution, the matrix structure of these elements is quite different. These elements are thin and porous. Spreading and analytical layers are less than several hundred micrometres thick and are generally composed of materials whose pore sizes are under $50\mu m$.

Fluid Considerations

Fluid Spreading

Spreading zones enhance the entry of fluids into these porous structures. In their absence, an applied drop of fluid tends to form a bead which does not penetrate the surface of the element. Spreading zones work by counteracting the surface tension of the applied fluid and by providing a wettable capillary matrix into which the fluid is drawn by capillary forces (Berke, 1988). The result is that the applied fluid very rapidly enters the zone, spreads laterally, and is self-metered to a uniform sample volume per unit volume of the element. This provides a reservoir from which the underlying layers can obtain fluid (Figure 2). Liquid can be drawn into lower gel layers because the osmotic pressure of rehydration there greatly exceeds the capillary retention forces in the more porous spreading layer.

Fluid Volume Constraints

Sample volume is constrained by the size of the thin-film element. Berke (1988) has estimated that a 1-mm-thick-film with an 80% void volume and 1 cm² detection area leads to a maximum sample aliquot of 80 µl. In practice, the volumes applied are usually smaller.

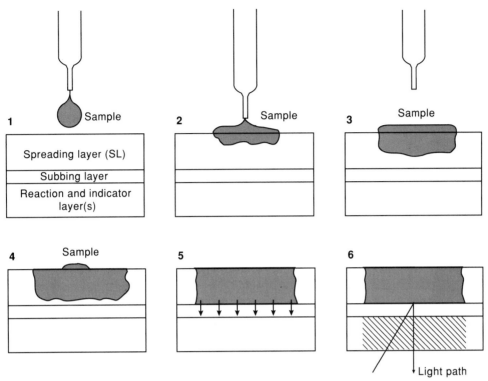

Figure 2 Sample spreading in a porous spreading layer. Reprinted with permission from Elsevier Science Inc. from T. Shirey (1983).

Diffusion Times

Berke (1988) has also estimated that the diffusion time for an IgG molecule traversing a 100µm thin film is 20 seconds. This estimate is based on the Einstein equation for Brownian motion and a diffusion coefficient for IgG of 5×10^{-7} cm^2 s^{-1}. However, diffusion distances are often less than this because capillary action draws the sample quickly throughout the spreading layer so that diffusion distances may be only those of the pore dimensions or interlayer dimensions. Thus, diffusion-controlled reactions occur quickly in thin films even in the absence of mixing, and consequently commercially developed thin-film immunoassays are rapid (usually under 10 minutes from sample application to final result).

Separation of Immunoreactive Materials

Generally, care must be taken in manufacturing to ensure that immunoreactive species, such as an antibody and an analyte label, do not react before application of the sample. If they do react, dissociation of this complex must occur before equilibrium is reached. This could lead to unacceptably long reaction times (greater than 30 minutes) because dissociation is usually a slow process. Several approaches have been developed to avoid this problem. For single-layer elements, multiple saturation steps using a succession of solvents are used that do not dissolve previously impregnated reagents (Rupchock *et al.*, 1985). For multilayer elements, a number

551

of techniques are available. Lamination allows preformed layers containing incompatible reagents to be integrated into a device without reactions occurring prematurely. Film-casting techniques can be used to build up successive layers of a multilayer element if appropriate solvent choices are made for each layer. Finally, low-wet laydown processes such as ink-jetting or gravure coating (Dappen *et al.*, 1992) have been used. These processes allow only a partial penetration of the applied material into an underlayer thereby physically separating the immunomaterials.

Homogeneous versus Heterogeneous Methods

The small size of the single- and multilayer elements suggests they are ideally suited for homogeneous immunoassays because there is no need for a bound/free separation step. In homogeneous assays, application of the liquid sample reconstitutes the reagents and initiates the binding reactions which in turn modulate the signal-generating reactions as a function of analyte concentration. The Bayer Corporation's (Elkhart, IN) ARIS system (Tyhach *et al.*, 1981) uses this methodology The adaptaton of heterogeneous immunoassays to thin films has required the development of specialised bound/free separation technology. Several commercial systems (Dade, Miami, FL (Geigel *et al.*, 1982); Johnson & Johnson Clinical Diagnostics, Rochester, NY (Danielson *et al.*, 1992); and Behring, Westwood, MA (Lehrer *et al.*, 1992)) have incorporated low-volume wash steps, made necessary by the limited device capacity, in their assay protocols. This is possible because the wash step is very efficient, a result of bulk fluid movement being the primary mode of molecular movement within the porous spreading layer as fluid is applied (Berke, 1988) and the small capillary structure within the spreading layer which directs fluid flow away from the point of application. Thus, unbound molecules are carried away in the direction of fluid flow from their immobilised counterparts . There is little or no difference in movement between high and low molecular mass materials. The spreading layer media must be either chosen or treated so the surface adsorption of any of the reagents, particularly those of high molecular mass, is minimised.

Analysis of High-concentration, High Molecular Mass Analytes

Many high molecular mass analytes that are present at high concentrations in serum (e.g. IgG, IgM, IgA) are measured by turbidimetric methods in solution assays. There is no comparable turbidimetric detection method currently available in thin films because of the scattering properties of the layers comprising these elements. Sandwich assays, which have been incorporated into thin films (Lehrer *et al.*, 1992; Wu *et al.*, 1994), offer an alternative approach for the analysis of this class of analytes. However, samples containing analytes at these high concentrations generally have to be substantially diluted before being applied to an element. This is because of the limitation on incorporation of suitable amounts of capture antibodies within the reaction zone of a thin-film necessary to obtain a sufficient reportable range and to avoid the high-dose hook effect (Fernando and Wilson, 1992). An alternative approach both to turbidimetric and to sandwich methods for these types of molecules has been described by Ashihara *et al.* (1991).

FABRICATION OF ANALYTICAL AND REFLECTIVE LAYERS

The analytical and reflective layers are prepared either by entrapping reagents (Liotta, 1984; Greenquist, 1989) into preformed porous matrices (saturation techniques) or by simultaneously forming the matrix and entrapping the reagents (film casting).

Saturation of Preformed Matrices

Saturation techniques are compatible with preformed porous matrices including paper, woven fabric and porous membranes made from a variety of materials. In this technique, the matrix is saturated with a solution of the desired reagents and then dried, leaving the reagents impregnated in the matrix. Additional reagents can be applied by repeating the saturation using solvents that do not dissolve the originally applied reagents. This approach allows construction of a single-layer element that contains reagents that otherwise might be incompatible (Greenquist *et al.*, 1984). The amount of reagents incorporated depends on the thickness and porosity of the matrix, on the concentration of the reagents in the saturating solution, and on the absorptivity of the solution by the matrix material. Several matrices can be laminated together to use this technique to form multilayer elements.

Entrapping Reagents Using Film-casting Techniques

Film-casting techniques have been developed by the photographic industry in which multi-layers, each serving a different physical or chemical function, are coated simultaneously using hopper coating technology. Discrete layers, in which component migration is minimised or eliminated, can be formed with the proper selection of materials for each layer, including solvent and dispersing medium.

Hopper Coating

Film-casting techniques for immunoassays must result in a water-insoluble but rehydratable layer that becomes porous once an aqueous sample is applied (Berke, 1988; Walter, 1988). These layers are prepared by a metered application of a viscous polymer solution through a slot-extrusion orifice (hopper) to underlayers that are moving past the orifice at a constant velocity. Drying occurs at a downstream location. Gelatin (denatured collagen) is a natural polymer which has been adapted for use in layer creation based on technology developed in the photographic industry. Other polymers that have been used include polyacrylamide, polyvinyl alcohol, hydroxypropyl methylcellulose, methylcellulose, polyvinyl acetate, agarose, alginate and carrageenan. Hydrophilic additives can be included in the coated liquid mixture to act as a solid diluent once the water is removed. These additives often make up the majority of the coating solution with the gelling polymer present only at a high enough concentration to generate a discrete layer. In addition, crosslinking agents may be added to the coating melt to increase the integrity of the cast layers.

The film porosity is directly dependent on water content and is controlled by such factors as the molecular mass of the polymer, the degree of crosslinking, and the concentration of the polymer in the casting medium. The quantities of reagents available during analysis are controlled by their concentration in the coating mixture, the thickness of the film wetted by the sample, and their solubility in the sample. The composition and thickness of the layers can be used to adjust reaction times to a certain degree. The primary mode of fluid transport in these layers is diffusion. Most gel media are not suitable for facilitating interaction of large molecules, such as high molecular mass analytes, antibodies and immune complexes because they are insufficiently porous at the levels of polymer required to maintain structural integrity of the coated layer.

Multilayer Coatings

The ability to produce coatings with multiple layers of different functionality creates interesting possibilities in designing immunoassays (and other assays as well). For example, in layered coatings, physical and chemical reactions can be physically separated (Shirey, 1983). The products of one reaction layer can proceed to another layer where subsequent reactions can occur. Each layer of a multilayer coating can provide a unique environment that makes possible reactions comparable to those occurring in solution as well as reactions that would not be possible in solution. Interferents can be left behind, altered or inactivated in upper layers. Reactions or signals can be enhanced by optimising the chemical environment in the appropriate layer. This layered format makes possible a multistep sequence of reactions with no operator involvement or expensive automation.

SPREADING LAYERS

The sample is applied to the spreading layer which is designed to allow rapid and uniform sample entry into its porous matrix. Although bulk fluid transfer is the main mode of molecular movement in this zone, reagents with binding functions can be immobilised within this layer to modulate the movement of some materials. Compositions of spreading layers range from filter paper to porous membranes to polymeric and particulate structures prepared by film-casting techniques. Novel spreading layers are important proprietary technologies of the companies that developed them and are usually protected from general usage by appropriate patents. The spreading-layer material is one of the distinguishing characteristics of a diagnostic company's thin-film elements.

Preformed Spreading Layers

Preformed spreading layers are those porous materials that have sufficient structural integrity to be produced and handled independently of a support layer or that serve as a support layer themselves. Filter paper (Rupchock *et al.*, 1985), glass-fibre matrices and woven fabric (Kitajima *et al.*, 1981a) are specific examples. Fluid dynamics within the pores of these materials are improved by impregnating them with wetting reagents using saturation or spraying techniques.

Fabric Spreading Layers

Kitajima *et al.* (1981a) have described a number of preformed fabric spreading layers prepared from both natural fibres (such as cotton, kapok, flax, hemp, silk) and synthetic fibres (viscose rayon, cupro-ammonium rayon, cellulose acetate). These fabrics are processed to introduce the desired degree of hydrophilicity by the incorporation of surfactants, wetting agents (e.g. glycerine or polyethylene glycol) or hydrophilic polymers (e.g. gelatin or polyvinyl alcohol). The proper level of reagent (usually from 0.1 to 10% per unit weight of fabric) for each fabric is determined experimentally. These fabric spreading layers are laminated to underlayers to create multilayer thin-film elements.

Additional reagents (e.g. for detection reactions) can also be impregnated into these fabric layers and, because the lamination process is not harsh, sensitive reagents can be included without loss of reactivity. The lamination process also prevents migration of reagents between the spreading layer and underlying layers prior to sample applications so that incompatible reagents remain separate. Adhesive layers, such as a hydrophilic polymer, can be used to strengthen the integrity of the laminated layers. Kitajima *et al.* (1981b) have described the production of a radiation blocking layer and a reflective layer by vacuum depositing a metal or metal alloy on the spreading fabric prior to lamination. The thickness of the deposited metal film layer is only about 5 to 50 Å. The layer is water permeable.

Plastic 'Spreader Grid'

Another preformed spreading zone is the plastic device used in the OPUS Immunoassay system (Behring). This device is described as a 'spreader grid' (Grenner, 1990) and is part of an injection-moulded plastic holder for the underlying thin film. It consists of multiple 100-µm-high pyramid-shaped projections which rise from a flat surface. When this structure is placed in contact with the top layer of the film, it results in a structure with a high degree of capillarity, thus achieving the same results as previously described spreading layers.

Film-cast Spreading Layers

Integral Blush Polymer Spreading Layer

The production of spreading layers by film-casting techniques was demonstrated in the early 1970s by Pryzbylowicz and Millikan (1976) of the Eastman Kodak Company. They were able to coat a polymer slurry over underlying reagent layers and form the spreading layer during the drying process. This resulted in the integral blush polymer spreading layer (Figure 3) that became the basis of the multilayer thin-film technology of Johnson & Johnson Clinical Diagnostics. This spreading layer is prepared by dissolving a nonswelling, water insoluble polymer, such as cellulose acetate, in a low-boiling solvent that is suitable for the polymer, such as acetone. A higher-boiling 'nonsolvent', such as toluene, which is a poor solvent for the polymer, is then added. This slurry is then coated onto the reagent layers and dried under controlled conditions. Following drying, an isotropically porous structure remains which is typically about 100 to 300 µm in thickness, with 60 to 90% void volume, and average pore sizes ranging from 1.5 to 3.0 µm. After incorporation of pigments such as TiO_2 or $BaSO_4$, these structures were found to have diffuse reflecting properties ideal for reflection densitometry. It was found that a variety of other materials could also be added to the formulation including carbon black for opacity, plasticisers to prevent cracking and surfactants to promote spreading (Pryzbylowicz and Millikan, 1976).

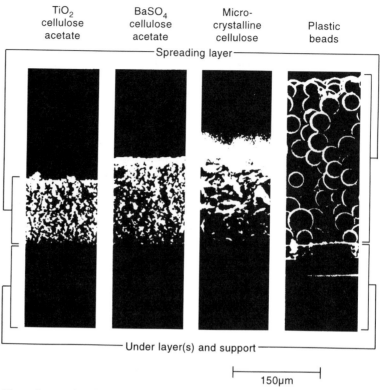

Figure 3 Photomicrographs of cross-sections of blush polymer and particulate bead spreading layers.

Particulate (Polymeric Bead) Spreading Layers

The direct incorporation of immunoreagents into a nonaqueous formula, such as the blush integral polymer layer described above, was found to present some problems because of the relative tendency of the immunoreagents to denature in the organic solvents used in this process. In addition, the tortuous flow patterns in these blush polymer layers created some difficulty in establishing a uniform distribution of very high molecular mass analytes, antibodies, labels and immune complexes. In an effort to produce a spreading layer with a higher degree of porosity that could be coated under aqueous conditions, it was discovered that mixtures of plastic spheres (diameter 1–100 μm) could be coated in the presence of certain types of adhesives to give coherent layers with the desired porosity and performance (Pierce and Frank, 1981). Liquid transport is facilitated in these spreading layers by the capillary action of the liquid being drawn through the interconnected spaces within the particulate structure of the layer. This approach results in the creation of sample spreading layers that are similar to the blush polymer spreading layer in their ability to distribute liquid sample uniformly in a constant volume per unit volume of matrix and also in their relative insensitivity to applied sample volume.

These particulate layers are generated *in situ* by coating and drying a metered coverage of an aqueous slurry of particles and adhesive over the reagent layers. The particles are inert, stable to the heat of drying, impermeable and do not swell in aqueous solutions. These properties ensure structural integrity and retention of the void spaces upon application of the sample. Beads that are near neutral buoyancy, such as polystyrene, are preferred because of their stabilisation of the coating slurry. The adhesive polymers typically have a glass transition temperature (T_g that is at least 30 °C lower than the heat stability temperature of the heat-stable particles). This allows the adhesive to flow without adversely affecting the particles. The attachment of the adhesive to the surface of the particles is facilitated in this state. As the drying process occurs, capillary pressure forces develop between adjacent particles, tending to draw adhesive to these regions (Pierce and Frank, 1981). This enhances the concentration of the adhesive at the junction of the particles, which results in the formation of a coherent particulate structure. The amount of binder must be sufficient to ensure adequate adhesive strength, but it cannot be present at levels high enough to decrease the void volume and impede fluid flow. In addition, the adhesive must remain insoluble following the initial drying in order to preserve the structural integrity of the spreading layer following rewetting by the applied sample. Photomicrographs of cross sections of blush polymer and particulate bead spreading layers are shown in Figure 3.

Particulates (Polymeric Beads) with Crosslinkable Groups

Koyama and Kikugawa (Konishiroku, Japan) (1984) have described the use of particulate polymer beads that contain crosslinkable reactive groups, such as glycidyl methacrylate, in order to form isotropically porous spreading layers which do not require the separate addition of adhesive. The crosslinking can occur between epoxide groups on adjacent beads or between different kinds of reactive groups (e.g. epoxide groups and amino groups) on adjacent beads. In addition to epoxide groups, other reactive groups are available for the formation of chemical bonds between adjacent particles having the same reactive group, including aziridyl, formyl, hydroxymethyl, thiol and carbamoyl groups. These particles have diameters of 1 to 350 μm and generate spreading layers containing void volumes of 25 to 85%. The preferred polymer particles are heat stable with T_gs of 40 °C or higher. The bound particulate structure has been designed to be impermeable and not to swell in the presence of aqueous fluids. These particulate layers are generated by coating a stable dispersion of reactive particles in a solvent which does not dissolve the particles. This is followed by removing the solvent at a temperature below the T_g of the polymers and, at the same time, promoting the chemical crosslinking of adjacent particles. Surfactants can be added to aid in the stabilisation of the reactive particle dispersions. Catalysts such as acids and bases are often added to the dispersions to promote chemical bond formation.

Koyama and Kikugawa (1985) have also described an alternative approach in which reactive epoxide groups have been grafted onto cellulose or polypropylene fibres, resulting in the generation of crosslinkable fibres. These materials are then coated and dried in order to form porous spreading layers. Enzymes and antibodies can be covalently immobilised via the same reactive groups prior to formation of the coated particulate layer.

DETECTION METHODS

As with solution immunoassays, optical methods are the most convenient methods to monitor reactions for thin-film elements. However, the structure of these assays complicates the use of transmission optical techniques because of the high light-scattering nature and even the

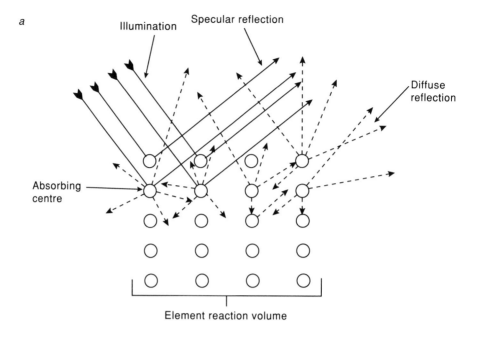

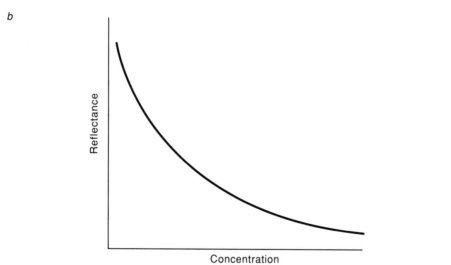

Figure 4 *a*, Principle of reflectance spectroscopy. *b*, Relationship of concentration to reflectance measurements. Reprinted with permission from Churchill-Livingstone Inc. from V. Marks and K. G. M. M. Alberit (eds) *Clinical Biochemistry Nearer the Patient* (1985).

opaqueness of the elements. Optical reflectance techniques (Walter, 1988) have been selected for use with these structures in all currently available commercial instrumentation.

Reflectance Densitometry

In reflectance techniques, the light source and the detector are located so that they both face the same side of an element. Reflectance densitometry uses either direct or diffuse light to irradiate the face of an element. In response, two types of reflected light are observed (Figure 4). One is specular reflectance, which is light that is scattered from the surface of the element at an angle equal to the angle of the incident radiation. Specular reflectance does not vary with the reactions occurring within the element. Thus, the geometry of the detector system is set so that the amount of specular reflectance reaching the detector is minimised. Light returned to the detector by diffuse reflectance (the other type of reflected light) is modulated by the chemistry occurring within the reaction volume of the element. Diffuse reflectance is a function of the absorption, transmission and scattering properties of the element and the absorption of chromophores developed within the element. Thus, the amount of diffusely reflected light reaching the detector is a measure of the extent of the registration chemistry.

The intensity of diffuse light reflected by the element and its reaction zone is usually compared to the reflectance from a standard reference reflector and is commonly expressed as per cent reflectance:

$$\%R = \left(\frac{I_s}{I_r}\right) R_f$$

where I_s is the reflected light from the sample, I_r is the reflected light from the reference reflector, and R_f is the per cent reflectivity of the standard. Per cent reflectance is analogous to transmittance measurements in absorption spectroscopy in that it is not directly proportional to concentration (Figure 4). However, algorithms to make linear the relationship between per cent reflectance and concentration have been derived. The application of either the Kubelka-Munk (1931) or the Williams-Clapper (1953) algorithm depends upon many factors including the optical properties of the element, the type of illuminating radiation and the detector geometry. The adaptation of the Williams-Clapper algorithm to multilayer thin films has been described elsewhere in more detail (Curme *et al.*, 1978).

Front-face Fluorometry

The second type of reflective spectroscopy that has been used to monitor thin-film elements is front-face fluorometry (Walter, 1983). As with reflectance densitometry, both the source of the probing radiation and, in this case, the detector for the emitted radiation are located on the same face of the element. Detection of specular reflectance is minimised both by the geometry of the optical system and by the use of filters or monochromators to reduce the amount of excitation radiation reaching the detector. This allows measurement of only the light produced by fluorescence of the sample which, like solution fluorescence, is proportional to the concentration of the emitting species in the absence of self-quenching or light-scattering phenomena.

559

Sensitivity Limitation

Both of these detection methodologies used to measure reactions in single- and multilayer elements are faced with the same limitation. The thin layers have only very short pathlengths (several hundred micrometres at most) available for reflectance densitometry or very small volumes from which emitted light can be sampled in front-face fluorometry. Thus, sensitivity can be a problem. This can be overcome to a certain extent by the use of dyes with high extinction coefficients and fluorophores with high quantum yields coupled with amplification methods (enzyme labels). However, more sensitive detection methods, such as chemiluminescence, must be incorporated in thin-film immunoassays in order to match the lowest concentrations currently measured with solution immunoassays (Ishikawa, 1987; Ishikawa *et al.*, 1991; Kricka, 1994).

SINGLE- AND MULTILAYER IMMUNOASSAY SYSTEMS

Up to this point this chapter has focused on the technologies available for the production of thin-film assays. The process of putting these techniques into practice has provided its own challenges. The solutions to these challenges have often been unique and creative, resulting in new materials and new approaches to immunoassays. By examining some of these systems (most of which are commercially available), the versatility and limitations of thin-film immunoassays will be illustrated.

Bayer ARIS Assays

The ARIS (apoenzyme reactivation immunoassay) method (Bayer Corporation, Elkhart, IN, USA (formerly Miles Laboratories Inc.)) is a homogeneous immunoassay method that has been incorporated into a single layer thin-film immunoassay. The ARIS system (Tyhach *et al.*, 1981) uses apoglucose oxidase (inactive) that can be reactivated by complexing with its cofactor, flavine adenine dinucleotide (FAD). The FAD is covalently linked to an analyte through a bridging group. Other reagents in the system include an anti-analyte antibody, the coupling enzyme peroxidase, and 3',3',5',5'-tetramethylbenzidine (TMB), a colorimetric substrate for peroxidase. The assay is based on a competition between the analyte and analyte-labelled FAD for anti-analyte antibody binding sites. Analyte-labelled FAD bound to the antibody cannot reactivate apoglucose oxidase whereas free analyte-labelled FAD can. Thus, the amount of reconstituted glucose oxidase increases with increasing analyte concentration. Peroxide formed as a product of the glucose oxidase catalysed reaction is converted to a coloured product by the coupling enzyme peroxidase. Reflectance densitometry is used to monitor the progress of the reaction.

Preparation of the Element

The ARIS element is prepared by the sequential saturation technique (Rupchock *et al.*, 1985). Cellulose paper is first impregnated with an acetone solution of TMB and then dried. This is followed by saturation with an aqueous buffer solution containing antibody, apoglucose oxidase, glucose, peroxidase, bovine serum albumin, polymers and wetting agents. TMB remains *in situ* because it is only slightly soluble in water. The dried paper is then impregnated a third time with a propanol solution containing the analyte-FAD conjugate. The use of propanol prevents premature interaction of the analyte-FAD conjugate with antibody or apoglucose oxidase. The dried paper is then cut into 0.5 × 1.0 cm pieces and mounted on a plastic layer.

Assay Protocol

The immunoassay reactions are initiated when a diluted (1:27) serum sample is applied to an element that has been placed on a temperature-controlled holder in the Seralyzer® reflectance photometer. The dilution results in the analyte concentration being in the range of the assay chemistry and also reduces the concentration of any interferents in serum. Reflectance is monitored for about one minute. The rate of increase of reflectance at 740 nm is correlated with the analyte concentration through a predetermined calibration curve. The element is stable at room temperature under proper storage conditions for 1 to 2 years (Thompson and Boguslaski, 1987) and the calibration is stable for several weeks. Reactivation of the glucose oxidase can occur if the element is hydrated by ambient moisture so there are time limits on the exposure of the element to room conditions. Tests for carbamazepine, phenobarbital, phenytoin, and theophylline (Ng, 1992) are currently available. ARIS assays have been found to have acceptable precision with within-run coefficients of variations (CVs) of <6% and between-run CVs of <8%.

Digoxin Assay

The glucose oxidase detection system is not sensitive enough for the measurement of digoxin whose detection limit needs to be about 0.5 µg l^{-1}, about 1,000-fold less than for the previously mentioned drugs. In order to accommodate a digoxin assay, Bayer has combined off-element separation steps (heterogeneous reaction) with the use of a single-layer registration element (Sommer *et al.*, 1990). All of the steps are done automatically by the Seralyzer® analyser. There is an initial addition of 30 µl of serum to a solution of β-galactosidase-anti-digoxin conjugate followed by mixing and an 8 minute incubation. This monoconjugate (one antibody binding site per enzyme prepared using a Fab′ fragment of a digoxin monoclonal antibody) binds the digoxin in the sample. After the incubation period, the instrument transfers the mixture to a vial containing a 'capture' phase (a digoxin analogue coupled to polyacrylamide beads) which removes any conjugate with a free digoxin binding site. The solid phase settles to the bottom of the vial and the supernatant is sampled. Application of an aliquot of the supernatant to a thin-film element, which contains the β-galactosidase substrate dimethylacridinone galactoside, initiates a colorimetric reaction monitored by reflectance densitometry. This method represents a coupling of conventional and thin-film technologies.

Dade International Stratus Immunochemistry Assays

Radial Partition Immunoassays

Like the Bayer digoxin assay, the Stratus (Dade International, Miami, FL, USA) immunoassay system uses a hybrid approach that combines features of thin-film immunoassays with other reagent addition mechanisms. All the assays adapted to the Stratus system are heterogeneous. They require a bound/free separation that is accomplished by the application of a wash/substrate solution to the element which removes unwanted, free label from the area of the element illuminated by the detection radiation. They call this technique radial partition immunoassay. The method has been applied to the measurement of about 30 large and small molecules in the areas of therapeutic drug monitoring, reproductive endocrinology, thyroid function, general endocrinology, cardiac disease, anaemia and allergy testing (Kahn and Bermes, 1992).

Methodology

The current system, Stratus II, is an automated batch immunoassay analyser which has on-board dilution. It contains three on-board dispensing stations for fluid handling (sample, conjugate and wash/substrate dispensers) which complement the functionality of the elements. The combination of these reagent dispensers with an element accommodates several different immunoassay methodologies including competitive and sequential saturation immunoassays for the measurement of low molecular mass molecules, and sandwich (immunometric) immunoassays for the measurement of high molecular mass molecules. In general, these assays have been found to have acceptable performance and correlate well with other commercially available immunoassays (Kahn and Bermes, 1992).

Glass-fibre Matrix

The element is composed of a glass-fibre matrix which was selected because of its favourable properties: porous, inert with minimal background absorbance and fluorescence, good fluid capacity, good dimensional wet stability, and a large surface area to facilitate immobilisation of the antibody. The glass-fibre membrane is contained in a plastic holder and together the unit is termed a reaction tab. An active immunoreactive tab is prepared by immobilising the antibody against the analyte on the glass-fibre matrix. This is done by first creating an immune complex of the analyte-specific antibody by titrating it with an appropriate secondary antibody. An aliquot of this complex is pipetted onto the glass-fibre matrix and allowed to dry, thus noncovalently immobilising the complex in a 10 × 15–mm reaction area.

Detection Enzymes

The detection enzymes used in these assays are either *Escherichia coli* or calf intestinal alkaline phosphatase (ALP). The substrate chosen was 4-methylumbelliferyl phosphate which is converted to the fluorescent 4-methylumbelliferone in the presence of ALP. Specific inhibitors of human alkaline phosphatase are added to the wash/substrate solution to eliminate interference from human ALP in serum samples.

Assay Protocol

The reaction is conducted on the glass-fibre matrix. For competitive immunoassays, the sample containing the antigen of interest is premixed with the enzyme-labelled antigen and is then spotted on the centre portion of the element. For sequential saturation immunoassays, the sample is prediluted if necessary and then spotted on the element. After an induction period during which the binding reaction takes place, the enzyme-labelled antigen is applied and binds to unoccupied antibody binding sites. For sandwich assays, sample is applied to the element, and then, following an incubation period, an enzyme-labelled second monoclonal antibody is applied. The final step, which separates free from bound label, is the same for all methods. An aliquot of a wash solution, which also contains substrate to initiate the enzyme reaction, is applied to the centre of the element. Unbound label is washed to the periphery of

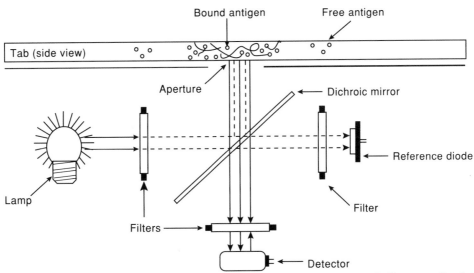

Figure 5 Front-face fluorometer used for analysis of Dade International STRATUS assays. Reprinted with permission from *Clinical Chemisty* from J. L. Giegel, *et al.* (1982).

the element, outside the area viewed by the detection system. The amount of conjugate remaining in the centre of the element following the wash is measured using front-face fluorometry (Figure 5).

Johnson & Johnson Clinical Diagnostics Assays

Dry Chemistry Clinical Chemistry Tests

Johnson & Johnson Clinical Diagnostics (formerly Eastman Kodak Company Clinical Diagnostics) thin-film coating technology was developed to adapt clinical chemical analysis to a dry-chemistry format (Curme *et al.*, 1978; Spayd *et al.*, 1978; Shirey, 1983). In this format, reagents are incorporated into one or more layers of hydrophilic polymer which are film-cast on a transparent plastic support. An isotropically porous, polymer spreading layer is coated over the reagent layer(s). For analysis, a 10–11 µl drop of serum is applied to the postage stamp-sized reaction chip. Upon application, the serum spreads uniformly and rapidly through the spreading layer by capillary forces. After this rapid spreading process occurs, the hydrophilic polymer underlayers take up fluid, rapidly swelling to several times their dry volume. This rehydration initiates the reactions that lead to colour formation. Colour formation is a function of analyte concentration and is measured by reflection densitometry. Tests for over 40 analytes are currently available in the thin-film format. Studies on the effects of interferences on various clinical chemistry systems for routine colorimetric and enzyme assays have shown that the VITROS (formerly EKTACHEM) system is least affected by haemolytic, icteric and lipaemic samples (Glick *et al.*, 1986).

Immuno-Rate Technology

Immunoassay capability has been added to the VITROS thin-film technology in a series of tests called Immuno-Rate assays (Danielson *et al.*, 1992). These are multilayer, thin-film elements that contain most of the reagents necessary for the measurement of a number of analytes in undiluted serum or plasma. These assays, designed for use on the VITROS 250 and VITROS 950 analysers, use both competitive and sandwich methodologies. Most elements are stable on the analyser for one week. A test is complete within 8 minutes of sample application.

Competitive Assays

Competitive assays have been described for phenytoin (Oenick *et al.*, 1993), phenobarbital (Hilborn *et al.*, 1993), digoxin (Kwong *et al.*, 1995), carbamazepine (Fyles *et al.*, 1995) and thyroxine (Danielson *et al.*, 1994b) in this format. All these assays have elements composed of a transparent plastic support layer over which there is a reagent layer, then an antibody layer, and uppermost, a porous reflective spreading layer consisting of 20–40-µm polymer beads. The reagent layer contains buffer and other reagents necessary for enzyme detection in a crosslinked gelatin matrix which is located directly on the support. The antibody layer contains specific antibody which has been immobilised on 1-µm beads. The antibody beads are incorporated in a thin polymer layer coated directly onto the reagent layer (or in some assays the antibody beads are incorporated directly in the spreading layer). The leuco dye, which is oxidised by a peroxidase label, is located in either the antibody layer or in the spreading layer. An analyte-peroxidase label, which has been designed to compete with the analyte in the serum sample for a limited number of immobilised antibody binding sites, is located in a thin layer on top of the spreading layer so that it does not react with the antibody prior to sample application.

The ability to keep the analyte- enzyme label in a thin zone at the top of the bead spreading zone is the result of a new approach to applying materials to thin-film elements developed by Dappen *et al.* (1992). They describe the use of a gravure coating process followed by rapid drying to coat the analyte-enzyme label. In this process, the gravure coating cylinder, which has micrometre-sized cells inscribed on its surface, transfers a solution of analyte-enzyme label to the bead spreading layer surface. The result is a low-wet laydown of the label solution so that the solution is only partially able to penetrate the spreading layer. This minimises the label's interaction with immobilised antibody already contained in the element.

Assay Protocol

Immuno-Rate assays (Figure 6) are initiated by the application of 11 µl of undiluted serum or plasma. This dissolves the analyte-enzyme label (as well as other reagents used in the reaction) and initiates the competition of the analyte in the sample and the analyte-enzyme label for the immobilised antibody binding sites. Following a five minute incubation at 37 °C, a 12 µl aliquot of a wash/substrate solution is applied about 4 mm from the initial sample application site. This fluid washes unbound analyte-enzyme label from the detection area and initiates the enzyme reaction used for detection. Colour formation at 670 nm due to the oxidation of the leuco dye by the peroxidase is followed over the next 2.5 minutes with reflection densitometry. The rate of colour formation is inversely related to the amount of analyte in the sample. The rate is correlated with analyte concentration using a standard curve. Within-run

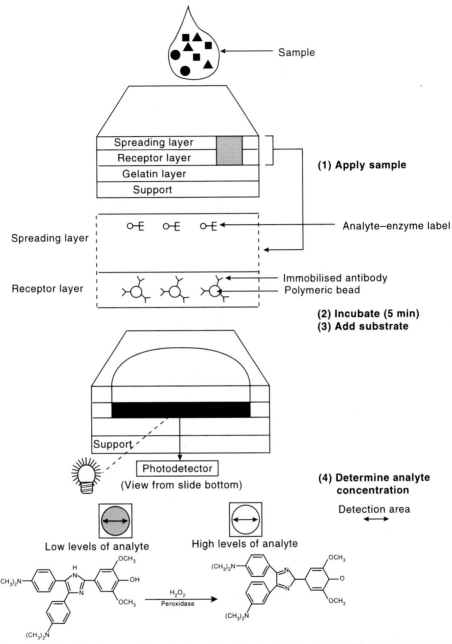

Figure 6 Principle of competitive binding Johnson & Johnson Clinical Diagnostics Immuno-Rate assays.

CVs of less than 5% have been reported for these assays, and the results have been found to correlate well with a variety of commercial assays (Hilborn *et al.*, 1993; Oenick *et al.*, 1993; Danielson *et al.*, 1994b; Fyles *et al.*, 1995; Kwong *et al.*, 1995).

Sandwich Assay

A sandwich assay for the high molecular mass analyte C-reactive protein (CRP) has also been developed in the Immuno-Rate thin-film format (Wu *et al.*, 1994). For this assay, a gelatin re-agent layer is first coated over the plastic support layer. On top of this layer is coated a poly-mer layer that contains both a monoclonal anti-CRP antibody conjugated with peroxidase and 'capture' beads, polystyrene beads to which a derivative of phosphorylcholine (PC) is co-valently bound. Over this is coated a bead spreading layer. The assay is initiated by the appli-cation of 11 µl of undiluted patient serum to the element. The element is incubated for 5 min-utes at 37°C during which the sandwich of PC beads/CRP/monoclonal antibody-peroxidase forms. After this incubation period, 12 µl of the substrate/wash solution is applied to remove unbound monoclonal antibody-peroxidase conjugate from the detection zone and to initiate the enzyme registration reaction. The amount of bound conjugate is measured using re-flectance densitometry. The results of this assay correlate well with the Behring nephelometric method. Within-run imprecision was found to be <7%. The assay range was 5 to 200 mg l^{-1} CRP with no high-dose hook effect up to 500 mg l^{-1} CRP (Wu *et al.*, 1994).

New Haptens, Linkers and Conjugation Chemistries

In addition to a new method of incorporating the label into thin films to prevent premature binding of analyte-label to antibody as described above, new and improved haptens, linkers and conjugation chemistries were developed for the preparation of enzyme labels so that the correct balance of antibody affinity for label and analyte could be achieved to optimise the position of competitive immunoassay dose-response curves. For example, the traditional ap-proach for digoxin label preparation (oxidation of the terminal monosaccharide residue to a dialdehyde followed by attachment to an enzyme amine) did not generate satisfactory peroxi-dase labels for these undiluted thin-film assays (Danielson *et al.*, 1987). Traditional ap-proaches resulted in preparations that contained a substantial fraction of label (>80%) which could not be bound by digoxin antibody. This contributed to higher than acceptable back-ground rates in a methodology that was constrained to use minimal volumes of wash solution to remove unbound peroxidase from the detection zone. Successful digoxin labels, however, were prepared using a new digoxin di-acid derivative. Introduction of additional reactive amines onto the peroxidase to which the new digoxin derivative could be covalently attached by mixed anhydride coupling chemistry further improved the label (Danielson *et al.*, 1987).

Novel extended linkers, which were designed to provide improved recognition of analyte-labels by analyte-specific antibodies, were used to generate labels for a variety of drugs in-cluding phenytoin, phenobarbital and carbamazepine (Danielson *et al.*, 1994a). Labels pre-pared from 4 or 5 carbon atom linkers between analyte and enzyme did not bind tightly en-ough to antibodies for the correct balance of affinity constants for analyte-label and analyte. However, when the linker between analyte and enzyme length was increased to 13 atoms, the binding of labels to a variety of antibodies improved. Optimisation of the coupling chemistry and the analyte/enzyme substitution ratio also improved the performance of the labels in these assays.

Particles for Immobilising Antibodies

The Immuno-Rate technology also requires immobilised antibodies to be incorporated into the thin-film element. Covalent attachment of antibody to the solid support is preferable to adsorption because of the potential of displacement by surfactants that are added to the element to promote spreading of the sample. Small (1 μm), uniform-sized copolymeric latex particles have been found to offer a very reactive substrate for immobilisation of antibodies (Sutton *et al.*, 1992). These particles are prepared by surfactantless emulsion polymerisation from styrene and a variety of novel monomers containing carboxylic acid. The structure of these monomers has been modified to provide hydrolytic stability and to achieve the desired hydrophobic/hydrophilic balance. These beads are hydrophobic and thus have a high protein adsorption capacity and are nonporous in aqueous media. This ensures that all reactions will occur at the surface of the beads. Covalent coupling protocols for the attachment of antibodies to these particles were developed so that 100% of the antibody was covalently bound to the beads. These new beads were compared to beads prepared using acrylic acid as the reactive monomer in thin-film immunoassays for thyroxine, phenytoin, phenobarbital and digoxin. The new carboxylic acid beads were 10-fold more immunoreactive with an equivalent amount of bound antibody (Danielson *et al.*, 1992).

In addition to the carboxyl group, a variety of other novel reactive copolymers have been incorporated into beads. This has made possible the efficient coupling of antibodies under mild conditions, thus maximising the retention of antibody activity. Copolymeric latex particles have been prepared from styrene and polymerisable monomers that contain pendant 2-substituted ethylsulphonyl and vinylsulphonyl groups (Sutton and Danielson, 1993). These beads and coupling chemistries have been optimised such that a very high percentage (>90%) of the offered antibody is covalently bound. This approach provides the added advantage of not requiring a separate reagent for activation of the beads.

Behring Diagnostics OPUS Assays

The thin-film immunoassay technology developed by Behring Diagnostics, Westwood, MA, USA (Velaquez, 1991; Lehrer *et al.*, 1992) has single-unit test modules that contain both a thin film and any solution reagents necessary for a single test. Two types of methodologies are used. For the analysis of most small molecular mass analytes (Jandreski *et al.*, 1991), including thyroid function assays (Lehrer *et al.*, 1992), multilayer film technology using heterogeneous competitive binding immunoassay principles has been incorporated into the test module. The bound/free separation of the label is accomplished by a thin-film design which effectively combines diffusion, compartmentalisation, and radiation blocking layers so that an additional separation step (e.g. a wash step) is not required (Grenner *et al.*, 1989). In addition, the design of this assay eliminates the need to keep the antibody and the analyte-label separate during the manufacturing process. Fluorescent detection is used. For the measurement of higher molecular mass analytes or antibodies and some low-concentration small drugs, a second type of test module is used that incorporates fluorogenic enzyme-linked immunosorbent assay (ELISA) methodology. This methodology incorporates a single-layer matrix with sequential reagent additions to achieve the desired sensitivity. The additional reagents are contained in each individual test module. The test modules for both the competitive methodology and the fluorescent ELISA methodology have the same external dimensions so that they can be processed similarly by an automated instrument.

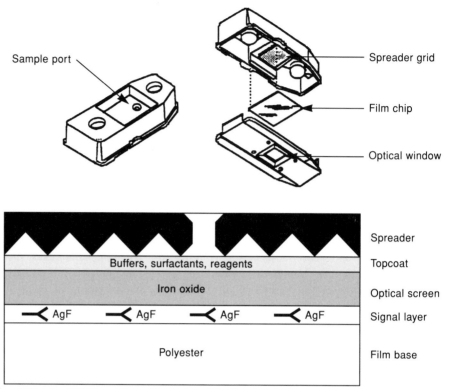

Figure 7 Behring OPUS multilayer film test module. Reprinted with permission from Academic Press, Inc. from Chan, D. W. (ed.) *Immunoassay Automation: A Practical Guide* (1992).

Competitive Assay Test Modules

The multilayer thin-film competitive assay, which requires no additional steps other than sample application, is based on a ligand displacement assay principle (Grenner *et al.*, 1989). The structure is shown in Figure 7. A very thin (<1 µm) signal generating layer is coated over a transparent plastic support. This layer contains an immobilised antibody along with a fluorescent-labelled analyte in an agarose matrix. Over this layer is coated a thicker radiation blocking layer (10 µm) which contains the pigment ferric oxide in an agarose matrix. This layer prevents the probing excitation radiation, which impinges on the element through the transparent plastic support, from penetrating to the upper layers of the element. Over the radiation blocking layer is coated another 10-µm-thick agarose layer which contains any buffers, detergents, displacement agents, or other reagents necessary for the reaction. This top layer also acts as a filter so that proteins and other high molecular mass molecules cannot penetrate to the signal layer and interfere with the immunoreaction. A preformed plastic spreading layer, described previously, is placed on top of the uppermost agarose layer.

For the competitive assays which use this multilayer structure, the reaction is initiated when 10 µl of an undiluted serum sample is applied to the spreading zone. After spreading, the sample rehydrates the underlying agarose layers. Small molecular mass analytes diffuse down through the reagent and radiation, blocking layers to the signal layer where they can displace the fluorescent-labelled analyte from antibody binding sites. The antibodies have been carefully selected for these assays to have very fast dissociation kinetics so that the competition reactions can reach equilibrium quickly (Grenner *et al.*, 1989). For example, the assay for theophylline has been reported to reach equilibrium in under 4 minutes at 37 °C, with the resultant signal remaining constant for more than 20 minutes. The thyroxine assay is slower, reaching 90% of equilibrium after 12 minutes, because of the slower dissociation rate of the more strongly binding antibody required for this assay. The displaced label is now free to diffuse throughout the thin-film structure. Because only 2% of the void volume of the element resides in the signal layer, this diffusion results in an effective bound/free separation. The radiation blocking layer prevents label other than that in the signal layer from contributing to the radiation which is detected by front-face fluorometry. As with other competitive mechanisms, the amount of bound labelled analyte is inversely proportional to the amount of analyte in the sample.

Fluorescent ELISA Test Modules

The test protocols for the higher molecular mass analytes and for some low-concentration small molecules are more complicated because they require the use of specific liquid reagents incorporated into these test modules. Both sandwich and sequential binding methodologies are available. In both cases, specific capture of analytes is required of the thin film. This is accomplished by incorporating immobilised antibody on a fibrous glass matrix which constitutes the single layer of these elements (Lehrer *et al.*, 1992; Velaquez, 1991). This glass matrix is then incorporated into the test module such that one end is under a wash port, the area containing immobilised antibody is under the central sample port, and the other end is in contact with an absorbent. The assay is initiated when the sample is pipetted through the sample port onto the element and allowed to incubate so that binding occurs between the analyte and the immobilised antibody. The next step occurs when the enzyme (alkaline phosphatase) conjugate solution (contained within each test module) is pipetted onto the reaction area through the sample port and allowed to complete the sandwich (or fill uncomplexed antibody binding sites in the sequential binding methodology). Following an incubation period, wash/substrate solution (also contained in each test module) is applied at the wash port. This solution migrates through the reaction zone towards the absorbent by capillary action, washing away unbound enzyme conjugate and initiating the detection reaction. The enzyme conjugate converts the substrate (4-methylumbelliferyl phosphate) into a fluorescent product (4-methylumbelliferone) which is measured by front-face fluorometry. Quantitative tests have been developed in this format for digoxin, human chorionic gonadotrophin (hCG), thyroid-stimulating hormone (TSH), and follicle-stimulating hormone (FSH) while qualitative tests for cytomegalovirus and toxoplasma are available. An analysis of whole blood samples would be possible by using these elements in combination with a filter device that has been described (Grenner, 1990).

Novel Materials

Several novel materials and approaches have contributed to the successful development of the OPUS system. One is the ferric oxide radiation blocking layer that enables the effective bound/free separation of analyte-label without a wash step. A second is the selection of antibodies with appropriate reaction kinetics to enable ligand displacement to occur in sufficiently short times for convenient assays. A third is the development of highly efficient fluorophores as direct labels (Grenner *et al.*, 1989) which overcome several of the problems associated with using undiluted serum samples and thin-film assays. These problems include the substantial intrinsic fluorescence of human serum and plasma, the high background fluorescence that is encountered from impurities and additives in the transparent plastic base which acts as the support layer, and the propensity of fluorescent labels to bind to serum proteins. The first two problems (intrinsic serum fluorescence and background fluorescence from the plastic film base) were minimised by the selection of certain xanthine dyes (e.g. rhodamine B and rhodamine 6G) which have absorption maxima at higher wavelengths (near 550 nm or higher) than the serum or film base interferents. In order to increase the fluorescent efficiency of these dyes, rotation of their amino groups was eliminated by ring closure which resulted in a fluorophore with a quantum yield of 0.9 in aqueous solution and with absorption and emission maxima at 550 and 580 nm, respectively. The third problem (nonspecific binding) was addressed by reducing the hydrophobicity of the fluorophore. The placing of two sulphonic acid groups and a hydrophilic spacer between the fluorophore and the hapten had the effect of reducing 10-fold the albumin-binding constant of a theophylline derivative relative to a theophylline-fluorescein conjugate.

The result of these developments has been the OPUS Magnum immunoassay analyser. Tests are currently available for therapeutic drug monitoring, endocrinology, fertility panels, infectious disease markers and cardiac markers. Test modules are stored at 2–8 °C with a shelf-life of at least 6 months. Reagents can be stored on board for at least 2 weeks for the fluorogenic ELISA assays and for 6 weeks for the multilayer film immunoassays. Test times range from 6 to 18 minutes. The OPUS Magnum allows storage on the instrument of up to 36 separate assays (360 test modules) and a throughput of up to 190 assays per hour (Auxter, 1995).

Fuji Thin-film Assays

A number of approaches for the adaptation of immunoassays to thin-film technology have been published in patents by workers from the Fuji Photo Film Company (Minami-Ashigara, Japan). Many of them use a preformed fabric spreading layer as the uppermost zone for sample introduction into the element. A novel homogeneous thin-film immunoassay for CRP has been commercialised by Fuji.

Photochemical Detection

One of the earliest thin-film immunoassays described by Fuji workers (Hiratsuka *et al.*, 1982) used a photochemical detection element for the analysis of insulin. The detection (lowest) layer consists of silver halide coated on top of a transparent support. Over this is coated a polyacrylamide bound/free separation layer. A spreading layer is laminated to this multilayer structure. Prior to being spotted on the element, insulin, labelled insulin, and anti-insulin antibody previously treated with a second antibody are mixed and incubated. The insulin is labelled with a carbocyanine dye that acts as a photographic spectral sensitiser or fogging agent. After the incubation period, the reaction mixture is applied to the thin-film element. The unbound labelled insulin penetrates the separation layer and comes in contact with the silver halide layer. The element is then exposed to light after which the resulting optical density is measured using densitometry.

Competitive Assay with a Capture Layer

A Fuji multilayer thin-film immunoassay for thyroxine has been described (Walter, 1988) which uses competitive ELISA methodology. A thyroxine-peroxidase conjugate is the enzyme label. The element is composed of a detection layer of glucose oxidase and a chromogen cast in gelatin over a support layer. Above this is a reflective layer of gelatin and $BaSO_4$ which also contains glucose. Next, a capture layer consisting of anti-thyroxine antibodies immobilised in a paper fabric is laminated over the lower layers. The uppermost layer is a paper fabric containing the thyroxine-peroxidase conjugate. The assay is initiated when a sample containing thyroxine is applied to the uppermost layer. The thyroxine-peroxidase conjugate is dissolved and competes with thyroxine for immobilised antibody binding sites in the next layer. Unbound conjugate continues to migrate to the gelatin registration layer where hydrogen peroxide is generated by the glucose and glucose oxidase. The colour formed as a result of chromogen production by the thyroxine-peroxidase label is detected by reflectance densitometry and can be correlated with the amount of analyte in the sample.

Competitive Assay Using Spatially Separated Substrate

Yet another competitive multilayer immunoassay format has been described by Fuji (Sudo *et al.*, 1990). In this format, a detection layer is coated onto the support layer. This detection layer is capable of coupling a reaction product produced in upper layers with a colorimetric detection scheme. The immunoreactions take place above this layer in a spreading layer. The spreading layer contains analyte-specific antibody immobilised on one set of agarose beads and an enzyme substrate immobilised on a second set of the agarose beads. The analyte-enzyme label can react with the immobilised substrate only when it is not bound to the immobilised antibody. It is the product of this enzymatic reaction that is detected in the lower layer.

A thyroxine (T_4) assay was developed using this approach. The assay is initiated when a sample containing thyroxine that has been spiked with a T_4-β-galactosidase label and a displacement agent is applied to the element. The spreading layer of the element is a glass fibre filter imbibed with agarose-immobilised T_4 antibody and a galactose oligomer. Only free label produces galactose which migrates through a thin radiation blocking layer (gelatin and TiO_2) to a galactose detection layer (gelatin containing galactose oxidase, peroxidase, 1,7-dihydroxynaphthalene, 4-aminoantipyrine and surfactants). The amount of colour formed is directly proportional to the amount of thyroxine in the sample.

Homogeneous Assay

The homogeneous immunoassay developed by Fuji (Ashihara *et al.*, 1988, 1991) depends upon the modulation of the activity of an analyte-specific antibody conjugate towards a high molecular mass substrate. When the antibody-enzyme conjugate is bound to a high molecular mass analyte, the enzymatic reaction towards the large substrate is inhibited. The free antibody-enzyme conjugate's activity is not inhibited. Thus the enzymatic activity is inversely proportional to the amount of high molecular mass analyte present in the sample. Assays for low molecular mass analytes use the same format except that a polymerised analyte competes with the analyte in the sample for binding to the antibody-enzyme conjugate (Sudo *et al.*, 1992). In these assays, the enzymatic activity is directly related to the concentration of the small ana-

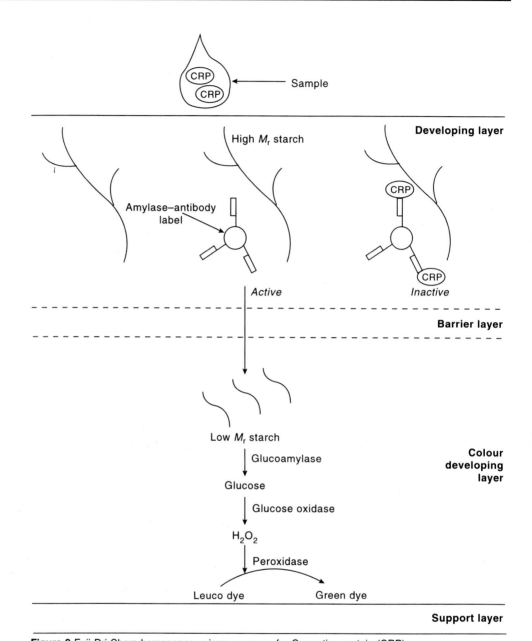

Figure 8 Fuji Dri-Chem homogeneous immunoassay for C-reactive protein (CRP).

lyte. Specifically, the high molecular mass substrate is insoluble starch and the enzyme used in the antibody-enzyme conjugate is α-amylase from *Bacillus subtilis*.

The thin-film format used in these assays (Figure 8) has a detection layer coated over the support layer. This layer contains glucoamylase (for converting low molecular mass starch into glucose), glucose oxidase, peroxidase and a leuco dye. Above this layer is a barrier zone through which the low molecular mass starch can migrate. The preformed spreading layer contains the antibody-amylase label and starch. A serum sample is first diluted 20 to 220-fold with a diluent buffer which contains a specific inhibitor to human serum amylase. This dilution also reduces endogenous glucose levels. The diluted sample (10μl) is applied to the thin-film element. Absorbance readings are taken at 4 and 6 minutes after sample application from which a two-point rate is calculated. Tests for CRP, ferritin, α-fetoprotein and theophylline have been described using this approach. The commercialised CRP assay has been compared to the Behring turbidimetric method and the theophylline assay with the Syva EMIT assay, demonstrating good correlation in both cases (Ashihara *et al.*, 1991).

Konishiroku Assays

Multilayer elements described in patents by Konishiroku Photo Industry Company (Tokyo, Japan) are based on the porous, bead layers produced using beads that have reactive groups to stabilise the layer structure (described previously). These layers are used in combination with other film-cast layers to produce the functionality necessary for the thin-film immunoassays. These assays have not been commercialised.

Yasoshima *et al.* (1986) describe an immunoassay method using a multilayer element which consists of three porous layers of particulate beads coated over a transparent support. The bottom layer consists of polystyrene-co-*n*-butyl methacrylate-co-glycidyl methacrylate particles (diameter 21 μm), which have been dried at an elevated temperature to form a cross-linked, porous layer. The second layer, which is designed to be a blocking layer, consists of the same beads which have been impregnated with a fluorescence blocking dye or pigment. The same particles are also used in the top layer with analyte-specific antibody adsorbed onto them prior to coating. A test for α-fetoprotein is described that uses fluorescein-conjugated α-fetoprotein as the label. The assay is conducted by applying a 10 μl aliquot of a sample containing a fixed concentration of the label onto the element. Following incubation at 37 °C for 20 minutes, the fluorescence is measured on either the top or bottom of the element to get a measurement of either the antibody bound or the free label. Results are given that show discrimination in levels of α-fetoprotein between 5×10^{-8} mol l^{-1} and 2×10^{-6} mol l^{-1} by either measurement.

Ito *et al.* (1989) describe another variation that is used for a human IgG assay, employing a fluorescein-labelled human IgG. The element is constructed by coating a reagent layer consisting of fluorescein-labelled human IgG and crosslinked gelatin over a transparent support. Laminated to this is a preformed porous particulate spreading layer comprising three sets of epoxide-containing beads: one set on which an anti-IgG antibody has been immobilised; another set on which anti-fluorescein antibody has been immobilised; a third set having immobilised bovine serum albumin. These beads are combined in appropriate ratios. The anti-fluorescein antibody has been selected for its ability to quench fluorescein. This spreading layer has been preformed on a separate transparent support from which it is peeled and laminated onto the gelatin detection layer of the immunoassay element. The assay for human IgG begins with the application of a 10 μl serum sample to the analytical element. After a 20 minute incubation at 37 °C, the fluorescence is measured from the spotted side of the element. At low levels of IgG, the label is bound preferentially to the IgG antibody and the measured fluorescence intensity is high. At high levels of IgG, more of the label is bound to the fluorescein antibody which quenches its signal so that the measured fluorescence intensity is low.

CONCLUSION

The impetus for developing unitised, thin-film elements for immunoassays is the ease of use and cost-effectiveness experienced by the analysts who use these assays. Because of the uniformity requirements for the unitised elements, the specialised equipment needed to produce them and the unique instrumentation used in detecting the signal from each element, thin-film immunoassays have become the province of commercial diagnostic companies. By virtue of their multilayer structure and the variety of materials and reagents that can be incorporated into these layers, specific embodiments of immunoassays are quite varied in the approach they take to solve the technical problems that are encountered. Manufacturers have been inventive in developing unique solutions to produce the various functional zones required in these elements. In general, thin-film immunoassays are more rapid, more stable, and less wasteful of reactive materials than their solution counterparts. Conversely, up to this point, thin-film immunoassays have not achieved the same level of sensitivity as solution immunoassays. Although the ideal thin-film assay contains within its element all the reagents necessary to carry out an assay, many of today's commercially available assays are hybrids of both wet and dry chemistries. This approach gives flexibility in order to optimise reaction conditions but it does place increased demands on either the operator or the instrument to carry out the additional steps. The objective of developing self-contained dry reagent immunoassays for analytes that span a very wide range of concentrations and molecular masses has not yet been completely achieved. However, the rewards for attaining this goal are great enough that technology will continue to be invented until that goal is reached.

REFERENCES

Ashihara, Y., Hiraoka, T., Makino, Y. *et al.* (1991) Immunoassay for determining low- and high-M_r antigens with a dry multilayer format. *Clin. Chem.* **37**, 1525–1526.

Ashihara, Y., Nishizono, I., Tanimoto, T. *et al.* (1988) Enzyme inhibitory homogeneous immunoassay for high molecular weight antigen (I). *J. Clin. Lab. Anal.* **2**, 138–142.

Auxter, S. (1995) Exposition offers glance at newest lab products. *Clin. Chem. News* September 12.

Berke, C. M. (1988) A primer for multilayer immunoassay. In: *Nonisotopic Immunoassay* (ed. Ngo, T. T.) pp. 303–12. (Plenum Press, New York).

Curme, H. G., Columbus, R. L., Dappen, G. M. *et al.* (1978) Multilayer film elements for clinical analysis: General concepts. *Clin. Chem.* **24**, 1335–1342.

Danielson, S. J., Brummond, B. A., Oenick, M. D. B. *et al.* (1994a) Labelled drug hapten analogues for immunoassays. *US Patent* No. 5,298,403.

Danielson, S. J., Daiss, J. D., Hilborn, D. A. *et al.* (1992a) Development of enzyme immunoassay in thin film format. In: *18th National Meeting of the Chemical Ligand Assay Society* (ed. Hawker, C. D.) pp. 105–107 (Associated Regional and University Pathologists, Inc., Salt Lake City).

Danielson, S. J., Detty, M. R. & Alexandrovich, S. K. (1987) Improved labels for use in digoxin multilayer enzyme immunoassays. *Clin. Chem.* **33**, 923(A).

Danielson, S. J., Ponticello, I. S., Sutton, R. *et al.* (1992b) Novel carboxylic acid copolymer beads and their use in thin-film immunoassays for thyroxine, phenytoin, phenobarbital, and digoxin. *Clin. Chem.* **38**, 1096(A).

Danielson, S. J., Warren, K., Birecree, J. *et al.* (1994b) Measurement of total thyroxine in serum using a thin-film slide enzyme immunoassay. *Clin. Chem.* **40**, 1024(A).

Dappen, G. M., Hassett, J. W. & Heinle, J. F. (1992) Analytical element coated by a gravure process. *European Patent Application* 517,338.

Fernando, S. A. & Wilson, G. S. (1992) Studies of the 'hook' effect in the one step sandwich immunoassay. *J. Immunol. Meth.* **151**, 47–66.

Free, A. H., Adams, E. C., Kercher, M. L. *et al.* (1957) Simple specific test for urine glucose. *Clin. Chem.* **3**, 163–168.

Free, H. M., Collins, G. F. & Free, A. H. (1960) Triple-test strip for urinary glucose, protein, and pH. *Clin. Chem.* **6**, 352–361.

Fyles, J., Byrne, D., Chambers, D. *et al.* (1995) Multilayer slide immunoassay for the measurement of carbamazepine in human serum. *Clin. Chem.* **41**, S57(A).

Geigel, J. L., Brotherton, M. M., Cronin, P. *et al.* (1982) Radial partition immunoassay. *Clin. Chem.* **28**, 1894–1898.

Glick, M. R., Ryder, K. W. & Jackson, S. A. (1986) Graphical comparisons of interferences in clinical chemistry instrumentation. *Clin. Chem.* **32**, 470–475.

Greenquist, A. C. (1989) Multizone analytical element having labeled reagent concentration zone. *US Patent* No. 4,806,311.

Greenquist, A. C., Rupchock, P. A., Tyhach, R. J. *et al.* (1984) Preparing homogeneous specific binding assay element to avoid premature reaction. *US Patent* No. 4,447,529.

Grenner, G. (1990) Biological diagnostic device and method of use. *US Patent* No. 4,906,439.

Grenner, G., Inbar, S., Meneghini, F. A. *et al.* (1989) Multilayer fluorescent immunoassay technique. *Clin. Chem.* **35**, 1865–1868.

Hilborn, D. A., Oenick, M. B., Danielson, S. *et al.* (1993) Measurement of phenobarbital in serum by multilayered slide immunoassay. *Clin. Chem.* **39**, 1232(A).

Hiratsuka, N., Mihara, Y., Masuda, N. *et al.* (1982) Method for immunological assay using multilayer analysis sheet. *US Patent* No. 4,337,065.

Ishikawa, E. (1987) Development and clinical application of sensitive enzyme immunoassays for macromolecular antigens: A review. *Clin. Biochem.* **20**, 375–385.

Ishikawa, E., Hashida, S. & Kohno, T. (1991) Development of ultrasensitive enzyme immunoassay reviewed with emphasis on factors which limit sensitivity. *Mol. Cell. Probes* **5**, 81–95.

Ito, T., Kawakatsu, S. & Onishi, A. (1989) Analytical element and method for determining a component in a test sample. *US Patent* No. 4,868,106.

Jandreski, M. A., Shah, J. C., Garbinclus, J. *et al.* (1991) Clinical evaluation of five therapeutic drugs using dry film multilayer technology on the OPUS immunoassay system. *J. Clin. Lab. Anal.* **5**, 415–421.

Kahn, S. E. & Bermes, E. W. Jr. (1992) Stratus II immunoassay system. In: *Immunoassay Automation: A Practical Guide* (ed. Chan, D. W.) pp. 293–316 (Academic Press, San Diego).

Kitajima, M., Arai, F. & Kondo, A. (1981a) Multilayer analysis sheet for analyzing liquid samples. *US Patent* No. 4,292,272.

Kitajima, M., Arai, F. & Kondo, A. (1981b) Multilayered integral element for the chemical analysis of the blood. *US Patent* No. 4,255,384.

Koyama, M., & Kikugawa, S. (1984) Analytical element and method of use. *US Patent* No. 4,430,436.

Koyama, M., & Kikugawa, S. (1985) Analytical element. *US Patent* No. 4,551,307.

Kricka, L. J. (1994) Selected strategies for improving sensitivity and reliability of immunoassays. *Clin. Chem.* **40**, 347–357.

Kubelka, P. & Munk, F. (1931) Ein Beitrag zur Optik der Forbenstriche. *Z. Tech. Phys.* **12**, 593–601.

Kwong, T., Meiklejohn, B., Bodman, V. *et al.* (1995) Performance of a new digoxin thin-film immunoassay in a hospital setting. *Clin. Chem.* **41**, S196(A).

Lehrer, M., Miller, L. & Natale, J. (1992) The OPUS system. In: *Immunoassay Automation: A Practical Guide* (ed. Chan, D. W.) pp. 245–267 (Academic Press Inc., San Diego).

Liotta, L. A. (1984) Enzyme immunoassay with two-zoned device having bound antigens. *US Patent* No. 4,446,232.

Mazzaferri, E. L., Lanese, R. R., Skillman, T. G. *et al.* (1960) Use of test strips with colour meter to measure blood-glucose. *Lancet* **1**, 331–333.

Ng, R. H. (1992) Immunoassay systems for the physician's office. In: *Immunoassay Automation: A Practical Guide* (ed. Chan, D. W.) pp. 351–363 (Academic Press, San Diego).

Oenick, M., Hilborn, D., Danielson, S. *et al.* (1993) Measurement of phenytoin in human serum by multilayered slide enzyme immunoassay. *Clin. Chem.* **39**, 1234(A).

Pierce, Z. R. & Frank, D. S. (1981) Element, structure and method for the analysis of transport of liquids. *US Patent* No. 4,258,001.

Przybylowicz, E. P. & Millikan, A. G. (1976) Integral analytical element. *US Patent* No. 3,992,158.

Rupchock, P., Sommer, R., Greenquist, A. *et al.* (1985) Dry reagent strips used for determination of theophylline in serum. *Clin. Chem.* **31**, 235–241.

Shirey, T. L. (1983) Development of a layered-coating technology for clinical chemistry. *Clin. Biochem.* **16**, 147–155.

Sommer, R. G., Belchak, T. L., Bloczynski, M. L. *et. al.* (1990) A unitised enzyme-labeled immunometric digoxin assay suitable for rapid testing. *Clin. Chem.* **36**, 201–206.

Spayd, R. W., Bruschi, B., Burdick, B. A. *et al.* (1978) Multilayer film elements for clinical analysis: Applications to representative chemical determinations. *Clin. Chem.* **24**, 1343–1350.

Sudo, Y., Ashihara, Y., Hiraoka, T. *et al.* (1992) Dry-type analytical element for immunoassay. *US Patent* No. 5,093,081.

Sudo, Y., Masuda, N. & Miura, K. (1990) Multilayered immunoassay for quantitative analysis of immunoreactant. *US Patent* No. 4,975,366.

Sutton, R. C. & Danielson, S. J. (1993) Water-insoluble reagents, elements containing same and methods of use. *US Patent* No. 5,177,023.

Sutton, R. C., Danielson, S. J., Findlay, J. B. *et al.* (1992) Biologically active reagents prepared from carboxy-containing polymer, analytical element and methods of use. *US Patent* No. 5,147,777.

Thompson, S. G. & Boguslaski, R. C. (1987) Homogeneous dry reagent immunoassay strips for the determination of therapeutic drugs in human serum or plasma. *J. Clin. Lab. Anal.* **1**, 293–299

Tyhach, R. J., Rupchock, P. A., Pendergrass, J. H. *et al.* (1981) Adaptation of prosthetic-group-label-homogeneous immunoassay to reagent-strip format. *Clin. Chem.* **27**, 1499–1504.

Velaquez, F. R. (1991) The P. B. Diagnostics' OPUS immunoassay system. *J. Clin. Immunoassay* **14**, 126–132.

Walter, B. (1983) Dry reagent chemistries. *Anal. Chem.* **55**, 498A–514A.

Walter, B. (1988) Construction of dry reagent chemistries: Use of reagent immobilisation and compartmentalisation techniques. *Meth. Enzymol.* **137**, 394–420.

Williams, F. C. & Clapper, F. R. (1953) Multiple internal reflections in photographic color prints. *J. Opt. Soc. Amer.* **43**, 595–599.

Wu, A., Harmoinen A., Chamber, D. *et al.* (1994) Comparison of a thin-film immunoassay for C-reactive protein (CRP) with a turbidimetric method. *Clin. Chem.* **40**, 1018(A).

Yasoshima, S., Koyama, M. & Okaniwa, K. (1986) Immunoassay method for measuring immunological antigen in fluid sample. *US Patent* No. 4,613,567.

Chapter 22

Disposable Integrated Immunoassay Devices

Christopher P. Price, Garry H. G. Thorpe, Jan Hall and Roger A. Bunce

INTRODUCTION

The perception that point-of-care testing can benefit the diagnosis and management of disease, or alternatively that central laboratory tests cannot meet the needs of today's clinical practice (Hilton, 1990; Santrack and Burritt, 1995; Hicks, 1996), has led to an explosion in the development of analytical devices for use by people who do not have a training in analytical techniques. The environment in which such a test might be used ranges from the home, the pharmacist's shop or the primary care health centre to various sites in the hospital (e.g. emergency room, outpatient clinic, intensive care unit or ward side-room). Indeed, such devices may be used in the laboratory when a rapid result is required, e.g. the diagnosis of an ectopic pregnancy.

The idea of a single-use, disposable analytical device is not particularly new, litmus paper for the measurement of pH being perhaps one of the earliest examples. Early point-of-care testing, which was confined to urine, involved the use of simple wet chemistry procedures in a test tube, the reagent being stored in liquid form in bottles and later produced as tablets. However, as the chemical reactions became more complicated, involving both multiple reactions and labile reagents (e.g. enzymes) and the need to analyse whole blood samples, the development of reliable tests that allowed improved convenience became a significant challenge. As a result, development scientists looked to encapsulation of reagents in a solid matrix, and with this came the reagent strip or stick test exemplified by the glucose test. There have been many subsequent developments in the measurement of glucose, yet the chemistry of the reactions needed to provide a visual reading are still fairly straightforward and typically involve up to three reaction sequences that can all be allowed to progress in the same phase (i.e. a homogeneous reaction). However, immunoassays can present a far greater challenge, because certain reagent concentrations may be critical to the performance of the assay and reactions may not reach equilibrium.

Requirements of a Disposable Immunoassay Device

Although there are many different formats of immunoassay for the measurement of small or large antigens or antibodies, there are basically two approaches: (1) a competitive assay or limited-reagent assay, and (2) an immunometric, sandwich or excess-reagent assay.

Sample and Reagent Metering

The competitive assay involves the use of a defined and limiting amount of both antibody and labelled antigen (in the case of an assay for antigen), the sensitivity and analytical range of the assay being strongly influenced by the proportion of these two reagents. The affinity constant of the antibody will also influence assay performance, influencing the rate of immunoreaction and consequently the sensitivity of the assay, particularly when a short incubation period is required (by definition an absolute requirement for a point-of-care application).

Thus, in addition to accurate metering of sample, accurate metering of reagents for a competitive immunoassay is an absolute requirement. In this respect it is interesting to note that the majority of disposable devices use the immunometric style of assay. In this situation, accurate metering of sample is necessary whereas the use of excess reagent conditions makes the metering of reagent less critical, albeit still requiring care. It goes without saying that the reproducible synthesis of labelled antigen or antibody is important for any assay.

Incubation Period. In order to achieve a short reaction time (i.e. time to result), most immunoreactions will not reach completion and consequently an accurate definition of the incubation period is important. In particular, if a device does not carry on-board calibration the incubation period must be reproducible across the batch of devices encompassed within a calibration procedure (e.g. calibration across a complete manufactured batch).

Mixing. Adequate mixing of constituents will define the commencement of an immunoreaction and, as such, it is vital that it is rapid and reproducible from device to device to ensure good within- and between-batch precision. Key determinants of this function will be the way liquid interacts with reagents within the porous matrix, and the matrix structure and geometry.

Temperature. It is now generally accepted that, in practical terms, the antigen-antibody reaction is temperature dependent, although it is not always found to be as responsive to temperature changes as an enzyme-mediated reaction. If, however, an immunoassay uses an enzyme label, the colorimetric end point may be influenced by the temperature of the environment in which the assay is performed. Despite this, most disposable immunoassay devices, particularly if internally calibrated, appear to operate satisfactorily over a reasonable, defined temperature range. It is, however, important from a practical standpoint to ensure that devices stored in a refrigerator are brought up to room temperature before use.

Endpoint Detection. The choice of endpoint will depend on whether to use visual detection or some form of photometric device, and the sensitivity requirements of the assay. The choice of label should take into account the extinction coefficient of the label, or a product of the label, and the visual accuracy of the observer. Reproducibility of performance will be influenced by the ratio of label to reagent antigen or antibody in the conjugates used, and the ability to manufacture devices consistently. In addition there is an important ethical consideration of the need to generate a permanent record of the result.

Calibration. Assays may be qualitative or quantitative, both requiring careful attention to calibration. In the case of a qualitative assay where a cutoff is defined, the issue of calibration revolves round the accurate definition of the cutoff point and the reproducibility of reagent production and device fabrication to ensure this. In the case of a quantitative assay, the result may be defined in semi- or fully quantitative terms but must encompass a lower limit, accuracy within a given analytical range, and an upper limit. The reproducibility of performance within and between batches of devices will in part depend on the technology used and will determine whether internal (i.e. on-board) calibration is necessary.

Quality Control. The control of the quality of a result produced by a disposable device is determined by the reproducibility of manufacture and the care of the operator in following instructions. The more steps that can be built into a device, the less will performance depend upon the operator. The operator in this context must include the person responsible for delivery and storage of the device because inappropriate delivery/storage conditions may degrade the viability of reagents.

Ideally a device should also carry a means of checking steps in the process that are vulnerable to operator-dependent error, e.g. storage conditions, sample addition and reaction timing. This is important when considering the regulatory requirements in the provision of tests, particularly for those sold over the counter, and the product liability issues for manufacturers.

The Ideal Device

Although devices such as glucose meters and pregnancy tests are widely used by the public, experience with a variety of single-use disposable devices outside the laboratory environment has shown that training (and possibly certification) of users is an important prerequisite for reliable performance of point-of-care testing; regular quality assurance testing and continuing education are important for maintaining good performance (Price *et al.*, 1988; Burnett and Freedman, 1994). Despite these procedures, which may be difficult and costly to maintain, particularly in the context of home testing, problems may still occur. This said, there have been very few studies published on the reliability of point-of-care testing.

The ideal device should produce a rapid result, be simple to use, and attempt to minimise variability in analytical performance, in particular operator-initiated steps, while also encompassing quality control procedures that check the viability of the system.

CLASSIFICATION OF DEVICES

There are four main types of integrated device that encompass various components of an analytical system:

Encapsulated Wet Chemistry. All of the components, including diluents, are encapsulated in a complex disposable plastic unit that only requires addition of sample. The devices generally require an instrument for reading a photometric end point of the reaction (Klotz, 1993; Pope *et al.*, 1993).

Simple Immobilised Analyte Capture. Typically a capture antibody is immobilised on a solid porous matrix to which sample is added. Additional reagents are added to detect captured antigen analyte (a capture antigen is used if the analyte of interest is an antibody) (Norman *et al.*, 1985; Valkirs and Barton, 1985). These may also be termed 'cross-flow' or 'flow-through' devices.

Chromatographic and Liquidic Circuits. All reaction components are impregnated or immobilised on a porous solid phase and are brought into contact with the sample in sequence after addition of a diluent (Zuk *et al.*, 1985; Bunce *et al.*, 1991; May, 1994). These may be termed 'lateral-flow' devices.

Immunosensors. The addition of sample to the sensor surface leads to capture of the antigen and a change in property of the immediate environment of the sensor surface (North, 1985; Robinson, 1991; Morgan *et al.*, 1996; see also Chapter 20).

Although this is a simple classification, it encompasses most of the devices that have been described. Importantly, it recognises the key features of: (1) manufacturing a complex plastic disposable unit to mimic, in a direct way, the fluidics of a wet-chemistry immunoassay; (2) trapping of the liquid phase in a porous matrix with immobilisation of a capture reagent and impregnation of the other components to obviate the need for addition of critical reagents; and (3) direct detection of antigen binding to capture antibody (or the reverse in the case of antibody detection).

At the heart of this technology is the need to fabricate a device and its constituent reagents in a way that minimises the need for equipment and a skilled operator. These criteria are not dissimilar to those discussed by Gorman *et al.* (Chapter 13) in the case of automated immu-

Field of Use	Analyte
Pregnancy/fertility	
Pregnancy	hCG
Ovulation prediction	LH, FSH
Contraception	Simultaneous LH and oestrone-3-glucuronide
Diabetic	
	Albumin
	Lipoprotein (a)
	HbA1c
Infectious diseases	
	Antigen or antibody (IgG or IgM)
Streptococcus A and B	Antigen
Chlamydia	Antigen
Herpes simplex virus 1 and 2	Antigen
HIV-1, HIV-2	Antibodies
Infectious mononucleosis	Antibody
Periodontal bacteria	Antigens
Helicobacter pylori	Antibody
Respiratory syncytial virus	Antigen
Rotavirus	Antigen
Malaria	*Plasmodium falciparum* antigen
Hepatitis B e	Antigen and antibody
Hepatitis B core	Antibody IgM and IgG
Influenza virus A	Antigen
Adenovirus	Antigen
Rubella	Antigen
Lyme	Antibody
Salmonella	Antigen
Cardiac	
	Creatine kinase MB
	Myoglobin
	Myosin light chain
	Troponin I
	Troponin T
	Multiple cardiac panels
	CK-MB/myoglobin
	CK-MB/myoglobin/troponin I, myosin light chains

Table 1 A list of some of the analytes measured by solid porous matrix devices.

noassay systems; however, here the operational requirements are different. Several of the features discussed earlier are also to be found in the analytical systems described by Daniellson and Hilborn (Chapter 21), although again the focus is more on devices for the central laboratory environment. Kricka and Wilding (Chapter 23), in their chapter on microfabrication, while again describing some of the devices that lie within the classification outlined above, point the way forward to the next generation of integrated devices in which miniaturisation is seen as a means of reducing costs, minimising sample volume and creating more flexibility of usage (by reducing the need for complex instrumentation). Immunosensors reviewed by Purvis, Pollard-Knight and Lowe (Chapter 20) allude to a device of minimal complexity

Field of Use	Analyte
Allergy	Total and specific IgEs
Drugs of abuse screen and therapeutic drug monitoring	
	Single or panel
	Amphetamine
	Metamphetamine
	Opiates
	Methadone
	Heroin
	Morphine
	Cocaine
	Cannabinoids
	Tetrahydrocannabinoid THC
	Barbiturates
	Benzodiazepine
	Phenytoin
	Theophylline
Cancer markers	
	Prostate-specific antigen
	Faecal occult blood
	Alphafetoprotein
Proteins	
	C-reactive protein (CRP)
	α_1-Microglobulin (urine)
	Albumin (urine)
	Rheumatoid factor

LH, Luteinising hormone; FSH, follicle-stimulating hormone.

Table 1 (cont.) A list of some of the analytes measured by solid porous matrix devices.

that could be achieved through direct detection of analyte capture: not yet achieved in practice although proved in concept (Morgan *et al.*, 1996).

Although encapsulated wet-chemistry devices effectively provide a reproducible formulation of established methods, all of the strengths and weaknesses of these systems pertain. The major feature of the remaining devices, and indeed the area in which there is currently most commercial realisation in this field, is the use of a porous solid matrix. The use of a porous matrix provides four key features: (1) a means of containing the liquid phase; (2) a means of immobilising antibody (and antigen reagent) in a dry state, thereby enhancing the stability of the reagents (Zipp and Hornby, 1984); (3) providing a large surface area and short diffusion distances (Mason and William, 1980; Stenberg and Nygren, 1988); and (4) assay parameters, e.g. reagent flow that can be modified by choice of matrix chemistry.

DISPOSABLE IMMUNOASSAY DEVICES

The early disposable immunoassay devices focused on the diagnosis of pregnancy using a urine sample and were designed for home use (the over-the-counter or OTC market). These assays typically involved a multistep assay based on latex agglutination or colorimetrically

Sample type	Analyte	Sample preparation	Product	Company
Whole blood	Troponin T antigen	No	TropT	Boehringer Mannheim
	H. pylori antigen	No	QuickVue (onestep)	Quidel
	Myoglobin + CKMB	No	Cardiac Status	Spectral Diagnostics
Serum/plasma	PSA	Blood separation	Biosign	Princeton Biomeditech
	Lp(a)	Blood separation	(Research)	Abbott Diagnostics
	HIV 1+2 antibodies	Blood separation	DoubleCheck	Orgenics
Serum	*H. pylori* antibody	Blood separation	FlexSure HP	Smithkline Diagnostics
	hCG	Blood separation	TestPack Plus Combo	Abbott Diagnostics
	Hepatitis B antigen	Blood separation	Hepator	Bionike
Urine	hCG	No	Clearview hCG	Unipath Ltd
		No	Precise	Becton Dickinson
		No	Predictor	Chefaro
	LH	No	Clearplan Onestep	Unipath Ltd
	Cocaine	No	Verdict	Diagnostix Inc.
	Drugs of abuse (panel)	No	Triage	Biosite Diagnostic (Merck)
	Microalbumin	No	Micral II	Boehringer Mannheim
Saliva	*H. pylori* antibody	No	Omniscan	Saliva Diagnostics Systems
	HIV 1+2 antibodies	No	Saliva Card	Trinity Biotech
Faeces	Haemoglobin	Faeces extraction	Hem-check-1	Veda Labs
	Adenovirus	Faeces extraction	Onestep	SA Scientific
Swab	*Streptococcus* A antigen	Swab extraction (In-line)	QuickVue	Quidel
	Chlamydia (LPS antigen)	Swab extraction	Clearview	Unipath Ltd

CKMB, creatine kinase (MB isoenzyme); PSA, prostate specific antigen; LPS, lipopolysaccharide

Table 2 Types of samples used in various devices.

monitored enzyme-labelled conjugates, with the assay being undertaken in a test tube or on a tile, and interpretation of the results being very operator-dependent (Thomas *et al.*, 1986). Advances in porous solid phase and developments such as plastics chemistry and fabrication technology, together with reagent developments such as monoclonal antibodies and nonradioactive labels, have led to a wide variety of systems for an ever-increasing range of analytes (some examples are given in Table 1).

Although early point-of-care testing used urine samples, as the perceived need for this type of testing increased, so did the requirements for the type of sample. As a consequence, the presentation of the sample to the device had to be taken into account. Examples of the use of different sample types are given in Table 2. In some cases the need to accommodate a complex sample such as whole blood has required an additional innovative step in the design of the device; the return on the investment, by obviating the need to separate cells from plasma with its concomitant safety issues and reducing of analytical time, is obvious.

The ingenuity that is built into many of the devices on the market today reflect considerable intellectual and financial investment. Consequently, a great deal of the theory behind the device is hidden in patent literature. Inexplicably, there is also only a limited amount of literature in the public domain on the performance (and any limitations) of these devices. In the remainder of this review we will focus on the fabricated total-reaction wet chemistry, flow-through and lateral-flow devices; the reader is referred to other chapters in this book dealing with other types of devices.

FABRICATED TOTAL-REACTION CELLS

The idea of premetering all reagents and encapsulating them in a reaction cell is not new, the DuPont (now Dade International) aca being one of the first examples, demonstrating reproducibility of performance, reducing the need for daily calibration and minimising the need for constant operator intervention (Maclin and Young, 1994). There are other examples where unique packaging of reagents has been used to minimise reagent preparation (Driscoll *et al.*, 1983); however, there are few examples where these features have been combined with whole blood sampling. This has been achieved with the Abbott Vision™ System (Abbott Laboratories, Chicago, USA) which uses centrifugation to facilitate movement of liquids through a complex network of channels in a precisely moulded plastic cassette (Schultz *et al.*, 1985).

There are at least two examples where complex plastic moulded cassettes have been developed for use with small photometers capable of reading the amount of light scattering produced in the reaction chamber. The DCA 2000® (Bayer Diagnostics, Tarrytown, USA) test for haemoglobin A1c (HbA1c) requires addition of 1 µl of whole blood; the remaining reagents needed to perform a latex-labelled immunoinhibition assay and haemoblogin measurement are contained in the cassette. Sample is drawn first into a lysing solution, and the HbA1c released competes with glucopeptide on a latex particle for a specific monoclonal antibody. A system of capillaries draws sample and reagents into the reaction cell, and the instrument provides temperature control, photometric reading and calculation of the result. The method compares with established methods with a coefficient of variation (CV) of less than 5% (Pope *et al.*, 1993).

The Biotrak 516 (Boehringer Mannheim, Germany) has been used in the measurement of several analytes, including therapeutic drugs. Again, the cassette meters an exact amount of sample into a lysing solution, mixing being achieved with an oscillating magnet and steel ball in the cassette. The lysed diluted blood is drawn by capillary action into a measuring chamber to quantify the haemoglobin, then drawn into a second chamber where a conventional latex immunoinhibition assay takes place, the reagents being stored initially in the second reaction chamber in dry form. An assay for theophylline gave coefficients of variation of less than 5% across the analytical range (Klotz, 1993). The design of the two cassette systems discussed are illustrated in Chapter 23.

POROUS MATRIX, LIQUID-PHASE ASSAYS

Most current disposable immunoassays rely on at least one reagent bound to a solid support. This is generally a membrane such as nitrocellulose, although reagents can be coupled to small particles which are themselves entrapped within the matrix of porous solid supports such as glass-fibre paper. These disposable devices can be broadly divided into 'flow-through' or 'lateral-flow' devices.

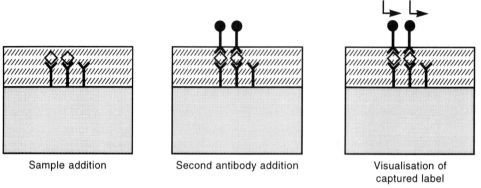

Sample addition	Second antibody addition	Visualisation of captured label

Figure 1 Schematic diagram of a flow through device comprising a membrane impregnated with capture antibody(hatched) and an absorbent reservoir (shaded). Visualisation of the enzyme label is by addition of substrate producing a coloured product (arrow).

Flow-through Devices

Although still multistep assays that involve several liquid reagents, 'flow-through' immunoassays have been extremely successful both in the laboratory, outpatient clinic and primary care environments. These devices are primarily heterogeneous immunometric assay systems based on a capture antibody immobilised onto a membrane attached to an absorbent reservoir. The sample is flowed through the membrane followed sequentially at specified times by defined volumes of reagents; including labelled antibody conjugate, wash solution and label location solution. The presence of analyte is indicated by a coloured response on the membrane. The intensity of the colour change can be proportional to the concentration of the analyte captured; alternatively, the response can be used to indicate the presence or absence of the analyte. A schematic diagram describing the concept is shown in Figure 1.

In the original Icon™ device from Hybritech (San Diego,USA)(Valkirs and Barton, 1985), first described for the detection of human chorionic gonadotrophin (hCG) in serum or urine, sample is added to the membrane, followed by a second antibody labelled with enzyme, a wash step and then the substrate. All additions are made by a dropper pipette. Urine samples with 50 IU l^{-1} hCG were always detected, the figure being 25 IU l^{-1} for serum samples. The sensitivity could also be improved by increasing the urine sample volume; using 5 ml instead of the usual 250 μl reduced the sensitivity to 1 IU l^{-1} (Hussa *et al.*, 1985). The sensitivity could also be increased by increasing the incubation times, with both antibody conjugate and enzyme substrate.

The Murex SUDS™ test cartridge features a reaction vessel that has absorbent pads as sides and a capture membrane as its base. Sample, together with latex particle-coupled capture antibody and enzyme-labelled antibody, is added to the vessel, followed by wash solution and then enzyme substrate. The latex provides a high surface area for rapid antigen capture and the latex particles are captured by the membrane, into which the coloured product diffuses. The sensitivity of the assay device depends on sample volume and incubation time, with values as low as 10 IU l^{-1} hCG being demonstrated (Marshall and Bush, 1987).

An alternative approach to the visual interpretation of a 'dot' was the creation of a plus sign for a positive result. In this format, the negative sign area is formed from material that binds the enzyme conjugate (or is made up of the enzyme coupled to the matrix) while the other 'vertical bar' to form the plus sign is formed from the capture antibody bound to the matrix. One example of this device gave a 'positive response' with five drops of urine with an hCG value of 50 IU l^{-1} (Brown *et al.*, 1992).

Similar devices have also been described for other analytes, e.g. the Quidel assay for *Heliobacter pylori* antibody (Pronovost *et al.*, 1994). In this device, 30 μl plasma is used in an assay taking about 8 min to complete. The 'negative sign capture material' is nonimmune human IgG while the 'positive capture material' is *H. pylori* antigen (Pronovost *et al.*, 1994). The device was shown to give 92.3% sensitivity and 88.1% specificity in a study of 256 patient samples.

An alternative approach, which has allowed the use of a whole blood sample, includes a blood-solubilising dilution system and a card containing holes to receive sample over a porous membrane containing immobilised monoclonal antibody positioned over an absorbent pad (Urdal *et al.*, 1992). A diluted sample (25 μl whole blood) is added to the test card followed by a second antibody preparation coupled to colloidal gold; the amount of analyte present is proportional to the colloidal gold captured. In an assay for C-reactive protein, between-series imprecision varied between 10.1 and 14.7% with a detection limit of 12 mg l^{-1} and good correlation ($r = 0.95$) with an established immunoassay.

These devices may be used with visual detection for a qualitative result, or even a semiquantitative result using a calibrated colour comparison chart. Alternatively, their use with a reflectance meter could give a quantitative result (Anderson *et al.*, 1986), and also provide for internal reference or calibration. Several types of flow-through devices have been developed and a range of assays are available commercially (see Table 3). These include simple plastic 'tubs' or membranes simply attached above absorbent material. The reagents can even be flowed into a credit card-like solid support. The type of label used as detector varies and can include an enzyme label requiring the addition of an appropriate substrate to produce a response or labels that can be visualised directly, including colloidal gold, selenium or dyed latex particles.

A novel homogeneous immunoassay device has been described (Merenbloom and Oberhardt, 1995) in which analyte-labelled thrombin is sterically hindered by an antibody to the analyte, and the free analyte releases the inhibition of the label caused by the antibody. The activity of thrombin in a coagulation cassette is monitored by the assessment of mobility of paramagnetic particles using UV light illumination. An assay for biotin demonstrated a detection limit of 0.026 nmol l^{-1}. The assay could be used with whole blood samples and it has been argued that the low detection limit was a consequence of using a cascade label (i.e. amplification).

Lateral-flow Devices

The use of antibody-coated coloured particles (such as latex or colloidal gold particles) that can be moved along membranes and captured by an antigen – itself captured by an antibody immobilised in small areas of the membrane, effectively concentrating the coloured particles – has enabled the development of simple-to-use disposable immunoassay devices based on immunochromatography. A range of devices for different analytes are available commercially (see Table 4). A schematic diagram to illustrate the concept is shown in Figure 2.

Sample type and volume	Sample preparation	Number of steps	Analytes measured	Procedural controls	Technology
Whole blood (25µl)	None	6 steps (1 min)	C-reactive protein	No	Nycocard (Nycomed) Semiquantitative immunometric assay. Diluted sample added to card followed by conjugate and wash. Resulting colour intensity compared to reference card.
Whole blood (20µl)	None	5 steps (20 min)	*H. pylori* antibody	Yes	Helisal Rapid Blood Test (Cortecs) Qualitative membrane immunoassay using coloured particle endpoint. Mix capillary blood sample with buffer. Add diluted blood to card and allow to drain. Wipe membrane clean with cotton bud to remove blue colour. Add colour reagent and allow to drain. Read result: 2 spots (+ve), 1 spot (−ve)
Serum/plasma (30µl)	Blood separation	8 steps (7 min)	*H. pylori* antibody IgG	No	QuickVue (Quidel) Qualitative membrane-based ELISA (using alkaline phosphatase).
Serum/plasma (50µl)	Blood separation	10 steps (10 min)	HIV 1+2 antibody	Yes	SUDS (Murex) Qualitative ELISA using microfiltration of latex particles through a membrane.
Urine (5 drops)	None	5 steps (5 min)	hCG	Yes	Icon II (Hybritech) Semiquantitative ELISA. Add sample, enzyme conjugate, substrate + wash. Compare colour of test zone with reference zone.
Urine (or saliva) (7 drops)	None	5 steps (6 min)	Amphetamine Cocaine Opiates Phencyclidine Cannabinoids	Yes	Fingerprint DOA (Fingerprint Biotech Inc.) Qualitative multianalyte test for DOA using ligands immobilized onto membrane mounted onto absorbent pad.
Faeces	Filtration	6 steps (<10 min)	Rotavirus antigen	Yes	Testpack (Abbott Laboratories) Qualitative immunofiltration assay. Positive results indicated by a purple cross versus a lighter background.

Table 3 Flow-through devices.

Format and Construction of Lateral-flow Devices

These devices can be constructed in a variety of ways that partly depends on the way in which they are to be used. Devices may be held directly in the urine stream, dipped directly into a sample contained in a collection vessel, or have samples applied to a strip contained in a plastic cassette or platform. The amount of sample taken up will depend on the absorbency of the matrix and the time of exposure (to a lesser extent) but it is clear that the sampling technique must determine overall design.

One example of a lateral-flow device is the Unipath (Bedford, UK) Clearview pregnancy test (Davidson, 1992; May, 1994) which comprises a chromatographic test strip that contains a line of immobilised anti-β-hCG monoclonal antibodies and a line of anti-mouse immunoglo-

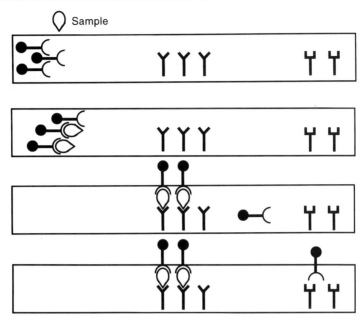

Figure 2 Schematic diagram of a lateral-flow device; and labelled second antibody (filled circle) carried along the device.

bulin antibodies as a reagent control. Close to the application zone is an impregnated zone (not immobilised) of coloured latex particles coupled to anti-α-hCG monoclonal antibody. The application of urine carries the latex particles along the strip, coupled to hCG if there is any present, until captured by the immobilised antibody; the excess latex particle-coupled antibody migrates until captured by the reagent control zone antibody. The assay takes 3 minutes with a sensitivity and specificity of 99%. In the evaluation of the Clearview device by Kingdom *et al.* (1991) in 130 women suspected of early complications of pregnancy, 79 women had a positive test including 12 women with an ectopic pregnancy who all had positive tests, even though the hCG varied between 19 and 47,800 IU l^{-1}, indicating an impressive detection limit and analytical range (absence of hook effect). One woman had a faintly positive result and was not found to be pregnant; the sensitivity and specificity were 100 and 98% respectively.

Clearview involves the addition of a few drops of sample or extract to the device and the qualitative result can be read in a few minutes. In the case of the ClearBlue concept, the device is held directly in the urine stream, an alternative approach using the same basic technology. The performance of an assay device for *Chlamydia trachomatis* has been described (Arumainayagam *et al.*, 1990; Stratton *et al.*, 1991; Young *et al.*, 1991) with sensitivity and specificity of 85.7–95.0% and 98.0–99.0%, respectively, and 76.0–90.0% and 98.6–99.7% predictive value for a positive and negative result, respectively, in studies on over 1,000 samples. The advantages of the device over current laboratory procedures were considered to be the ability to transport a dry sample, the need for only one reagent (extraction diluent) and a heating block, together with the assay time of 30 minutes. Similar performance has been shown with the Kodak Surecell flow-through device (Hammerschlag *et al.*, 1990) and the Abbott TestPack (Coleman *et al.*, 1989). Wilsmore and Davidson (1991) described similar performance for a Clearview-style device for *Chlamydia pittaci (ovis)* from a vaginal swab or foetal membranes. Roberts (1994) described another application for the detection of *Listeria* species in foodstuffs.

Sample type and volume	Sample preparation	Number of steps	Analytes measured	Procedural controls	Technology
Whole blood (7 drops)	None	3 steps (15 min)	Myoglobin + CKMB	Yes	Point of Care (Spectral Diagnostics) Sandwich immunoassay using colloidal gold-conjugated antibody labels. Simultaneous detection of two analytes by addition of sample, removal of separation membrane and addition of developer.
Whole blood (50µl) or Serum/plasma (25µl)	None Blood separation	1 step (12–15 min) (8–10 min)	Lipoprotein a	Yes	Research paper (Abbott Laboratories) Competitive semiquantitative immunochromatographic assay using colloidal selenium as a label to colour a series of bars depending upon concentration.
Whole blood (150µl)	None	1 step (20 min)	Troponin T	Yes	TropT (Boehringer Mannheim) Sandwich immunoassay using streptavidin bound biotin-labelled antibody and a coloured second labelled antibody.
Serum/plasma (350µl sample +) 350µl of diluent) or Urine (700µl)	Blood separation None	2 steps (4 min) 1 step (4 min)	hCG	Yes	Auratek hCG (Organon Teknika) Sample dip and read (urine) or pipette and read (serum). Sandwich immunoassay using colloidal gold particles in a simple format using a reactive strip and reagent sink pad.
Serum/plasma (6 drops)	Blood separation	1 step (10 min)	Hepatitis B s antigen	Yes	Stat-Pak (Chembio Diagnostics) Sandwich immunoassay using colloidal gold particles. Simply pipette sample and read result.
Serum/plasma (5µl)	Blood separation	2 steps (3–8 min)	Infectious mononucleosis antibody	Yes	Biosign (Princeton Biomeditech) Sandwich immunoassay using colloidal gold particles. Add sample, developer solution and read test result.
Serum (1 drop)	Blood separation	3 steps (4 min)	*H. pylori* antibody	Yes	FlexSure HP (Smithkline Diagnostics) Bidirectional chromatographic immunoassay using colloidal gold as an antibody label. Add buffer and sample to separate pads on a folding card. Close card and read.

Table 4 Lateral-flow devices.

An alternative form of lateral-flow device has been described using antibody labelled with colloidal carbon in place of the coloured latex (van Amerongen *et al.*, 1994). In this example, image analysis using a video camera enabled quantification; the between-run coefficient of variation was less than 5% across the concentration range studied (50–450 IU l^{-1} of hCG) with a detection limit of 10 IU l^{-1}. The analysis time was less than 5 minutes.

Immobilised antigen on the surface of latex particles embedded in a fibre matrix wick enabled the production of an assay for human immunodeficiency virus (HIV) antibody in serum.

Sample type and volume	Sample preparation	Number of steps	Analytes measured	Procedural controls	Technology
Urine (Dipstick)	None	1 step (2 min)	Microalbumin	Yes	Micral II (Boehringer Mannkeim). Dip into sample and read.
Urine (3–4 drops)	None	1 step (5 min)	Drugs of abuse: multiple panel THC Opiates Cocaine Amphetamines	Yes	First Check Panel 4 (Worldwide Medical) One-step simultaneous assay.
Urine (3 drops)	None	1 step (5 min)	hCG	Yes	Visualline II (Hanson Hong Biomedical) Sandwich immunoassay using coloured label.
Urine (3 drops)	None	1 step 2–3 min (>250 mIU ml^{-1}) 4–6 min (<250 mIU ml^{-1})	hCG	Yes	TestPack Plus (Abbott) Sandwich immunoassay using colloidal label. Pipette sample and read result.
Urine (Hold sample wick in urine)	None	1 step (3 min)	LH	Yes	Clearplan Onestep (Unipath) Sandwich immunoassay using blue latex as a label. Hold sample wick in urine stream and read result after 3 min comparing colour of test and control line.
Urine (5–7 drops)	None	1 step (10 min)	FSH	Yes	SAS-1-Step FSH (SA Scientific) Simple pipette sample and read test.
Microbiological swab (endocervical) or Early morning urine (7 drops extract/urine)	Swab extraction	2 steps (20 min)	*Chlamydia* (LPS antigen)	Yes	Stat-Pak (Chembio Diagnostic Systems) Sandwich immunoassay using colloidal gold as a label. Single reagent used to extract swab. Add extract to test cassette and read result.
Microbiological swab (Throat)	In line swab extraction	2 steps (5 min)	*Streptococcus* (Group A antigen)	Yes	QuickVue (Quidel) Sandwich immunoassay with in-line swab extraction. Use of two different coloured labels to distinguish test.
Saliva	None	1 step	*H. pylori* antibody	Yes	In development (Saliva Diagnostic Systems)
Faeces (5–7 drops extract)	Sample extraction	2 steps (10 min)	Adenovirus	Yes	SA Scientific Sandwich immunoassay using a coloured conjugate. Add extracted sample and read result.

Table 4 (cont.) Lateral-flow devices.

Addition of diluted serum leads to concentration of any antibody by capture with antigen. The antibody is detected with protein A peroxidase, glucose oxidase being impregnated on latex particles that flow into the antibody capture zone. The substrate glucose is released from a reservoir sponge. The colour is read with a fibre-optic reflectance meter. The assay can be completed in 15 minutes. Whole blood can also be used, and avoiding the need for sample preparation is an attractive safety feature (Dafforn *et al.*, 1990).

TropT (Boehringer Mannheim, Germany) a commercially available assay for troponin T, uses a whole blood sample; the device incorporates separation of plasma from red cells and is not suitable for use with serum (Collinson *et al.*, 1996). The troponin T combines with both biotinylated and gold sol particle-labelled anti-troponin T antibodies to form a sandwich. The mixture flows along the chromatographic support, the biotin binding with avidin immobilised in a line on the strip at the read zone. The intensity of the gold sol particle line is proportional to the analyte concentration. The excess gold sol-labelled antibody migrates beyond the read zone and is captured by immobilised troponin T thereby providing a reagent control. The detection limit of the device is claimed to be 0.2 μg l^{-1} (Antman *et al.*, 1995).

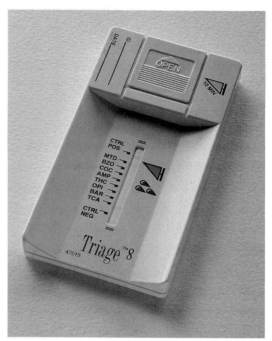

Figure 3 An example of a conventional multianalyte device for testing for drugs of abuse (Triage™, Biosite Diagnostics).

Multianalyte devices have also been described for the simultaneous detection of several molecules, e.g. drugs of abuse (Buechler *et al.*, 1992). In the Triage™ panel (Biosite Diagnostics Inc., San Diego, USA), urine sample is mixed with antibodies directed against the drugs and drugs bound to gold particles. After incubation for 10 minutes, the mixture is added to a membrane device on which is immobilised more antibody against the respective drugs, in lines. In the absence of drug, or in the presence of drug up to a threshold value, the quantity of antibody coupled is sufficient to bind all of the gold-labelled drug and none of the labelled drug is left to bind to the membrane; more drug in the sample (i.e. a positive) displaces labelled drug from the free antibody which binds to the membrane line indicating a positive result. In this way, the amount of high-affinity antibody (monoclonal) can be used to set a threshold value for a positive result, i.e. a cutoff value. Examples of the threshold values were 300 μg l^{-1} for barbiturates and 1,000 μg l^{-1} for amphetamines. The ability to maintain reliable performance at the threshold value is dependent on the type of high-affinity antibody selected and the drug loading in the gold sol particles. An example of this device is shown in Figure 3.

An alternative approach to achieve a more quantitative result is the use of immunochromatography. In one example that uses an immunometric format in which a sample is applied to a chromatographic strip, the analyte migrates through a conjugate pad which contains a sol particle or enzyme-labelled antibody. The analyte-antibody complex then migrates into a region of immobilised antibody (directed against another epitope). The extent of binding measured as distance or number of individual lines of immobilised antibody coupled is equivalent to the concentration of analyte; such a device was described by Lou *et al.* (1993) for quantification of lipoprotein (a) (Lp(a)). These authors used a selenium sol label and the assay was designed to provide a semiquantitative answer. There were some discrepancies between the results from this device and those from assays based on a microtitre plate. In the Acculevel™ system (Behring/Syva, San Francisco, USA) originally described for the hapten theophylline (Zuk *et al.*, 1985), fully quantitative results were achieved using a continuous band of immobilised antibody. In the case of haptens, sample is mixed with labelled hapten (for Acculevel the label is an enzyme); the more sample analyte present the further the labelled analyte moves along the strip before being captured by immobilised antibody; substrate impregnated in the strip enables visualisation of the amount. A fully quantitative assay for hCG was described by Birnbaum *et al.* (1992) with a coloured latex-labelled monoclonal antibody as the mobile reagent; in this case the intensity of the colour immobilised by the presence of antigen was logarithmically proportional to the antigen concentration. These authors calculated that they had used 8 µg immobilised and 6 µg mobile antibody, with the assay capable of visual detection of 1 fmol antigen corresponding to 100 IU l^{-1} (or 10 µg l^{-1}) in a 4 µl sample.

Chemical and Mechanical Considerations

Porous materials should not be considered inert as their surfaces and structures play an important part in the rate of flow of reagents, and also allow nonspecific binding (of analyte, reagents and other sample constituents). Thus, the choice of solid phase and the pretreatment of its surface will help to achieve the desired flow of reagent (and therefore reaction time between exposure of sample and reagent constituents), the resuspension of impregnated mobile reagents, the mixing of constituents and the minimisation of nonspecific binding. In addition, the chemistry of the solid phase will determine the strategy for immobilisation of the capture reagent while also influencing the release rate of the impregnated (temporarily immobilised) mobile reagents.

Devices can also be fabricated from several different materials in contact via overlapping regions. Different materials may facilitate spreading of the sample, mixing with temporarily bound (i.e. impregnated) conjugates and movement of reagents over immobilised materials, and they may act as a reservoir to ensure movement of liquid along the device. In addition, there are now new materials available that will facilitate separation of red blood cells from plasma or provide a more homogeneous material along which liquids and reagents flow. Differential capillarity of overlapping regions can be used to temporarily prevent the flow of liquid into certain regions of strip-type devices. This principle is exemplified in devices that separate plasma from whole blood and that automatically define the volume used in analysis (Bunce, 1995). Klimov *et al.* (1995) attempted to address perceived problems of poor sensitivity, nonuniform colour development and flooding of strips by placing anti-drug antibody-labelled microparticles in a separate membrane strip. Urine is diverted into the second membrane attached part way along the device, some liquid continuing along the main strip.

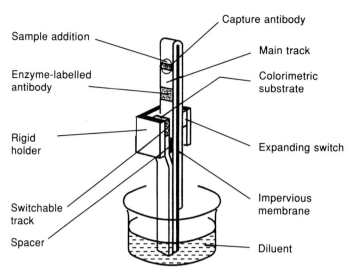

Figure 4 Schematic diagram of a device incorporating a liquid-operated switch.

This was considered to lead to more uniform rehydration of reagent and use of more labelled particles, thereby improving sensitivity; the prewetting of the membrane ahead of the movement of antibody was also thought to be important.

Assay design and performance requirements can influence the design of the housing. Plastic housings are used for protection and to hold porous tracks in precise positions to enable appropriate interaction with the sample when it is added. It is also necessary to enable venting, flow of liquid and collection of excess liquid while allowing access for visualisation of the end points. The whole device must also be capable of storage in desiccant to ensure the dry state necessary for retention of reactivity after long-term storage.

Reagent Sequence and Variation Times

Several approaches have been investigated to allow automatic timing and sequential delivery of multiple reagents flowing along a porous matrix. The properties of individual reagents can be exploited to produce differential flow, and hence timed delivery of reagents. Alternatively, multiple reagents can be incorporated into a series of partially overlapped porous media as in the Micral-Test for α_1-microglobulin and albumin in urine (Boehringer Mannheim, Germany) (Jung *et al.*, 1993; Kutter *et al.*, 1995). The Micral II test for albumin provides a semiquantitative assay with the lowest colour bar being at 0–20 mg l^{-1}; evaluators found some variation in response at the lowest detectable level but good correlation with a reference method at higher levels.

A variation adopted by Bradshaw *et al.* (1995) employed a single chromatographic strip, but with a reservoir pad at each end. Serum added to one end flows up the strip with capture of antigen by immobilised antibody. Buffer added to the reservoir at the end farthest from the point of application rehydrates colloidal gold antibody conjugate and initiates flow in the reverse direction. The strip is held in a device such that when closed it initiates the back flow aided by the contact with the absorbent pad which assists metering. A unidirectional mode was also demonstrated with a detection limit of 5 ng haemoglobin in a faecal occult blood test with the sample dissolved in a reaction buffer.

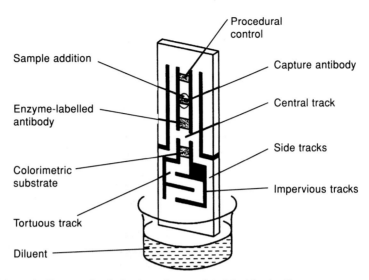

Figure 5 Schematic diagram of a device based on a printed liquidic circuit.

Simpler and potentially more readily adaptable systems may be possible using specific configurations of the porous media support (Bunce *et al.*, 1991, 1993, 1994; Bunce and Starsmore, 1993, 1994; Bunce, 1994). These are exemplified by two concepts: (1) switch devices in which the analytical sequence is achieved by 'switching' porous tracks together by the hydration and subsequent expansion of a foam switching element; and (2) printed liquidic circuits where the analytical sequence is achieved by the track geometry achieved by hydrophobic printing of a single layer of porous material. The analytical sequence is determined physically rather than chemically, and allows reagent additions, timing and wash steps to be defined and determined independently. Diagrammatic representations of these two approaches are shown in Figures 4 and 5. The feasibility of the concept has been demonstrated using dyes to visualise reagent flow and the incorporation of a colorimetric enzyme immunometric assay for hCG in urine. Modification of both concepts can produce systems enabling several immunoassays for different analytes to be performed simultaneously in the same device. Equally, the concepts should be applicable to immunoassays using various labels and, in conjunction with developments allowing incorporation of liquid diluent and the use of whole blood samples, may form the basis of a more flexible analytical system for disposable integrated immunoassay devices. An example of a conventional multianalyte device is shown in Figure 6.

ANALYTICAL PERFORMANCE

As pointed out earlier, much of the fundamental technology underlying integrated immunoassay devices is protected by patents and information not readily available in the public domain. Furthermore, although many of the systems have been developed for the measurement of hCG in urine as a pregnancy test, there are few evaluations of this essentially qualitative assay system in the literature.

There are several publications that have evaluated a wide range of quantitative assays for hCG in urine (Gelletile and Bleber Nielsen, 1986; Thomas *et al.*, 1986; Alfthan *et al.*, 1993).

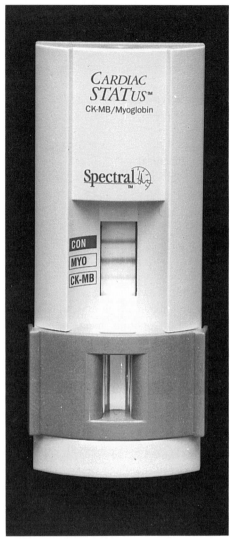

Figure 6 An example of a multianalyte device for cardiac markers in whole blood (Spectral Diagnostics).

The earlier paper compared tube-based assays, slide agglutination tests and flow-through devices. The detection limits varied between 25–50 and 2,200 IU l^{-1}; the accuracy, defined as the proportion of correct results (positive and negative) varied between 89 and 99% with some of the earlier assays affected by blood and protein. In the earlier methods the specificity of the antibodies varied, as did the reference calibration material. In the more recent evaluation (Alfthan *et al.*, 1993), 10 different assays were evaluated, including one cross-flow and three lateral-flow devices. All of the assays took 5 minutes or less to complete, with detection limits of between 20 and 50 IU l^{-1}. The authors found that all the assays performed according to the manufacturers' claims, but drew attention to the influence of urine density on the analytical result, the correlation between the serum and urine results being improved by correction for density. This observation illustrates the importance of preanalytical factors on the performance and interpretation of results because the concentration of the urine samples in the study varyied by up to 10-fold.

There is an inherent problem in attempting to evaluate the performance of a point-of-care testing device, in part because one is applying a scientific and technical discipline to an environment where it may not necessarily pertain; evaluation of a point-of-care device should also include determining its operator dependency and any potential frailty of the system, i.e. the potential for obtaining an incorrect result. This emphasises a point made earlier, that successful use of a device depends on reliable fabrication and proper operator performance. This said, the published evaluations of qualitative 'positive/negative' devices have been shown to perform well against reference laboratory procedures, albeit the evaluations having been undertaken by laboratory personnel. Furthermore, there is no doubt that these devices are increasing in number and versatility, and make a valuable contribution to diagnosis in the point-of-care testing environment.

Analyte	Lowest reliable detectable amount	Sample	Precision (%)	Assay time (min)	Reference
Albumin	20 mg l^{-1}	Urine	–	5	Kutter *et al.*, 1995
Amphetamines	1,000 µg l^{-1}	Urine	–	10	Buechler *et al.*, 1992
C-reactive protein	12 mg l^{-1}	Whole blood	10–15	3	Urdal *et al.*, 1992
Barbiturates	300 µg l^{-1}	Urine	–	10	Buechler *et al.*, 1992
Haemoglobin	76 µg l^{-1}	Faeces	–	5	Bradshaw *et al.*, 1995
Chorionic gonadotrophin	2.5 µg l^{-1}	Serum	–	5	Valkirs & Barton, 1985
Chorionic gonadotrophin	5.0 µg l^{-1}	Urine	–	5	Valkirs & Barton, 1985
Chorionic gonadotrophin	5.0 µg l^{-1}	Urine	–	5	Brown *et al.*, 1972
Chorionic gonadotrophin	1.0 µg l^{-1}	Urine	–	10	Marshall & Bush, 1987
Chorionic gonadotrophin	1.0 µg l^{-1}	Urine	<5	10	Van Amerangen *et al.*, 1994
Chorionic gonadotrophin	1.9 µg l^{-1}	Urine	–	3	Kingdom *et al.*, 1991
Chorionic gonadotrophin	2.5 µg l^{-1}	Urine	<15	5	Anderson *et al.*, 1986
Lipoprotein (a)	40 mg l^{-1}	Serum	–	15	Lou *et al.*, 1993
Theophylline	2.5 mg l^{-1}	Whole blood	<8	15	Zuk *et al.*, 1985
Troponin T	0.2 µg l^{-1}	Whole blood	–	20	Antman *et al.*, 1995

Table 5 An overview of the performance characteristics of some integrated immunoassay devices.

Experience to date suggests that these devices perform well where a qualitative or semi-quantitative response is required. Most current devices use a dilute sample such as urine, the sample providing the reconstitution fluid for the assay. A range of systems also use more viscous samples such as plasma either alone or in conjunction with a liquid diluent, and devices that use only a whole blood sample are increasingly becoming commercially available

(Tables 3 and 4). The breadth of application of these devices has been illustrated earlier; the sensitivity of several assays is shown in Table 5.

CONCLUSIONS

The disposable integrated immunoassay device is designed to provide a diagnostic test at the point-of-decision/care, be it in the home, health centre, outpatient clinic or ward. Devices based on porous media dominate the field and have been combined with improvements in immunoassay technology, and innovations that minimise the number of operator-dependent steps. Appropriate specimen collection and handling, and proper performance of the assay are obviously still required to produce clinically useful results.

It is clear that the availability of highly sensitive labels (e.g. amplified enzyme systems, colloidal gold and carbon) when linked to the ability to capture all of the label in a small area, can provide a very high sensitivity of detection. Some systems, particularly those that include diluent and a means of quantifying the response, can produce accurate and precise results equal to those produced in a central laboratory.

Qualitative and semiquantitative devices have been shown to compare well against reference procedures where a cutoff point or outcome has been clearly defined. There is little doubt when used appropriately they can improve the efficiency of diagnosis whether it be for the convenience of the patient, the nurse or the doctor.

Over the years, much time and many resources have been dedicated to the development of simple-to-use immunoassays for hCG and whole blood glucose. Very impressive systems are currently available and the number of immunoassay devices is increasing both in application and sophistication. It is expected that this trend will continue with further innovations in technology and an increasing array of applications including more for whole blood samples.

Although it is important to review disposable immunoassay technology critically against established analytical criteria, it is also important to recognise the environment in which it is used and thus review it against the needs of that environment. This provides the challenge for the future, not solely for the development scientist and the analyst, but also for the clinician, to determine how best to use the benefits and convenience of the point-of-care testing technology.

REFERENCES

Alfthan, H., Bjorses, U. M., Titinen, A. *et al.* (1993) Specificity and detection limit of ten pregnancy tests. *Scand. J. Lab. Clin. Invest.*, **53**, 105–113.

Anderson, R. R., Lee, T. T., Saewert, D. C. *et al.* (1986) Internally referenced immunoconcentration™ assays. *Clin. Chem.* **32**, 1692–1695.

Antman, E. M., Grudzien, C. & Sacks, D. B. (1995) Evaluation of a rapid bedside assay for detection of serum cardiac troponin T. *J. Amer. Med. Assoc.* **273**, 1279–1282.

Arumainayagam, J. T., Matthews, R. S., Uthayakumar, S. *et al.* (1990) Evaluation of a novel solid phase immunoassay, Clearview Chlamydia, for the rapid detection of *Chlamydia trachomatis. J. Clin. Microbiol.* **28**, 2813–2814.

Birnbaum, S., Uden, C., Magnusson, C. G. M. *et al.* (1992) Latex based thin layer immunoaffinity chromatography for quantitation of protein analytes. *Anal. Biochem.* **206**, 168–171.

Bradshaw, P., Fitzgerald, D., Stephens, L. *et al.* (1995) Flexsure® test device: Qualitative immunochromatographic test format. *Clin. Chem.* **41**, 1360–1363.

Brown, W. E., Clemens, J. M., Devereaux, S. M. *et al.* (1992) Solid phase analytical device and method for using same. *US Patent* No. 5,149,622.

Buechler, K. F., Moi, S., Noar, B. *et al.* (1992) Simultaneous detection of seven drugs of abuse by the Triage™ panel for drugs of abuse. *Clin. Chem.* **38**, 1678–1684.

Bunce, R. A. (1994) Analytical device. *UK Patent Application* GB 2276 002 A.

Bunce, R. A. (1995) Liquid transfer device. UK Patent Application GB 2284 479 A.

Bunce, R. A. & Starsmore, S. J. (1993) Liquid transfer device for diagnostic assays. *UK Patent Application* GB 2261 283 A.

Bunce, R. A., Starsmore, S. J. (1994) Liquid transfer devices. *PCT Patent Application* Int. Pub. No. WO 94/22579.

Bunce, R. A., Thorpe, G. H., Gibbons, J. E. C. *et al.* (1993) Liquid transfer devices. *US Patent* No. 5,198,193.

Bunce, R. A., Thorpe, G. H., Gibbons, J. E. C. *et al.* (1994) Liquid transfer devices. *US Patent* No. 5,354,538.

Bunce, R. A., Thorpe, G. H. & Keen, L. (1991) Disposable analytical devices permitting automatic, timed sequential delivery of multiple reagents. *Anal. Chim. Acta* **249**, 263–269.

Burnett, D. & Freedman, D. B. (1994) Near-patient testing: The management issues. *Health Services Management*, March, 10–13.

Coleman, P., Varitek, V., Mushahwar, I. K. *et al.* (1989) Testpack Chlamydia, a new rapid assay for the direct detection of *Chlamydia trachomatis*. *J. Clin. Microbiol.* **27**, 2811–2814.

Collinson, P. D., Gerhardt, W., Katus, H. A. *et al.* (1996) Multicentre evaluation of an immunological rapid test for the detection of TroponinT in whole blood samples. *Eur. J. Clin. Chem. Clin. Biochem.* **34**: 591–598.

Dafforn, A., Irvine, J. D., Kurn, N. *et al.* (1990) Rapid simple and reliable doctors office test for antibodies to human immunodeficiency virus-1 in serum. *Clin. Chem.* **36**, 1312–1316.

Davidson, I. (1992) Rapid immunoassays. *Anal. Proc.* **29**, 459–460.

Driscoll, R. C., Edwards, R. B., Liston, M. D. *et al.* (1983) Discrete automated chemistry system with tableted reagents. *Clin. Chem.* **29**, 1609–1615.

Gelletile, R. & Bleber Nielsen, J. (1986) Evaluation and comparison of commercially available pregnancy tests based on monoclonal antibodies to human choriogonadotrophin. *Clin. Chem.* **32**, 2166–2170.

Hammerschlag, M. R., Gelling, M., Roblin, P. *et al.* (1990) Comparison of the Kodak Surecell Test Kit wih culture for the diagnosis of chlamydia conjunctivitis in infants. *J. Clin. Microbiol.* **28**, 1441–1442.

Hicks, J. M. (1996) Near patient testing: Is it here to stay? *J. Clin. Path.* **49**, 191–193.

Hilton, S. (1990) Near patient testing in general practice: A review. *Brit. J. Gen. Pract.* **40**, 32–36.

Hussa, R. O., Barnes, C., Schweitzer, P. G. *et al.* (1985) Semiquantitative visual

TANDEM® hCG tests for trophoblastic disease follow up. In: *National Cancer Institute Monographs.* (ed. Rice, J.) Washington.

Jung, K., Pergande, M., Priem, F. *et al.* (1993) Rapid screening of low molecular mass proteinuria: Evaluation of the first immunochemical test strip for the detection of α_1 microglobulin in urine. *Eur. J. Clin. Chem. Clin. Biochem.* **31**, 683–687.

Kingdom, J. C. P., Kelly, T., MacLean, A. B. *et al.* (1991) Rapid one-step urine test for human chorionic gonadotrophin in evaluating suspected complications of early pregnancy. *Brit. Med. J.* **302**, 1308–1311.

Klimov, A. D., Tsai, S. C. J., Towt, J. *et al.* (1995) Improved immunochromatographic format for competitive type assays. *Clin. Chem.* **41**, 1360.

Klotz, U. (1993) Comparison of theophylline blood measured by the standard TD_x assay and a new patient-side immunoassay cartridge system. *Ther. Drug Monit.* **15**, 462–464.

Kutter, D., Thomas, J., Kremer, A. *et al.* (1995) Screening for oligoalbuminuria by means of Micral Test® II: A new immunological test strip. *Eur. J. Clin. Chem. Clin. Biochem.* **33**, 243–245.

Lou, S. C., Patel, C., Chung, S. *et al.* (1993) One-step competitive immunochromatographic assay for semiquantitative determination of lipoprotein (a) in plasma. *Clin. Chem.* **39**, 619–624.

Maclin, E. & Young, D. S. (1994) Automation in the clinical laboratory. In: *Tietz Textbook of Clinical Chemistry* 2nd edn (eds Burtis, C. A. & Ashwood, E. R.) pp. 313–382 (W. B. Saunders & Co., Philadelphia).

Marshall, D. L. & Bush, G. A. (1987) Latex particle enzyme immunoassay. *Amer. Biotech. Lab.* **May/June**, 48–53.

Mason, D. W. & William, A. F. (1980) The kinetics of antibody binding to membrane antigens in solution and at the cell surface. *Biochem. J.* **187**, 1–20.

May, K. (1994) Unipath ClearBlue One Step™, Clearplan One Step™ and Clearview™. In: The *Immunoassay Handbook*, (ed. Wild, D.) pp. 233–235. (Macmillan Press, London).

Merenbloom, B. K. & Oberhardt, B. J. (1995) Homogeneous immunoassay of whole-blood samples. *Clin. Chem.* **41**, 1385–1390.

Morgan, C. L., Newman, D. J. & Price, C. P. (1996) Immunosensors: Technology and opportunities in laboratory medicine. *Clin. Chem.* **42**, 193–209.

Norman, R. J., Lowings, C. & Chard, T. (1985) Dipstick method for human chorionic gonadotrophin suitable for emergency use on whole blood and other fluids. *Lancet*, **i** 19–20.

North, J. (1985) Immunosensors. *Trends Biotechnol.* **3**, 180–186.

Pope, R. M., Apps, J. M., Page, M. D. *et al.* (1993) A novel device for the rapid in-clinic measurement of haemoglobin A1c. *Diab. Med.* **10**, 260–263.

Price, C. P., Burrin, J. M. & Nattrass, M. (1988) Extra-laboratory blood glucose measurement: A policy statement. *Diab. Med.* **5**, 5705–5709.

Pronovost, A. D., Rose, S. L., Pavlak, J. W. *et al.* (1994) Evaluation of a new immunodiagnostic assay for *Helicobacter pylori* antibody detection: Correlation with histopathological and microbiological results. *J. Clin. Microbiol.* **32**, 46–50.

Roberts, P. (1994) An improved cultural/immunoassay for the detection of *Listeria* species in foods and environmental samples. *Microbiol. Eur.* **2**, 18–21.

Robinson, G. A. (1991) Optical immunosensing systems: Meeting the market needs. *Biosens. Bioelectron.* **6**, 183–191.

Santrack, P. J. & Burritt, M. F. (1995) Point of care testing. *Mayo Proc.* **70**, 493–494.

Schultz, S. G., Holen, J. T., Donohue, J. P. *et al.* (1985) Two dimensional centrifugation for desk top clinical chemistry. *Clin. Chem.* **31**, 1457–1463.

Stenberg, M. & Nygren, H. (1988) Kinetics of antigen-antibody reactions at solid-liquid interfaces. *J. Immunol. Meth.* **113**, 3–15.

Stratton, N. J., Hirsch, L., Harris, F. *et al.* (1991) Evaluation of the rapid Clearview Chlamydia test for direct detection of Chlamydia from cervical specimens. *J. Clin. Microbiol.* **29**, 1551–1553.

Thomas, C. M. G., Segers, M. F. G., Leloux, A. M. *et al.* (1986) Comparison of the analytical characteristics of ten urinary hCG tests for early pregnancy diagnosis. *Ann. Clin. Biochem.* **23**, 216–222.

Urdal, P., Borch, S. M., Landaas, S. *et al.* (1992) Rapid immunometric measurement of C-reactive protein in whole blood. *Clin. Chem.* **38**, 580–584.

Valkirs, G. E. & Barton, R. (1985) ImmunoConcentration™: A new format for solid phase immunoassays. *Clin. Chem.* **31**, 1427–1431.

van Amerongen, A., van Loon, D., Berendsen, B. J. M. *et al.* (1994) Quantitative computer image analysis of a human chorionic gonadotrophin colloidal carbon dipstick assay. *Clin. Chim. Acta* **229**, 67–75.

Wilsmore, A. J. & Davidson, I (1991) 'Clearview' rapid test compared with other methods to diagnose chlamydial infection. *Vet. Record* **128**, 503–504.

Young, H. Moyes, A. Lough, H. *et al.* (1991) Preliminary evaluation of 'Clearview Chlamydia' for the rapid detection of chlamydia antigen in cervical secretions. *Genitourin. Med.* **67**, 120–123.

Zipp, A. & Hornby, W. E. (1984) Solid phase chemistry: Its principles and application in clinical analyses. *Talanta* **31**, 863–877.

Zuk, R. F., Ginsberg, V. K., Houts, T. *et al.* (1985) Enzyme immunochromatography: A quantitative immunoassay requiring no instrumentation. *Clin. Chem.* **31**, 1144–1150.

Chapter 23

Microfabricated Immunoassay Devices

Larry J. Kricka and Peter Wilding

INTRODUCTION

Immunoassays come in many forms. These can range from test tubes (or microwells) on large analysers to small devices for qualitative or quantitative assays. A recent trend has been to fashion immunoassay tests into small disposable devices that are processed on a dedicated analyser. Development of immunoassay devices has also been directed towards point-of-care applications such as the doctor's office, the home, workplace or bedside. This has given rise to a variety of small self-contained and self-indicating devices. Most of the new immunoassay devices are in the millimetre to centimetre size range, but an emerging trend is towards microfabricated devices that incorporate components with micrometre-sized and eventually possibly nanometre-sized dimensions (Drexler *et al.*, 1991).

In this chapter we offer a critical appraisal of microfabricated immunoassay devices. Devices are categorised on the basis of their analytical functions and features, and range from low-complexity single-function devices, such as a dipstick, to the highly complex multifunction, multifeature cassette- and cartridge-type devices (Table 1). Many aspects of the technology, development and production of immunoassay devices remain unpublished because of their proprietary nature, and thus descriptions of such devices are often incomplete. In the final section of this chapter we discuss in detail the technology underlying the emerging area of micromachined immunoassay devices.

Motivation behind the development of most immunoassay devices is either to exploit a new and automatable technology (e.g. radial separation of bound and free fractions on a porous tab, or multilayer reagent films (Grenner *et al.*, 1989; McClellan and Plaut, 1994)), or to make the assay suitable for point-of-care applications. There are a number of problems encountered when configuring or formatting an immunoassay as a small disposable device. The technical demands of devices that are used in conjunction with an analyser are considerably less than those for self-contained, self-indicating devices that only require the addition of the sample. In the former, the analyser implements the usual tasks of sample and reagent addition, mixing, incubation, signal detection and analysis, and the normal calibration and quality control can be performed. In a self-contained device a series of controls and monitoring features must be incorporated to ensure that reliable results are obtained. These include positive, negative and procedural controls, interference controls and end-of-test indicators (Kricka, 1992).

LOW-COMPLEXITY DEVICES

The simplest devices incorporate a single analytical function, that of capturing the analyte of interest by means of an immobilised antibody. A sandwich assay format is most commonly used. This is because in a sandwich assay the key reagents are in excess, hence metering of reagents is not critical. In contrast, a competitive immunoassay has the added difficulties of careful timing and accurate sample and reagent metering.

The long-established dipstick qualitative assay format is the least complex, and varying degrees of sophistication have been achieved in dipstick design and fabrication. Many are simply a strip of nylon, polycarbonate, nitrocellulose (Snowden and Hommel, 1991; Rabello *et al.*, 1993) or polyvinylidine difluoride (PVDF) membrane (Kim and Doyle, 1992) onto which reagents are dotted and dried. This strip can then be affixed to a cellulose-acetate stick for greater rigidity and for ease of handling. The immunoassay then involves sequential incu-

	Immunoassay device															
	A	B	C	D	E	F	G	H	I	J	K	L	M	N	O	P
Function																
Sample preparation	−	−	−	−	−	−	−	−	−	−	−	−	+	+	−	−
Analyte capture	+	+	+	+	+	+	+	+	+	+	+	+	+	+	+	+
Reagent addition																
Conjugate	−	−	−	−	+	+	+	−	−	−	−	−	+	+	+	+
Detection reagent(s)	−	−	−	−	−	+	−	−	−	−	−	−	+	+	−	−
Flow control	−	+	+	+	+	+	−	+	+	−	−	−	+	+	+	+
Sump	−	+	+	+	+	+	−	+	+	−	−	−	+	+	+	+
Sample metering	+	−	−	−	+	−	+	−	−	−	−	−	+	+	−	+
Cuvette	+	−	−	−	+	−	+	−	−	−	−	−	+	+	−	−
Active mixing	−	−	−	−	−	−	−	−	−	−	−	−	+	+	−	−
Feature																
Immobilised capture reagent	+	+	+	+	−	+	+	+	+	+	+	+	−	−	+	+
Multiple capture reagents	+	−	−	−	−	−	−	−	−	+	+	−	−	−	+	−
Positive control	+	−	+	+	−	−	−	+	−	−	−	−	−	−	−	+
Low control	−	−	−	+	−	−	−	−	−	−	−	−	−	−	−	−
Negative control	+	−	−	−	−	−	+	−	−	+	−	−	−	−	−	+
Interference control	−	−	+	−	−	−	−	−	−	−	−	−	−	−	−	−
Procedural control	−	−	+	−	−	−	−	−	−	−	−	−	−	−	+	+
Duplicate test zones	−	−	−	+	−	−	−	−	−	−	+	−	−	−	−	−

A, MAST Immunosystems Inc., MASTpette™; B, Hybritech ICON® I; C, ICON® II; D, ICON® QSR®; E, PB Diagnostics, OPUS® (Behring Diagnostics, Westwood, MA) dry-film competitive assay; F, OPUS® ELISA; G, Serono (Woking, Surrey, UK) fluorescent capillary fill device; H, Kodak (Rochester, NY) SureCell®; I, Baxter (Miami, FL) Stratus®; J, Quidel allergy screen; K, Abbott Laboratories MATRIX; L, Adeza Biomedical Corp. (Sunnyvale, CA) OBA™; M, Ames DCA 2000®; N, Ciba-Corning Diagnostics BioTrack 516; O, Biosite Diagnostics (San Diego, CA) Triage™ Ascend™; P, Abbott Laboratories TestPack™ Plus.

Table 1 Analytical functions and features of some immunoassay dipstick, cassette and cartridge devices.

bation in sample, conjugate and signal-generation solution, with the appropriate intermediate washing steps.

A specific benefit of formatting an immunoassay into a device is the facility for simultaneous multianalyte immunoassay (Ekins and Chu, 1991; Kricka, 1992). Available surface area on a dipstick can be sufficiently large to accommodate a number of test zones, thus allowing analysis of a series of substances in a test sample. For example, the Quidel (San Diego, CA) allergen screen (Figure 1*a*) tests for IgE antibodies to *Dermatophagoides pteronyssinus*, *Dermatophagoides farinae*, Japanese cedar, ragweed, cat dander, sweet vernal grass, egg white

a

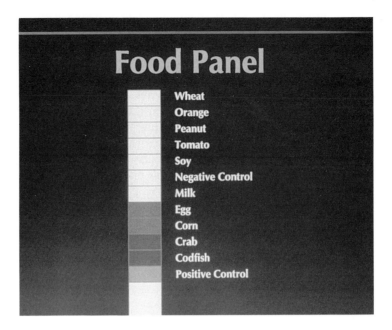

b

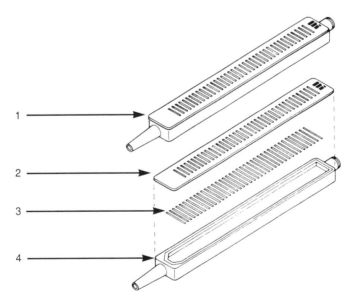

Figure 1 Multianalyte immunoassay test devices. *a*, Quidel allergy screen. *b*, MASTpette™ test chamber. (1) Intact test chamber; (2) black silk-screened polystyrene cover slip; (3) individual cellulose threads; (4) polystyrene test chamber body. (Reproduced courtesy of American Association for Clinical Chemistry (Brown *et al.*, 1985.)

and two different house dusts (Iwamoto *et al.*, 1990). The different allergens are coated onto discrete test zones formed by paper pads. The multizone dipstick is then incubated successively with the serum sample, an alkaline phosphatase mouse monoclonal anti-human IgE conjugate, and enzyme substrate (5-bromo-4-chloro-3-indolyl phosphate). Positive results are indicated by the deposition of a blue indoxyl dye at specific test zones.

The size of discrete test zones in different products spans the micrometre to millimetre range. In the Abbott (Chicago, IL) MATRIX™ device for detecting viral antibodies (e.g. HIV-1 and HIV-2 antibodies) (Donohue *et al.*, 1989) the individual zones in the 5 × 6 test array are formed by islands 2.5 mm in diameter embossed into a nitrocellulose membrane using an ultrasonic horn. In contrast, the 'microspot' assay zones occupy an area of 100 μm^2 and are produced by spotting capture antibody labelled with Texas red onto a flat piece of polystyrene (Ekins and Chu, 1991). The captured analyte is reacted with a fluorescein-labelled specific antibody and bound fluorescein label is detected using a confocal microscope.

The MASTpette™ (MAST Immunosystems, Mountain View, CA) (Figure 1*b*) illustrates another type of device with multiple discrete test areas that also serves as a pipette for sample metering, and as a cuvette for the detection reaction. This is a plastic pipette that contains a parallel array of cellulose threads onto which individual allergens have been covalently attached. Each pipette (1.3 ml) contains up to 38 threads and can be used to test for 35 allergens (plus positive and negative controls). The device is filled with serum, incubated, emptied, washed and the cycle of incubation, emptying and washing is repeated with conjugate and a chemiluminescent substrate solution containing luminol. Light emission from positive reactions on individual threads is recorded on instant photographic film (Miller *et al.*, 1984; Brown *et al.*, 1985).

MODERATELY COMPLEX DEVICES

Several different analytical functions can be combined in an immunoassay device. The most common combination is analyte capture together with a means of drawing fluid through the analyte capture region. The general design is a membrane in close contact with an absorbent pad. The reagent is immobilised onto the central part of the membrane, and the pad serves as a reservoir for excess sample and reagents applied to the membrane. The wicking action of the pad efficiently draws liquids through the membrane. The ICON® (Hybritech, San Diego, CA) and its many variants (Payne *et al.*, 1994) exemplify this type of device.

Fluid flow can be lateral as opposed to the vertical flow used in the ICON® type of devices. This combination of a lateral radial diffusion and analyte capture is used effectively in the Stratus™ tab. In this device, radial diffusion through a paper/glass fibre pad effectively removes excess reagents from a central analyte capture area and this simplifies the washing steps in this analyser-based assay (McClellan and Plaut, 1994).

Analyte capture and a component of the detection system has also been combined in an optical biosensor device for the measurement of human chorionic gonadotrophin (hCG) (Tsay *et al.*, 1991). This device is fabricated from a highly polished piece (4 mm × 5 mm) of a silicon wafer. The surface of the silicon is activated with aminopropyltriethoxysilane, and then the activated surface reacted with an anti-hCG antibody. Short wavelength ultraviolet illumination through a quartz photomask (regular pattern of opaque and clear lines) creates a surface grating pattern comprising immunologically active and inactive antibody. The chips are then mounted onto dipsticks. Reaction of the active antibody on the surface of the silicon chip with hCG forms a biological diffraction grating. Illumination of the highly reflective surface of the reacted chip with a diode laser (670 nm) produces a diffraction signal that is proportional to the hCG concentration in the sample (detection limit 5 IU l^{-1}).

MULTIFUNCTION AND MULTIFEATURE DEVICES

The cassette or cartridge device represents the most sophisticated type of unitised immunoassay device. Diverse combinations of the analytical steps in an immunoassay have been combined, including analyte capture, sample metering, flow control and reagent addition. Examples of three devices of differing degrees of complexity are described below.

Analyte capture, sample metering and reagent delivery are combined in the fluorescence capillary fill device (FCFD). This is constructed from two 30-mm-long pieces of glass spaced 100 μm apart to form a 25-μl reaction chamber. Capture antibody is immobilised onto the inside surface of the glass and a fluorescently labelled conjugate microdosed into the device. Analyte (e.g. prostate-specific antigen or hCG) in the sample reacts with the specific antibodies to form sandwiches on the surface of the glass, and these are detected by an evanescent wave technique (Deacon *et al.*, 1991; Fletcher *et al.*, 1993).

The DCA 2000® (Bayer, Tarrytown, NY) test for haemoglobin A1c (HbA1c) in whole blood combines sample preparation, reagent addition, mixing, measurement and calculation (% HbA1c) (Figure 2*a*). A capillary prefilled with 1 μl whole blood from a fingerstick is placed into the 55 × 55 × 12-mm cassette. The cassette is then inserted into the DCA 2000® analyser and this provides temperature control and initiates the sequence of reagent addition,

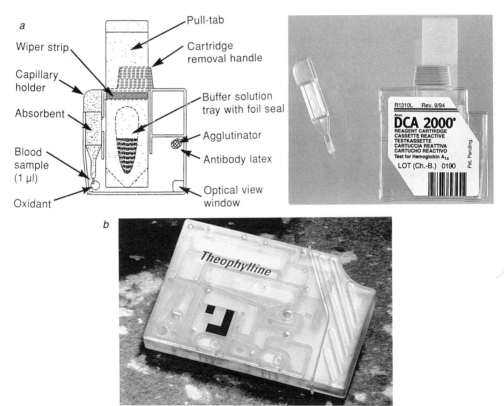

Figure 2 Multifunction, multifeature immunoassay cartridges. *a*, AMES DCA 2000® test device for haemoglobin A1c (left-hand panel, schematic; right-hand panel, photograph of device and associated pipette). (Reproduced courtesy of *Diabetes Care* (1992) 15, 1047.) *b*, Biotrack 516 test device for theophylline. (Courtesy of Boehringer Mannheim Corporation.)

mixing, incubation and the spectrophotometric readings for this 9-minute test (Pope *et al.*, 1993). The key assay reagent is a synthetic polymer containing HbA1c glucopeptide hapten which causes agglutination of anti-HbA1c-coated latex beads. HbA1c in the sample inhibits the agglutination and the degree of agglutination is measured spectrophotometrically. Total haemoglobin is measured by first oxidising haemoglobin to methaemoglobin using ferricyanide, and then measuring the absorbance at 530 nm. HbA1c is then determined as a percentage of the total haemoglobin. The intra-assay coefficient of variation (CV) for this device for HbA1c concentrations of 5.2% and 13% is 1.6% and 2.4%, respectively.

The Biotrack 516 (Boehringer Mannheim, Indianapolis, IN) illustrates one of the most complex immunoassay cassette devices (Klotz, 1993). It combines sample metering, sample treatment, dilution, mixing, reagent addition and optical measurements, and provides a rapid (<3 min) assay for theophylline (range 2.5–40 μg ml^{-1}) in an unmeasured drop (at least 20 μl) of whole blood. The design of the 9 × 8 × 0.9-cm three-part injection-moulded device is shown in Figure 2*b*. After application of a drop of blood to the well, it is taken up by a metering capillary which fills to a preset volume (6.4 μl) based on surface tension forces (surplus blood flows into a capillary drain). The cassette is inserted into the monitor which initiates the sequence of analytical events. Diluent containing a Lubrol® detergent, potassium ferricyanide and azide (to lyse red blood cells and convert haemoglobin to methaemoglobin) is released from a glass ampoule in the cassette. This washes the metered sample of blood from the capillary into the first measuring chamber (volume 156 μl) where it is mixed by agitation (20 s at 7 Hz) with a steel ball (0.24 cm diameter) contained in the chamber. Haemoglobin content in the lysate is determined from an absorption measurement at a wavelength of 565 nm. The haemoglobin concentration is used to correct the immunoassay result for haematocrit effects and provide plasma levels of theophylline.

Next, the haemolysed sample is transferred to a second measurement capillary (9 μl) and excess fluid is drawn into a drain. A second diluent displaces the metered haemolysate (1:18 dilution) into a second reaction chamber (volume 158 μl) coated with the dried reagents: theophylline-labelled latex particles (0.1 μm diameter) and monoclonal anti-theophylline antibody. After a brief mixing step (4 s at 7 Hz) by agitation of a steel ball, turbidity measurements are made for a period of 10 s. In this turbidimetric latex-agglutination inhibition assay, drug present in the haemolysed blood sample inhibits the antibody-mediated agglutination of the particles by competing for binding sites. Bubble formation that would compromise the operation of the device is precluded by the shape and internal surface properties of the chamber.

The external monitor provides light-emitting diode optics for optical measurements and verification of fluid flow, solenoids to release diluent from the glass ampoules inside the cassette and control the valve, a magnet to activate mixing, and a heater. The valve inside the cassette is formed from a latex film sandwiched between the body and back cover of the cassette. It is opened and closed by a solenoid that pushes the latex against the cassette body to form a seal. Quality control cartridges with known theophylline levels are used to check overall system performance, and comparative studies have confirmed the validity and reproducibility of the assay (theophylline 11.5–25 μg ml^{-1}, intra-assay CV 2.8–4.0%, interassay CV 3.7–4.7%).

MICROMACHINED AND MICROFABRICATED DEVICES

Micromachined devices have a number of potential advantages and benefits compared to the macrosized immunoassay devices described in the previous sections. Total analytical system (TAS) integration is one of the most compelling advantages. Available micromachining technology permits the construction of complex micrometre-sized interconnecting structures with diverse functions (valves, filters, diaphragms, pumps, motors) (Angell *et al.*, 1983) and the integration of electronic sensors and control, all on a single microchip to form a micro-total analytical system (μTAS) (Manz *et al.*, 1990, 1991).

To date there are no examples of fully integrated immunoassay microchips, but individual elements in the total analytical system have been achieved and some simple chip-based immunoassays have been described. In this section we examine micromachining and review the current status of microchip immunoassay.

Micromachining and Microfabrication

Micromachining involves the controlled removal or deposition of material at a micrometre scale. A range of techniques and materials are available for micromachining (Table 2) and simple wet etching of silicon is the most extensively developed technology (Petersen, 1982; Bard, 1994). However, there is an expanding interest in micromachining of glass (soda glass and Pyrex) because of its transparency and insulating properties.

Feature sizes of approximately 1 μm are achievable using conventional photolithography and wet etching of silicon. Other fabrication methods allow structures with feature sizes of

Materials	
Alumina	Glass (Pyrex, soda)
Aluminium	Gold
Ceramics	Indium phosphide
Copper	Quartz
Diamond	Rubidium molybdenum oxide
Fluorocarbon polymers	Silicon
Gallium-arsenide	Silicon carbide.

Method	
Atomic force microscope	Laser
Anisotropic etching	Reactive ion etching
Electron-beam	Scanning probe microscope
Embossing	Scanning tunnelling microscope
Focused ion-beam	Solvent softening
Isotropic etching	

Table 2 Materials and methods for microfabrication.

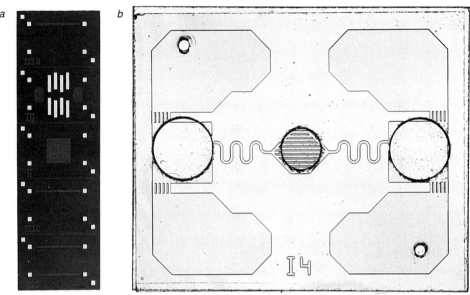

Figure 3 Silicon and glass-glass microchips. *a*, Section of a wafer showing examples of silicon microchips illustrating a range of channel and chamber structures. Individual chips are labelled IIIB, IV, V, IIIC, IIC and are shown prior to capping with glass. Square holes through the silicon are the entry and exit ports. Holes at the upper left and lower right of each chip are locator holes for the chip holder. *b*, Glass-glass microchip comprising a series of chambers linked by channels (centre) and barriers (left and right). Holes pierce the glass cover to provide access to three of the chambers. The small holes upper left and lower right are air-vent holes.

<1 μm to be produced (e.g. minimum feature sizes: 0.3 μm, deep UV (230–260 nm); 0.1 μm, X-ray and electron-beam; <1 nm, scanning tunnelling microscope) (Petersen, 1982; Sze, 1988; Garfunkel *et al.*, 1989; Shoji and Esashi, 1993). Sacrificial-layer techniques provide a further dimension to microfabrication. A sacrificial layer is an intermediate layer that can be selectively removed to release an overlying structure. In this way complex multicomponent devices with moving parts such as motors can be produced (Fan *et al.*, 1988). Components can be bonded together to form multilayer structures and holes introduced by laser drilling (Shoji and Esashi, 1995). Some examples of silicon and glass-glass microchips are shown in Figure 3 above.

Advantages of Microfabrication

Microfabrication offers increased flexibility in design and ease of manufacture compared to the manufacturing techniques used to produce macroscale devices. For devices made from silicon, existing microelectronics industry manufacturing processes are already geared to high-volume low-cost production (millions of wafers per year). Device density on a 4-inch or a 6-inch wafer is high, and thus many different microchip designs can be simultaneously fabricated on the same wafer. This leads to rapid design cycles and the potential for many more design iterations than would normally be possible for a macroscale device. Similarly, a change in the design of a microfabricated product is easier and cheaper, because it may only involve relatively simple modifications to the photolithographic mask.

The internal volume of microchip analysers is low (microlitres to picolitres). This leads to an economic benefit because the reagent consumption per test is greatly reduced, and to a clinical benefit because the volume of sample required for analysis is minimal, e.g. nanolitre to picolitre volumes as compared to the microlitre volumes used in current analysers. In a clinical setting this is beneficial to the patient and more convenient for the phlebotomist (finger-stick versus venepuncture). It is also especially advantageous for neonatal and paediatric patients where total blood volume is relatively small and removal of large samples is medically contra-indicated. The small sample size also reduces the exposure of health workers to potentially hazardous specimens. The low capacity of devices minimises the volume of waste fluids, and it is also possible to entomb the contents of a device (unreacted sample, reagents and reaction mixture) for safe disposal.

The small size of microfabricated devices allows faster response times, and the production of compact hand-held analysers that are suitable for point-of-care testing and environmental testing (e.g. stream-side). In addition, multiple test sites for simultaneous multiplicate assays can be designed on one microfabricated device. This built-in redundancy provides an analytical safeguard not easily achieved in a conventional macroscale system, where duplicate assays represent the normal extent of repetitive assay of a specimen. Also, encapsulated microscale devices may provide extended operation over a wider range of environmental conditions of humidity and temperature.

Finally, the design flexibility of a microfabricated device does not lock the chip into a single assay design. Development of single-principle immunoassay devices suitable for assaying large or small analytes (sandwich or competitive assay designs) has been fraught with difficulties; such limitations do not apply to microfabricated devices.

System Integration

Microfabrication provides a route to total system integration for a multistep analytical method such as immunoassay. Table 3 lists some of the micromechanical devices that have been fabricated and could be used in the design of an immunoassay microchip. These could be used in combination with on-chip sensors (ion selective electrodes, ion-sensitive field-effect transistors, heaters (strip heaters or Peltier elements) (van Gerwen *et al.*, 1995) and optical devices (lamps, filters) (Muller and Mastrangelo, 1994). Table 4 lists some recent examples of micro-total analytical system devices. The progress made in total analytical system integration for other applications suggests that the production of an immunoassay microchip will eventually be successful.

Microchip Immunoassays

Examples of microchip immunoassays are currently very limited (Table 5) and the micromachined devices restricted to relatively simple channels, chambers and filters. Qualitative ABO blood typing has been accomplished in glass-capped silicon microchambers (5 mm × 5 mm × 40 μm deep) (Figure 4*a*). Application of a blood sample to a chamber containing anti-A or anti-B antiserum produced agglutination of the red blood cells and this was monitored visually using a microscope. Likewise, IgG has been detected using a microchannel or a microchamber (150 μm wide × 40 mm deep) filled with anti-IgG-coated 4.55-μm-diameter

Device/function	Reference
Diffraction grating	(Chen, 1993)
Electrode	(Suzuki and Sugama, 1994)
Filter	(Kittisland and Stemme, 1990; Wilding *et al.*, 1994)
Flow cell	(Verpoorte *et al.*, 1992)
Fluid injector	(Fiehn *et al.*, 1995)
Heat Exchanger	(Friedrich and Kang, 1994)
Lamp	(Mastrangelo *et al.*, 1992; Muller and Mastrangelo, 1994)
Light-emitting diode	(Granstrom *et al.*, 1995)
Liquid transport	(Columbus, 1980)
Mirror	(Buser *et al.*, 1992)
Motor	(Paratte *et al.*, 1991)
Optical filter	(de Frutos *et al.*, 1994; Gebhard and Benecke, 1995)
Peltier heater/cooler element	(van Gerwen *et al.*, 1995)
Pressure sensor	(Buser and de Rooij, 1991)
Pressure switch	(de Bruin *et al.*, 1990)
Pump	(Fuhr *et al.*, 1992; Schomburg *et al.*, 1993)
Refrigerator	(Little, 1984)
Valve	(Gordon, 1991)

Table 3 Micromechanical elements available for micro-total analytical system devices.

Device/analyser	Reference
Multi–analyte analyser (Na+, K+, urea, etc.)	(Erickson and Wilding, 1993)
Mass spectrometer	(Feustel *et al.*, 1995)
Gas–liquid chromatograph	(Bruns, 1994)
Liquid chromatograph	(Cowen and Craston, 1995)
Flow microreactor	(Mensinger *et al.*, 1995)
Amperometric analyser (glucose)	(Forssen *et al.*, 1995)
Modular ISFET analyser (phosphate)	(van der Schoot *et al.*, 1995)
Flow injection analyser	(Karube, 1995)
Capillary zone electrophoresis analyser	(Effenhauser *et al.*, 1993; Harrison *et al.*, 1993a,b)
Blood gas analyser	(Shoji *et al.*, 1988)

Table 4 Examples of micro-total analytical system devices.

fluorescent beads. Agglutination was assessed visually using a fluorescence microscope (Figure 4*b*).

Analyte	Device	Material	Immunological reaction on or off chip	Detection limit	Reference
α-fetoprotein	Microchip	Glass	On	10 pg ml^{-1}	(Song *et al.*, 1994)
Blood typing	Microchip	Silicon/glass	On	Qualitative	(Wilding *et al.*, 1994)
BSA	Microchip CE	Glass, quartz or fused silica	On	2 µg	(Harrison *et al.*, 1995)
Cortisol	Microchip CE	Fused silica	Off	10 ng ml^{-1}	(Koutny *et al.*, 1996)
Human IgG	Microchip	Silicon/glass	On	Qualitative	(Wilding *et al.*, 1994)
Mouse IgG	LAPS	Silicon	Off	25 pg	(Briggs and Fanfili, 1991)

BSA, Bovine serum albumin; CE, capillary electrophoresis; IgG, immunoglobulin G; LAPS, light-addressable potentiometric sensor.

Table 5 Immunoassays in devices micromachined in silicon or glass.

More sophisticated fluorescent bead latex-agglutination immunoassays for α-fetoprotein have been performed in a series of four microchannels (0.4 µl; 10 mm long, 80 µm deep, 500 µm wide) etched in Pyrex glass (Song *et al.*, 1994) (Figure 5). An alternating electric field was used to increase the rate of agglutination of the beads (1.66 µm diameter) and agglutination assessed using a fluorescent microscope and an image analyser. This 1-minute assay detected α-fetoprotein down to 10 pg ml^{-1}.

Micromachined silicon pits that incorporate a pH-sensitive light-addressable potentiometric sensor (LAPS) (Molecular Devices, Sunnyvale, CA) (Figure 6) have been adapted to immunological assays (Briggs and Fanfili, 1991; Owicki *et al.*, 1994). A model two-site immunoassay for mouse IgG illustrates the general principle of this type of assay. The immunological assay is performed on a biotinylated membrane using a biotinylated anti-mouse antibody, a fluorescein-labelled anti-mouse antibody, an anti-fluorescein-urease conjugate, and avidin. Sample is reacted with these reagents in solution, then the biotinylated membrane captures the immune complexes (avidin:biotin–anti-mouse IgG antibody:IgG:anti-mouse IgG antibody–fluorescein:anti-fluorescein– urease). The membrane bearing the immune complexes is then placed in contact with the LAPS containing 0.5 µl of a urea substrate. Changes in pH due to the action of the bound urease label on the urea substrate are detected by the LAPS. This assay was linear over the range 25–5,000 pg of mouse IgG. Assays for potential contaminants of recombinant protein products (e.g. *Escherichia coli* protein, protein A), hormones (e.g. hCG) and infectious agents (e.g. *Yersinia pestis*) have also been developed using the LAPS detector (Briggs, 1991; Briggs and Fanfili, 1991).

An emerging trend is the use of microchip capillary electrophoresis to measure the concentration of bound and free species in competitive immunoassays (Harrison *et al.*, 1995; Koutny *et al.*, 1996). Capillary electrophoresis (CE) coupled with laser-induced fluorescent detection is fast, sensitive and requires only a few nanolitres of sample. In one approach, the immunoassay is performed off-chip in a conventional tube, and then the reaction mixture transferred to a CE microchip (17 mm × 60 mm), and analysed in a 28-µm-deep × 66-µm-wide × 2.5-cm-long separation channel. Preliminary results for a cortisol assay are favourable (analytical range 10–600 µg l^{-1}) and the separation of bound and free fluorescein-labelled cortisol was accomplished in 30 s using an injection volume of 0.75 nl (Koutny *et al.*, 1996).

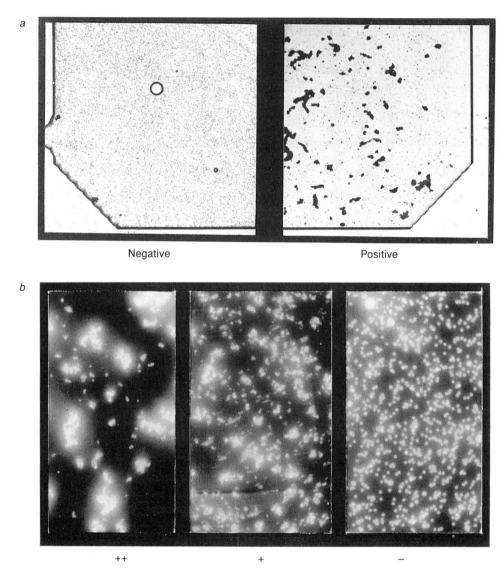

Figure 4 Agglutination immunoassays in silicon-glass microchambers. *a*, Blood grouping in 5 mm × 5 mm × 40-μm-deep chamber showing positive agglutination of A-type red blood cells with anti-A antibodies. *b*, Assay for human IgG using anti-IgG antibody-coated fluorescent microparticles (4.55 μm diameter) in a 150-μm-wide × 40-μm-deep microchannel. Results are shown for a negative (−), weakly positive (+), and strongly positive (++) sample.

Another approach combines the immunological reaction and the CE separation on a chip (Harrison *et al.*, 1995). A fluorescein label is used and the immunological assay takes place in a 3.6 nl mixing chamber. A model assay for bovine serum albumin has demonstrated the proof-of-principle for this integrated immunoassay microchip.

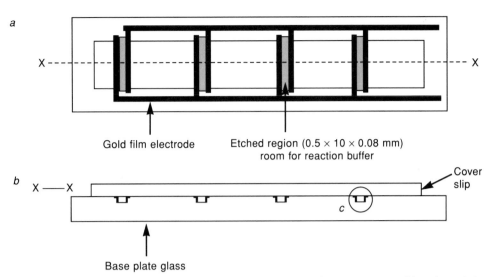

Figure 5 Microreactor for an alternating-current field-enhanced immunoassay. *a*, Top view of the microreactor; *b*, Front view of the microreactor; *c*, etched region of the base plate. (Reproduced courtesy of *Analytical Chemistry* (Song *et al.*, 1994).)

CALIBRATION

Different strategies have been adopted for calibration of disposable microfabricated analytical devices. Most rely on the simple qualitative calibration afforded by a positive and negative control (e.g. MASTpette for IgE analysis) (Brown *et al.*, 1985). Some devices use electronic calibration. For example, the reagent cartridges for the DCA 2000 HbA1c analyser are calibrated by the manufacturer and the lot-specific calibration parameters stored as a bar code on a calibration card. The analyser is programmed by simply passing the card past the instrument's reader (Marrero *et al.*, 1992). For disposable biosensor-based devices it is possible to calibrate the sensor directly by first passing a calibrator solution over the active surface. In the i-STAT (Princeton, NJ) cartridge the calibrator solution is stored in a small pouch and when the cartridge containing the blood sample is placed in the analyser this is punctured and the calibrator fluid flows over the sensor array for calibration prior to assay of the blood sample. The issue of calibrating disposable micromachined immunoassay devices has not been addressed authoritatively. Various strategies may be possible. The available surface area on a microchip could accommodate several test zones and these could be used for performing analysis of standards alongside the test sample. Precalibration of a batch of devices may also be an option and this will depend on the reliability of the production techniques chosen to mass-produce immunoassay microchips.

CONCLUSIONS

There is a general trend towards qualitative and quantitative unitised, disposable immunoassay devices, and varying degrees of sophistication have been achieved. Many of the functions and features required for either a competitive or a sandwich immunoassay have been

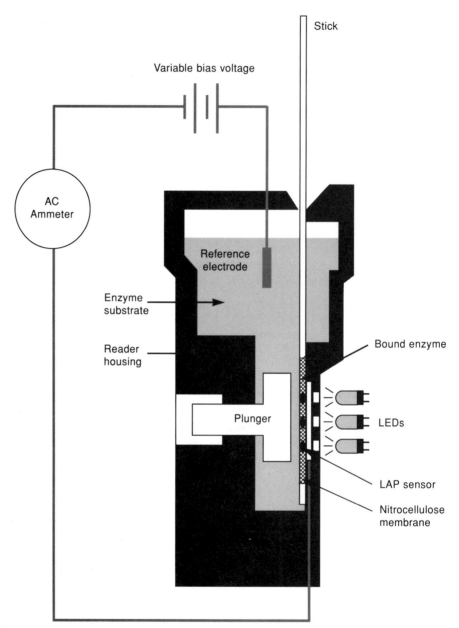

Figure 6 Light-addressable potentiometric sensor (LAPS). (Illustration kindly provided by Molecular Devices Corporation, Sunnyvale, CA.)

successfully formatted into a small disposable device. Further refinement by miniaturisation is the next most likely step in the development of immunoassay devices. The concept of an immunoassay, or even a complete immunoassay analyser on a microchip is appealing, and the preliminary results with the microchip combining an immunological reactor and capillary electrophoretic separation underscores the feasibility and potential of microchip immunoassay. The building blocks for more sophisticated devices already exist and are a result of

the work of the micromachinist and the developers of micro-total analytical systems. Continued development of microchips for immunoassay is anticipated because micromachining techniques offer a level of system integration (chemistry, detection, read-out, etc.) not readily achievable with current macroscale devices. Routine implementation of immunoassay microchips still faces many legislative, technical and economic hurdles, including calibration, reliability, and cost-effectiveness in routine practice.

REFERENCES

Angell, J. B., Terry, S. C. & Barth, P. W. (1983) Silicon micromechanical devices. *Scient. Amer.* **248**, 44–55.

Bard, A. (ed.) (1994) *Integrated Chemical Systems* (Wiley, New York).

Briggs, J. (1991) Sensor-based system for rapid and sensitive measurement of contaminating DNA and other analytes in biopharmaceutical development and manufacturing. *J. Parenteral Sci. Technol.* **45**, 7–12.

Briggs, J. & Fanfili, P. R. (1991) Quantitation of DNA and protein impurities in biopharmaceuticals. *Anal. Chem.* **63**, 850–859.

Brown, C. R., Higgins, K. W., Frazer, K. *et al.* (1985) Simultaneous determination of total IgE and allergen-specific IgE in serum by the MAST chemiluminescent assay system. *Clin. Chem.* **31**, 1500–1505.

Bruns, M. W. (1994) High-speed portable gas-chromatograph-silicon micromachining. *Erdol. Kohle Erdgas. Petrochem.* **47**, 80–84.

Buser, R. & de Rooij, N. F. (1991) Silicon pressure sensor based on a resonating element. *Sens. Actuators* **A25–27**, 717–722.

Buser, R. A., de Rooij, N. F., Tischhauser, H. *et al.* (1992) Biaxial scanning mirror activated by bimorph structures for medical applications. *Sens. Actuators* **A31**, 29–34.

Chen, T. (1993) Wavelength-modulated optical gas sensor. *Sens. Actuators* **B13–14**, 284–287.

Columbus, R. L. (1980) Liquid transport device. *US Patent* No. 4,233,029.

Cowen, S. & Craston, D. H. (1995) The challenge of developing μTAS. In: *Micro Total Analytical Systems* (eds van den Berg, A. & Bergveld, P.) pp. 295–298 (Kluwer Academic Publishers, Dordrecht).

de Bruin, D. W., Allen, H. V., Terry, S. C. *et al.* (1990) Electrically trimmable silicon micromachined pressure switch. *Sens. Actuators* **A21–23**, 54–57.

de Frutos, J., Rodriguez, J. M., Lopez, F. *et al.* (1994) Electrooptical infrared compact gas sensor. *Sens. Actuators* **B18–19**, 682–686.

Deacon, J. K., Thomson, A. M., Page, A. L. *et al.* (1991) An assay for human chorionic gonadotropin using the capillary fill immunosensor. *Biosens. Bioelectron.* **6**, 193–199.

Donohue, J., Bailey, M., Gray, R. *et al.* (1989) Enzyme immunoassay system for panel testing. *Clin. Chem.* **35**, 1874–1877.

Drexler, E., Peterson, C. & Pergamit, G. (1991) *Unbounding the Future: The Nanotechnology Revolution* (William Morrow & Co., New York).

Effenhauser, C. S., Manz, A. & Widmer, H. M. (1993) Glass chips for high-speed capillary electrophoresis separations with submicrometer plate heights. *Anal. Chem.* **65**, 2637–2642.

Ekins, R. & Chu, F. W. (1991) Multianalyte microspot immunoassay: Microanalytical 'compact disk' of the future. *Clin. Chem.* **37**, 1955–1967.

Erickson, K. A. & Wilding, P. (1993) Evaluation of a novel point-of-care system: The i-STAT portable clinical analyzer. *Clin. Chem.* **39**, 283–287.

Fan, L.-S., Tai, Y.-C. & Muller, R. S. (1988) Integrated movable micromechanical structures for sensors and actuators. *Inst. Elect. Electron. Engrs Trans. Electron. Devices* **35**, 724–730.

Feustel, A., Muller, J. & Relling, V. (1995) A microsystem mass spectrometer. In: *Micro Total Analytical Systems* (eds van den Berg, A. & Bergveld, P.) pp. 299–304 (Kluwer Academic Publishers, Dordrecht).

Fiehn, H., Howitz, S., Pham, M. T. *et al.* (1995) Components and technology for a fluidic-ISFET-microsystem. In: *Micro Total Analytical Systems* (eds van den Berg, A. & Bergveld, P.) pp. 289–293 (Kluwer Academic Publishers, Dordrecht).

Fletcher, J. E., O'Neil, P. M., Stafford, C. G. *et al.* (1993) Rapid, biosensor-based, assay for PSA in whole blood. *Tumor Marker Update* **5**, 99–101.

Forssen, L., Elderstig, H., Eng, L. *et al.* (1995) Integration of an amperometric glucose sensor in a µTAS. In: *Micro Total Analytical Systems* (eds van den Berg, A. & Bergveld, P.) pp. 203–207 (Kluwer Academic Publishers, Dordrecht).

Friedrich, C. R. & Kang, S. D. (1994) Micro-heat exchangers fabricated by diamond machining. *Prec. Engng J. Amer. Soc. Prec. Engrs* **16**, 56–59.

Fuhr, G., Hagedorn, R., Müller, T. *et al.* (1992) Pumping of water solutions in microfabricated electrohydrodynamic systems. *Proc. Micro Electro Mechanical Systems Conference (MEMS '92)* pp. 25–30 (Inst. Elect. Electron. Engrs, New York).

Garfunkel, E., Rudd, G., Novak, D. *et al.* (1989) Scanning tunneling microscopy and nanolithography on a conducting oxide, $Rb_{0.3}MoO_3$. *Science* **246**, 99–100.

Gebhard, M. & Benecke, W. (1995) Concept of a miniaturised system for multicomponent gas analysis based on non-dispersive infrared techniques. In: *Micro Total Analytical Systems* (eds van den Berg, A. & Bergveld, P.) pp. 279–282 (Kluwer Academic Publishers, Dordrecht).

Gordon, G. B. (1991) Thermally-actuated microminiature valve. *US Patent* No. 5,058,856.

Granstrom, M., Berggren, M. & Inganas, O. (1995) Micrometer- and nanometer-sized polymeric light-emitting diodes. *Science* **267**, 1479–1481.

Grenner, G., Inbar, S., Meneghini, F. A. *et al.* (1989) Multilayer fluorescent immunoassay technique. *Clin. Chem.* **35**, 1865–1868.

Harrison, D. J., Fluri, K., Chiem, N. *et al.* (1995) Micromachining chemical and biochemical analysis and reaction systems on glass substrates. *Transducers '95: Eurosensors* **IX**, 752–755.

Harrison, D. J., Fluri, K., Seiler, K. *et al.* (1993a) Micromachining a miniaturized capillary electrophoresis-based chemical analysis system on a chip. *Science* **261**, 895–897.

Harrison, D. J., Glavina, P. G. & Manz, A. (1993b) Towards miniaturized electrophoresis and chemical analysis systems on silicon: An alternative to chemical sensors. *Sens. Actuators* **B10**, 107–116.

Iwamoto, I., Yamazaki, H., Kimura, A. *et al.* (1990) Comparison of a multi-allergen dipstick IgE assay to skin-prick test and RAST. *Clin. Exp. Allergy* **20**, 175–179.

Karube, I. (1995) µTAS for biochemical analysis. In: *Micro Total Analytical Systems* (eds van den Berg, A. & Bergveld, P.) pp. 37–46 (Kluwer Academic Publishers, Dordrecht).

Kim, M. S. & Doyle, M. P. (1992) Dipstick immunoassay to detect enterohemorrhagic *Escherichia coli* O157:H7 in retail ground beef. *Appl. Environ. Microbiol.* **58**, 1764–1767.

Kittilsland, G. & Stemme, G. (1990) A sub-micron particle filter. *Sens. Actuators* **A21–23**, 904–907.

Klotz, U. (1993) Comparison of theophylline blood measured by the standard TD_x assay and a new patient-side immunoassay cartridge system. *Ther. Drug Monit.* **15**, 462–464.

Koutny, L. B., Schmalzing, D., Taylor, T. A. *et al.* (1996) Microchip electrophoretic immunoassay for serum cortisol. *Anal. Chem.* **68**, 18–22.

Kricka, L. J. (1992) Simultaneous multianalyte immunoassays. *In-service Train. Contin. Educat.* **10**, 7–11.

Little, W. (1984) Microminiature refrigeration. *Rev. Scient. Instrum.* **55**, 661–680.

Manz, A., Graber, N. & Widmer, H. M. (1990) Miniaturized total analysis systems: A novel concept for chemical sensors. *Sens. Actuators* **B1**, 244–248.

Manz, A., Harrison, D. J., Verpoorte, E. M. J. *et al.* (1991) Miniaturization of chemical analysis systems: A look into next century's technology or just a fashionable craze? *Chimia* **45**, 103–105.

Marrero, D. G., Vandagriff, J. L., Gibson, R. *et al.* (1992) Immediate HbA1c results. *Diab. Care* **15**, 1045–1049.

Mastrangelo, C. H., Yeh, J. H. J. & Muller, R. S. (1992) Electrical and optical characteristics of vacuum-sealed polysilicon microlamps. *Inst. Elect. Electron. Engrs Trans. Electron. Devices* **39**, 1363–1374.

McClellan, W. N. & Plaut, D. (1994) Baxter Stratus immunoassay systems. In: *The Immunoassay Handbook* (ed. Wild, D.) pp. 149–154 (Stockton Press, New York).

Mensinger, H., Richter, T., Hessel, V. *et al.* (1995) Microreactor with integrated static mixer and analysis system. In: *Micro Total Analytical Systems* (eds van den Berg, A. & Bergveld, P.) pp. 237–243 (Kluwer Academic Publishers, Dordrecht).

Miller, S. P., Marinkovich, V. A., Riege, D. H. *et al.* (1984) Application of the MAST immunodiagnostic system to the determination of allergen-specific IgE. *Clin. Chem.* **30**, 1467–1472.

Muller, R. S. & Mastrangelo, C. H. (1994) Vacuum-sealed silicon incandescent light. *US Patent* No. 5,285,131.

Owicki, J. C., Bousse, L. J., Hafeman, D. G. *et al.* (1994) The light-addressable potentiometric sensor. *Ann. Rev. Biophys. Biomol. Struct.* **23**, 87–113.

Paratte, L., Racine, G., de Rooij, N. F. *et al.* (1991) Design of an integrated stepper motor with axial field. *Sens. Actuators* **A25–27**, 597–603.

Payne, G. P., Saewert, M. & Harvey, S. (1994) Hybritech ICON and TANDEM ICON QSR. In: *The Immunoassay Handbook* (ed. Wild, D.) pp. 175–178 (Stockton Press, New York).

Petersen, K. E. (1982) Silicon as a mechanical material. *Proc. Inst. Elect. Electron. Engrs* **70**, 420–456.

Pope, R. M., Apps, J. M., Page, M. D. *et al.* (1993) A novel device for the rapid in-clinic measurement of haemoglobin A1c. *Diab. Med.* **10**, 260–263.

Rabello, A. L. T., Garcia, M. M. A., Dias Neto, E. *et al.* (1993) Dot-dye-immunoassay and dot-ELISA for the serological differentiation of acute and chronic schistosomiasis mansoni using keyhole limpet haemocyanin as antigen. *Trans. R. Soc. Trop. Med. Hyg.* **87**, 279–281.

Schomburg, W. K., Fahrenberg, J., Maas, D. *et al.* (1993) Active valves and pumps for microfluidics. *J. Micromech. Microengng* **3**, 216–218.

Shoji, S. & Esashi, M. (1993) Microfabrication and microsensors. *Appl. Biochem. Biotechnol.* **41**, 21–34.

Shoji, S. & Esashi, M. (1995) Bonding and assembling methods for realizing a µTAS. In: *Micro Total Analytical Systems* (eds van den Berg, A. & Bergveld, P.) pp. 165–179 (Kluwer Academic Publishers, Dordrecht).

Shoji, S., Esashi, M. & Matsuo, T. (1988) Prototype miniature blood gas analyser fabricated on a silicon wafer. *Sens. Actuators* **14**, 101–107.

Snowden, K. & Hommel, M. (1991) Antigen detection immunoassay using dipsticks and colloidal dyes. *J. Immunol. Meth.* **140**, 57–65.

Song, M. I., Iwata, K., Yamada, M. *et al.* (1994) Multisample analysis using an array of microreactors for an alternating-current field-enhanced latex immunoassay. *Anal. Chem.* **66**, 778–781.

Suzuki, H. & Sugama, A. (1994) Micromachined glass electrode. *Sens. Actuators* **B20**, 27–32.

Sze, S. M. (1988) *VLSI Technology* 2nd edn (McGraw Hill, New York).

Tsay, Y. G., Lin, C. I., Lee, J. *et al.* (1991) Optical biosensor assay (OBA). *Clin. Chem.* **37**, 1502–1505.

van der Schoot, B. H., Verpoorte, E., Jeanneret, S. *et al.* (1995) Microsystems for analysis in flowing solutions. In: *Micro Total Analytical Systems* (eds van den Berg, A. & Bergveld, P.) pp. 181–190 (Kluwer Academic Publishers, Dordrecht).

van Gerwen, P., Baert, K., Slater, T. *et al.* (1995) Temperature controller for µTAS applications. In: *Micro Total Analytical Systems* (eds van den Berg, A. & Bergveld, P.) pp. 263–266 (Kluwer Academic Publishers, Dordrecht).

Verpoorte, E., Manz, A., Ludi H. *et al.* (1992) A silicon flow cell for optical detection in miniaturized total chemical analysis systems. *Sens. Actuators* **B6**, 66–70.

Wilding, P., Kricka, L. J. & Zemel, J. N. (1994) Fluid handling in mesoscale analytical devices. *US Patent* No. 5,304,487.

Chapter 24

Microspot®, Array-based, Multianalyte Binding Assays: The Ultimate Microanalytical Technology?

Roger P. Ekins and Frederick Chu

INTRODUCTION

Particular attention has been drawn in Chapter 9 to the existence of myths in the immunoassay field stemming from fallacious concepts of assay design, including the false notion that use of an antibody concentration approximating $0.5/K$ (where K is the equilibrium constant) maximises the sensitivity of conventional labelled antigen immunoassays. Such 'mythology' has frequently impeded immunoassay development in the past. For example, it prevented general recognition of the principles underlying so-called 'ultrasensitive' immunoassays, thus leading to the widespread failure by immunoassay practitioners and kit manufacturers immediately to perceive the immense significance of Köhler and Milstein's (1975) development of *in vitro* methods of monoclonal antibody production.

A more recent example of this phenomenon is provided by the development of array-based Microspot® immunoassay and DNA analysis techniques. (Microspot® is a registered trade mark of Boehringer Mannheim GmbH, with whom the authors are collaborating in developing microarray-based immunoassay and DNA analysis technologies.) This miniaturised, ultrasensitive, technology (which is likely to constitute the next, possibly the ultimate, major development in the binding assay field) relies on the use of amounts of antibody (or oligonucleotide in the case of DNA-directed arrays) so small as to be confinable within a 'microspot' on a solid probe such that, in principle at least, some 50–100 separate spots can be located within the cross-sectional area of a human hair. The possible development of microarray technology of this kind was delayed by its obvious non-adherence to widely accepted (albeit specious) assay design principles (for example, that referred to above), leading many in the field initially to conclude that the use of such small amounts of antibody would yield assays of low sensitivity requiring prolonged incubation times. (As indicated later in this chapter, antibody concentrations used in microarray technologies are generally in the order of $0.01/K$ and lower, and yield superior sensitivity to conventional assay designs.) This perception has been shown to be incorrect, and microarray technologies now represent the focus of some of the most heavily financed research programmes ever established in the biomedical field. Thus, although they are still in the development stage, their conceptual basis represents an appropriate subject for discussion in this volume.

Our own experimental studies in this area (also those subsequently conducted jointly with Boehringer Mannheim) have related primarily to 'immunoarrays', albeit we have long been conscious of the potential long-term importance of 'oligoarrays' for DNA analysis, and certain of our studies have therefore centred on this topic.

Antibody-based array technologies are clearly likely to be of particular value in certain fields, e.g. in the identification of specific allergies, of viral antigens in transfusion blood, etc. Indeed, even when a diagnostic test requires determination of only a limited panel of analytes (such as in the diagnosis of thyroid disease), the requirement by a miniaturised technology for only very small blood samples, and the savings in time and cost of laboratory personnel consequent upon simultaneous measurement of all clinically-relevant parameters in a single test, are likely to prove compellingly attractive to hospital laboratories under increasing pressure to reduce health-care costs.

Meanwhile, interest in microarray technologies in the USA has primarily focused on the development of oligonucleotide arrays for DNA testing. Francis Collins of The National Institute of Health, Director of the Human Genome Project in the USA, has, for example, drawn attention to the importance of the array-based DNA-analysis technology currently being developed by the Genosensor consortium (established in 1992 as part of the US National Institute of Standards and Technology's Advanced Technology Program). (Members of the consortium include Beckman Instruments, Genometrix Inc., Genosys Biotechnologies, MicroFab Technologies, Laboratories for Genetic Services, Triplex Pharmaceuticals, Houston Advanced Research Center, Baylor College of Medicine and the Massachusetts Institute of Technology. It is supported by grants in excess of $50 million from the National Institute of Standards and Technology, the National Center for Human Genome Research and the Department of the (US) Air Force, matching funds deriving from participating manufacturers.) Certain participating manufacturers have envisaged the localisation (in discrete areas) of each of the 65,536 possible 8-base oligonucleotide strands in the form of an array on the surface of a 1-cm^2 chip, the binding of complementary DNA strands to individual oligonucleotides being signalled by optical or electronic detectors. (Note: in practice members of the consortium appear to be relying on confocal microscopy (see below) or charge-coupled device (CCD) detectors to scan oligoarrays, essentially emulating array-scanning methods originally developed by Boehringer Mannheim and ourselves.)

Genetic analysis raises a number of well-known ethical issues that are currently the subject of discussion in scientific journals, national legislatures, etc., and that are inappropriate to discuss here. Although only 2–3% of human disease is monogenic in origin, it nevertheless appears likely that DNA analysis relying on oligonucleotide arrays to detect specific gene defects (such as those giving rise to cystic fibrosis, thalassaemia, etc.) will feature increasingly prominently in the diagnostic armamentarium as the Human Genome Project nears completion in the year 2003 or earlier (see, e.g. Evans, 1996). Moreover DNA analysis is of diagnostic importance for a number of other reasons, for example for tissue typing for transplantation surgery, 'DNA fingerprinting' for forensic purposes, and the detection or identification of infectious agents (e.g. viruses) in human blood and tissues.

However, before discussing array-based technologies in greater detail, a basic analytical concept underlying our own studies in this field must first be examined.

AMBIENT ANALYTE IMMUNOASSAY

The recognition that all immunoassays essentially rely on measurement of antibody occupancy (see Chapter 9) leads to a potentially important type of assay, termed 'ambient analyte immunoassay' (Ekins, 1983). This term is intended to describe assay systems that, unlike conventional methods, measure the analyte concentration in the medium to which an antibody is exposed, being independent both of sample volume, and of the amount of antibody present. The possibility of developing such assays follows from the mass action laws which lead to the following equation, representing the fractional occupancy (F) of antibody binding sites by analyte (at equilibrium):

$$F^2 - F\left(\frac{1}{[Ab]} + \frac{[A]}{[Ab]} + 1\right) + \frac{[A]}{[Ab]} = 0 \tag{1}$$

where [A] = analyte concentration and [Ab] = antibody concentration (both expressed in units of 1/K).

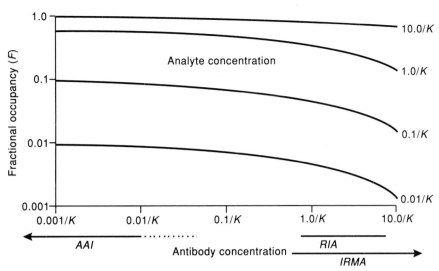

Figure 1 Fractional antibody binding-site occupancy (*F*) plotted as a function of antibody binding-site concentration for different values of analyte (antigen) concentration [A]. All concentrations are expressed in units of $1/K$. For antibody concentrations of less than $0.01/K$ (approximately), fractional binding-site occupancy is essentially unaffected by variations in antibody concentration extending over several orders of magnitude, being governed solely by the ambient analyte concentration (ambient analyte immunoassay (AAI)). Radioimmunoassays (RIA) and other 'competitive' immunoassays are conventionally designed using antibody concentrations approximating $0.5/K–1/K$ or above (implying binding of analyte concentrations close to zero (B_0) of $< 30\%$) in accordance with the precepts of Yalow and Berson. Conventionally designed sandwich assays (e.g. sandwich IRMAs) use capture antibody concentrations considerably in excess of $1/K$.

From this equation it may readily be shown that, for antibody concentrations tending to zero, $F \simeq [A]/(1 + [A])$. This conclusion is illustrated in Figure 1 in which the fractional occupancy of ('monospecific' or 'monoclonal') antibody binding sites in the presence of varying analyte concentrations, plotted against antibody concentration, is portrayed. This figure shows that, when an amount of antibody less than (say) 0.01 (i.e. $0.01/K$ when expressed in conventional molar units: preferably, but not essentially, coupled to a solid support, is exposed to an analyte-containing medium, the resulting (fractional) occupancy of antibody binding-sites solely reflects the ambient analyte concentration in the surrounding medium, and is independent of the total amount of antibody in the system (Note: if, for example, $K = 10^{11}$ l mol^{-1}, a binding site concentration of $0.01 \times 1/K$ represents 0.01×10^{-11} mol l^{-1}, or $0.01 \times 10^{-11} \times 10^{-3} \times 6.02 \times 10^{23} = 6.02 \times 10^7$ binding sites per ml). For example, if a solid probe bearing 10 antibody molecules on its surface is placed in a medium containing antigen at such concentration that, in accordance with equation (1). 1, 5 of the antibody molecules become occupied (i.e. when $[A] \simeq 1$, or $1/K$ if expressed in molar units), then, when a similar probe on which 100 antibody molecules are located is placed in the same medium, 50 of the binding sites will become occupied; when 1,000 molecules are on the surface, 500 will become occupied, and so on. (Note: these predictions disregard statistical variations arising from the small molecular numbers involved.)

Clearly, analyte sequestration by antibody causes depletion of (unbound) analyte in the medium, but because the amount bound is small, the resulting reduction in the ambient analyte concentration is insignificant. For example, if the sensor-antibody concentration is less than $0.01/K$, analyte depletion in the medium is invariably less than 1% (irrespective of the initial analyte concentration in the medium), and the system is therefore effectively sample volume independent.

A close similarity exists between these concepts and the operation of a simple thermometer. A small thermometer, when placed in a liquid in a container, extracts heat from the liquid until it reaches thermal equilibrium, at which time the ambient temperature of the liquid will be displayed. Provided the thermometer is small (and its thermal capacity is therefore insignificant) the temperature recorded will be essentially independent of thermometer size. However, the introduction of a large thermometer into the liquid will cause a drop in temperature, so that the final temperature recorded by the thermometer will differ from the original liquid temperature, and will, *inter alia*, depend on the thermometer's size and thermal capacity.

This simple analogy is also instructive in other ways. For example, it is evident that the smaller the thermometer, the faster it will reach thermal equilibrium, and the sooner the temperature of the liquid will be recorded. Similarly, considerations of molecular diffusion show that the smaller the amount of antibody on the probe, the sooner the fractional occupancy of antibody binding sites will provide a measure of the analyte concentration in the sample. Likewise, the lower limit on thermometer size is essentially determined by its ability to emit a readable signal (albeit statistical effects would clearly obviate its use as a temperature-measuring device were it so reduced in size as to assume molecular dimensions). Analogous limitations apply to the amount of antibody that can be located on a probe, i.e. those arising from the requirement to determine the fractional occupancy of antibody binding sites (this being a function of the specific activity of the label used in the system), and statistical variations when molecular numbers become very small.

These theoretical considerations lead to two further novel concepts. First, the antibody may be confined to a 'microspot' on a solid support, the total number of antibody molecules within the microspot being less than $v/K \times 10^{-5} \times N$ (where v = the sample volume to which the microspot is exposed (in ml) and N = Avogadro's number (6×10^{23})). (For example, if v = 1 and $K = 10^{12}$ l mol^{-1}, then the maximum number of antibody binding sites that will cause negligible depletion (<1%) of the ambient analyte concentration is 6×10^6, this number being greater for lower-affinity antibodies. Note: this prediction presupposes the attainment of thermodynamic equilibrium in the system. Because, in practice, incubations are generally terminated before equilibrium is reached, the value of the equilibrium constant applicable in this context (as in many other similar contexts) is the 'apparent' or 'effective' affinity constant determined at the end of the incubation period. This implies that a larger amount of antibody may be located within the microspot than permitted by the above formula if the true equilibrium constant is used as a parameter.) The second concept relates to the measurement of antibody occupancy. Occupancy may be determined by a number of different methods; however, the perception that the ratio of occupied (or unoccupied) to total binding sites is solely dependent on the ambient analyte concentration leads to the idea of dual-label, 'ratiometric', microspot immunoassay.

DUAL-LABEL MICROSPOT IMMUNOASSAY

Following exposure of an antibody microspot (located on a suitable probe) to an analyte-containing fluid (Figure 2), the probe may be removed and exposed to a solution containing a relatively high concentration of a 'developing' antibody directed against either a second epi-

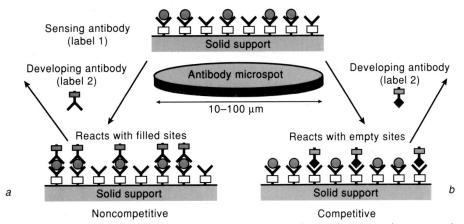

Figure 2 Microspot immunoassay. Following exposure of the antibody microspot to the test sample, the fractional occupancy of antibody binding sites reflects the ambient analyte concentration. Exposure of the microspot to a second 'developing' antibody (or other labelled material) reactive with either occupied sites ('non-competitive assay') or unoccupied sites ('competitive assay') reveals sensor antibody binding site occupancy. Note that both developing and sensor antibodies may be labelled.

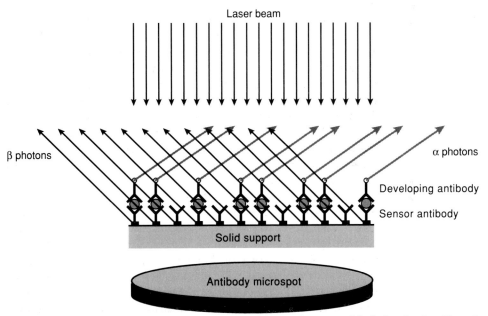

Figure 3 Dual-label, ambient-analyte immunoassay relying on fluorescent-labelled antibodies. The ratio of α and β fluorescent photons emitted reflects the fractional occupancy of antibody binding sites and is solely dependent on the analyte concentration to which the probe has been exposed.The ratio is unaffected by the amount or distribution of antibody coated (as a monomolecular layer) on the probe surface.

tope on the analyte molecule if this is large (i.e. the occupied site, Figure 2*a*), or against unoccupied antibody binding sites in the case of small analyte molecules (Figure 2*b*). An estimate of sensor-antibody fractional occupancy may be derived by measurement of the ratio of sensor and developing antibodies forming the dual-antibody 'couplets'. This can be readily achieved by labelling the 'sensor' and 'developing' antibodies with different labels, for example, a pair of radioactive, enzyme or chemiluminescent markers (or even labels of entirely different type). (It should be noted that it is necessary to label only a small proportion of sensor antibodies located within the microspot, thus obviating significant interactive effects that might occur between sensor and developing antibody labels.) Fluorescent labels are potentially particularly useful in this context because, by the use of appropriate optical techniques (Figure 3), they permit arrays of antibody 'microspots' distributed over a surface (each microspot directed against a different analyte) to be scanned, thereby permitting multiple analyte assays to be simultaneously performed on the same sample.

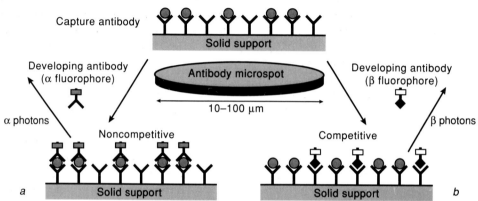

Figure 4 Both occupied and unoccupied sensor antibody binding sites may be determined using developing antibodies labelled with different fluorophores, yielding an assay that is both competitive (*b*) and noncompetitive (*a*). (The sensor antibody is not labelled in these circumstances.)

An alternative dual-label approach relies on the use of two (labelled) developing antibodies, one directed against occupied sites, the second against unoccupied sites (Figure 4). If the total number of antibody binding sites is n, and assuming an ambient analyte concentration [A], $F_A n$ sites will be occupied, and $(1-F_A)n$ sites will be unoccupied (F_A being the antibody fractional occupancy at an analyte concentration [A]). If the measurement efficiency of the signal generated by occupied sites is ε_1, and of the signal generated by unoccupied sites is ε_2, the ratio ($R_A n$) of the signals generated from occupied and unoccupied sites is $\varepsilon_1 F_A / \varepsilon_2 (1-F_A)$, or $CF_A/(1-F_A)$, where $C = \varepsilon_1/\varepsilon_2 =$ constant. Because F_A is solely dependent on the ambient analyte concentration, and because C is constant for both unknown samples and standards, measurement of R_A yields a measure of [A] irrespective of the value of N. A system operating in this manner can be described as both 'competitive' and 'non-competitive' and is advantageous in that it yields high precision at both low and high analyte concentrations (i.e. when ε_1 and ε_2, respectively, are small). In other words such a strategy extends the working range of the assay.

Several advantages stem from adopting a dual fluorescence-measurement approach. For example, neither the amount nor the distribution (i.e. the surface density) of the sensor-antibody within the detector's field of view are of importance, because the ratio of the emitted fluorescent signals is unaffected. Likewise the effects of any fluctuations in the intensity of the incident (exciting) light beam are thereby reduced or eliminated. Nevertheless it should be emphasised that, if the techniques for manufacturing microspot arrays are very well controlled (such that, for example, the surface density and/or amount of sensor antibody located in each microspot is identical) and the efficiency of signal detection is constant or otherwise monitored, the use of a dual-label approach may not be necessary.

MICROSPOT IMMUNOASSAY SENSITIVITY

Because 'microspot immunoassay' challenges concepts that have dominated immunoassay design theory in the past two to three decades, consideration of the sensitivity attainable by this approach is obviously of primary importance. In particular, the proposition that very low sensor-antibody concentrations (some 100- or 1,000-fold lower than conventionally used) are not incompatible with high sensitivity may generate scepticism amongst those accustomed to conventional ideas, and has certainly been claimed by many commentators to be 'nonintuitive'. However, the validity of this proposition may readily be demonstrated by consideration of a simple model system.

Let us postulate that sensor-antibody molecules are attached to the surface of a solid support in such a manner that their binding sites remain exposed to the analyte, and that their affinity vis-a-vis the analyte is thereby unchanged. (The antibody concentration in the system – given by the number of molecules on the support divided by the incubation volume – is unaffected by such attachment, and antibody occupancy by analyte at equilibrium will be identical to that occurring were the antibody distributed uniformly throughout the incubation mixture.) Let us also suppose that the antibody molecules exist as a monolayer of maximal surface density on the support. Thus a change in the antibody concentration implies a corresponding change in the surface area over which antibody is distributed. (If, for example, the antibody affinity constant is 10^{11} l mol^{-1}, the total incubation volume is 1ml, and the antibody surface density is 6,000 molecules per μm^2, then a surface area of 10^5 μm^2 (i.e. 0.1 mm^2) accommodates antibody molecules corresponding to a concentration of $0.1/K$; an area of 0.01 mm^2 corresponds to an antibody concentration of $0.01/K$, etc.) Let us further postulate that, following sensor-antibody exposure to a medium containing analyte at a concentration of $0.01/K$ (i.e. 6×10^7 molecules per ml), we measure 'noncompetitively' the resulting antibody occupancy (e.g. by exposure to a second, labelled, antibody directed against the analyte, forming a typical antibody sandwich. (Note: although the amount of sensor-antibody located in the microspot area may be very small, the sites *occupied* by analyte are determined in this example (using a relatively high concentration of labelled antibody to recognise occupied sites). The system thus relies on the 'noncompetitive' approach. Finally, let us suppose that all occupied sites react with the labelled antibody, the latter also binding 'nonspecifically' to the solid support itself at a surface density of 1 molecule per μm^2.

We may now consider the effects of progressive reduction of the antibody-coated surface area from, for example, 1mm^2 (effective antibody concentration $1/K$) through 0.1mm^2 ($0.1/K$) to 0.01 mm^2 ($0.01/K$) and below. From equation (1), the value of F for the 1mm^2 microspot area is 4.98×10^{-3}. Thus the number of analyte and labelled antibody molecules specifically bound to the area = 2.99×10^7 (i.e. about 50% of the total analyte molecules present), while the number of labelled antibody molecules nonspecifically bound = 10^6. Thus, assuming the 'field of view' of the detecting instrument is restricted to the area on which the sensor antibody is deposited, and (provisionally) assuming the background of the instrument itself to be zero (i.e. the only source of background is the nonspecifically-bound labelled antibody within the instrument's field of view), the signal/background ratio observed for the 1mm^2 area is approximately 30. Similarly, the value of F for a 0.1mm^2 area is 9.02×10^{-3}, the number of

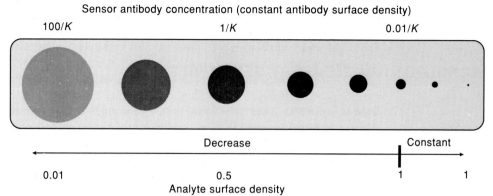

Figure 5 Assuming sensor antibody is coated at a constant surface density, increasing the diameter of the coated area increases the amount of analyte bound to sensor antibody, but decreases the analyte surface density. The signal generated per unit area by a second (developing) antibody binding to captured analyte (and the signal/background ratio) thus falls. This figure illustrates this phenomenon diagrammatically, the larger spots fading into the background as their diameter increases.

labelled antibody molecules specifically bound to the area = 5.41×10^6, the number nonspecifically bound = 10^5, and the signal/background ratio is approximately 54. Likewise the signal/background ratio for a 0.01 mm² area can be shown to be approximate 59. In short, the signal/background ratio increases as the antibody-coated surface area is decreased, approaching a maximal (plateau) value of 60 as the area of sensor-antibody falls below 0.01 mm² and approaches zero. These concepts are illustrated diagrammatically in Figure 5.

If, on the other hand, reduction in the antibody-coated area were not accompanied by a corresponding reduction in the detecting instrument's field of view, the resulting reduction in 'signal' would not lead to a corresponding fall in background emitted by nonspecifically bound labelled antibody. So although reduction in the coated area would increase sensor-antibody fractional occupancy, the signal/background ratio might either remain constant or fall. In these circumstances it might be advantageous to increase the coated area. Likewise if the surface density of sensor-antibody were decreased (the microspot area being held constant), the same conclusion would be reached.

Meanwhile, if the background signal generated within the detecting instrument itself – e.g., from the photocathode of a photomultiplier tube used to detect photons emitted from the antibody-coated area – were not zero, and remained constant regardless of the instrument's field of view, then a maximum signal/background ratio would likewise be attained at some optimal value of the antibody-coated area, below which the ratio would fall. However, because it is possible to reduce the size of the detector (and hence the detector-generated background) *pari passu* with that of the signal-emitting area, there is no reason, in principle, for the signal/background ratio to diminish as the antibody-coated area is progressively reduced towards zero. Thus if, albeit somewhat simplistically, we accept the signal/background ratio as indicative of the precision of the antibody-occupancy measurement, these considerations suggest that it is advantageous to reduce the antibody-coated surface area (and hence the sensor-antibody concentration) towards zero, even though it is evident that (assuming equilibrium is reached in the system) little advantage is likely to accrue from reducing the area below 0.01 mm² (and hence the sensor-antibody concentration below 0.01/K).

An obvious flaw in these simple arguments is that, were the antibody-coated area indeed reduced to zero, both signal and background would likewise fall to zero (the ratio between them nevertheless remaining constant), implying that no signal of any kind would be recorded. In practice, statistical factors come into play when the number of individual events observed by a detecting instrument is very low (as indicated above), thus prohibiting reduction of the sensor-antibody concentration to zero in the manner suggested above. The point at which reduction in the antibody-coated area causes such loss of detectable signal that the precision of the antibody-occupancy measurement significantly deteriorates depends, *inter alia*, on the specific activity of the labelled antibody used to measure occupied binding sites: the higher the specific activity, the smaller the permissible area. Another constraint on minimal microspot size is the number of analyte molecules that ultimately become bound to sensor antibody within the microspot area. Clearly, statistical fluctuations in the measured signal will increase and become significant when this number falls below about 1,000, albeit the point at which such fluctuations become unacceptable depends on the particular use to which the assay is put.

It is nevertheless evident that, given very high specific activity labels, circumstances can be envisaged in which, even in a 'noncompetitive' system, the optimal sensor-antibody concentration may be exceedingly low, lying well within the range encompassed by 'ambient analyte' immunoassay. A more general conclusion is that a variety of factors, including the characteristics of instruments used for labelled antibody (or labelled analyte) measurement, influence microspot immunoassay design, implying, *inter alia*, that it is virtually impossible to construct general rules in this area. For example, reagent concentrations that are optimal using isotopically-labelled reagents and a conventional radioisotope counter (possessing a fixed background dependent on its basic construction) are likely to be entirely different when very high specific activity labels are used and freedom exists to 'tailor' the measuring instrument to samples of any size. In short, certain conclusions based on experience of radioimmunosaay (RIA) and immunoradiometric assay (IRMA) techniques may prove misleading when applied to nonisotopic methodologies and should be treated with circumspection.

A more detailed theoretical consideration of (noncompetitive) microspot immunoassay sensitivity (Ekins *et al.*, 1990) suggests that (assuming thermodynamic equilibrium):

$$C_{min} = D^*_{min} \times \frac{(6 \times 10^{20})(1 + [Ab^*])}{DK[Ab^*]} \tag{2}$$

where D = sensor antibody monolayer surface density (molecules per μm^2), K = sensor antibody affinity (l mol^{-1}), $[Ab^*]$ = labelled antibody concentration in developing solution (expressed in units of $1/K^*$, where K^* = labelled antibody affinity), D^*_{min} = minimum detectable developing antibody surface density (molecules per μm^2), and C_{min} = assay detection limit (molecules per ml). For example, if $[Ab^*] = 1$, $D = 10^5$ molecules per μm^2, $K = 10^{11}$ l mol^{-1} and $D^*_{min} = 20$ molecules/per μm^2, then $C_{min} = 2.4 \times 10^6$ molecules per ml = 4×10^{-15} mol l^{-1}, the fractional occupancy of sensor antibody binding sites by the minimum detectable analyte concentration being 0.04%. Figure 6 shows theoretical assay sensitivities attainable using sensor antibodies of varying affinities, plotted as a function of D^*_{min}.

Similar analysis of competitive microspot assays indicates that potential sensitivities are essentially identical to those attainable with conventional competitive methodologies. In summary, such considerations indicate *inter alia* that the attainment of high microspot sensitivity requires close packing of sensor-antibody molecules within the microspot area,

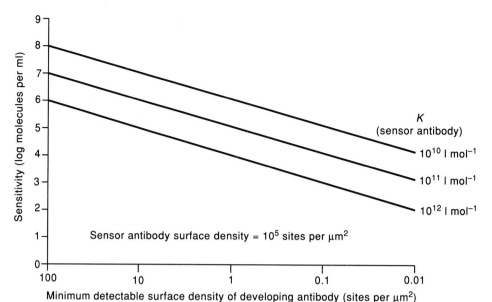

Figure 6 Theoretically-predicted noncompetitive microspot immunoassay sensitivity plotted as a function of the minimum developing antibody density detectable within the microspot area. Values of capture antibody surface density of 10^5 molecules per μm^2, and of developing antibody concentration of $1/k^*$, have been assumed. Note that currently available instruments permit detection of between 10 and 1 molecules of fluorescein-labelled antibody per μm^2.

combined with the use of an instrument capable of accurately measuring very low surface densities of developing antibodies. They also suggest:

1 that microspot assay sensitivities considerably higher than those obtainable by conventional isotopically-based immunoassays are achievable;

2 that sensitivities yielded by noncompetitive microspot assays are likely to be considerably greater than those of corresponding competitive assays.

MICROSPOT IMMUNOASSAY KINETICS

The theoretical considerations summarised above – based on the assumption that measurements are carried out at equilibrium – lead to the conclusion that reduction of the microspot area below that required to accommodate sensor antibody yielding a concentration of about $0.01/K$ does not increase fractional occupancy of antibody binding sites by analyte, and hence causes no improvement in final signal/background ratios. However, when molecular diffusion effects are taken into consideration, it is demonstrable that further reduction in microspot area is likely to be advantageous in consequence of the resulting increase in antigen/antibody reaction rates.

This proposition, and the conclusion that a microspot format is capable of yielding assays that are more rapid than conventional methodologies, may cause surprise because it is widely accepted that the use of high concentrations of antibody in a noncompetitive assay implies more rapid binding of analyte (and hence attainment of equilibrium) in accordance with the mass action laws. The theoretical basis of the latter view is illustrated in Figures 7 and 8,

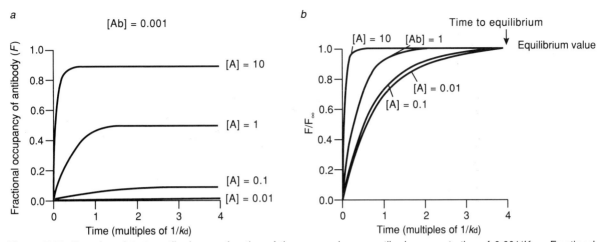

Figure 7 Binding of analyte to antibody as a function of time, assuming an antibody concentration of 0.001/K. *a*, Fractional occupancy of antibody binding sites. *b*, Fractional occupancy expressed in terms of the final equilibrium value (F_∞). Note that equilibrium is essentially reached within a time of about $4/k_d$ for all analyte concentrations.

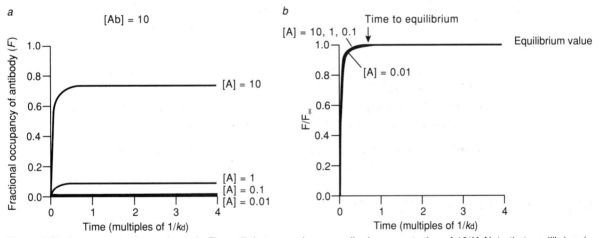

Figure 8 Similar curves to those shown in Figure 7, but assuming an antibody concentration of 10/K. Note that equilibrium is reached in a time of about $0.5/k_d$.

which show antibody-bound analyte concentrations (both in absolute terms and as fractions of the final equilibrium value) as a function of reaction time (the latter being expressed in units of $1/k_d$ where k_d = the dissociation rate constant of the antibody/analyte complex; expressing time in $1/k_d$ units makes the curves applicable to any binding reaction). Figure 7 relates to an antibody concentration (in a homogeneous liquid phase) of 0.001/K; Figure 8 relates to a concentration of 10/K. The rate at which equilibrium is reached is, in both cases, dependent on the analyte concentration; however, for all concentrations, equilibrium is essentially reached in a reaction time of about $0.5/k_d$ or less using an antibody concentration of 10/K, whereas reaction times some eightfold longer (i.e. in the order of $4/k_d$) are necessary when the antibody concentration is 0.001/K.

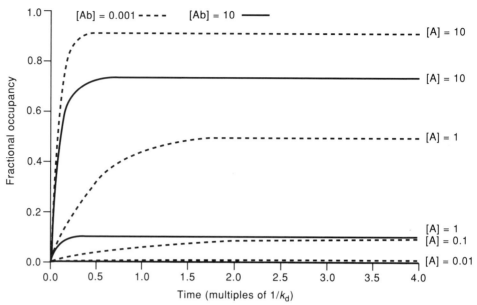

Figure 9 Curves shown in Figures 7*a* and 8*a* combined, demonstrating that fractional occupancy of antibody binding sites is greater at all times in the case of the lower antibody concentration.

Calculations of this kind underlie accepted ideas regarding, the advantages, in regard to binding reaction kinetics, of the use of large amounts of antibody in a liquid phase (non-competitive) immunoassay. However, a different picture emerges if the same data are expressed in terms of changes in fractional occupancy of antibody with time, as shown in Figure 9. This demonstrates that fractional occupancy (and implicitly the final signal/background ratio in a microspot system) is at all times greater for the lower antibody concentration. Thus, if – temporarily disregarding the diffusion constraints that apply to a system in which one of the reactants is linked to a solid support – we visualise the antibodies to be localised as microspots on a surface, one microspot 100-fold greater in diameter (i.e. 10,000-fold greater in area) than the other, the analyte surface density will *at all times* be greater in the case of the smaller spot. Thus the signal/background ratio is always higher in the latter case despite the larger spot's more rapid attainment of equilibrium. In other words, a higher sensitivity is likely to be reached in a shorter time when using the smaller amount of antibody located on the smaller spot.

But this simplified analysis clearly disregards the diffusion constraints on the rate of the binding reaction if sensor-antibody molecules are linked to a solid support. These constraints on the migration rates of analyte molecules to and from the solid support reduce both the effective association and dissociation rates of the reaction prior to the attainment of equilibrium, albeit (assuming that linking the sensor antibody to the solid support neither alters the antibody's structure nor affects its physicochemical microenvironment) the final equilibrium state is thereby unaffected (i.e. the equilibrium constant of the reaction remains unchanged). However, it should be noted that, in the limiting case of a microspot containing only a single antibody molecule, the kinetics of antibody reaction with analyte are essentially identical to those that would be observed were the antibody moving freely in solution. This suggests that the smaller the microspot area, the closer the velocity of the binding reaction

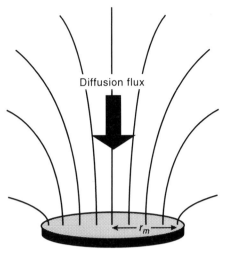

Diffusion flux

Under diffusion controlled conditions:

- Antigen diffusion flux is proportional to r_m
- Antibody on spot is proportional to r_m^2
- Rate of antibody binding site occupation by antigen is proportional to $1/r_m$

Antibody microspot

Figure 10 Diffusion of molecules into a circular sink.

will approximate to the one that would be obtained were the reagents in solution in a homogeneous single-phase system.

Analysis of the diffusion of (analyte) molecules (Crank, 1975) present in a solution towards a circular absorber or 'sink' confirms this conclusion. This reveals that the diffusion flux (molecules per second) is given by $4Dr[A]$, where D = diffusion coefficient (cm^2/s^{-1}), r = radius (cm) and [A] is the analyte concentration (molecules per ml). Assuming uniformity of the antibody surface density (d_{Ab} (molecules per cm^2)) within the microspot area, the migration rate of analyte molecules to a circular microspot of radius r_m is thus proportional to r_m, whereas the number of analyte molecules that must be bound to reach a specified occupancy level of antibody located within the microspot is proportional to the microspot area, i.e. πr_m^2, and hence to r_m^2 (Figure 10). Hence – assuming the reaction is diffusion controlled – the rate of antibody occupancy within the microspot is proportional to $1/r_m$.

More detailed consideration of the rate at which analyte molecules migrate towards, and bind to, an antibody microspot reveals that the (initial) antibody occupancy rate (OR) per unit area of microspot is given by:

$$OR = \frac{4r_m k_a D[A] d_{Ab}}{\pi r_m^2 k_a d_{Ab} + 4Dr_m} \quad \text{molecules per second per cm}^2 \tag{3}$$

where k_a = association rate constant (ml per sec per molecule) and [A] = ambient analyte concentration (molecules per ml). This expression reveals that, as r_m tends to zero, the term $\pi r_m^2 k_a d_{Ab}$ becomes small compared with $4Dr_m$, and equation (3) approximates OR = $k_a[A]d_{Ab}$. In other words, the kinetics of the reaction increase with reduction in r_m, ultimately approximating those observed in solution, as illustrated in Figure 11.

Computer models revealing the full sequence of events following the introduction of antibody microspots of varying diameters into an analyte-containing solution, and embracing the kinetics of the analyte-antibody reaction, the initial establishment of concentration gradients

639

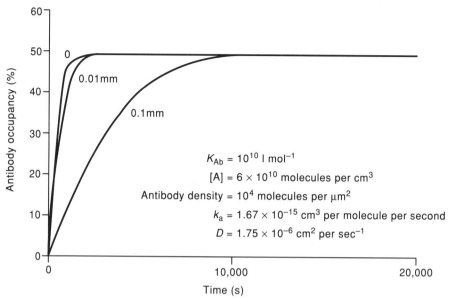

Figure 11 Calculated increase with time of analyte bound to an antibody microspot, assuming parameter values shown.

within the solution, etc., have likewise confirmed that the smaller the microspot area, the lower the diffusion constraints on the rate of analyte binding to antibody, and the more closely will the kinetics of the reaction approximate to those seen in a homogeneous liquid-phase system.

In summary, these considerations suggest that higher signal/background ratios are attained in a shorter time using an antibody microspot format, implying that microspot assays are likely to prove at least as rapid as assays of conventional macroscopic design. The use of relatively small amounts of sensor antibody nevertheless implies that thermodynamic equilibrium is reached somewhat more slowly. This implies that equilibrium may not be reached within a very short incubation time, leading to assay drift unless incubation times are carefully standardised. However, in practice, using automatic equipment, this phenomenon is unlikely to constitute a major problem.

MICROSPOT IMMUNOASSAYS AND DNA ANALYSIS TECHNIQUES: IMPLICATIONS AND PRACTICAL ASPECTS

It is neither appropriate nor useful at this stage to discuss in detail the practical implementation of the concepts and physicochemical theory underlying microarray techniques outlined above; nevertheless it is necessary briefly to indicate the manner in which these concepts have been applied in our own experimental work lest they be dismissed as purely speculative and of only academic interest. It should, of course, be emphasised that – assuming the ultimate emergence of commercial instruments and arrays onto the market – far more sophisticated techniques and (purpose-built) instrumentation will be used than those that we have relied on in our initial 'feasibility' studies.

Although a variety of high specific activity antibody labels are potentially usable in this context, our experimental studies have, in practice, relied largely on the use of conventional fluorophores (although the use of lanthanide chelates or cryptates and time-resolution techniques of fluorescence measurement constitute a possible alternative when the highest sensitivity is required, given development of appropriate time-resolving equipment). The simultaneous measurement of dual fluorescence from small areas is, of course, a well established technique, and the availability from commercial sources of suitable instrumentation (e.g. the laser scanning confocal microscope), albeit not specifically designed for the present purpose, proved useful in demonstrating the validity of the microspot approach.

Laser scanning confocal fluorescence microscopes are increasingly being used for the scanning of microarrays (see Figure 12), and a brief description of their mode of operation is therefore warranted here. In such microscopes, a small area of the specimen is illuminated by a focused laser beam, fluorescence photons emitted from this area being focused in turn onto a detector, typically a low dark-current photomultiplier (Ploem, 1986; White *et al.*, 1987). At the 'confocal' point, the projection of the illumination pinhole and the back-projection of the detector pinhole coincide. Fluorescence photons emitted at other points thus possess a low

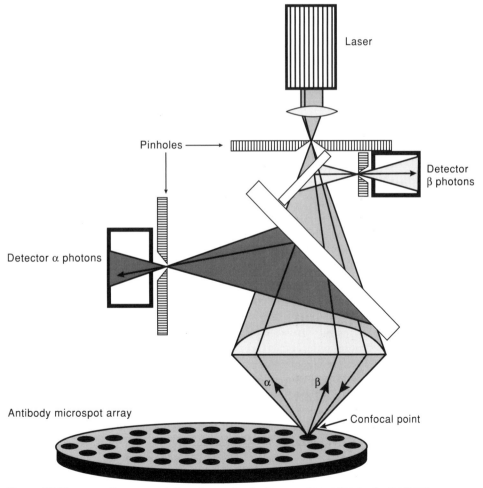

Figure 12 Diagrammatic representation of a confocal microscope scanning a microspot array.

probability of reaching the detector. Such systems contrast with conventional epifluorescence microscopes, in which the specimen is exposed to an essentially uniform flux of illumination, and, *inter alia*, yield much sharper images of fluorescent emitters situated in a defined plane of a tissue sample. They can therefore be used for three-dimensional imaging of thick tissue sections, albeit this is of limited value in the present context, in which fluorescent microspots are distributed in a planar array. Electrons spontaneously emitted by the photomultiplier photocathode contribute to the background signal of the instrument, and must – for highest microspot assay sensitivity – be minimised. Fortunately the design of such instruments permits the photocathode to be very small in area, and this source of background can be expected to diminish with future improvements in photomultiplier design. Other sources of background include fluorescence emitted by components of the optical system, which may not have been constructed with background reduction as a prime consideration. Nevertheless current instruments display high sensitivity of detection of fluorescent signals. For example, one commercially-available microscope is claimed to detect fluorescein at a density of 10 molecules per μm^2. Most commercially available fluorescein isothiocyante (FITC)-labelled IgG exhibits a fluorophore:protein ratio of about 4, implying an antibody surface density detection limit (D^*_{min}) of about 2–3 FITC-labelled IgG molecules per μm^2. This implies in turn a theoretical sensitivity of ~ 2–3×10^5 analyte molecules per ml for a two-site immunoassay, assuming identical parameter values as above, or 2–3×10^4 molecules per ml using a 'sensing' antibody with an affinity of 10^{12} l mol^{-1}.

Studies of 'ratiometric' assays in our own laboratory have relied on a less sensitive microscope, albeit one possessing facilities for dual fluorescence measurement. Its argon laser emits two excitation lines at 488 and 514 nm. It is thus particularly efficient in exciting blue/green-emitting fluorophores such as FITC (excitation maximum 492 nm), but is less efficient in exciting fluorophores such as Texas red (excitation maximum 596 nm). However, the ratiometric assay principle permits considerable variation in detection efficiencies of the two labels because, *inter alia*, the specific activities of the labelled antibody species forming the antibody couplets can be chosen to yield signal ratios approximating unity. Inefficiency of the argon laser in exciting Texas red is thus not a major handicap in the present context. Although this instrument relies on a conventional microscope and not on a purpose-designed optical system (and is implicitly less sensitive), it permits quantification of fluorescence signals generated from microspots of any selected area. Initial studies revealed that, under conditions that are not optimal, the instrument was capable of detecting about 25 FITC-labelled and/or 150 Texas red-labelled IgG molecules per μm^2, scanning an area of about 50 μm^2. (It should, of course, be emphasised in this context that manufacturers (such as the Californian company Affymetrix (Kozal *et al.*, 1996)) presently engaged in the development of purpose-built microarray-based analysers are incorporating advanced confocal systems for array scanning that are of smaller dimensions and with characteristics superior to the original general-purpose confocal microscopes used in our own studies.)

The development of microspot immunoassays has also necessitated closer scrutiny of the mechanisms involved in the coupling of antibodies to solid supports. In the present context, these should display a capacity to adsorb (in the form of a monolayer) – or to link covalently – a high surface density of antibody combined with low intrinsic signal-generating properties (e.g. low intrinsic fluorescence) thus minimising background. We initially examined a number of candidate materials, such as polypropylene, Teflon®, cellulose and nitrocellulose membranes, microtitre plates (black, white and clear polystyrene plates), glass slides and quartz optical fibres coated with 3-(aminopropyl)triethoxy silane, etc., and a number of alternative protocols for the achievement of high densities of monolayer coating. These studies exposed phenomena neither evident nor of importance when antibody binding to solid supports is examined at a macroscopic level. In practice, black Dynatech Microfluor microtitre plates – formulated for the detection of low fluorescence signals, and yielding high signal/background ratios and high coating densities of functional antibodies (about 5×10^4 IgG molecules per μm^2) – were used for assay development, albeit such plates are not ideal, often showing significant interbatch variations.

More recently, plastic sample holders specifically manufactured by Boehringer Mannheim for use in the present context have been used. These possess highly standardised characteristics and quality, yielding, *inter alia*, negligible (and constant) background fluorescence across the entire surface on which the microspot array is deposited. Boehringer Mannheim has also developed elegant technology (relying on ink-jet spotting techniques) permitting the production on a large scale of arrays comprising 196 antibody microspots located on the flat circular base (3 mm in diameter) of these sample holders. These arrays can be produced at a rate of approximately 5,000 per hour, each array being individually quality controlled as part of the production process.

A somewhat different approach has been adopted by Affymetrix for the construction of oligonucleotide arrays (Fodor *et al.*, 1991). This relies on the use of so-called 'combinatorial chemical techniques' to construct *in situ* the different oligonucleotide sequences within the individual spots that make up the oligonucleotide array. The technique (illustrated in Figure 13) involves sequential masking and exposure of selected areas on a silicon base using photolitho-

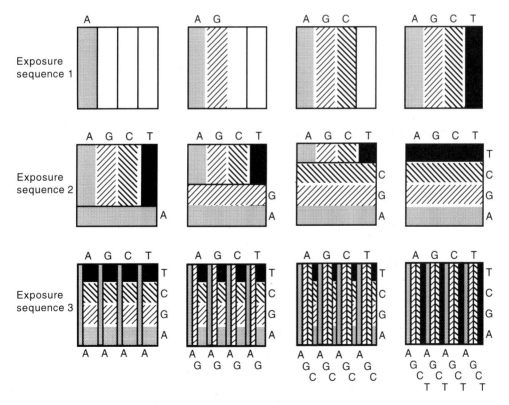

Figure 13 Construction of oligonucleotide array by combinatorial techniques (see Fodor *et al.*, 1991). Repeated masking and exposure to selected nucleosides progressively creates oligonucleotides of increasing length. The three exposure sequences illustrated result in the formation of an array of the 64 different 3-mers.

graphic techniques similar to those used in the electronics industry for the construction of semiconductor chips. Such technology – although applicable to binding agents such as oligo-nucleotides and polypeptides which can be built up sequentially in such a manner – are obviously not directly applicable to antibodies, which cannot be synthesised *in situ* in this particular fashion.

Nevertheless, such techniques are of potential relevance to the construction of antibody arrays. Mindful of the possibility that certain users of the technology may wish to construct immunoarrays relevant to their own specialised needs, we have constructed arrays made up of (18-mer) oligonucleotides, thereby creating 'protoarrays' or array templates to which the users may attach antibodies (to which complementary oligonucleotides have been coupled) of their own choice (Ekins, 1994). Antibody-oligonucleotide complexes migrate specifically to assigned positions in the array, and thereafter function perfectly as sensor antibodies in the usual way.

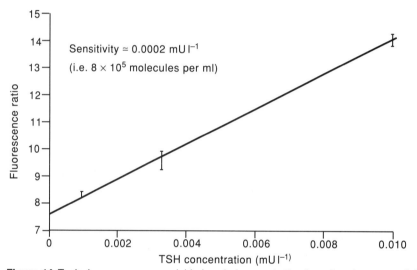

Figure 14 Typical response curve yielded early in our studies in a (hand-processed) TSH microspot ratiometric assay following overnight incubation. Sensitivity currently achieved using 15-minute incubation times in prototype automatic analysers is somewhat lower, but entirely sufficient for clinical purposes.

Notwithstanding the limitations of our original instrumentation (which, *inter alia*, does not permit the use of time-resolving techniques to distinguish two individual fluorescence signals either from each other or from background fluorescence), and the crudeness of our own methods for coupling antibodies onto small areas, the theoretical concepts outlined above were soon verified by comparing the performance of several assays when constructed in microspot format and when conventionally designed. Although unoptimised, ratiometric microspot assays have yielded sensitivity values superior to those of conventional, optimised IRMAs. As an example, typical results of an overnight thyroid-stimulating hormone (TSH) microspot assay are shown in Figure 14. The TSH sensor (or 'capture') antibody used in these early studies possessed a relatively low affinity (about 10^9 l mol^{-1}); this value, combined with other data, indicated that the minimal detectable TSH density within the microspot area approximated 1 molecule per 15 μm^2. These results were obtained using a multiple labelling technique, thereby increasing the specific activity of the developing antibody; nevertheless, bearing in mind the well known limitations of 'conventional' fluorophores when used as immunoassay reagent labels, such results were encouraging. Further work using higher-affinity antibodies, improved fluorophores and antibody microspotting techniques, and purpose-built instrumentation are ultimately likely to yield even higher sensitivities. For example, Boehringer Mannheim claims – using current scanning technology – to detect as little as 1 analyte molecule per 100 μm^2, scanning a complete array in less than 15 seconds.

Although antibody microspot arrays comprising more than 200 microspots are unlikely ever be required for conventional diagnostic purposes, the ability to measure panels of analytes simultaneously in the same sample can be anticipated to have revolutionary consequences in medicine and other similar areas. Such techniques may also, *inter alia*, ultimately permit the individual analysis of the multiple isoforms of certain 'heterogeneous' analytes (e.g. the glycoprotein hormones), such molecular heterogeneity presenting a major obstacle to the standardisation and interpretation of many immunological measurements (Ekins, 1991). Meanwhile, in the case of genetic analysis, arrays comprising much larger numbers of oligonucleotide microspots are obviously likely to be necessary.

SUMMARY AND CONCLUSION

As emphasised earlier, microarray techniques are still in the process of intense development. We have therefore primarily focused here on their underlying principles rather than practical details, the latter being clearly the subject of continued investigation by major manufacturers in Europe and the USA.

In this chapter's title, the question is posed: do such techniques constitute the ultimate microanalytical technology? It is obviously rash to predict future technological developments, and impossible to foresee future inventions. Nevertheless there are valid grounds for speculating on the possibility that such miniaturised binding assay systems represent a development that, if successful, is unlikely to be superseded for many years to come. Among the fundamental grounds for this belief is the proposition that recognition of individual molecular species in complex biological mixtures primarily relies on the observation of molecular shape, i.e. on the ability of a detector molecule to recognise (and bind to) target molecules. Nature has developed exquisitely specific systems of this kind for molecular recognition and it therefore seems unlikely that binding assays – which rely on the exploitation of such systems – will be replaced within the foreseeable future. Moreover, contrary to previously accepted views, the use of a vanishingly small amount of the binding agent (e.g. antibody or oligonucleotide) on a barely-visible spot yields higher sensitivity and faster assays than any other approach. It also permits, in principle, the determination of a virtually unlimited number of different substances in a small sample, such as a single drop of blood. Indeed it is difficult to visualise analytical objectives (i.e. the rapid, ultrasensitive determination of multiple analytes in the same microsample) beyond those that are now being addressed using microarray technologies, or any alternative approach whereby such objectives are likely to be achieved. Thus, bearing in mind the worldwide interest such technologies have aroused, there can be little doubt of their emergence and widespread use within the foreseeable future.

REFERENCES

Crank, J. (1975) *The Mathematics of Diffusion.* 2nd edn. (Oxford University Press, Oxford).

Ekins, R. P. (1983) Measurement of analyte concentration. *British Patent* No. 8224600.

Ekins, R. P. (1991) Immunoassay standardization. *Scand. J. Clin. Lab. Invest.* **51** (**Suppl 205**), 33–46.

Ekins, R. P. (1994) Binding assay using binding agents with tail groups. *British Patent* No. 9404709.9.

Ekins, R. P., Chu, R. & Biggart, E. (1990) The development of microspot, multi-analyte ratiometric immunoassay using dual fluorescent-labelled antibodies. *Anal. Chim. Acta.* **227**, 73–96.

Evans, G. A. (1996) Commercial implications of the human genome project. *Trends Biotechnol.* **14**, 143–144.

Fodor, S. P. A., Read, J. L., Pirrung, M. C. *et al.* (1991) Light-directed, spatially addressable parallel chemical synthesis. *Science* **251**, 767–773.

Köhler, G. & Milstein, C. (1975) Continuous culture of fused cells secreting specific antibody of predefined specificity. *Nature* **256**, 495–497.

Kozal, M. J., Shah, N., Shen, N. *et al.* (1996) Extensive polymorphisms observed in HIV-1 clade B protease gene using high density oligonucleotide arrays. *Nature Med.* **2**, 753–759.

Ploem, J. S. (1986) New instrumentation for sensitive image analysis of fluorescence in cells and tissues. In: *Applications of Fluorescence in the Biological Sciences.* (eds Tayer, D. L., Waggoner, A. S., Lanni, F. *et al.*) pp. 289–300 (Alan R. Liss, New York).

White, J. G., Amos, W. B. & Fordham, M. (1987) An evaluation of confocal versus conventional imaging of biological structures by fluorescence light microscopy. *J. Cell. Biol.* **105**, 41–48.

Chapter 25

Future Developments in Immunoassay

David J. Newman and Christopher P. Price

INTRODUCTION

In our Introduction (Chapter 1) we traced the development of immunodiagnostics as an analytical approach. In the 1950s there were semiquantitative assays and through the late 1950s and early 1960s there were the first fully quantitative assays; these were followed by the developments both of solid-phase technologies and of the sandwich assays, in the late 1960s. The 1970s saw the introduction of hybridoma technology and the start of the great advances in assay specificity, continuing through the 1980s with an increasing variety of detection technologies and ever-decreasing detection limits. The 1990s have given us great advances in automation, reducing assay times without compromising assay sensitivity, along with further improvements in antibody technology with the introduction of antibody engineering. But what of the 21st century? Will that bring the end, or the triumph of immunosensors? Will the homogeneous assay replace the heterogeneous while maintaining performance? What new technologies will come forward? What or who will drive these developments?

DEVELOPMENTS IN ANTIBODY TECHNOLOGY

The mid-1980s and early 1990s saw the advent of recombinant antibody techniques with extensive claims for the impact they were to have. The main interests of the early workers in this field was *in vivo* therapeutics and it is still only in this area that any real impact for this technology has been felt (Boulianne *et al.*, 1984; Winter and Milstein, 1991). The costs involved in antibody engineering and the complexities of the techniques bring to mind the early days of monoclonal antibodies. Hybridoma technology took about a decade to have a major effect on *in vitro* immunodiagnostics, but it does seem unlikely that engineered antibodies are going to make an equivalent impact unless there are real advances made in the manipulation of specificity and kinetics. Aside from the CEDIA™ technology there has been very little use of molecular biological engineering in commercialised assays; hybridoma technology and direct chemical conjugation of antibody-enzyme conjugates remaining the preferred techniques. The development of CRABs (bivalent antibody fragments generated by linking together two sFvs with different specificities) does seem an interesting possibility as a means of generating higher-affinity and more-specific immunoreagents. However, these would only be an advantage for analytes with multiple epitopes (Chapter 4).

Phage display as a means of expressing sFvs was first demonstrated in 1985 and has developed into a powerful tool (Smith, 1985). The use of naive phage libraries containing a complete set of human (or any other species) variable region genes has been proposed as an alternative to the use of animal immunisation (Gram *et al.*, 1992). A library could be screened for the desired specificities and the selected phages grown and investigated further. Antibody engineering could be used to improve upon affinity and specificity characteristics and the resultant DNA sequence could be linked to that of the chosen enzyme-label (Olabiran *et al.*, 1994). This is the proposed scenario, and with improved knowledge about antibody structure, designer changes may become possible by the use of molecular modelling to reduce the time (and costs) involved in producing the desired characteristics. Avoiding the use of animals could have ethical, regulatory and cost benefits. Removing all animal involvement in the production process does make the consideration of the use of recombinant antibodies in an *in vitro* diagnostic setting seem more attractive but the technology does need considerable development before this can be realistically considered. Within the next 5 years we should have a clearer idea.

As mentioned in Chapter 6, there has recently been more discussion concerning the use of receptor assays, particularly for drugs (Jin *et al.*, 1992; Soldin, 1995). There is the possibility of using molecular biology techniques to clone drug receptors and express the sequence responsible for binding specificity in such a way that it could be used as a binding agent. This reawakens the discussion of the relative merits of biological versus structural information. However, in this case it would be the structural specificity of the receptor that was being used and not the biological response linked to it, as was previously the case. The DNA sequence of the receptor binding site could be little different to that of an immunoglobulin variable region from an antibody generated against the ligand. However, the surrounding structurally supportive regions could be significantly different and this could either be advantageous or disadvantageous with regards to their respective usefulness in an assay.

Then there is the possibility of totally synthetic polymers to produce binding agents devoid of any biological origin, the antibody mimics (Andersson, 1996; Ansell *et al.*, 1996; Chapter 7). As a concept these have also been around for a decade or more but have yet to achieve a working nonextraction assay, let alone a commercial product. The possibility of an infinitely stable reagent, that could be moulded into intricate structures may find application in nanotechnology devices. There are clearly enough haptens to measure that an inability to develop protein-specific reagents need not be an ultimate limitation, but it is likely that in an increasingly competitive environment this will remain a significant disincentive to widespread assay development using antibody mimics.

Control of the Antigen-Antibody Reaction

Over recent years the use of molecular biology techniques for mutating antibody binding sites, allied with an ever greater understanding of molecular structure and intermolecular forces, has developed into a powerful tool for studying the antigen-antibody reaction. Application of this knowledge may enable a more theoretical approach to be developed for immunoassay optimisation (Newman and Price, 1996). Recombinant antibodies and molecular modelling could enable the predominant intermolecular forces that control a particular epitope-paratope reaction to be determined. This understanding could then be used to select the pH, ionic strength and chaotropic constitution of an appropriate assay buffer for the optimisation of an immunoassay.

PCR versus Immunodiagnostics

The introduction of qualitative and semiquantitative polymerase chain reaction (PCR) technologies has been considered to pose a challenge to immunodiagnostics in screening for inherited disorders and in the identification of infective organisms. For instance, should the genetic defect that causes muscular dystrophy be screened for using molecular biology techniques or by immunoassay quantifying the levels of circulating dystrophin (Morandi *et al.*, 1995)? The underlying difficulty is that genetic defects can produce less, more, or functionally altered protein. If it is the latter then an antibody would have to discriminate between the native and altered protein form, which is certainly possible if an oligonucleotide hybridisation reaction can do so. However, immunodiagnostics would be preferable if the mutation caused quantifiable differences in protein expression.

For identification of infective organisms, PCR technology offers some significant benefits over immunodiagnostics and culture techniques. The main difficulties lie with rapidly mutating organisms and endemic or constitutive infections. The former would make probe design difficult and the latter poses the difficult question as to whether any amount of infection is harmful.

If considered as a binding interaction, DNA hybridisation and the specificity of its interaction needs to be assessed in a similar manner to antigen-antibody binding. Careful control of reaction conditions is needed to obtain reproducible results; nonspecific reactions are a major concern and precise quantification of the starting sequence is dependent upon reproducible amplification. PCR as a diagnostic tool has excellent possibilities in the area of identification of risk (either genetic or infective), all-or-nothing measurements and diseases where the protein expressed is unknown, but it is likely to have little impact on quantitative immunodiagnostics.

Detection Technologies

Assay detection limits have steadily reduced over the past decade with the introduction of better antibodies and detection technologies. Homogeneous technologies have achieved excellent success in the nanomolar and above concentration range, and many different possibilities exist for developing assays that take anywhere between 1 and 5 minutes. In the concentration range below this there is already the capability to measure thyroid-stimulating hormone (TSH) in the atto- to femtomolar range in 5–10 minutes. Theoretical detection of a few hundred molecules (zeptomolar) has now been reached, with claims of even less (Cook and Self, 1993; Kricka, 1994). Not all of these technologies have achieved reliability in clinical samples but some may yet do so. The most sensitive systems do now seem to be those that use some form of luminescence, either chemical or biological (Bronstein *et al.*, 1989; Smith *et al.*, 1991; Ullman *et al.*, 1996). One interesting recent development is that of Immuno-PCR, combining the amplification of the polymerase chain reaction with the immunological specificity of DNA-labelled antibodies (Hendrikson *et al.*, 1995). However, overall it seems unlikely that this will be an area of dramatic change over the next few years, although the potential for enhancing homogeneous immunoassays seems good e.g. LOCI™ (Ullman *et al.*, 1996).

Immunosensors

What can be said for biotechnology can also be considered true for immunosensor technology. As described by Treloar *et al.* (Chapter 19) and Purvis *et al.* (Chapter 20), immunosensor technology contains many exciting analytical tools; however, the biological specimen is proving to be too difficult a matrix for many of them. As described in our review, immunosensors may have left it too late, 'despite huge innovations and investments, however, immunosensors fill the pages of our literature rather than the benches of our laboratories' (Morgan *et al.*, 1996). The advancements in 'conventional' immunoassay technologies in terms of both instrumentation and detection technologies have provided an enormous spectrum of systems that can achieve many of the potential advantages that immunosensors appeared to offer a decade ago (Blackburn *et al.*, 1991; Hendrikson *et al.*, 1995; Hoyle *et al.*, 1996). In combination with miniaturisation, as described by Kricka and Wilding, sensors may yet find a place, but they will be competing against some technologies that will already have a proven track record, e.g. fluorescence and chemiluminescence (Chapter 23).

Nanotechnology

This is the engineering discipline that designs devices in which every atom is known and is in a selected position. It offers some interesting possibilities to produce very high performance systems first hinted at by Richard Feynman as far back as 1959 (Feynman, 1992; Kaehler, 1994). This approach to miniaturisation is reaching the early development stage with the use of silicon chip micromachining (as discussed by Kricka and Wilding in Chapter 23). Miniaturisation has benefits as an end in itself, enabling more flexible siting of analytical devices, but to make a significant impact it seems likely that either performance enhancements or significant cost savings will be required. The experience with immunosensors must temper our enthusiasm for this technology. Proof of concept is a long way from a commercial product. Reliably producing a consistent product at a reasonable price is essential, but extremely difficult to achieve.

Simultaneous Multianalyte Methods

Multiple analyte technologies were first developed in the early 1980s for the simultaneous measurement of two analytes, e.g. triiodothyronine and thyroxine (Blake *et al.*, 1982). Measurement of more than two analytes has developed a little more recently (Ekins *et al.*, 1990; Hendrikson *et al.*, 1995). Roger Ekins, in particular, has suggested that, using ambient analyte immunoassay technology, this will be an important innovation that will challenge accepted concepts of assay standardisation and diagnostic investigation (Ekins *et al.*, 1990 and Chapter 24). Although there has been a significant investment in this type of technology over the past few years there is little sign yet of a working technology for clinical practice. Whether there is a real future for this potentially very exciting approach should become clear in the next 5 years. Multiple analyte technologies have been successfully developed for semi-quantitative measurement. Several examples have been described in the chapters by Price *et al.* (Chapter 22) and Kricka and Wilding (Chapter 23). These types of device, aimed at a particular diagnostic question, such as diagnosis of myocardial infarction, should become more widely available in the near future. Other potential diagnostic questions to be approached could be the unconscious patient (drugs of abuse), screening for diabetic complications or for osteoporosis, identification of the causes of food poisoning, etc., although the clinical and economic benefits of doing so have not yet been established.

Automation and Laboratory Organisation

There has been a significant growth in the number of laboratories using automated immuno-analysis systems, driven by improvements in instrument choice and reliability, in combination with an increased need to reduce staffing budgets in health service laboratories. There has been a worldwide effort, across governments of different political persuasions, to reduce the healthcare costs, with *in vitro* diagnostics being an easily targeted area. This has led to work-station consolidation both within and across laboratory disciplines. Technological developments enable an analyser to be used for the automation of haematology, biochemical and endocrinological investigations as described by Gorman *et al.* in Chapter 13. At the same time the eye of the health service manager is looking at turnaround time, not just in the laboratory, but also in the out-patient clinic and hospital ward. Thus although improved central laboratory automation can combine disciplines and test menus, there is an alternative approach requiring simplified and robust instruments to perform immunoassays at the bedside and in the clinic, if not the home such as described by Price *et al.* in Chapter 22 (Kost, 1996). It is clear that there are opportunities in both these areas and this has stimulated the nanotechnology revolution and the improvements in main laboratory automation simultaneously.

The past few years have also seen significant consolidation occurring in the diagnostics industry with the resultant reduction in the numbers of leading companies (Anon., 1995). Economically driven, these amalgamations should provide a smaller number of better financed and more viable companies. The next 5–10 years will show whether this will be at the cost of reduced investment in research and development. This may act as a continuing spur to smaller high-technology companies to provide the technologies that the larger companies select from and develop further. Some of the high-risk investments in protein engineering and novel detection systems will be required to be successfully commercialised and to give a return on the investors' capital. The biotechnology revolution still seems to be living on promise, rather than product at the present.

Standardisation

Improved calibration of methods has long been agreed to be essential for the greater harmonisation of analytical results. An excellent example of this is the development of the serum protein calibrant CRM470 by an international committee (Whicher *et al.* 1994). The main thrust towards achieving this aim has been to develop internationally agreed standards; however, in a few cases reference methods have been developed that can take the process one step further than harmonisation and establish 'true' values for analytes (particularly mass-spectrophotometric methods for drugs).

A recent Bergmeyer conference has suggested that this may not be sufficient and that reference or internationally recognised antibodies should be established, with fully defined specificities, and a reference assay format (Albert, 1991; *see also* chapter 11). As a result manufacturers would then be required to demonstrate agreement with the reference assay, rather than with the market leader. It could even be extended to require all manufacturers to use the reference antibody, or antibodies, and the differences between manufacturers would then be based on system attributes. There would be significant problems in introducing this form of standardisation in a competitive diagnostic market and in any case it could not eliminate the differences that can be introduced into the binding characteristics of an antibody by conjugating it to different solid phases or labelled molecules (*see* Chapter 6).

Regulation and Regulatory Approval

The devolved laboratory is now a real possibility, with robust technologies in small boxes placed in out-patient clinics and doctors' offices avoiding the need for patients and or samples to travel long distances. The instruments will be electronically linked to a central laboratory computer to ensure adequate quality assurance and data interpretation; with the same central laboratory providing bulk sample analysis for the hospital in-patients. The same technology and reagents could be used in both the outlying and central laboratories, formatted in a high-throughput mode with a single automated, multidisciplinary laboratory with specialist subsections. Developments in laboratory accreditation, and health services funding, can both play roles in driving laboratory consolidation and the development of increased turnaround time and 'patient friendliness' (Burnett, 1996). The successful companies will be those that have integrated sample handling, data entry and analysis for immunochemistry with a technology or technologies that are fully compatible and able to meet the above needs (Kost, 1996).

The regulatory authorities will have ensured that there are recognised international calibrators for all assays and there will be an increasing drive towards the use of reagent standards with defined clones of monoclonals stored for reference with fully characterised specificity and affinity. Any new method for the same analyte would have to use the same antibody or prove equivalence.

New Diagnostics Markers

One ever-increasing area of progress linked to new immunodiagnostic methods is the development of novel diagnostic markers. Refinements in antibody and detector technology continue to aid the researcher in the search for more sensitive and specific markers of disease. Molecular biology techniques such as subtractive hybridisation and differential display may facilitate the identification of cell-disease, or organ-specific DNA sequences. However, without the development of specific antibodies for the proteins encoded within those sequences, it is not possible to investigate whether the gene product is released into the peripheral circulation. If a marker is to be useful in a diagnostic sense, then it has to be present in a body fluid that is reasonably accessible. If it is not, then a biopsy and histopathological investigation will be required. These approaches are inappropriate both for population screening and for routine disease monitoring: essential attributes of a successful *in vitro* immunodiagnostic.

CONCLUSION

There is always a danger in crystal ball gazing and the only certainty is that in 5 years time there will have been considerable change in the technology and application of *in vitro* immunodiagnostics. This exciting and diverse field built around the elegant simplicity of the antigen-antibody reaction has matured over the past 40 years, but does not seem to have reached any kind of 'mid-life crisis' yet. We look forward to continuing developments in this vibrant technology that links so many academic and clinical disciplines. A technology that will not be superseded by the advent of PCR and molecular biology but has assimilated these self-same tools to continue its development (Hendrikson *et al.*, 1995).

REFERENCES

Albert, W. H. W. (1991) The antibody/antiserum as an analytical reagent in quantitative immunoassays. *Scand. J. Clin. Lab. Invest.* Suppl. **205**, 51, 79–85.

Andersson, L. I. (1996) Application of molecular imprinting to the development of aqueous buffer and organic solvent based radioligand binding assays for (s)-propranolol. *Anal. Chem.* **68**, 111–117.

Anon. (1995) Managing the future in a changing healthcare environment. *Clinica* **648**, 9.

Ansell, R. J., Ramström, O. & Mosbach, K. (1996) Towards artificial antibodies prepared by molecular imprinting. *Clin. Chem.* **42**, 1506–1512.

Blackburn, G. F., Shah, H. P., Kenten, J. H., *et al.* (1991) Electrochemiluminescence detection of immunoassays and DNA probe assays for clinical diagnostics. *Clin. Chem.* **37**, 1534–1539.

Blake, C., Al Baisan, M. N., Gould, B. J., *et al.* (1982) Simultaneous enzyme immunoassay of two thyroid hormones. *Clin. Chem.* **28**, 1469–1473.

Boulianne, G. L., Hozumi, N. & Shulman, M. J. (1984) Production of functional chimaeric mouse/human antibody. *Nature* **312**, 643–646.

Bronstein, I., Voyta, J. C., Thorpe, G. H. G., *et al.* (1989) Chemiluminescence assay of alkaline phosphatase applied in an ultra sensitive enzyme immunoassay of thyrotropin. *Clin. Chem.* **35**, 1441–1446.

Burnett, D. (1996) *Understanding Accreditation in Laboratory Medicine* (ACB Venture Publications, London).

Cook, D. B. & Self, C. H. (1993) Determination of one thousandth of an attomole (1 zeptomole) of alkaline phosphatase: application in an immunoassay of proinsulin. *Clin. Chem.* **39**, 965–971.

Ekins, R. P., Chu, R. & Biggart, E. (1990) The development of microspot multi-analyte ratiometric immunoassay using dual fluorescent-labelled antibodies. *Anal Chim. Acta* **227**, 73–96.

Feynman, R. (1992) There's plenty of room at the bottom: An invitation to enter a new field of physics. In: *Nanotechnology, Research and Perspectives* (eds Randall B. C. & Lewis J.) MIT Press (Cambridge, MA) pp. 347–363.

Gram, H., Marconi, L. A., Barbas, C. F., *et al.* (1992) *In vitro* selection and affinity maturation of antibodies from naive combinatorial immunoglobulin library. *Proc. Natl Acad. Sci. USA* **89**, 3576–3580.

Hendrickson, E. R., Truby, T. M., Joerger, R. D. *et al.* (1995) High sensitivity multianalyte immunoassay using covalent DNA-labelled antibodies and polymerase chain reaction. *Nucleic Acids Res.* **23**, 522–529.

Hoyle, N. R., Eckert, B. & Kraiss, S. (1996) Electrochemiluminescence: leading edge technology for automated immunoassay analyte detection. *Clin. Chem.* **42**, 1576–1578.

Jin, Y. J., Burakoff, S. J. & Bierer, B. E. (1992) Molecular cloning of a 25 kDa high affinity rapamycin binding protein FKBP-25. *J. Biol. Chem.* **267**, 10942–10945.

Kaehler, T. (1994) Nanotechnology: Basic concepts and definitions. *Clin. Chem.* **40**, 1797–1799.

Kost, G. J. (ed.) (1996) *Clinical Automation, Robotics, and Optimisation* (John Wiley & Sons, New York).

Kricka, L. J. (1994) Strategies for improving sensitivity and reliability of immunoassays. *Clin. Chem.* **40**, 347–357.

Morandi, L., Mora, M., Confalonieri, V. *et al.* (1995) Dystrophin characterization in BMD patients: Correlation of abnormal protein with clinical phenotype. *J. Neur. Sci.* **132**, 146–155.

Morgan, C. L., Newman, D. J. & Price, C. P. (1996) Immunosensors: Technology and opportunities in laboratory medicine. *Clin. Chem.* **42**, 193–209.

Newman, D. J. & Price, C. P. (1996) Molecular mechanisms in immunoassay for drugs. *Ther. Drug Monit.* **18**, 493–497

Olabiran, Y., Koumi, P., George, A. J. T. *et al.* (1994) Engineering of antibodies to bone/liver alkaline phosphatase for improved discrimination of these isoenzymes in monitoring of metabolic bone disease. *Proc. 5th Int. Conf. Antibody Engineering.* (La Jolla, CA, USA).

Smith, D. F., Stults, N. L., Rivera, H. *et al.* (1991) Applications of recombinant bioluminescent proteins in diagnostic assays. In: *Bioluminescence and Chemiluminescence: Current Status* (eds Stanley, P. E. and Kricka, L. J.) pp. 529–532 (John Wiley & Sons, Chichester).

Smith, G. P. (1985) Filamentous fusion phage: Novel expression vectors that display cloned antigens on the virion surface. *Science* **228**, 1315–1317.

Soldin, S. J. (1995) Receptor (immunophilin-binding) assay for immunosuppressive drugs. *Ther. Drug Monit.* **17**, 574–576.

Ullman, E. F., Kirakossian, H., Switchenko, A. C. *et al.* (1996) Luminescent oxygen channeling assay (LOCI™): Sensitive, broadly applicable homogeneous immunoassay method. *Clin. Chem.* **41**, 1518–1526.

Whicher, J. T., Ritchie, R. F., Johnson, A. M., *et al.* (1994) New international reference preparation for proteins in human serum (RPPHS). *Clin. Chem.* **40**, 934–938.

Winter, G. & Milstein, C. (1991) Man-made antibodies. *Nature* **349**, 293–299.

Subject Index

501, 548, 552, 561, 567,
588, 649
Heterogeneous and
homogeneous assays, 5,
155, 156, 301–305, 311
Heterogeneous
fluoroimmunoassay (see
Fluorescence immunoassay),
256, 257, 311, 391, 395,
396
Heterohybridoma, 48, 133,
165
Heterophilic antibodies, 254,
365
Hofmeister series, 457, 469
Homogeneous
fluoroimmunoassay (see
Fluorescence immunoassay),
391, 415
Homogeneous immunoassay,
8, 301, 302, 306–308, 311,
318, 319, 334, 404, 452,
483, 490, 491, 496, 497,
499, 500, 548, 552, 560,
570–572, 581, 639, 640,
649, 651
Hook effect (see also Antigen
Excess detection), 6, 7, 228,
256, 552, 566, 591
Hormones, 175, 213, 230,
232, 248, 249, 251, 472
polypeptide hormones,
246, 251, 263
prohormones, 255
steroid hormones, 247,
251–253, 259, 369
thyroid hormones, 247,
251, 252, 369
Horseradish peroxidase
(HRP), 231, 351, 356, 357,
361, 362, 364, 367,
373–375, 377–379, 400,
434, 437, 492
Human chorionic
gonadotrophin (hCG), 133,
247, 248, 253, 255, 257,
258, 292, 306, 379, 398,
399, 402, 495, 497, 500,

569, 588–591, 595,
597–600, 610, 611, 617
free β-subunit, 258, 401
Human placental lactogen
(HPL), 397, 410
Hybridoma, 41, 47–49,
52–55, 87
Hybridoma technology, 4,
37, 68, 83, 87, 88, 125,
636, 649
nonsecreting hybridomas,
75
production, 40, 41, 47–50
Hydrophilicity, 25, 26, 553,
555, 563, 567, 570
Hydrophobicity, 20, 21, 26,
48, 106, 144, 147, 468,
498, 567, 570, 597
Hydrophobicity/
hydrophilicity plots, 25, 31,
396
Immobilised onto a
membrane, 191, 192, 245,
278, 379, 588, 589, 594,
610
Immobilisation (see also
Conjugation chemistries),
101, 107–111, 113, 114,
117, 127, 136, 309, 370,
377, 378, 495, 496, 500,
503, 504, 513, 518, 521,
523, 524, 527–532, 536,
537, 549, 554, 557, 562,
564, 566, 571, 573, 583,
585, 590, 591, 594–596,
607
Immune complex formation
(see also
Immunoprecipitate), 333,
439, 449, 451, 453–457,
459, 463, 496, 503, 505,
536, 556, 562
Immunisation (see also
Antibody preparation), 23,
39–45, 56, 68, 84, 254,
257, 649
DNA immunisation, 45,
46

immunogen, 40–42
immune response, 39–42,
45, 54, 74
in vitro, 46, 47
Immunoassay classification,
190, 261, 302, 303, 583
Immunoassay design, 9, 118,
183, 185–188, 191, 192,
194, 195, 197–199,
202–205, 245, 256, 302,
305, 306, 312, 464, 554,
596, 607, 627, 633, 635,
644
Immunoassay optimisation,
194, 197, 198
Immunochromatography,
217, 247, 377, 378, 447,
589, 595
Immunofluorometric assay
(IFMA), 311, 312, 391,
392, 394, 395, 397, 399,
401, 402, 404
Immunogenicity, 15, 21, 41,
44–46, 72, 73, 78, 254
Immunoglobulins, 15–18, 21,
44, 46, 48, 67, 69, 72, 74,
75, 80, 134, 159, 162, 254,
255, 307, 370, 373, 397,
403, 404, 450, 463, 513,
536, 650
immunoglobulin A, 17, 18,
42, 162, 262, 552
immunoglobulin E, 17, 43,
162, 380, 608, 609, 619
immunoglobulin G, 15–18,
43, 44, 47, 48, 67, 68,
72, 76, 82, 111, 159,
160, 254, 262, 282, 358,
364, 370, 379, 410, 454,
459, 467, 471, 501, 524,
528, 536, 537, 551, 552,
589, 615–617, 642
immunoglobulin M, 17,
18, 39, 44, 46, 162, 262,
370, 461, 471, 552, 573
structure, 16–18, 69
fragments, 68, 72, 80, 135
F(ab')₂, 18, 52, 82, 134,